Medicine in a Day 2: Case Presentations

Medicine in a Day 2: Case Presentations

EDITORS:

PROFESSOR MARCUS DRAKE

(BM BCH, MA, DM, FRCS (UROL))

Professor of Neurological Urology, Imperial College and
Charing Cross Hospital, London, UK

DR ALEXANDER ROYSTON

(MB CHB, BA, MSC)

Internal Medical Trainee, Bristol Royal Infirmary, Bristol, UK

DR GREGORY OXENHAM

(MB CHB, BA)

Junior ED Registrar, Palmerston North Hospital, Mid Central DHB, NZ

DR HOLLIE BLABER (ILLUSTRATOR)

(MB CHB, BSC)

Trust Grade Doctor, Milton Keynes University Hospital , UK

DR BERENICE AGUIRREZABALA ARMBRUSTER

(MB CHB, BSC)

Ear, Nose and Throat SHO, University Hospitals Coventry and
Warwickshire, Coventry, UK

ELSEVIER

ISBN 978-0-323-84769-8

Content Strategist: Clodagh Holland-Borosh
Content Project Manager: Shivani Pal
Designer: Brian Salisbury

Printed in India

Last digit is the print number: 9   8   7   6   5   4   3   2   1

CONTENTS

HOW TO USE THIS BOOK

Medicine in a Day 2: Case Presentations covers all presentations stated by the UKMLA, plus more! We included things that we thought are essential for your medical training. Table 2 lists the UKMLA presentations, which you can tick off as you revise them. We sometimes combined two UKMLA presentations into the same chapter if there was extensive overlap. For example, the presentations 'Eye Trauma' and 'Foreign body in eye' are dealt with together in Chapter 34, while 'Diplopia' and 'Ptosis' are both covered in Chapter 30. A few chapters, denoted by including 'outline' in the title, cover comparatively small topics which do not need the same amount of description as the other chapters. Because conditions commonly contribute to more than one presentation, we generally cross-refer between chapters rather than repeating description of a condition multiple times. Relevant page numbers in *Medicine in a Day: Revision Notes*, shortened to "Book 1", are also given in Table 2 if you need a more detailed description of any condition mentioned in the presentations.

The structure of each presentation is as follows:

- Presentation title
- Vignette, describing an example of this type of presentation
- Questions, based on the presentation (not necessarily the vignette)
- Answers to questions
- Table of differentials for the presentation title (not necessarily the vignette), covering key features, investigations and management
- Image or diagram relevant to the presentation
- Commentary, giving things to consider and explaining the diagnosis in the vignette
- Revision tips

Please note the following:

- **Table of differentials:** This table covers the most common differentials to the presentation title, emphasising the ones not to miss. This is not an exhaustive list, but it helps you think about potential differentials to each presentation

- **Features:** Risk factors (RFs), with history and examination (Hx & O/E) findings, are the main ones, but others may be included. RFs are sometimes given in another column to even up the amount of text
- **Investigations:** Baseline bloods may include FBC (full blood count), U&Es (urea and electrolytes), LFTs (liver function tests), CRP (C-reactive protein) and clotting. Pre-operative bloods may include baseline bloods + group and save ± crossmatch (G&S, CM)
- **Management:** Antibiotics (Abx) mentioned are based on BNF recommendations (UK), but you should always check local guidelines. Management guidelines may be updated over time, so ensure you keep up to date with them
- **For more details regarding conditions**, please refer to **MEDICINE IN A DAY: *Revision Notes*** for *Medical Exams, Finals, UKMLA and Foundation Years*
- **Please keep up to date:** Guidelines and knowledge about conditions and presentation may be updated over time

A NOTE ON REFERENCE RANGES

Interpretation of a laboratory test relates the patient's results with the laboratory 'reference range'. The reference range is the average value for a 'normal population', and a range (often ±2 standard deviations) to allow for natural variation. The range covers 95% of the reference group, so a result will lie outside the reference range for around 5% of people, even in a normal population. Hence 'reference range' is a more appropriate term than 'normal range'. Normal for one group does not necessarily apply to another, and for some tests (e.g. cholesterol) it may be more appropriate to think in terms of target values. Reference ranges may be affected by age and sex. For example, alkaline phosphatase is expected to be high in children because of bone growth. Creatinine and creatine kinase (CK) can be affected by ethnicity and muscle mass, which varies considerably between individuals, and is lower if someone is paraplegic. Results for some tests can be affected by circadian cycle, diet (e.g. vegetarian, alcohol, supplements), fasting (lipids), position, interventions (e.g. PSA after DRE) and vigorous exercise (e.g. CK, AST, LDH). In Europe, most tests use the International System of Units - e.g. moles (mol) and litres (L). The US laboratories often use mass units – e.g. milligrams in decilitre volumes (mg/dL). The reference ranges are specific to the laboratory, and *haematology test results particularly rely on provision of reference ranges by the laboratory*, as each uses different equipment and testing methods.

Some typical adult reference ranges for commonly requested tests are given in Table 1. Please note that for the reasons stated above, reference ranges will vary and, depending on which source you are using for your revision, you may find slightly different reference ranges. Ideally, reference ranges should be stated in your exams to help you answer the question. However, please clarify with your medical school if these will be given in your exams and if not given which ones you should be memorising.

TABLE 1

Test	Range (for 95% of people) and units
Serum sodium*	133–146 mmol/L
Serum potassium*	3.5–5.3 mmol/L
Serum urea*	2.5–7.8 mmol/L
Serum creatinine (adult)**	Male 59–104 µmol/L Female 45–84 µmol/L
Serum chloride*	95–108 mmol/L
Serum bicarbonate*	22–29 mmol/L
Serum phosphate*	0.8–1.5 mmol/L
Serum magnesium*	0.7–1.0 mmol/L
Serum albumin*	35–50 g/L
Serum total protein*	60–80 g/L
Serum osmolality*	275–295 mOsm/kg
Hb (adult age ≥15)**	Male 130–170 g/L Female 120–150 g/L
Haematocrit (adult)**	Male 0.40–0.52 L/L Female 0.37–0.45 L/L
Platelets (adult)*	150–450 × 10^9/L
WBCs (adult)*	4.0–11.0 × 10^9/L

*Labtestonline.org.uk
**North Bristol NHS Trust

TABLE 2   UKMLA Presentations and Where to Find Them

Patient presentations	Case number	Page	Relevant pages in Book 1	Revised?
Abdominal distension	68	197	232–5, 251, 434	
Abdominal mass	70	203	231–2, 236–7, 246–51, 434	
Abnormal cervical smear result	137	392	378–9	
Abnormal development/developmental delay	147	422	4–5, 411–2	
Abnormal eating or exercising behaviour	173	500	447–8	
Abnormal involuntary movements	106	307	317–8, 450–1	
Abnormal urinalysis	198	581	406–7, 502, 363–4, 508–9, 183–4, 201, 202	
Acute abdomen	67	193	225–8, 373	
Acute and chronic pain management	159	462	432–4, 634–5	
Acute change in or loss of vision	37	104	158–62	
Acute joint pain/swelling	186	544	549–54, 560–2, 588–91	
Acute kidney injury	176	508	270–2, 502, 508–10, 650–6	
Acute rash	15	44	111, 106–7, 124–5, 125–6, 101	
Addiction	169	490	180–1, 185–7, 433	
Allergies	146	420	105–8, 111–2, 175	

TABLE 2 UKMLA Presentations and Where to Find Them

Patient presentations	Case number	Page	Relevant pages in Book 1	Revised?
Altered sensation, numbness and tingling	108	314	318–21	
Amenorrhoea	114	333	201–2, 214–6, 358, 413	
Anaphylaxis	53	151	111–2, 175	
Anosmia	26	74	140	
Anuria/acute or chronic urinary retention	195	572	376–7, 605–9, 613, 619–20	
Anxiety, phobias, OCD	167	484	442–4	
Ascites	83	239	250–1, 508–9	
Auditory hallucinations	166	481	440–2, 439	
Back pain	192	563	295, 349–52, 430	
Behaviour/personality change	172	497	180, 312–3, 439–41, 445–7	
Behavioural difficulties in childhood	155	450	417–9, 448	
Bites and stings	54	153	105, 190, 299–300	
Blackouts and faints	46	132	51, 55–6, 59–71, 183	
Bleeding antepartum	126	364	364–5	
Bleeding from lower GI tract	71	206	228–9, 235–8	
Bleeding from upper GI tract	50	143	181, 219–20, 244–6	
Bleeding postpartum	129	372	369–70	
Bone pain	158	459	29, 279, 425, 432–3, 557–60	
Breast lump	3	7	25–9	
Breast tenderness/pain	2	4	25–29	
Breathlessness	40	113	176–8, 538–45	
Bruising	89	257	274–81	
Burns	55	156	12–4, 191	
Cardiorespiratory arrest	43	123	178–9	
Change in bowel habit	84	242	254–8	
Change in stool colour	69	200	222–7, 246, 254	
Chest pain	11	32	36, 46–9, 36, 176–8, 227–8, 472, 485–9	
Child abuse	156	452	595–7, 417–9	
Chronic abdominal pain	81	232	221–2, 227–8, 244–6	
Chronic joint pain/stiffness	187	547	549–53, 560–1	
Chronic kidney disease	177	511	407–8, 508–15	
Chronic rash	16	47	104–5, 108–111, 112–114, 243–4	
Cold, painful, pale, pulseless leg/foot	5	14	32–5	
Complications of labour	128	369	366–70	
Confusion	47	135	312–3	
Congenital abnormalities	152, 153	443, 446	392–6	
Constipation	85	245	402, 434, 634	
Contraception request/advice	116	339	371–3	
Cough	185	541	244–5, 537–40, 545–6, 464	
Crying baby	144	413	402, 405–6	
Cyanosis	150	436	394–6, 397–8	

Continued

TABLE 2   UKMLA Presentations and Where to Find Them—cont'd

Patient presentations	Case number	Page	Relevant pages in Book 1	Revised?
Death and dying	160, 161	464, 467	431–5	
Decreased appetite	78	225	219–220	
Decreased/loss of consciousness	46	132	51, 55–6, 59–71, 183	
Dehydration	175	505	183–4, 190, 200–1, 212–4	
Deteriorating patient	41	116	9–21, 175–190	
Diarrhoea	86	247	254–8, 290–4	
Difficulty with breastfeeding	130	375	26	
Diplopia	30	84	148–52, 204, 322–3	
Dizziness	12	37	67–8, 55–6, 263–8, 309, 136–8, 320–1	
Driving advice	62	180	308	
Dysmorphic child	148	425	412, 557–8	
Ear and nasal discharge	20	58	133–6	
Elation/elated mood	165	478	439–40, 445–6, 312–3	
Elder abuse	162	470	312–315	
Electrolyte abnormalities	61, 178–181	176, 515–525	515–527	
End-of-life care/ symptoms of terminal illness	161	467	431–5	
Epistaxis	27	76	140–141, 564, 274, 625	
Erectile dysfunction	201	589	214–6, 615–7	
Eye pain/discomfort	36	100	160–7, 562–3	
Eye trauma	34	95	160–6	
Facial pain	107	311	305–6, 103	
Facial weakness	102	296	311–2, 322–3	
Facial/periorbital swelling	39	110	163–4, 416	
Faecal incontinence	75	217	351–2, 402	
Falls	48	137	136–8, 514	
Family history of possible genetic disorder	149	433	412	
Fasciculation	109	317	321–2, 518–27	
Fatigue	188	550	142–3, 203–4, 327	
Fever	90	261	288–9	
Fit notes	190	556	348–51, 438–9, 444–5	
Fits/seizures	100	290	306–8	
Fixed abnormal beliefs	170	493	441–2	
Flashes and floaters in visual fields	33	93	158–160, 303–5	
Food intolerance	79	227	255	
Foreign body in eye	34	95	160	
Frailty	157	456	136, 244–5, 314	
Genital Ulcers/warts	139	399	381–3	
Gradual loss of vision	38	107	152–8	
Gynaecomastia	65	188	202, 620–1	
Haematuria	199	584	358, 406–7, 500–2, 605–6, 617–9	
Haemoptysis	95	276	57–8, 294–7, 564–5	
Head injury	49	140	335–7, 480–2	
Headache	99	287	303–6, 345–6	

TABLE 2   UKMLA Presentations and Where to Find Them

Patient presentations	Case number	Page	Relevant pages in Book 1	Revised?
Hearing loss	22	63	134–8	
Heart murmur	9	26	54–8, 49–51	
Hoarseness and voice change	29	81	141–2, 203, 322–3	
Hyperemesis	117	342	373–4	
Hypertension	7	20	42–5	
Immobility	157	456	136, 244–5, 314	
Incontinence	75, 200	217, 587	351–2, 402–7, 500–2, 605–9	
Infant feeding problems	143	410	402–3, 406–7	
Intrauterine death	122	355	372–4	
Jaundice	94	273	247–9	
Labour	127	367	366–9	
Laceration	56	159	…	
Large for gestational age	123	357	361–4	
Learning disability	154	448	448	
Limb claudication	4	11	32–8, 349–50	
Limb weakness	110	320	206–7, 323	
Limp	151	440	587–95	
Loin pain	196	575	406–7, 500–2, 605–6, 617	
Loss of libido	64	185	201–2, 215–6, 376–8	
Loss of red reflex	32	90	166–8, 152, 158–160	
Low blood pressure	42	119	12–6	
Low mood/affective problems	164	475	438–442, 312–4	
Lump in groin	72	209	236–7	
Lymphadenopathy	91	264	146, 294–6, 297, 384–5, 275–9, 396–7	
Massive haemorrhage	44	126	35–6, 369–70, 570–9	
Melaena	50	143	181, 219–20, 244–6	
Memory loss	103	299	312–4, 335	
Menopausal problems	115	337	214–6, 376, 379	
Menstrual problems	133	382	358–9	
Mental capacity concerns	174	503	449	
Mental health problems in pregnancy or post partum	163	472	370–1	
Misplaced nasogastric tube	76	220	19, 464	
Muscle pain/myalgia	189	553	554–5, 631	
Musculoskeletal deformities	193	566	560, 584–5, 595	
Nail abnormalities	19	56	109, 119, 263–5	
Nasal obstruction	25	72	140	
Nausea	80	230	183–4, 293–4, 373–4, 402, 632–4	
Neck lump	60	173	143–7	
Neck pain/stiffness	93	270	289–90, 312, 349–51, 337–9	
Neonatal death or cot death	141	404	392–7, 404	
Neuromuscular weakness	110	320	206–7, 323	
Night sweats	91	264	277, 384–5, 396–7, 425	
Nipple discharge	1	1	26–9, 201–2, 450, 483	

Continued

TABLE 2   UKMLA Presentations and Where to Find Them—cont'd

Patient presentations	Case number	Page	Relevant pages in Book 1	Revised?
Normal pregnancy and antenatal care	120	349	358–60	
Oliguria	176	508	502–5	
Organomegaly	92	267	275–81, 250–1, 299, 297	
Overdose	52	148	185–7	
Pain on inspiration	11	32	36, 46–9, 36, 176–8, 227–8, 472, 485–9	
Painful ear	21	61	134–6	
Painful sexual intercourse	131	378	374–5	
Painful swollen leg	45	129	39–40, 101, 194–5	
Pallor	87	250	263–70, 275–77	
Palpitations	10	29	65–70, 442, 204, 185, 211	
Pelvic mass	134	385	375–6, 380–1	
Pelvic pain	133	382	358–9, 374–6, 382	
Perianal symptoms	73	212	102–3, 235–6, 383–4	
Peripheral oedema and ankle swelling	8	23	49–51, 250–1, 508–10	
Petechial rash	88	254	564–5, 270–2, 289–90	
Pleural effusion	184	538	49–50, 250–1, 545–6, 542–44	
Poisoning	51	146	185–8, 628–36	
Polydipsia (thirst)	175	505	183–4, 190, 201–2	
Post-surgical care and complications	66	191	12–4, 543, 632–4	
Pregnancy risk assessment	120	349	358–63	
Prematurity	140	401	397, 403–4, 411–2	
Pressure of speech	165	478	312–4, 439–44	
Pruritus	82	236	104–108	
Ptosis	30	84	180–1, 204, 303–4, 322–3	
Pubertal development	63	182	392–3	
Purpura	88	254	270–3, 564–5	
Rectal prolapse	74	215	231–6	
Red eye	35	98	160–6	
Reduced/change in foetal movements	125	362	…	
Scarring	14	42	…	
Scrotal/testicular pain and/or lump/swelling	197	578	236–7, 609–12, 620–1	
Self-harm	171	494	446–7	
Shock	42	119	12–6	
Skin lesion	17	50	115–124	
Skin or subcutaneous lump	18	53	27, 425, 109, 112	
Skin ulcer	6	17	30–4	
Sleep problems	112	325	142, 327–9, 439–444	
Small for gestational age	124	359	361–4	
Snoring	57	164	140–3, 199	
Soft tissue injury	191	559	572–8, 589	
Somatisation/medically unexplained physical symptoms	168	487	444–5	
Sore throat	28	79	141–2, 297	
Speech and language problems	101	293	308–11	

TABLE 2   UKMLA Presentations and Where to Find Them

Patient presentations	Case number	Page	Relevant pages in Book 1	Revised?
Squint	31	87	148–52	
Stridor	182	531	142, 399–400	
Struggling to cope at home	157	456	136, 244–5, 314	
Subfertility	119	339	214–6, 374–5, 382	
Substance misuse	121	352	180–1, 185–7, 360, 433	
Suicidal thoughts	171	494	438–48	
Swallowing problems	77	223	218–221	
The sick child	145	415	183–4, 312, 400, 406, 413–7	
Threats to harm others	172	497	180, 312–3, 439–41, 445–7	
Tinnitus	23	66	137–8, 133–5	
Trauma	44, 194	126, 569	10–12, 35–6, 179, 369, 572–9, 589, 595	
Travel health advice	98	284	290–4, 299	
Tremor	105	304	253, 325, 316–7	
Unsteadiness	111	323	180–1, 325	
Unwanted pregnancy and termination	118	345	373–4	
Urethral discharge	138, 139	395,399	381–3	
Urinary incontinence	200	587	406–7, 500–2, 605–9	
Urinary symptoms	200	587	406–7, 500–2, 605–9	
Vaccination	97	283	289, 294, 312, 401, 413	
Vaginal discharge	138	395	102–3, 381–3	
Vaginal prolapse	132	380	376–7	
Vertigo	24	69	136–9, 309	
Viral exanthems	96	279	413–7	
Visual hallucinations	104	302	303, 306, 441	
Vomiting	80, 117	330, 342	183–4, 293–4, 373–4, 402, 632–4	
Vulval itching/lesion	136	390	104, 375, 378	
Vulval/vaginal lump	135	387	375, 378, 383–4	
Weight gain	59	59	203, 206-7, 438-9	
Weight loss	58	167	204-6, 254-7, 438-9, 184-5	
Wellbeing checks	142	407	35-6, 231-3, 425	
Wheeze	183	535	535-40, 542-3, 175-7	

PREFACE

This book is the companion volume to *Medicine in a Day: Revision Notes for medical exams, finals, UKMLA and foundation years*, covering all the conditions required for the United Kingdom Medical Licensing Assessment (UKMLA). This new volume helps you develop the key skill of an effective doctor: the ability to deal with the typical presentations seen in the clinical setting.

The chapters build on knowledge of the conditions, by applying it to circumstances seen in practice. Patients do not attend with a ready-made diagnosis, so the symptoms and signs need to be considered, and appropriate evaluations used to recognise the possible causes. Diagnosing the underlying condition requires alertness and acumen so that the situation can be dealt with promptly, enabling appropriate treatment for each individual.

In many circumstances, several conditions can present in a rather similar way, so beware of dangers that will trap the unwary. The underlying cause may not be obvious at first presentation, or the initial impression may have been wrong, so the working diagnosis must be kept under review. Bear in mind that sometimes referrals are based on limited information and can be slow to reach the relevant specialty, so the cause is often not clear and the seriousness might only emerge once homeostatic mechanisms begin to decompensate. And, of course, pain referred away from the causative organ directs attention to the wrong place and is perfect for testing in exams.

When one starts in practice, it can seem a bit baffling. Nonetheless, there is generally a key pointer or two that can quickly direct the focus appropriately. In this second volume, we distil the essence of the presentations to bring out the potential contributory conditions, and the key points of each that could reveal the cause for an individual case. All the presentations in the UKMLA syllabus are covered, and some additional ones. The book stays true to the succinct and practical ethos of *Medicine in a Day*. It does not attempt to mention every possible fact, as that would make it unwieldy for revision; vital knowledge is prioritised over detail.

As with the first volume, we have partnered with Don't Forget The Bubbles (DFTB) Skin Deep, and we are very grateful for their high-quality photographs of medical conditions illustrated in a range of skin tones. Again, Dr Hollie Blaber has provided characterful and engaging illustrations. We are deeply grateful to our many authors, who come from a wide spectrum of the entire medical profession. Working with each one has been a privilege.

Please use this book to hone your intellectual familiarity with the conditions into relevant and practical knowledge suited to solving this broad sweep of clinical presentations. We hope that, once again, you enjoy revising the whole of medicine in a day (indeed, whatever timeframe you choose).

Marcus, Sandy, Greg, Hollie, and Berenice

CONTRIBUTORS

The editors acknowledge and offer grateful thanks for the input of all contributors, without whom this book would not have been possible.

Dr Oliver Agutu
Dr Viren Ahluwalia
Dr Leia Alston
Dr Omar Amar
Miss Katherine Anderson
Dr Lucy Andrews
Dr Christian Aquilina
Dr Ann Archer
Dr Denize Atan
Dr Lelyn Osei Atiemo
Dr Harriet Ball
Dr Richard Barlow
Mr Shivam Bhanderi
Ms Alka Bhide
Dr Rachael Biggart
Dr Francesca Blest
Dr Caroline Bodey
Mr Matthew Boissaud-Cooke
Dr Juliet Brown
Dr Claudia Burton
Dr Alexander Calthorpe
Dr Michael Campbell
Dr Alex Carrie
Miss Emma Carrington
Dr Ela Chakkarapani
Dr James Chataway
Dr Hannah Clark
Mr Jonathan Cobley
Dr Emma Corke
Dr Eleanor Courtney
Dr Megan Crofts
Dr Laura Crosby
Mr Vincent Cumberworth
Dr Jon Dallimore
Dr Lowri Foster Davies
Dr Alex Digesu
Dr Harriet Diment
Dr Sofia Eriksson
Dr Benjamin Faber
Dr Judith Fox
Dr Margarita Fox
Dr Ben Gibbison
Dr Connie Glover
Dr David Grant
Dr Francesca Guest
Dr Emma Gull
Dr Natalia Hackett

Dr Lucy Harrison
Dr Rachel Hawthorne
Dr Emily Henderson
Dr Stella Hristova
Dr Ioan Llwyd Hughes
Dr Emmanuella Ikem
Dr Rada Ivanov
Dr Annapurna Jagadish
Mr Abraham John
Dr Nwaorima Kamalu
Dr Zoe Kay
Dr Sophie Kellman
Dr Henna Khattak
Dr Sung-Hee Kim
Dr Kirstie Kirkley
Dr Chetna Kohli
Miss Angeliki Kosti
Mr For Tai Lam
Dr Kathleen Levick
Dr Nicole Lundon
Dr Marie-Louise Lyons
Dr Sian Maguire
Mr Aditya Manjunath
Dr Louise Mathias
Dr Kate McCann
Dr Ciara McClenaghan
Mr Angus McNair
Mr James Miller
Dr Felix Miller-Molloy
Dr Damien Mony
Dr Dafydd Morgan
Dr Hamish Morrison
Dr Aldoph Nanguzgambo
Dr Kavita Narula
Dr Tejas Netke
Dr Rebecca Newhouse
Miss Lydia Newton
Ms Peta Nixon
Dr Thomas Nutting
Dr Abigail Nye
Dr Anna Ogier
Miss Shilpa Ojha
Dr Kaobi Okongwu
Dr Joseph Page
Dr Eva Papaioannou
Dr Alice Parker
Dr Katherine Parker

Dr Mital Patel
Dr Elizabeth Perry
Dr Alice Pitt
Dr Hannah Podger
Dr Jennifer Powell
Professor Athimalaipet Ramanan
Dr Alexander Reed
Dr Nicholas Rees
Dr Dalilah Restrepo
Professor Matthew Ridd
Dr Alex Ridgway
Dr David Roberts
Dr Hannah Rodgers
Dr Lindsey Rowley
Dr Anya Rutherfurd
Dr Aws Sadik
Dr Shruthi Sankaranarayanan
Dr Simon Scheck
Dr Sanchita Sen
Dr Maximilian Shah
Dr Vidit Singh
Dr Laura Skinner
Dr Matthew Smith
Dr Tirion Smith
Dr Amelia Stockley
Dr Amber Syed
Dr Dylan Thiarya
Dr Graham Thornton
Dr Simon Thornton
Dr Katie Turner
Dr Jonathan Tyrell-Price
Dr Udaya Udayaraj
Dr Stephanie Upton
Mr Natarajan Vaithilingam
Miss Jajini Susan Varghese
Dr Emily Vaughan
Dr Manuj Vyas
Dr Emily Warren
Dr James Wiggins
Professor Michael Whitehouse
Dr Oliver Whitehurst
Dr Mariella Williams
Dr Julia Wolf
Dr Katie Wong
Dr Lara Yorke
Dr Meijia Mary Xie

ACKNOWLEDGEMENTS

To our friends and family for their love and support, and for believing in us.

Especially to Arthur, Berenice's baby, who cuddled mum for so many hours whilst working on this book, and to our co-editors for their never-ending enthusiasm, motivation and guidance.

To all those who contributed to this book – we are so proud of all of you.

And finally ... To all those who dream to become the best doctor; we hope this book helps you make that dream come true!

ABBREVIATION LIST

Abbreviation	Term
2WW	Two week wait
A&E	Accident and emergency
AAA	Abdominal aortic aneurysm
ABA	Applied behavioural analysis
ABCDE	Airway, Breathing, Circulation, Disability, Exposure
ABG	Arterial blood gas
ABPI	Ankle brachial pressure index
ABPM	Ambulatory blood pressure monitoring
ABs	Antibodies
Abx	Antibiotics
AC	Abdominal circumference
ACA	Anterior cerebral artery
ACE	Angiotensin-converting enzyme/ Adverse childhood experience
ACE-i/ACE-I	Angiotensin-converting enzyme inhibitor
ACE-III	Addenbrooke's cognitive examination III
AChE	Acetylcholinesterase
AChR	Acetylcholine receptor
ACL	Anterior cruciate ligament
ACR	Albumin:creatinine ratio
ACS	Acute coronary syndrome
ACTH	Adrenocorticotropic hormone
AD	Autosomal dominant/ Antidepressant/ Alzheimer's disease
ADAMTS13	A disintegrin and metalloproteinase with a thrombospondin motif 13
ADH	Anti-diuretic hormone
ADHD	Attention deficit hyperactivity disorder
ADL	Activities of daily living
AF	Atrial fibrillation
AFP	Alpha-fetoprotein
AHI	Apnoea/hypopnoea index
AIDS	Acquired immune deficiency syndrome
AKI	Acute kidney injury
ALARM	Anaemia, Loss of weight, Anorexia, Recent dysphagia, Melaena/ haematemesis
ALD	Alcoholic liver disease
ALL	Acute lymphoid leukaemia
ALP	Alkaline phosphatase
ALS	Advanced life support
ALT	Alanine aminotransferase
AMA	Anti-mitochondrial antibody

Abbreviation	Term
AMD	Age-related macular degeneration
AML	Acute myeloid leukaemia
AMT(S)	Abbreviated mental test (score)
AN	Anorexia nervosa
ANA	Antinuclear antibody
ANCA	Antineutrophil cytoplasmic antibody
Anti-CCP	Anti-cyclic citrullinated peptide antibody
Anti-dsDNA	Anti-double stranded DNA antibody
Anti-GBM	Anti-glomerular basement membrane
Anti-HBc IgG	IgG Antibodies against Hepatitis B core antigen
Anti-HBc IgM	IgM Antibodies against Hepatitis B core antigen
Anti-HBS	Antibodies against Hepatitis B Surface Antigen
Anti-HCV	Anti-Hepatitis C antibody
Anti-LKM	Anti-liver-kidney microsomal antibody
Anti-SRP	Anti-signal recognition particle antibody
Anti-TNF	Anti-tumour necrosis factor antibody
Anti-TTG	Anti-tissue transglutaminase antibody
AOM	Acute otitis media
AP	Antero-posterior
APGAR	Appearance, Pulse, Grimace, Activity, Respiration
APH	Antepartum haemorrhage
APTT	Activated partial thromboplastin time
AQ	Autism spectrum quotient test
AR	Aortic regurgitation
ARB	Angiotension II receptor blocker
ARDS	Acute respiratory distress syndrome
ARM	Artificial rupture of membranes
AS	Aortic stenosis
ASA	American Society of Anesthesiologists
ASAP	As soon as possible
ASD	Atrial septal defect/ Autism spectrum disorder
AST	Aspartate aminotransferase
ATLS	Advanced trauma life support
AUDIT	Alcohol use disorders identification tool
AUR	Acute urinary retention
AV	Atrioventricular/ Arterio-venous
AVM	Atrioventricular malformation/ Arterio-venous malformation
AVN	Avascular necrosis

Abbreviation	Term
AVNRT	Atrioventricular nodal re-entrant tachycardia
AVPU	Alert, Voice, Pain, Unresponsive
AVR	Aortic valve replacement
AVSD	Atrioventricular septal defect
AXR	Abdominal x-ray
BAC	Blood alcohol content
BASDAI	Bath ankylosing spondylitis disease activity index
BCC	Basal cell carcinoma
BCG	Bacillus Calmette-Guérin
BD	Twice a day (bis in die)
BDI-II	Beck's depression inventory 2
β-HCG	β-human chorionic gonadotrophin
BLO	Bowels last open
BM	Blood glucose measurement
BMAT	Bone marrow aspirate and trephine
BMD	Bone mineral density
BMI	Body mass index
BNF	British National Formulary
BNP	Brain natriuretic peptide
BOAST	British Orthopaedic Association standards for trauma and orthopaedics
BP	Blood pressure
BPAD	Bipolar affective disorder
BPD	Bronchopulmonary dysplasia
BPE	Benign prostatic enlargement
BPH	Benign prostatic hyperplasia
bpm	Beats per minute
BPPV	Benign paroxysmal positional vertigo
BRCA	Breast cancer gene
BS	Bowel sounds
BSO	Bilateral salpingo-oophorectomy
BTS	British Thoracic Society
BXO	Balanitis xerotica obliterans
Ca++/Ca	Calcium/ Carcinoma
Ca125	Cancer antigen 125
Ca19-9	Cancer antigen 19-9
(C)ABCDE	Catastrophic haemorrhage, Airway, Breathing, Circulation, Disability, Exposure
CABG	Coronary artery bypass graft
CAD	Coronary artery disease
CAH	Congenital adrenal hyperplasia
CAI	Carbonic anhydrase inhibitor
CAM	Confusion assessment method
CAMHS	Child and adolescent mental health services
CAP	Community acquired pneumonia

Abbreviation	Term
CARS	Childhood autism rating scale
CAST	Childhood Asperger syndrome test
CBD	Corticobasal degeneration
CBG	Capillary blood glucose
CBT	Cognitive behavioural therapy
CCB	Calcium channel blocker
CCF	Congestive cardiac failure
CCU	Coronary care unit
CDH	Congenital diaphragmatic hernia
CEA	Carcinoembryonic antigen
CES	Cauda equina syndrome
CF	Cystic fibrosis
CFTR	Cystic fibrosis transmembrane conductance regulator
CFU	Colony forming units
CHF	Congestive heart failure
CHL	Conductive hearing loss
CI	Contraindication
CIN	Cervical intraepithelial neoplasia
CIS	Carcinoma in situ
CIWA	Clinical institute withdrawal assessment for alcohol
CK	Creatinine kinase
CKD	Chronic kidney disease
CLL	Chronic lymphocytic leukaemia
CM	Crossmatch
CML	Chronic myeloid leukaemia
CMPA	Cow's milk protein allergy
CMV	Cytomegalovirus
CN	Cranial nerve
CNS	Central nervous system
CO	Carbon monoxide
COCP	Combined oral contraceptive pill
COHb	Carboxyhaemoglobin
COMT	Catechol-O-methyltransferase
COPD	Chronic obstructive pulmonary disease
CPA	Cerebellopontine angle/ Chronic pulmonary aspergillosis
CPAP	Continous positive airway pressure
CPR	Cardiopulmonary resuscitation
CRP	C-reactive protein
CRT	Capillary refill time
CrUSS	Cranial ultrasound scan
CS	Caesarean section
CSF	Cerebrospinal fluid
CSW	Cerebral salt wasting
CT	Computed tomography
CTA	CT angiogram
CT CAP	CT chest/ abdomen/ pelvis
CTG	Cardiotocograph

Abbreviation	Term
CTH	CT head
CTPA	CT pulmonary angiogram
CT TAP	CT Thorax, abdomen and pelvis
CURB65	Pneumonia severity calculator
CVD	Cardiovascular disease
CVE	Cerebrovascular event
CVS	Cardiovascular system/ Chorionic villus sampling
CXR	Chest xray
D&C	Dilation and curettage
DA	Dopamine
DaT	Dopamine active transporter
DBP	Diastolic blood pressure
DBS	Deep brain stimulator
DBT	Dialectical behavioural therapy
DCCT	Direct current cardioversion therapy
DDH	Developmental dysplasia of the hip
DDx	Differential diagnosis
DEXA/ DXA	Dual-energy X-ray absorptiometry (bone densitometry)
DHS	Dynamic hip screw
DHx	Drug history
DI	Diabetes insipidus
DIC	Disseminated intravascular coagulation
DIP	Distal interphalangeal joint
DKA	Diabetic ketoacidosis
DLCO	Diffusing capacity of the lungs for carbon monoxide
DM	Diabetes mellitus
DMARD(s)	Disease-modifying anti-rheumatic drug(s)
DMSA	Dimercaptosuccinic acid
DNA	Did not attend
DOAC	Direct oral anticoagulant
DRE	Digital rectal exam
dsDNA	Double-stranded deoxyribonucleic acid
DSM	Diagnostic and Statistical Manual of Mental Disorders
DVLA	Driver and Vehicle Licensing Agency
DVT	Deep vein thrombosis
D/W	Discuss with
DWI	Diffusion weighted imaging
Dx	Diagnosis
DXA/ DEXA	Dual X-ray absorptiometry (bone densitometry)
EAC	External auditory canal
EAM	External auditory meatus
EASI	Eczema area and severity index
EBV	Epstein Barr virus
ECG	Electrocardiogram

Abbreviation	Term
Echo(CG)	Echocardiogram
ECMO	Extra-corporeal membrane oxygenation
ECT	Electroconvulsive therapy
ECV	External cephalic version
ED	Emergency Department/ Erectile dysfunction/ Extensor digitorum
EDH	Extra dural haemorrhage
EEG	Electroencephalogram
EF	Ejection fraction
EFW	Estimated fetal weight
eGFR	Estimated glomerular filtration rate
EGFR	Epidermal growth factor receptor
EGPA	Eosinophilic granulomatosis with polyangiitis
ELISA	Enzyme linked immunosorbent assay
EM	Erythema multiforme
EMDR	Eye movement desensitization and reprocessing
EMG	Electromyogram
EN	Erythema nodosum
ENT	Ear, nose and throat
EoL	End of life
EPI	Exocrine pancreas insufficiency
EPO	Erythropoietin
EPU	Early pregnancy unit
ERCP	Endoscopic retrograde cholangiopancreatography
ESDM	Early Start Denver Model
ESM	Ejection systolic murmur
ESR	Erythrocyte sedimentation rate
ESRF	End stage renal failure
ESWL	Extracorporeal shockwave lithotripsy
ET	Essential thrombocythaemia/ Endotracheal
EtOH	Alcohol
ETT	Endotracheal tube
EUA	Examination under anaesthetic
EUPD	Emotionally unstable personality disorder
EVD	Extra-ventricular drainage
FA	Friedrich's ataxia
FAP	Familial adenomatous polyposis
FAS	Fetal alcohol syndrome
FAST	Focused assessment with sonography for trauma
FB	Foreign body
FBC	Full blood count
FCU	First catch urine
FDR	First degree relative
FESS	Functional endoscopic sinus surgery

Abbreviation	Term
FEV1	Forced expiratory volume in one second
ffDNA	Free fetal DNA
FFP	Fresh frozen plasma
FGM	Female genital mutilation
FGR	Fetal growth restriction
FH	Familial hypercholesterolaemia/ Family history
FHx	Family history
FiO$_2$	Fraction inspired O$_2$
FIT	Faecal immunochemical test
FLAIR	Fluid-attenuated inversion recovery
FNAC	Fine needle aspiration cytology
FODMAP	Fermentable oligosaccharides, disaccharides, monosaccharides and polyols
FRAX	Fracture risk algorithm
FSGS	Focal segmental glomerulosclerosis
FSH	Follicle stimulating hormone
FTD	Frontotemporal dementia
FTT	Failure to thrive
FVC	Forced vital capacity
G6PDH	Glucose-6-phosphate dehydrogenase
G&S	Group and save
GA	General anaesthetic
GABA	Gamma-aminobutyric acid
GAD	Generalised anxiety disorder
GAD-7 score	Generalised anxiety disorder score
GBM	Glomerular basement membrane
GBS	Group B streptococcus/ Guillain-Barré syndrome
GCA	Giant cell arteritis
GCS	Glasgow Coma Scale
GDM	Gestational diabetes mellitus
GGT	Gamma-glutamyl transferase
GH(RH)	Growth hormone (releasing hormone)
GI	Gastrointestinal
GN	Glomerulonephritis
GnRH	Gonadotrophin releasing hormone
GORD	Gastro-oesophageal reflux disease
GP	General practitioner
GPA	Granulomatosis with polyangiitis
GTN	Glyceryl trinitrate
GU	Genitourinary
GUM	Genito-urinary medicine
HADS	Hospital anxiety and depression scale
HAS	Human albumin solution
HAV	Hepatitis A virus
Hb	Haemoglobin
HbA1c	Haemoglobin A1C (glycosylated Hb)
HBPM	Home blood pressure monitoring

Abbreviation	Term
HBV	Hepatitis B virus
HBsAG	Hepatitis B surface antigen
HCC	Hepatocellular carcinoma
HCG	Human chorionic gonadotrophin
HCO$_3$	Bicarbonate
HCM	Hypertrophic cardiomyopathy
HCV	Hepatitis C virus
HDU	High dependency unit
HELLP	Haemolysis, elevated liver enzymes and low platelets
HER2	Human epidermal growth receptor 2
HFNO	High flow nasal oxygen
HG	Hyperemesis gravidarum
HHT	Hereditary haemorrhagic telangiectasia
Hib/ HiB	Haemophilus influenzae type B
HIDA	Hepatobiliary iminodiacetic acid
HINTS	Head impulse, nystagmus, and test of skew
HIV	Human immunodeficiency virus
HLA	Human leukocyte antigen
HPC	History of presenting complaint
HPOA	Hypertrophic pulmonary osteoarthropathy
HPV	Human papilloma virus
HR	Heart rate
hrHPV	High risk HPV
HRS	Hepato-renal syndrome
HRT	Hormone replacement therapy
HS	Heart sounds
HSCT	Hematopoietic stem cell transplant
HSG	Hysterosalpingogram
HSP	Henoch-Schönlein purpura
HSV	Herpes simplex virus
HTN	Hypertension
HUS	Haemolytic uraemic syndrome
HVA	Homovanillic acid
HVS	High vaginal swab
Hx	History
iADL	Instrumental activities of daily living
IAM	Internal auditory meatus
IAPT	Improving access to psychological therapies
IBD	Inflammatory bowel disease
IBS	Irritable bowel syndrome
IC	Intermittent claudication
ICD	Implantable cardioverter defibrillator
ICD-10	International Statistical Classification of Diseases and Related Health Problems
ICH	Intracranial haemorrhage

Abbreviation	Term
ICP	Intracranial pressure
ICS	Inhaled corticosteroid
ICSI	Intracystoplasmic sperm injection
ICU	Intensive care unit
IDDM	Insulin dependent diabetes mellitus
IEM	Inborn errors of metabolism
IF	Intrinsic factor
IgA	Immunoglobulin A
IGC	Inhaled glucocorticoid
IGF1	Insulin like growth factor 1
IHD	Ischaemic heart disease/ Intermittent haemodialysis
IIH	Idiopathic intracranial hypertension
IL4R	Interleukin-4 receptor
IL5/R	Interleukin-5/ IL5 receptor
ILD	Interstitial lung disease
ILS	Intermediate life support
IM	Intramuscular
IMB	Intermenstrual bleeding
iNO	Inhaled nitric oxide
INR	International normalised ratio
IOL	Induction of labour
IOP	Intracocular pressure
IPSS	International prostate symptom score
IRT	Immunoreactive trypsinogen
ITP	Immune thrombocytopenic purpura
IUD	Intrauterine device
IUGR	Intrauterine growth restriction
IUI	Intrauterine insemination
IUS	Intrauterine system
IV	Intravenous
IVC	Inferior vena cava
IVDU	Intravenous drug usage
IVF	In-vitro fertilisation
IVH	Intraventricular haemorrhage
IVI	Intravenous infusion
IVIG	Intravenous immunoglobulin
JASPER	Joint attention, symbolic play, engagement & regulation
JIA	Juvenile idiopathic arthritis
JVP	Jugular venous pressure
K+/KCl	Potassium/ Potassium chloride
KDIGO	Kidney disease improving global outcomes
kg	Kilogram
KUB	Kidney ureter bladder
LA	Local anaesthetic
LABA	Long acting beta 2 agonist
LACS	Lacunar stroke
LAMA	Long-acting muscarinic antagonist

Abbreviation	Term
LBBB	Left bundle branch block
LBD	Lewy body dementia
LBO	Large bowel obstruction
LD	Learning disability
LDH	Lactate dehydrogenase
LEMS	Lambert Eaton myasthenic syndrome
LFTs	Liver function tests
LGA	Large for gestational age
LH(RH)	Luteinizing hormone (releasing hormone)
LL	Lower limb
LLETZ	Large loop excision of the transformation zone
LLSE	Lower left sternal edge
LLQ	Lower left quadrant
LMP	Last menstrual period
LMN	Lower motor neurone
LMWH	Low molecular weight heparin
LN	Lymph Node
LOC	Loss of consciousness
LP	Lumbar puncture/ Lichen planus
LPA	Lasting power of attorney
LRTA	Leukotriene receptor antagonist
LRTI	Lower respiratory tract infection
L/S	Lumbar/ sacral
LSCS	Lower segment caesarean section
LTOT	Long term oxygen therapy
LUTS	Lower urinary tract symptoms
LVAD	Left ventricular assist device
LVEF	Left ventricular ejection fraction
LVF	Left ventricular failure
LVH	Left ventricular hypertrophy
LVSD	Left ventricular systolic dysfunction
MAHA	Microangiopathic haemolytic anaemia
MAOB	Monoamine oxidase type B
MAOI	Monoamine oxidase inhibitor
MAP	Mean arterial pressure
MBT	Mentalization-based therapy
MC&S	Microscopy, culture and sensitivity
MCA	Middle cerebral artery
MCD	Minimal change disease
M-CHAT	Modified checklist for autism in toddlers
MCL	Medial collateral ligament
MCP	Metacarpophalangeal
MCV	Mean cell volume
MCUG	Micturating cystourethrogram
MDMA	3,4-Methylenedioxymethamphetamine (ecstasy)
MDT	Multidisciplinary team

Abbreviation	Term
odm	Model of end stage liver disease
MEN	Multiple endocrine neoplasia
MEq	Milliequivalents
mg/ Mg	Milligram/ Magnesium
MGUS	Monoclonal gammopathy of undetermined significance
MHA	Mental health act
MHI	Mental health illness
MI	Myocardial infarction
MM	Multiple myeloma
MMF	Mycophenolate mofetil
mmHg	Millimetres of mercury
MMR	Measles, mumps and rubella
MMSE	Mini mental state examination
MN	Membranous nephropathy
MND	Motor neurone disease
MOCA	Montreal cognitive assessment
MOsm	Milliosmoles
MPH	Mean parental height
MR	Mitral regurgitation
MRA	Mineralocorticoid receptor antagonist
MRCP	Magnetic resonance cholangiopancreatography
MRI	Magnetic resonance imaging
MRI IAM	MRI of internal auditory meatus
MS	Mitral stenosis/ Multiple sclerosis
MSA	Multiple system atrophy
MSE	Mental state examination
MSK	Musculoskeletal
MSM	Men who have sex with men
MST	Morphine slow-release tablet
MSU	Mid stream urine
MSUD	Maple syrup urine disease
MTC	Major trauma center
MTX	Methotrexate
MUST	Malnutrition universal screening tool
N/A	Not applicable
N&V	Nausea and vomiting
Na^+	Sodium
NAAT	Nucleic acid amplification tests
NAC	N-acetylcysteine
NAFLD	Non-alcoholic fatty liver disease
NAI	Non accidental injury
NAS	Neonatal abstinence syndrome
NASH	Non-alcoholic steatohepatitis
NBM	Nil by mouth
NBS	Normal bowel sounds
Neb	Nebuliser
NEC	Necrotising enterocolitis
NEWS	National Early Warning Score

Abbreviation	Term
NG(T)	Nasogastric (tube)
NGU	Non-gonococcal urethritis
NHL	Non-Hodgkin lymphoma
NICE	National Institute for Health and Care Excellence
NICU	Neonatal intensive care unit
NIPE	Neonatal and infant physical examination
NIHSS	National Institutes of Health Stroke Severity
NIV	Non-invasive ventilation
NKDA	No known drug allergy
NMDA	N-methyl-D-aspartate glutamate receptor
NO	Nitric oxide
NOF(#)	Neck of femur (fracture)
NOK	Next of kin
NRT	Nicotine replacement therapy
NSAIDs	Non-steroidal anti-inflammatory drugs
NSTEMI	Non-ST elevation myocardial infarction
NT	Nuchal translucency
NT-pro-BNP	N-terminal pro B type naturetic peptide
NVD	Normal vaginal delivery
OA	Osteoarthritis/ Occiput anterior
OAB	Overactive bladder syndrome
OAE	Otoacoustic emissions
Obs	Observations
OC	Obstetric cholestasis
OCD	Obsessive compulsive disorder
OCP	Oral contraceptive pill
OCT	Optical coherence tomography
OD	Overdose/ Once daily
OE	Otitis externa
O/E	On examination
OGD	Oesophagogastroduodenoscopy
OGTT	Oral glucose tolerance test
OM(E)	Otitis media (with effusion)
OMP	Outer membrane protein
ORIF	Open reduction and internal fixation
OSA	Obstructive sleep apnoea
OT	Occupational therapy
OTC	Oxytocin/ Over the counter
PA	Postero-anterior
$PACO_2$	Partial pressure of carbon dioxide (alveolar)
$PaCO_2$	Partial pressure of carbon dioxide (arterial)
PACS	Partial anterior circulation stroke
PAD	Peripheral artery disease
PAH	Pulmonary arterial hypertension

Abbreviation	Term
PALB	Partner and locator of BRCA2
PAN	Polyarteritis nodosa
PaO_2	Partial pressure of oxygen (arterial)
PAO_2	Partial pressure of oxygen (alveolar)
PAP	Pulmonary artery pressure
PAPP-A	Pregnancy associated plasma protein-A
PASI	Psoriasis area and severity index
PBC	Primary biliary cholangitis
PCA	Patient controlled analgesia
PCB	Post-coital bleeding
PCD	Primary ciliary dyskinesia
PCI	Percutaneous intervention
PCKD	Polycystic kidney disease
PCL	Posterior cruciate ligament
PCNL	Percutaneous nephrolithotomy
PCOS	Polycystic ovarian syndrome
PCR	Polymerase chain reaction/ Protein:creatinine ratio
PCT	Procalcitonin
PD	Parkinson's disease/ Peritoneal dialysis/ Personality disorder
PDA	Patent ductus arteriosus
PDE-5	Phosphodiesterase-5
PDI	Protein disulphide isomerase
PE	Pulmonary embolism
PEA	Pulseless electrical activity
PEARL	Pupils equal and reactive to light
PEEP	Positive end expiratory pressure
PEFR	Peak expiratory flow rate
PEG	Percutaneous endoscopic gastrostomy
PESI	Pulmonary embolism severity index
PET	Pre-eclampsia
PFMT	Pelvic floor muscle training
pGALS	Paediatric gait, arms, legs, spine
PH	Pulmonary hypertension
PHA	Pseudohypoaldosteronism
PHE	Public Health England
PHQ-9	Patient health questionnaire-9
PICA	Posterior inferior cerebellar artery
PID	Pelvic inflammatory disease/ Prolapsed intervertebral disc
PIH	Post-inflammatory hyperpigmentation
PIP	Proximal interphalangeal joint
PKD	Polycystic kidney disease
PKU	Phenylketonuria
PMB	Post menopausal bleeding
PMC	Percutaneous mitral commissurotomy
PMF	Primary myelofibrosis
PMHx	Past medical history

Abbreviation	Term
PMR	Polymyalgia rheumatica
PMS	Pre-menstrual syndrome
PND	Paroxysmal nocturnal dyspnoea
PO	Per os (taken orally)
PO_4	Phosphate
POCS	Posterior circulation syndrome
POI	Premature ovarian insufficiency
POMC	Proopiomelanocortin
PONV	Post-operative nausea and vomiting
POP	Progesterone only pill/ Pelvic organ prolapse
PPE	Personal protective equipment.
PPH	Post-partum haemorrhage
PPHN	Persistent pulmonary hypertension of the newborn
PPI	Proton pump inhibitor
PPROM	Preterm premature rupture of membranes
PPV	Pneumococcal polysaccharide vaccine
PROM	Premature rupture of membranes
PR	Per rectum/ Progesterone receptor
PRISMA-7	Program of Research to Integrate Services for the Maintenance of Autonomy
PRN	As needed (pro re nata)
PRV	Polycythaemia rubra vera
PS	Pulmonary stenosis
PSA	Prostate-specific antigen/Psoriatic arthropathy
PSC	Primary sclerosing cholangitis
PSGN	Post-streptococcal glomerulonephritis
PSM	Pan systolic murmur
PSP	Progressive supranuclear palsy
PT	Physiotherapy/Prothrombin time
PTA	Pure tone audiogram
PTH(rP)	Parathyroid hormone (related peptide)
PTL	Preterm labour
PTSD	Post traumatic stress disorder
PTT	Partial thromboplastin time
PTX	Pneumothorax
PV	Per vaginam/ Polycythaemia vera
PVD	Periperal vascular disease/ Posterior vitreous detachment
PVL	Periventricular leucomalacia
PVR	Post void residual
QoL	Quality of life
QTc	Corrected QT interval
RA	Rheumatoid arthritis
RAD	Right axis deviation

Abbreviation	Term
RAMPS	Radical antegrade modular pancreatosplenectomy
RAPD	Relative afferent pupil defect
RAST	Radioallergosorbent test
RB	Retinoblastoma
RBBB	Right bundle branch block
RBC	Red blood cells
RBD	REM sleep behaviour disorder
RCA	Right coronary artery
RCC	Renal cell carcinoma
RCT	Randomised control trial
RDS	Respiratory distress syndrome
REM	Rapid eye movement
RF	Rheumatoid Factor
RFs	Risk factors
RFM	Reduced fetal movements
RhF	Rheumatoid factor
RHF	Right heart failure
RICE	Rest, ice, compression, elevation
RIPE	Rifampicin, isoniazid, pyrazinamide, ethambutol
RLQ	Right lower quadrant
r/o	Rule out
ROLA	Rapid onset long acting beta2-agonist
ROM	Range of movement/ Rupture of membranes
ROSC	Return of spontaneous circulation
RPE	Retinal pigment epithelium
RPGN	Rapidly progressive glomerulonephritis
RPR	Rapid plasmin reagin
RR	Respiratory rate/ Risk ratio
RRT	Renal replacement therapy
RS	Respiratory system
RSV	Respiratory syncytial virus
RTA	Road traffic accident/ Renal tubular acidosis
RTx	Radiotherapy
RUL	Right upper lobe
RUQ	Right upper quadrant
RVH	Right ventricular hypertrophy
SAAG	Serum-ascites albumin gradient
SABA	Short acting beta 2 agonist
SACE	Serum angiotension II converting enzyme
SAD	Syncope, angina, dyspnoea
SAH	Subarachnoid haemorrhage
SALT	Speech and language therapy
SAMA	Short-acting muscarinic antagonist
SAN	Sinoatrial node

Abbreviation	Term
SARC-F	Strength, Assistance in walking, Rise from a chair, Climb stairs, and Falls
SBO	Small bowel obstruction
SBP	Systolic blood pressure/ Spontaneous bacterial peritonitis
SBR	Serum bilirubin
SC	Subcutaneous
SCA	Spinocerebellar ataxia
SCC	Squamous cell carcinoma
SCD	Sickle cell disease
SCF	Supraclavicular fossa
SCLC	Small cell lung cancer
SDH	Subdural haemorrhage
SEs	Side effects
SFH	Symphysial fundal height
SGA	Small for gestational age
SGLT	Sodium glucose co-transporter
SHBG	Sex hormone binding globulin
SHx	Social history
SIADH	Syndrome of inappropriate anti-diuretic hormone
SIBO	Small intestinal bacterial overgrowth
SIDS	Sudden infant death syndrome
SJS	Stevens Johnson syndrome
SLE	Systemic lupus erythematous
SLNB	Sentinel lymph node biopsy
SLR	Straight leg raise
SNHL	Sensorineural hearing loss
SNRI	Seritonin-norepinephrine reuptake inhibitor
SNT	Soft non tender
SOB(OE)	Shortness of breath (on exertion)
SOGS	Schedule of growing skills
SOL	Space occupying lesion
SpO_2	Oxygen saturation
SR	Systems review
SRS	Stereotactic radiosurgery
SSRI	Selective serotonin reuptake inhibitor
SSSS	Staphylococcal scalded skin syndrome
STD	Sexually transmitted disease
STEMI	ST elevation myocardial infarction
STI	Sexually transmitted infection
SUFE	Slipped upper femoral epiphysis
SUI	Stress urinary incontinence
SUNA	Short-lasting, Unilateral, Neuralgiform headaches with cranial Autonomic symptoms
SUNCT	Short-lasting, Unilateral, Neuralgiform headaches with Conjunctival injection and Tearing

Abbreviation	Term
SVC(O)	Superior vena cava (obstruction)
SVD	Spontaneous vaginal delivery
SVT	Supraventricular tachycardia
Sx	Symptoms
T	Temperature
Ta/Tis/T1/....	Tumour histology stages
T1DM	Type 1 diabetes mellitus
T1RF	Type 1 respiratory failure
T2DM	Type 2 diabetes mellitus
T2RF	Type 2 respiratory failure
T3	Triiodothyronine/Stage T3 histology
T4	Thyroxine/Stage T4 histology
TAC	Trigeminal autonomic cephalgia
TACS	Total anterior circulation stroke
TAH	Total abdominal hysterectomy
TAUSS	Transabdominal Ultrasound
TAVI	Transcatheter aortic valve implantation
TB	Tuberculosis
TBI	Traumatic brain injury
TBII	Thyrotropin binding inhibiting immunoglobulins
TBSA	Total body surface area
TCA	Tricyclic antidepressant
TCC	Transitional cell carcinoma
TD	Traveller's diarrhoea
TDS	Ter die sumendum (three times daily)
TEACCH	Treatment and education of autistic and related communications handicapped children
TEN	Toxic epidermal necrolysis
TENS	Transcutaneous electrical nerve stimulation
TFTs	Thyroid function tests
TG	Triglyceride
TGA	Transposition of the great arteries
TGN	Trigeminal neuralgia
THR	Total hip replacement
TIA	Transient ischaemic attack
TIBC	Total iron binding concentration
TIPS	Transjugular intrahepatic portosystemic shunt
Tis	Tumour in situ
TM	Tympanic membrane
TMN	Toxic multi-nodular
TNF	Tumour necrosis factor
TOE	Transoesophageal echocardiogram
TOF	Tetralogy of Fallot
TORCH	Toxoplasmosis, other agents, rubella, cytomegalovirus, and herpes simplex
TPMT	Thiopurine methyl transferase

Abbreviation	Term
TPN	Total parenteral nutrition
TPO	Thyroid peroxidase
TR	Tricuspid regurgitation
TR-Ab	Thyrotropin receptor antibody
TRH	Thyrotropin releasing hormone
TS	Tricuspid stenosis/ Tuberous sclerosis
TSH	Thyroid stimulating hormone
TTE	Transthoracic echocardiogram
TTG	Tissue transglutaminase
TTP	Thrombotic thrombocytopenic purpura
TURBT	Transurethral resection of bladder tumour
TURP	Transurethral resection of prostate
TVUS(S)	Transvaginal ultrasound (scan)
TWOC	Trial without catheter
TXA	Tranexamic Acid
U&Es	Urea and electrolytes
UF-heparin	Unfractionated heparin
UC	Ulcerative colitis
UGI(B)	Upper GI (bleeding)
UI	Urinary incontinence
UKMEC	UK Medical Eligibility Criteria for Contraceptive Use
UL	Upper limb
ULSE	Upper left sternal edge
UMN	Upper motor neurone
UO, U/O	Urine output
UPSI	Unprotected sexual intercourse
URTI	Upper respiratory tract infection
US(S)	Ultrasound (scan)
UTI	Urinary tract infection
VA	Visual acuity
VATS	Video assisted thoracic surgery
VBAC	Vaginal birth after caesarean
VBG	Venous blood gas
VEGF	Vascular endothelial growth factor
VF	Ventricular fibrillation
VGCC	Voltage gated calcium channel
vHL	von-Hippel Lindau syndrome
VIN	Vulval intraepithelial neoplasia
VMA	Vanillylmandelic acid
V/Q	Ventilation-perfusion
VSD	Ventricular septal defect
VT	Ventricular tachycardia
VTE	Venous thromboembolism
vWF	von Willebrand Factor
VZV	Varicella Zoster virus
WBC	White blood cell
WCC	White cell count

Abbreviation	Term
WFNS	World Federation of Neurological Surgeons
WHO	World Health Organisation
WIU	Weeks in utero
WLE	Wide local excision
WOB	Work of breathing
WPW	Wolff-Parkinson-White syndrome
XR	X-ray
#	Fracture
+ve	Positive

Nipple Discharge

*Natalia Hackett, Margarita Fox, Alexander Royston,
Lydia Newton, and Kavita Narula*

**GP CONSULTATION, FEMALE, 55.
BILATERAL GREEN NIPPLE DISCHARGE**

HPC: 4 weeks history of green nipple discharge without improvement. No breast tenderness, no lumps, no other changes. **PMHx:** 2 NVD at age 26 and 28, asthma in childhood, osteoarthritis, depression. **DHx:** sertraline, ibuprofen. **SHx:** non-smoker, retired librarian.

O/E: slightly overweight, no palpable breast lump, no skin changes, inverted nipples bilaterally, green nipple discharge bilaterally when expressed, no tenderness, no lymphadenopathy on palpation.

---

1. What would be your top differential and first-line management if the patient:
   a. was breastfeeding, feeling feverish and now had a tender nipple?
   b. had an itchy rash on her nipple and had noticed some blood-stained discharge?
2. A 49-year-old male presents with milky discharge from both nipples. PMHx: hypertension (HTN), asthma, gastro-oesophageal reflux disease (GORD). DHx: spironolactone, salbutamol, fluticasone, metoclopramide, omeprazole. Which drug is probably responsible?
3. Acute severe headache, vomiting, visual impairment, ocular palsy may suggest what severe condition?

Answers: 1a. Mastitis, encourage breastfeeding and simple analgesia. If no improvement after 24 hours, exclude abscess. 1b. Paget disease, 2WW suspected breast cancer pathway. 2. Metoclopramide. Prolactin levels should normalise on cessation. 3. Acute haemorrhage or ischaemic infarction of a pituitary prolactinoma (pituitary apoplexy).

TABLE 1.1

	Features	Investigations	Management
Breast-Related Breast cancer (lobular or ductal carcinoma)	**RFs:** female, ↑oestrogen exposure (older, nulliparity, late menarche, early menopause, HRT, COCP, obese), smoking, FHx, BRCA 1/2. **Hx & O/E:** Lump (hard, painless, tethered). Skin changes includes 'peau d'orange'. Bloody discharge. Enlarged lymph nodes. Metastasis: dyspnoea, bone pain, weight loss, hepatomegaly	Triple assessment: 1. History and examination 2. Imaging (USS/mammogram) 3. Histology (core biopsy)/ cytology (FNAC). Genetic testing: (BRCA 1/2)	2WW breast referral. Surgery (conserving vs mastectomy), chemotherapy, radiotherapy, hormonal therapy

(Continued)

TABLE 1.1 (Cont'd)

	Features	Investigations	Management
Duct ectasia (Fig. 1.1)	**RFs:** post-menopausal, obesity. **Hx & O/E:** chronic blockage and dilation of ducts (benign). Green discharge from both nipples, inverted nipple/mass. Breast pain is possible (uncommon)	Triple assessment. **Mammogram:** dilated calcified ducts. **USS:** distended branching/ tubular structures (anechoic)	2WW. Watchful wait. If troublesome, microdiscectomy/duct excision
Intra-ductal papilloma	**RFs:** age (35–55 yo). **Hx & O/E:** one duct, clear discharge for <6 months. Benign lump, often asymptomatic/ incidental finding	Triple assessment. **Mammogram:** usually normal. May be dilated duct with benign-looking mass. **USS:** can show well-defined solid intra-ductal mass	2WW. Some consider this a high-risk precursor lesion; surgical excision
Paget disease of the breast	See *2. BREAST TENDERNESS*		
Mastitis	See *2. BREAST TENDERNESS*		
Galactorrhoea Prolactinoma	**RFs:** age (rare in childhood), FHx, MEN-1, Carney complex. **Hx & O/E:** galactorrhoea, bitemporal hemianopia, headaches, low libido, amenorrhoea/oligomenorrhoea, infertility, dyspareunia, reduced bone mineral density. Men: gynaecomastia, erectile dysfunction	**Bloods:** ↑↑Prolactin, ↓/↔LH, ↓/↔FSH, βhCG (to r/o pregnancy), TFTs, U&Es, LFTs **MRI with contrast:** pituitary <10 mm micro-, >10 mm macro-prolactinoma. **Visual fields:** r/o optic chiasm compression	Dopamine agonist; • Cabergoline first line • Bromocriptine in pregnancy Transsphenoidal surgery (if large, or drug treatment fails/intolerable)
Drug-induced	**Prolactin release stimulants:** H_2 antagonist, dopamine antagonist (antipsychotics, haloperidol, metoclopramide), verapamil, opioids, OCP, SSRIs	Often due to ↑ serum prolactin levels	Review medication if significant symptoms. Check prolactin returns to normal to exclude other causes
Non-functioning pituitary adenoma	Pituitary tumour compresses stalk; stops hypothalamic dopamine inhibiting prolactin. **RFs:** damage to pituitary stalk (surgery, MS, sarcoidosis, TB). **Hx & O/E:** bitemporal hemianopia, headaches, ± hypopituitarism	**Serum prolactin:** ↑(moderately: less than equivalent prolactinoma). **Pituitary profile:** GH, TSH, LH/ FSH, ACTH, Cortisol. **Short Synacthen Test** (SST). **Visual field testing**	**Small adenoma:** observe **Large/symptomatic:** trans-sphenoidal transnasal hypophysectomy. Hormone replacement if deficient. Substitute steroids if patient fails SST (Addison's)-life-threatening
Breastfeeding/ pregnancy	Most common perinatally: breastfeeding (physiological). Lactation can continue ≥2 years after finishing breastfeeding	History and examination of breasts	Reassurance. Bothersome: tissue/ maternity breast pad. Review if bloody

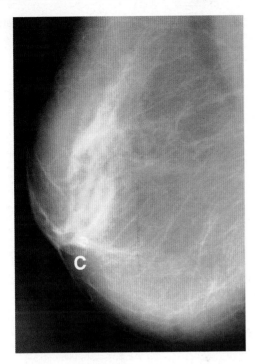

Fig. 1.1 Mammary Duct Ectasia. Radiopaque mass of dilated ducts with no features of malignancy. Large duct calcification (C) and skin indentation caused by fibrosis. Clinically, this condition can be mistaken for carcinoma. (Reproduced with permission from Quick CRG, Biers SM, Arulampalam THA. Disorders of the breast. In: *Essential Surgery: Problems, Diagnosis and Management.* 6th ed. Elsevier. UK; 2019:564–584.)

The top differential for the vignette is mammary duct ectasia. However, the most important differential not to miss would be carcinoma, which can present with discharge. Incidence of malignancy in patients presenting with abnormal nipple discharge is 7% to 15%, and higher when a lump is also present and the patient is aged >50. The key pointer to it not being cancer is that symptoms are bilateral. Furthermore, inverted nipples are typical for duct ectasia, as is the green colour to the discharge.

REVISION TIPS

- Discharge: green – duct ectasia, clear – papilloma, bloody – malignancy/inflammatory, milk – galactorrhoea/pregnancy, pain – mastitis
- The components of a triple assessment:
  - Clinical history and examination (breast surgeon)
  - Radiological imaging (USS <35 years, mammogram >35)
  - Core biopsy or fine-needle aspiration

Breast Tenderness

Tejas Netke, Alexander Royston, and Lydia Newton

GP PRESENTATION, FEMALE, 27.
SEVERAL MONTHS OF BREAST PAIN

HPC: Bilateral, intermittent, appears just before menstruation, severity of 6/10 in upper quadrants, dull ache with no radiation. No nipple changes/discharge, breast lumps or erythema. Otherwise well in herself, no fevers or unintentional weight loss. **PMHx:** Gravida 1, Para 1 (3-year-old son). **DHx:** microgynon 30. **FHx:** Grandmother had breast cancer at 64. **SHx:** Smokes 10 cigarettes per day, occasional alcohol.

O/E: Breasts look symmetrical with no obvious nipple changes. No signs of infection (erythema/warmth). No pain on palpation currently.

---

1. What is the recommended treatment and monitoring of the condition in the vignette?

2. Given your top differential, how would this change in a woman with nipple changes/discharge?

3. When do you refer women under the 2-week wait (2WW) pathway?

Answers: 1. Monitoring: pain diary. Treatment: check bra-fitting, paracetamol, topical NSAID. See commentary. 2. 2WW referral to rule out breast cancer. 3. 2WW referral indications (noting that locally they may vary);
a. Discrete hard lump ± fixation ± tethering
b. >30 years old with unexplained lump
c. Spontaneous unilateral bloody/blood-stained discharge
d. Nipple retraction/distortion of recent onset
e. Skin distortion/tethering/ulceration/peau d'orange
f. Unexplained axillary lump (e.g. lymphadenopathy)
g. Suspected recurrence of previous breast cancer
h. Other features with high index of suspicion

TABLE 2.1

	Features	Investigations	Management
Breast			
Cyclical breast pain (mastalgia)	Most common cause. **RFs:** age (20–40 years), stress, caffeine, smoking, lactation frequency, large breasts, poorly fitting bra. **Hx & O/E:** dull, achy pain ± diffuse lumpy breasts, associated with menstruation, bilateral	Pregnancy test. Breast diary: can help to identify pattern of pain. If >40: mammogram (screening opportunity). <40: localised USS (patient reassurance)	Reassurance. **Conservative:** well-fitted bra ± oral/topical analgesia
Fibrocystic disease	Common. Diffusely lumpy breasts in younger women. **RFs** (related to oestrogen levels): obesity, nulliparity, late first birth and late menopause	Mammogram, ultrasound or both to confirm cysts and rule out cancer. Aspiration could diagnose and treat	Reassurance, pain-relief. Mastalgia with associated symptoms/relevant FHx or personal history: 2WW

TABLE 2.1   (Cont'd)

	Features	Investigations	Management
Pre-menstrual syndrome	RFs: stopping OCP, depression, stress. Hx & O/E: mood swings, irritability associated with menstruation; breast tenderness, bloating, acne	Symptom diary for 2–3 cycles	Reassurance. Lifestyle – regular exercise and sleep. Analgesia if pain. **Definitive:** consider SSRI/oral contraceptive
Mastitis	RFs: previous mastitis, nipple cracking, stagnation in lactation (intermittent feeds), smoking, obesity, immunosuppression. Hx & O/E: unilateral, painful, erythematous, unwell (fever/malaise)	Usually *Staphylococcus aureus*. Clinical diagnosis. Can progress to an abscess. **USS** if suspecting abscess	Reassure. Continue breast-feeding if lactational. Analgesia. Consider antibiotics if symptoms persist ≥24 h/clear signs of infection (usually flucloxacillin)
Abscess	RFs: as for mastitis. Hx & O/E: fluctuant lump (beware if fluctuation is late/absent), hot erythematous skin, tender, signs of systemic infection	↑ inflammatory markers. **USS-guided aspiration.** (MC&S), treatment	Antibiotics (oral/IV). USS-guided aspiration ± repeated aspirations. Incision and drainage rarely done (risk of milk fistula)
Paget's disease of the breast (Fig. 2.1)	Uncommon: associated with invasive breast cancer. RFs: any previous breast cancer. Hx & O/E: Nipple/areola; itchy, erythema ± lump, yellow/bloody discharge, nipple inversion	Physical examination. Mammography and/or ultrasound. **Biopsy/cytology:** Paget cells (large cells with clear cytoplasm)	2WW breast clinic referral. **Definitive:** MDT. Surgery (conserving vs mastectomy), chemotherapy, radiotherapy, hormonal therapy
Extra-Mammary Costochondritis	RFs: hypermobility, persistent coughing/overuse (exercise). Hx & O/E: Unilateral, anterior chest pain, exacerbated on deep inspiration. Pain on costochondral palpation	Clinical diagnosis. Rule out other causes: ECG, CXR	NSAIDs + PPI cover
Mondor disease (superficial thrombophlebitis)	RFs: idiopathic, middle-age, F>>M. Hx & O/E: inflammation of the superficial veins. Uncommon. Raised, tender, cord-like lesion on the skin	Clinical diagnosis	Reassurance: self-limiting ± NSAIDs
Rib fracture	RFs: contact sports, chronic cough; exclude metastasis if low energy. Hx & O/E: swelling, bruising, pain (breathing/coughing)	CXR. CT	**Conservative:** analgesia + chest physiotherapy
Thoracic shingles	RFs: age (>50), autoimmune, immunocompromise. Hx & O/E: erythematous, painful vesicular lesions in a dermatomal distribution, do not cross midline	Reactivation of varicella zoster. Clinical diagnosis	Topical analgesia, cold compress, calamine lotion. **Definitive:** Oral anti-viral therapy (acyclovir)

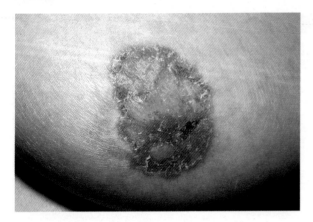

Fig. 2.1 Erythema and scale crust that had been treated as a dermatitis, showing partial destruction of the nipple; there was an underlying ductal breast carcinoma. (Courtesy Fitzsimons Army Medical Center teaching files.)

This case describes a typical presentation of cyclical mastalgia, without any discrete palpable lump. Mastitis/abscess are unlikely due to lack of lactation and absence of fever. Cyclical pain tends to increase from mid-cycle onwards, affecting the upper outer quadrant/lateral portion. The breast becomes tender, may increase in size and there may or may not be areas of increased lumpiness. The pain is usually relieved by menstruation. Fibrocystic disease is a similar presentation but with more convincing lumpiness found, often on self-examination. The presence of any lump will understandably cause alarm in both patients and doctors, and precautionary 2WW referrals are common.

REVISION TIPS

- Exclude infection, suggested by: localised breast swelling, redness, warmth, pain, fever
- Exclude lumps with a thorough examination sequence:
  - Inspection: scars, asymmetry, masses, nipple abnormalities, skin changes – hands pushed into hips/above head
  - Palpation: systematic – including axillary tail, nipple-areolar complex, lymph nodes

3

Breast Lump

Christian Aquilina and Natarajan Vaithilingam

BREAST CLINIC. FEMALE, 61. LUMP IN RIGHT BREAST

HPC: 6-weeks history of right breast lump, not painful, unsure if increasing in size. No previous breast history of lumps or cancer, nor FHx. Gravida 3 para 2, breast-fed all children, last menstrual period (LMP) 7 years ago, hormonal contraception for 15 years in past, never used hormone replacement therapy (HRT). Five cigarettes daily for 30 years, alcohol 12 units a week. She wears size 36C bra.

O/E: Looks well, high BMI. A 3-cm lump in the inferior pole of the right breast, firm, non-tender, not freely mobile within the breast, not attached to chest wall. No skin changes. No regional lymphadenopathy. Contralateral breast/axilla/supraclavicular fossa (SCF) nil remarkable.

1. If the woman was 25 and had the same lump on examination, would your top differential be different?
2. What drugs serve as endocrine treatments of breast cancer, and how do they work?
3. How common are breast cancers? Can men be affected?

Answers: 1. The top differential is cancer; red flags (hard irregular lump, tethering to muscle/skin, restricted mobility/non-mobile, fast growing, painless) needs triple assessment regardless of age. 2. Tamoxifen is a selective oestrogen receptor modulator (SERM); anastrozole/letrozole/exemestane are aromatase inhibitors (AIs) that block the adrenal and peripheral synthesis of oestrogen. 3. Risk: 1 in 8 lifetime risk for women; 0.6% of breast cancers occur in men.

TABLE 3.1

	Features	Investigations	Management
Breast Lump that can be Benign or Malignant			
Phyllodes tumour	Fibroepithelial neoplasm; mostly benign, local recurrence (low risk), metastasis (rare). Average age 40-50. **Hx & O/E:** unilateral painless mass, stretched skin, distended superficial veins, (bloody nipple discharge). Axillary lymphadenopathy- nodal mets rare.	**Biopsy:** intra-canalicular growth with leaf-like projections. USS: hypoechoic mass-cystic component suggests malignant. MRI: to evaluate chest wall invasion in malignant tumor	Wide local excision. Mastectomy. Adjuvant radiotherapy.

(Continued)

TABLE 3.1   (Cont'd)

	Features	Investigations	Management
Malignant Breast Lump			
Carcinoma	**RFs:** female, increasing age (80% post-menopausal), FHx, genetic predisposition (BRCA1, BRCA2, P53, PALB mutation, etc.), post-menopausal obesity, nulliparity, no breastfeeding Hx, early menarche/late menopause, HRT, smoking. **Hx & O/E:** <u>Systemic features</u> (metastatic): anorexia, asthenia, anaemia, cachexia/weight loss, bone pain, cough, shortness of breath, jaundice, headache. <u>Lump:</u> painless unless locally advanced or some invasive lobular carcinomas (ILCs), hard, gritty (ILC can be soft), ill defined, not mobile within breast (unlike fibroadenoma), occasionally tethered to skin or muscle/chest wall, may be regional lymph node enlargement (axilla, SCF). <u>Nipple changes:</u> recently inverted (particularly concentric rather than slit-like), deviated, bloody or clear discharge, Paget's disease (eczematous nipple areolar complex). <u>Skin:</u> tethering, puckering, peau d'orange (cutaneous lymph-oedema), nodules, ulceration and IBC (Inflammatory Breast Cancer – brawny induration of 1/3 or more of breast skin).	2WW referral. **Triple assessment:** 1. History + physical examination. 2. Imaging (mammogram/USS/MRI as required). 3. Tissue examination (core-needle biopsy/fine-needle aspiration cytology). **Staging CTTAP** and bone scan to rule out/confirm metastasis in Stage 3 disease (14% incidence of asymptomatic distant metastasis, ≤40% in IBC). <u>TNM classification and clinical staging:</u> **Early Breast Cancer (EBC)** Stage 1-2 (T1-2, N1). **Loco-regionally advanced breast cancer** (LABC) Stage 3 (T4, N2-3, T3N1). **Metastatic breast cancer** (MBC): Stage 4 (M1, any T/N).	**Breast Conservation Surgery** wide local excision ± onco-plasty/partial breast reconstruction. **Mastectomy** ± immediate/later reconstruction (implant/tissue). **SLNB** (sentinel LN biopsy) or **ANC** (axillary LN clearance). **Adjuvant therapy** for non-metastatic disease with curative intention. **Radiotherapy** whole/ partial breast/ intra-operative. **Endocrine:** anti-oestrogens in ER+ (80% of BC). Tamoxifen (any age), aromatase inhibitors (post-menopause). **Chemotherapy:** many regimes, 6–8 "thrice-weekly cycles", e.g. FEC-T (Taxol), AC-T. Carboplatin in triple-negative breast cancer (TNBC), gemcitabine in resistant cases. **Targeted therapy** (monoclonal Ab against HER2): Trastuzumab (Herceptin), pertuzumab. **Neo-adjuvant therapy:** endocrine/ chemotherapy and occasional radiotherapy downsizing/downstaging, assess prognosis (complete pathological response), potential better overall survival. **Palliative** in metastatic setting. **New personalised therapy CDK4/6 inhibitors** (e.g. palbociclib/ribociclib). **Immunotherapy** (e.g. pembrolizumab).

TABLE 3.1 **(Cont'd)**

	Features	Investigations	Management
Non-Malignant Breast Lump			
Fibroadenoma	**RFs:** peak age group 20–35 years. **Hx & O/E:** painless, mobile, discrete lump. Sometimes called 'breast mouse'	**USS** is usually conclusive. **Core needle biopsy** in women of age 25 and above to confirm diagnosis.	Reassurance. **Excision:** if symptoms, large and enlarging, women >35 years old (unlikely to resolve spontaneously), concerns over cosmesis or uncertainty in diagnosis (B3 lesion)
Cyst/ Fibrocystic changes	See *2. BREAST TENDERNESS*		
Abscess	A fluctuant lump (beware of late/absent fluctuation), hot erythematous skin, tender, systemic signs (tachycardia, fever, sweating, etc.)	**Bloods:** raised inflammatory markers. **US-guided aspiration** for microbiology and treatment.	Antibiotics, analgesia, US-guided aspiration (repeat as required), surgical drainage if devitalised skin/ multiloculated abscess/thick pus
Benign breast disease	Cyclical pain and swelling, lumpy breasts on examination	Triple assessment to rule out cancer	Reassurance. Topical NSAID gel, simple analgesics, hormonal manipulation (e.g. COCP), supportive bra. Low-dose (10 mg OD) **tamoxifen in luteal phase** for severe mastalgia.
Galactocele	Usually on stopping lactation. Clinically like cyst, firm mass under the areola or peripheral. Singular or multiple, bilateral or unilateral.	**USS** to confirm diagnosis. **Aspiration** if USS inconclusive, to identify secondary infection	Self-resolve over weeks to months. **Aspiration** if large. **Antibiotics** if secondary infection.

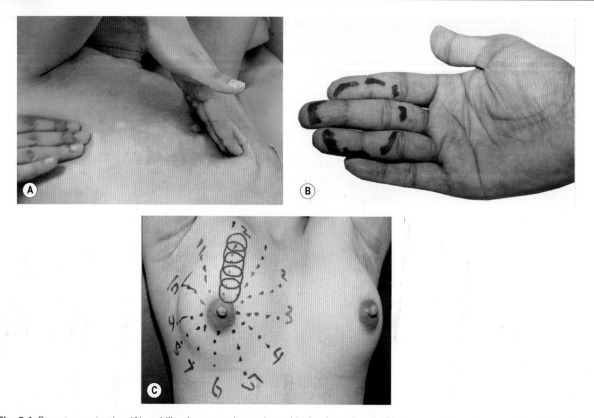

Fig. 3.1 Breast examination (A) stabilise breast and examine with dominant hand; (B) use area shown in green to palpate lump; (C) dial of a clock used to document location of mass. (Reproduced with permission from Lohani KR, Srivastava A, Jeyapradha DA, et al. "Dial of a clock" search pattern for clinical breast examination. *J Surg Res*. 2021;260:10–19.)

The most likely diagnosis is cancerous breast lump. When carrying out a breast examination (Fig. 3.1), examine both breasts and document lump characteristics (site, size, shape, consistency, mobility), nipple changes (discharge, inversion), skin changes (scaling, erythema, puckering, peau d'orange), lymph node changes (enlargement).

REVISION TIPS

- **Triple assessment:** Check nipple areolar complex, inframammary fold, axillary tail, axilla and SCF on both sides; assess risk factors for breast cancer; know national screening age.
- Triple-negative breast cancer oestrogen/progesterone receptors, HER2 negative; 10%–15% of breast cancers. More common if age <40, black ethnicity, or who have BRCA1 mutation.
- Refer using 2WW cancer pathway if age ≥30 with an unexplained breast lump, or age ≥50 with unilateral nipple discharge/retraction. Consider 2WW pathway if skin changes suggest breast cancer or age ≥30 with unexplained axillary lump. Consider non urgent referral if age <30 with an unexplained breast lump.

- **Other differentials;** Phyllodes tumour and sarcoma, lipoma, intramammary lymph node, sebaceous cyst, lymphoma and metastasis (contralateral breast, melanoma, small cell lung cancer, rhabdomyosarcoma, etc.).
- **NHS population breast screening programme:** mammogram every 3 years for women aged 47–73 (beyond 70–73, women can call NHS BSP to have screening MMG every 3 years).
- **Indications for mastectomy;** multi-centric or large tumour, contraindication for adjuvant radiotherapy, co-morbidity, patient choice, risk reduction.

4

Limb Claudication

James Chataway and Francesca Guest

HPC: 6 months 'cramp-like' calf pain when walking, worse on right, exacerbated by climbing stairs, relieved by rest. No relief of pain through sitting or stooping forward. PMHx: T2DM, HTN, stable angina. DHx: Amlodipine, atenolol, atorvastatin, gliclazide, GTN, metformin. FHx: Myocardial infarction (MI). SHx: Current smoker (45 pack years).

O/E: Small body habitus, tar staining. CVS: HR 98, BP 137/91, HS I+II+0. Chest: clear. Abdomen: SNT, NBS. Faint dorsalis pedis pulses, R>L. Ankle-brachial pressure index (ABPI) = 0.7

1. What are the ABPI differences between the three peripheral artery disease (PAD) subtypes?
2. What are the two medications that PAD patients should be prescribed?
3. What are the six P's for acute limb-threatening ischaemia?

Answers: 1. 0.6 to 0.9 intermittent claudication, <0.6 critical ischaemia, <0.3 limb-threatening ischaemia. 2. High-dose (80 mg) atorvastatin, antiplatelet (clopidogrel). 3. Pale, pulseless, painful, paralysed, paraesthetic, perishingly cold.

TABLE 4.1

	Features	Investigations	Management
Peripheral arterial disease (PAD)	**RFs:** smoker, diabetes, hypertension, hyperlipidaemia, CVD, >40 years. **Hx & O/E:** Aching/burning feeling in calf (thigh/buttock). Hanging legs out of bed. Diminished pulses. **Intermittent claudication:** pain relieved by rest. **Critical ischaemia:** pain at rest, ulcers. **Limb-threatening:** Pale, pulse-less, painful, paralysed, paraesthetic, perishingly cold	ABPI. Duplex USS. CT/MRI. Angiography	**Intermittent claudication:** atorvastatin 80 mg and clopidogrel. Naftidrofuryl oxalate (vasodilator). Exercise training, lifestyle advice. **Critical ischemia:** as above, revascularisation. **Limb-threatening:** ABCDE, urgent revascularisation. Amputation last resort

(Continued)

TABLE 4.1 (Cont'd)

	Features	Investigations	Management
Spinal stenosis (Fig. 4.1)	Back/buttock/bilateral leg pain, relieved by sitting, stooping forward. Easier to walk uphill than downhill. May be motor weakness	MRI spine	NSAIDs, physiotherapy. Laminectomy
Nerve root compression	Radiculopathy pain in dermatomal distribution, often worse sitting	MRI	NSAIDs and physiotherapy
Baker's cyst/ ruptured Baker's cyst	Popliteal fossa. May be associated with arthritis, sports injury, gout. Asymptomatic or pain, swelling, erythema in calf	Duplex USS; cystic mass in popliteal fossa	**Child:** usually resolve. **Adults:** treat underlying cause
Leriche syndrome	**RFs:** same as PAD. **Classic triad:** claudication of buttocks and thighs, decreased femoral pulses, erectile dysfunction.	ABPI reduced. Angiography is diagnostic.	Endovascular angioplasty, stenting of iliac occlusions
Buerger disease (thromboangiitis obliterans)	**RFs:** men aged 25–35, smoking. **Hx & O/E:** distal ischaemic change (e.g. pain/cyanosis in toes/fingers), may progress to ulcers and gangrene	Corkscrew collaterals on angiogram	Smoking cessation

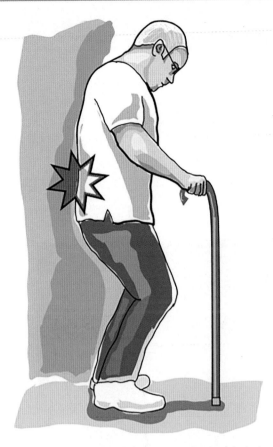

For acute leg pain, serious differentials include limb-threatening ischemia, DVT and compartment syndrome. Chronically, the main causes are vascular (PAD) or neurogenic (spinal stenosis). Calf pain which is worse on exertion (increased blood flow requirement), unaffected by back position, and with an abnormal ABPI suggests PAD. In the vignette, the pain is relieved by rest and the ABPI is >0.6, so the diagnosis is intermittent claudication rather than critical limb ischaemia.

Fig. 4.1 Patients with spinal stenosis may have a 'simian' posture (forward-flexed trunk, slightly bent knees when walking), to decrease symptoms of pseudoclaudication. (From Waldman SD. *Physical Diagnosis of Pain: An Atlas of Signs and Symptoms.* Philadelphia: Saunders; 2006:261.)

REVISION TIPS

- Likely clinical setting associated with given ABPI values:
  - >1.2: calcified arteries
  - 0.9-1.2: normal
  - 0.6-0.9: intermittent claudication
  - 0.3-0.6: critical limb ischaemia
  - <0.3: limb-threatening
- If there is a positional element to the pain, think lumbar spinal stenosis rather than claudication
- Young male smoker and distal limb ischaemia, consider Buerger disease (thromboangiitis obliterans)

5

Cold, Painful, Pale, Pulseless Leg/Foot

Christian Aquilina and Angeliki Kosti

EMERGENCY DEPARTMENT, MALE, 68.
COLD AND PAINFUL RIGHT LEG

HPC: 6 hours history of very painful leg, sudden onset. Two-year history of calf pain on exertion. **PMHx:** Stable angina and HTN.

O/E: Right leg is pale, cold to touch, pulses are impalpable. Left leg is warm to touch, with impalpable posterior tibial and dorsalis pedis arteries. BP 154/98, HR 101, pulse irregular.

1. What is the mortality rate of acute limb ischaemia?
2. What would be the most likely diagnosis if the symptoms came on over 3 months?
3. What does an ankle-brachial pressure index (ABPI) of >1.2 suggest?

Answers: 1. 20% mortality rate. 2. More likely to be acute on chronic limb ischaemia. 3. Arterial calcification.

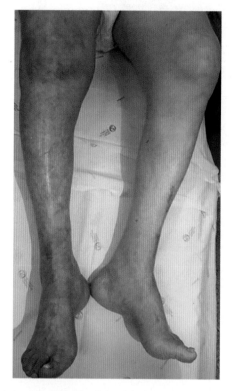

Fig. 5.1 Acute ischaemia of the right lower limb in lighter skin. (Reproduced with permission from Björck M, Earnshaw JJ, Acosta S, et al. Editor's Choice – European Society for Vascular Surgery (ESVS) 2020 clinical practice guidelines on the management of acute limb ischaemia. *Eur J Vasc Endovasc Surg.* 2020; 59(2):173–218.)

TABLE 5.1

	Features	Investigations	Management
Acute limb ischaemia	**Causes:** sudden decrease in limb perfusion which threatens the limb due to **emboli** (AF, previous MI/ventricular aneurysm. No previous claudication), **thrombosis** (more common, thrombosis of atherosclerotic vessel, previous claudication, reduced pulse in other leg, risk factors of CVD), **trauma**	FBC, clotting, glucose, troponin, lactate, group and save, U&E. **Urgent CT angiogram.** ECG	High-flow oxygen, IV fluid, opioid analgesia. Urgent vascular centre. IV heparin bolus and infusion. Ongoing: continue heparin or interventional therapy. Intra-arterial thrombolysis, bypass, angioplasty (if thrombotic), embolectomy. Amputation if irreversible
Chronic limb ischaemia	**Causes:** atherosclerosis. **RFs:** obesity/inactivity, smoking, diabetes, HTN, hyperlipidaemia, FHx. <u>Fontaine classification:</u> **Stage I** – asymptomatic. **Stage II** – intermittent claudication. **Stage III** – ischaemic rest pain. **Stage IV** – ulceration and/or gangrene	FBC and lipid profile. **ABPI:** • Normal: >0.9. • Mild: 0.8–0.9. • Moderate: 0.5–0.8. • Severe: <0.5. **Buerger's test.** Consider USS arterial duplex ± CTA	Supportive: exercise programme, smoking cessation, optimise co-morbidities (diabetes, HTN, raised cholesterol). Antiplatelets and statins. Regular vascular review. Consider surgery
Critical limb ischaemia	**RFs:** severe chronic limb ischaemia. **Hx & O/E:** rest pain **or** tissue necrosis including ulceration/gangrene (Stage III/IV) **or** ABPI <0.5. Pale/cold/pulseless leg	Same as for chronic limb ischaemia + USS arterial duplex and CTA	Urgent surgical intervention to revascularise limb
Deep vein thrombosis	See *45. PAINFUL SWOLLEN LEG*		
Lumbar radiculopathy	Usually unilateral leg pain radiating down into the foot, tingling, numbness, weakness, lower back pain. Increased symptoms on straight leg raise	Neurological examination. Rule out spinal cord compression	Analgesia, encourage normal activity, PT. Safety net for back pain red flags. May need spinal team input

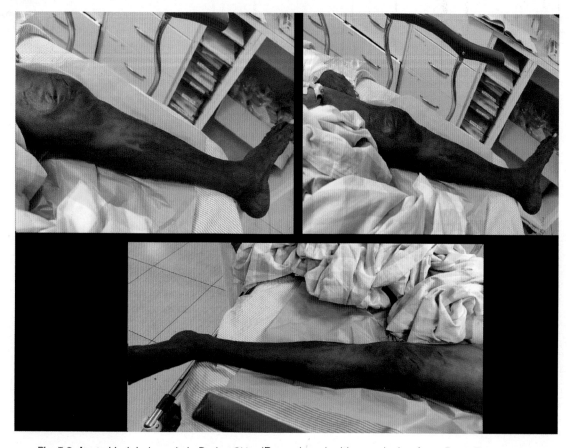

Fig. 5.2 Acute Limb Ischaemia in Darker Skin. (Reproduced with permission from Bose B, Daswaney A, Lath V. Infrarenal aortic thrombosis causing acute limb ischemia. *Vis J Emerg Med.* 2021;25:101099.)

The most likely diagnosis is acute limb ischaemia (Figs. 5.1, 5.2). *Typical features of acute limb ischaemia includes the six P's: pale, pulseless, painful, paralysed, paraesthetic, perishingly cold (not all need to be present for diagnosis). If ischaemia is due to an embolus, onset is acute and limb appears pale (lack of collaterals). If due to thrombosis, onset is more gradual, leg may not appear pale and symptoms may be less severe (collaterals have had time to develop). Check if the pulse is regular or irregular, as embolism from atrial fibrillation (AF) is a common factor in acute limb ischaemia. An ECG must be performed to confirm, and subsequent investigations will be required.*

REVISION TIPS

- CT angiogram is crucial if it can be done without delay
- Know the severity of an acutely ischaemic limb and how to manage it; you need to speak to a vascular centre immediately – delays lead to irreversible ischaemia and amputation
- If the patient is in AF, do not forget to treat this concurrently
- All patients with chronic arterial disease are started on antiplatelets and statins unless contraindicated

6

Skin Ulcer

Katherine Parker and Angeliki Kosti

GP CONSULTATION, FEMALE, 71. LEG ULCER

HPC: 6-week history of slowly enlarging ulcer, more painful at night. **PMHx** T2DM, poor diabetic control, HTN, ex-smoker.

O/E: Poor footwear, signs of self-neglect. Left foot: 2 cm diameter, well demarcated, deep ulcer on the sole-base is clean. Surrounding skin is cooler than that of the right foot. Some left-sided calf wasting. Peripheral pulses weak bilaterally. Crude touch sensation reduced bilaterally. Bloods: random capillary blood glucose (raised), HbA1C 53. FBC, CRP, B12 and cholesterol within normal range.

1. What are your differentials if a patient presents with **genital** ulcers?
2. What are your differentials if a patient presents with **oral** ulcers?

Answers: 1. Herpes simplex virus, Behcet's, syphilis, chancroid, lymphogranuloma venereum. 2. Aphthous mouth ulcers, herpes simplex virus, Behcet's, pemphigus vulgaris, and also hand, foot and mouth disease.

TABLE 6.1

	Clinical	Investigations	Management
Neuropathic ulcer	RFs: DM, B12 deficiency, PVD. Hx & O/E: painless or abnormal sensation. Well defined, 'punched out', with a deep sinus ± callus. Warm skin, normal pulses (weak if neuroischaemic). Site: pressure areas (e.g. soles, heel, metatarsal heads, toes)	↑BM, ↑HbA1c ± ↑inflammatory markers. ABPI: may be normal (0.8–1.2) or indicate arterial insufficiency (<0.8) or calcification (>1.2). X-ray to exclude osteomyelitis and soft tissue gangrene	Referral to diabetic foot clinic for MDT management. Glycaemic control and screening for complications. Monitor for Charcot's foot

(Continued)

TABLE 6.1   (Cont'd)

	Clinical	Investigations	Management
Venous ulcer	**RFs:** venous disease, varicose veins, DVT, obesity, pregnancy, DM, previous trauma. **Hx & O/E:** mild pain, heaviness, worse when *standing*. **Site** gaiter area. Large, shallow, irregular ulcer with exudative granulating base. Pulses palpable. Skin warm. Venous insufficiency – oedematous leg ± haemosiderin and melanin deposition, lipodermatosclerosis, atrophie blanche, venous eczema	Duplex USS (retrograde or reversed flow). ABPI may be normal (0.8–1.2) or show arterial insufficiency (<0.8)	Leg elevation. Graded compression bandaging – **contraindicated in arterial insufficiency.** Optimisation of RFs – nutrition, smoking cessation. Vascular referral if diagnostic uncertainty, rapid deterioration of ulcer, falls, non-healing with compression treatment
Arterial ulcer	**RFs:** vasculopathy, Hx arterial disease **Hx & O/E:** painful, especially at night (worse *lying down*). Small, sharply defined 'punched out', deep. Necrotic base. Site: areas of pressure/trauma, pretibial, submalleolar, distal (tips of toes, metatarsal heads). Cold, shiny, pale skin. Weak/absent pulses, slow CRT, loss of hair, gangrene ± night pain	ABPI – arterial insufficiency (<0.8, <0.5 *severe* arterial insufficiency). Arterial doppler studies, CT angiography. Inflammatory markers to rule out infected ulcer	Urgent revascularisation of limb. **Compression bandaging is contraindicated**
Pressure ulcer	Unrelieved **pressure**, plus shear, friction and moisture, worsened by poor tissue perfusion. **RFs:** immobility, impaired sensation, malnutrition, DM, PVD, cognitive impairment. **Site:** bony prominences (sacrum, coccyx, heels). Often infected	**Waterlow** Scale Risk assessment tool. Lesion variable from small and superficial to extensive and deep (down to bone) – assessment of grade; Fig. 6.1	Regular repositioning and assessment, skin care, pressure relieving devices, moisture reduction, nutritional support, carer education. Consider referral to tissue viability in community
Marjolin ulcer (SCC subtype)	Persistent ulcer **on site of prior scar**. Excessive granulation, foul odour, fragile ± painful. **RFs:** Age 40–60, chronic inflamed	**Site** legs, feet, head, neck. Biopsy	Wide local excision ± sentinel lymph node biopsy. MDT discussion
Pyoderma gangrenosum	**Painful.** Single or multiple erythematous papules that rapidly enlarge, becoming deep violaceous ulcers 2–20 cm. **RFs: IBD**, RA, haematological malignancy, Hepatitis C, GPA	**Site** anywhere. Clinical diagnosis. Consider bloods/biopsy (to identify associated disease/rule out alternative diagnoses)	Urgent dermatology. Immunosuppression (topical steroids), wound care ± antibiotics. Consider systemic immunosuppression

GPA, granulomatosis with polyangiitis

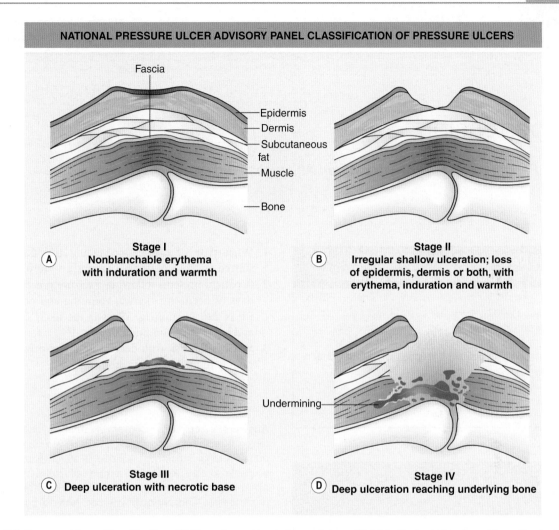

NATIONAL PRESSURE ULCER ADVISORY PANEL CLASSIFICATION OF PRESSURE ULCERS

Fascia

Epidermis
Dermis
Subcutaneous fat
Muscle

Bone

(A) Stage I
Nonblanchable erythema
with induration and warmth

(B) Stage II
Irregular shallow ulceration; loss
of epidermis, dermis or both, with
erythema, induration and warmth

(C) Stage III
Deep ulceration with necrotic base

Undermining

(D) Stage IV
Deep ulceration reaching underlying bone

Fig. 6.1 Pressure Ulcers Classification. (A) Stage I: non-blanchable erythema of intact skin, heralding impending skin ulceration. For darker-skinned individuals, other signs may be indicators and include warmth, oedema, discoloration of the skin, and induration. (B) Stage II: partial-thickness skin loss involving the epidermis, dermis, or both – abrasion, blister, or shallow crater. (C) Stage III: full-thickness skin loss, in which subcutaneous tissue is damaged or necrotic and may extend down to, but not including, the underlying fascia. (D) Stage IV: full-thickness skin loss and extensive tissue necrosis, destruction to muscle, bone, or supporting structures. Undermining or sinus tracts can be present. (Adapted with permission from Bolognia JL, Schaffer JV, Duncan KO, et al. Ulcers. In: *Dermatology Essentials.* 2nd ed. Elsevier; 2022:871–885.e2.)

The most likely diagnosis in the vignette is a **neuro-ischaemic ulcer**, where both diabetic nephropathy and peripheral arterial disease are contributory. Investigations include arterial duplex (likely to show arterial calcification and luminal narrowing, possible collaterals), ABPI and consider CT angiogram. Screen for diabetic complications. Other differentials are seen in Table 6.1.

REVISION TIPS
- Not all ulcers are clear cut and they can often be of mixed pathology
- Past medical history and risk factors are key

7

Hypertension

Alice Parker, Alexander Royston, Viren Ahluwalia, and Katie Wong

**GP CONSULTATION, WHITE MALE, 60.
CLINIC BP FOUND TO BE 165/101 MMHG**

HPC: Attends for annual review of T1DM. **PMHx:** Diagnosed with type 1 diabetes at 14 years old – poorly controlled CBG with ×4 hospital admissions for hypoglycaemia. Currently reasonably fit and well, but overweight and complains of fatigue. **DHx:** atorvastatin, detemir and novorapid. **SHx:** Ex-smoker.

O/E: CVS: HR: 84, BP: 165/101 mmHg, HS: I+II+0, swollen ankles. Fundoscopy shows exudates and microaneurysms, no peripheral neuropathy detected.

1. What type of medication should this patient be started on, considering his age and co-morbidities?
2. A patient presents following a seizure preceded by 2 days of headache, nausea, vomiting and confusion. BP is 226/112 mmHg. What is the likely diagnosis and how is this condition managed?
3. What is the risk with decreasing blood pressure too rapidly in malignant hypertension?

Answers: 1. Angiotensin-converting enzyme inhibitor/angiotensin II receptor blocker (ACE-i/ARB) – with dose adjustment for renal impairment + insulin + statin (± ezetimibe). If unable to achieve <140/90 mmHg, add calcium channel blocker, and/or thiazide-like diuretic, and/or β-blocker. 2. Hypertensive encephalopathy – can lead to coma. Use labetalol or sodium nitroprusside IVI. 3. May cause stroke: watershed infarcts. Aim to lower BP initially by ≤25% to reduce risk of cerebral, coronary or renal ischemia.

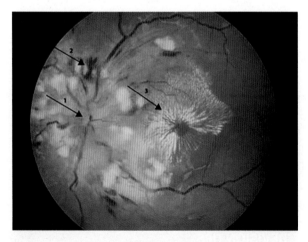

Fig. 7.1 Fundus photograph of the left eye showing optic disc swelling *(arrow 1)* with flame-shaped haemorrhages *(arrow 2)* and prominent macula exudates *(arrow 3)*. (Reproduced with permission from Tajunisah I, Patel DK. Malignant hypertension with papilledema. *J Emerg Med.* 2013;44(1):164–165.)

TABLE 7.1

	Features	Investigations	Management
Cardiovascular			
Primary hypertension	Most common cause. **RFs:** age, sex (M > F), ethnicity, genetics, lifestyle. **Hx & O/E:** Usually asymptomatic. If severe, can cause headache, blurred vision, chest/abdominal pain, dyspnoea, dizziness. Stage 1: 140/90 mmHg (>135/85 ABPM/HBPM). Stage 2: 160/100 mmHg (>150/95 ABPM/HBPM). Stage 3: >180/120 mmHg	Ambulatory/home BP. Monitoring (ABPM/HBPM) readings. Urinalysis-albumin:creatinine ratio (ACR). Fasting glucose, lipids, U&Es. Target clinic BP: <ul><li><140/90 mmHg</li><li>150/90 (>80) mmHg</li><li><130/80 mmHg (T1DM)</li></ul>	Lifestyle measures. Start drug if: HBPM > 150/95 mmHg, *or* HBPM > 135/85 mmHg + <80 years + ≥1 of; organ damage, CVD, renal disease, DM, QRISK > 10%. *First line:* >55/ Afro-Caribbean: **CCB** <55/ DM: **ACE-i** *Second line:* ACE-i + CCB OR thiazide. *Third line:* ACE-i + CCB + thiazide *Fourth line:* add α/β-blocker if K$^+$ < 4.5, or add spironolactone if < 4.5. **Statin** if: T1DM, age >40 years, DM for >10 years, established nephropathy, CVD risk factors.
Secondary hypertension	DM: diabetic nephropathy. Renal: chronic pyelonephritis, PCKD, glomerulonephritis, RCC. Vascular: renal artery stenosis, coarctation. Endocrine: Conn's, Cushing's, phaeochromocytoma, thyroid disease, hyperPTH, acromegaly. Drugs and alcohol.	**Urinalysis + ACR:** microalbuminuria and proteinuria. U&Es (↓K in Conn's and Cushing's), HbA1c. Consider: renal USS, 24 h urinary metanephrines, urinary cortisol, MR aorta and renal arteries.	Annual screening for diabetic nephropathy in T1DM. **Anti-hypertensives:** <ul><li>ACE-i in T1DM</li><li>Statin</li></ul>
Malignant hypertension	Elevated BP with target organ damage (headache, blurred vision, seizures, SOB, retinal haemorrhages, ± papilloedema (Fig. 7.1), ↑troponin, pulmonary oedema). Risks: heart failure, haemorrhagic stroke, AKI, encephalopathy.	U&Es, FBC (low Hb/Plts), blood film-schistocytes. ECG, Echo. Assess cardiovascular risk/organ damage (ACR, haematuria, fundoscopy).	**Labetalol**, nicardipine. Avoid precipitous fall in BP in first few hours. Consider secondary cause of HT (renal, pheochromocytoma).
Non-Cardiovascular			
White coat hypertension	Suspect if clinic BP > 20/10 mmHg above average ABPM/HBPM.	ABPM/HBPM	
Pregnancy-induced hypertension	New HTN (>140/90 mmHg) starting after 20 weeks gestation. No pre-eclamptic features	**Urine dipstick** (no proteinuria)	**Treatment:** BP remains >140/90 mmHg or immediately if >160/110 mmHg (admit)

(Continued)

TABLE 7.1   (Cont'd)

	Features	Investigations	Management
Pre-eclampsia (PET) *always consider: Could this patient be pregnant?*	**RFs (High)**: previous PET, CKD, DM, chronic HTN, SLE, anti-phospholipid syndrome. **(Moderate)**: first pregnancy, >40 years, BMI > 35 kg/m^2, 10 years between pregnancies, FHx PET, multiple pregnancy **Hx & O/E**: new hypertension (>140/90 mmHg) beyond 20 weeks gestation + proteinuria OR other dysfunction (renal, neurological, liver, haematological, uteroplacental). Severe headache, blurred vision, diplopia, flashes/floaters, abdo pain, vomiting, SOB, oedema	**Urine dipstick** (proteinuria). ACR (>8 mg/mmol) or PCR (>30 mg/mmol). FBC (anaemia, thrombo-cytopenia), clotting (↑PT+APTT). U&E (↑creatinine), LFTs (abnormal ?HELLP – see *Revision Tips*). USS: foetal growth restriction, oligohydramnios	**Admission:** BP > 160/110 mmHg (monitoring). Aspirin 75–150 mg OD from 12 weeks (if >1 high RF or >2 moderate RFs). **Treatment**: >140/90 mmHg or immediately if >160/110. First line: labetalol. Aim BP < 135/85 mmHg. Continue 6 weeks post-partum. Only cure: induction

The patient in the vignette has poorly controlled T1DM and is showing signs of hypertension. He is now at high risk of diabetic nephropathy and some early signs of this make secondary hypertension the most likely diagnosis. Peripheral oedema suggests low serum albumin and proteinuria (raised ACR), and diabetic retinopathy is frequently seen alongside nephropathy. The mechanism by which hypertension is exacerbated by failing kidney function is not well understood, but he needs aggressive treatment for both his hypertension and his glycaemic control.

REVISION TIPS

- Primary hypertension: BP > 140/90 mmHg (clinic) or > 135/85 mmHg (ABPM/HBPM) – no known cause
- First-line management: ACE-i/ARB (<55 years or DM) or CCB (>55 or Afro-Caribbean)
- Secondary hypertension: caused by other disease processes, e.g. diabetes mellitus, renal artery stenosis
- Pre-eclampsia is new hypertension **after** 20 weeks gestation plus proteinuria or other organ dysfunction
- HELLP (haemolysis, elevated liver enzymes, low platelets) syndrome is a life-threatening variant of PET

8

Peripheral Oedema and Ankle Swelling

Natalia Hackett, Alexander Royston, Katie Wong, and Viren Ahluwalia

GP CONSULTATION, MALE, 68.
LEG SWELLING

HPC: Fatigued, becoming more out of breath walking to the shops. Claims he's gained weight without eating more. **PMHx:** Myocardial infarction 1 year ago, angina, HTN, T2DM, hypercholesterolaemia. **DHx:** GTN spray PRN, bisoprolol, aspirin, ticagrelor, ramipril, amlodipine, atorvastatin, morphine, nicotine replacement. **SHx:** 30 units alcohol per week, ex-smoker.

O/E: BP: 98/82 mmHg, HR: 65 bpm, RR: 26, afebrile, JVP: elevated, S3 palpable at apex, coarse inspiratory crackles bilaterally (lower zones), abdomen soft non-tender, no organomegaly, pitting oedema to patella.

1. What are the signs on a chest radiograph suggestive of heart failure?
2. Heart failure is a complication of an MI; what other complications of MI can you think of?
3. An 8-year-old boy with scrotal/ankle oedema, nephrotic syndrome suspected and renal biopsy showed no complex deposition on light microscopy, podocyte fusion under electron microscopy; what disease is likely?

Answers: 1. ABCDE – <u>A</u>lveolar oedema, Kerley <u>B</u> lines (Fig. 8.1), <u>C</u>ardiomegaly, <u>D</u>ilated upper lobe veins, pleural <u>E</u>ffusions. 2. Cardiogenic shock, arrythmias, left ventricular free wall rupture/aneurysm, pericarditis, ventricular septal defect (VSD), acute mitral regurgitation. 3. Minimal change disease, the commonest cause of nephrotic syndrome in children.

TABLE 8.1

	Features	Investigations	Management
Heart failure	**RFs:** cardiac disease: previous MI, IHD, cardiomyopathies, arrhythmia, valvular disease, myocarditis. Also: high output state (anaemia/thyrotoxicosis), infection. **Hx & O/E:** Orthopnoea/SOBOE, ankle oedema, fatigue. Signs: peripheral oedema, ↑JVP, RV heave, S3. *LHF:* pulmonary oedema, orthopnoea, PND, wheeze, pink frothy sputum, nocturia. *RHF:* oedema, hepatosplenomegaly	**ECG** (arrhythmia/ischaemia). **CXR** (A–E). FBC (anaemia), U&Es, TFT, LFTs, CBG and HbA1C. **Transthoracic echocardiogram** (LVEF, ventricular dilation). BNP (not acute setting)	Acute Mx: sit patient up, A–E, oxygen, furosemide. Chronic Mx; • ACEi/Entresto • β-blocker • Mineralocorticoid receptor antagonist, SGTL2i dapagliflozin (all not only diabetics: if eGFR OK) Lifestyle (smoking cessation, annual flu vaccine, one-off pneumococcal vaccine). Diuretic (help symptoms)

(Continued)

TABLE 8.1   (Cont'd)

	Features	Investigations	Management
Liver cirrhosis (Fig. 8.2)	See *83. ASCITES*		
Glomerulonephritides (GN)	**RFs:** childhood, FHx, past/current renal impairment, DM, HTN, medications, toxin exposure. **Hx & O/E:** fatigue, HTN, oedema in face/hands/feet/abdomen, haematuria and proteinuria, oliguria. **Non-proliferative:** minimal change disease, membranous GN, focal segmental glomerulosclerosis. **Proliferative:** post-infectious GN, IgA nephropathy, membranoproliferative GN, rapidly progressive GN. Many other causes of GN: anti-GBM, complement-associated GN (rare)	**Urine:** ACR, urinalysis and MC&S (in GP). **PCR** (also detects light chains in myeloma: better screening test). FBC, ↑U&Es, LFTs (↓albumin), ↑INR. **Biopsy** (kidney)	Anti-hypertensives. Treat reversible cause(s) of AKI. Fluid restriction only if overloaded
Nephrotic syndrome	**RFs:** age (MCD 5–8 yo, FSGS 15–30 yo, membranous 50–60 yo), Secondary: DM, SLE, amyloidosis, infection (HIV, Hep B/C), NSAIDs. **Hx & O/E:** oedema, proteinuria, hypoalbuminaemia, thrombosis, hyperlipidaemia	**Urine:** ACR, urinalysis and MC&S (in GP). PCR. FBC, U&Es, ↑INR, LFTs (↓albumin), cholesterol, ↑INR. **Biopsy**	**Initial:** steroids, prophylactic ABx (in paeds, not adults). Therapeutic anticoagulation (albumin <20)
Dependent oedema	**RFs:** immobility (recent surgery/reduced functioning); venous stasis	Other causes excluded	Support mobilisation
Drugs	CCB, NSAIDs, prolonged steroid use, amlodipine (ankle swelling in 10%)	Medication review	Alternatives
Post-thrombotic syndrome	**RFs:** 6–12 months post-DVT. **Hx & O/E:** pain, oedema, hyperpigmentation, heavy legs, itch, cramps, ulcer	Signs of infection. ABPI	Compression stockings (once PAD excluded). Prevent recurrence
Malnutrition	**RFs:** NBM, stroke, increased frailty	BMI, assess nutrition. FBC, ↓albumin, haematinics	Dietitian input

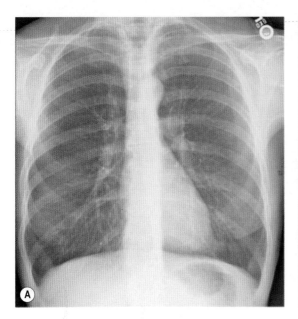
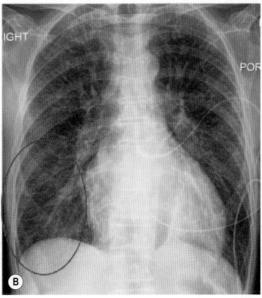

Fig. 8.1 59-year-old female with nonischemic cardiomyopathy, EF 10 % in a euvolemic state (a) and with interstitial edema (b) as demonstrated by interstitial prominence, Kerley A and B lines (red circle). (From: Maria Barile, Pulmonary Edema: A Pictorial Review of Imaging Manifestations and Current Understanding of Mechanisms of Disease, *European J of Radiology Open.* Elevier, 2020; 7: 100274.)

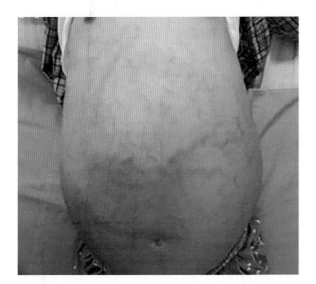

Fig. 8.2 Patients with cirrhosis-related portal hypertension may present with cutaneous manifestations such as visible varicose veins on the abdominal wall called caput medusae. (Reproduced with permission from Liu CH, Hsu CH. Caput medusa. *Clin Gastroenterol Hepatol.* 2011;9(9):A26–A26.)

The top differential in the vignette is decompensated congestive heart failure (CHF), though other factors must be initially also considered. With his diabetes, particularly if it is poorly controlled, he will be prone to renal impairment – which may cause nephrotic-level low albumin and peripheral oedema. He is on amlodipine (side effect of ankle swelling). He drinks more than twice the weekly recommendation, although history does not suggest liver failure and he has no clinical ascites. CHF is most likely here due to cardiovascular history, relative hypotension but elevated JVP, breathlessness, peripheral oedema, coarse crackles – all of which are characteristic if not diagnostic.

> **REVISION TIPS**
>
> - Peripheral oedema, consider hypoalbuminaemia
> - Nephrotic syndrome; risk of clots/thrombosis, infection, hypercholesterolaemia
> - GN triad: **Haematuria, AKI, HTN**
> - When pathological, S3 is due to LV distension
> - Gynaecomastia with spironolactone, hence eplerenone for men

9

Heart Murmur

Lucy Andrews, Alexander Royston, and Viren Ahluwalia

HPC: Symptoms worsening for 3 months. No syncope, no personal or familial cardiac history. **PMHx:** HTN, hypercholesterolaemia, GORD, ex-smoker. **DHx:** ramipril, atorvastatin.

O/E: CVS: HS I+II+ESM, radiates to carotids, BP 159/112, HR: 78, regular. RS: bibasal crackles, RR: 24, shallow breathing.

1. Which murmurs are diastolic and when in the cardiac cycle are they heard?
2. What is an innocent murmur?

3. If mitral regurgitation develops after a MI, which territory is the infarct likely to have affected?

Answers: 1. Tricuspid stenosis (mid-diastolic), mitral stenosis (mid-diastolic), aortic regurgitation (early diastolic), pulmonary regurgitation (early decrescendo, often associated with pulmonary hypertension). 2. Usually describes a paediatric murmur that does not represent underlying pathology: quiet, often position dependant. Examples are Still's murmur (mid-diastolic, buzzing) and venous hum (heard inferior to the clavicles, continuous sound). 3. Suspect papillary muscle damage, due to right coronary artery blockage causing inferior MI.

TABLE 9.1

	Features	Investigations	Management
Systolic Murmurs Aortic stenosis	**RFs:** degenerative senile calcification (age > 55: ↑prevalence with ↑age), congenital (age < 55) e.g. bicuspid valve, rheumatic heart disease (RHD). **Hx & O/E:** ESM → radiates to carotids. Symptoms: Syncope, Angina, Dyspnoea (SAD). Signs: slow rising pulse, narrow pulse pressure	**ECG:** signs of heart strain/failure. **FBC** (anaemia). **TTE** with ejection fraction: dysfunctional valve ± reduced EF depending on severity.	Most common murmur, asymptomatic → observe. Symptomatic → valve replacement **(or TAVI).** Asymptomatic + valve gradient > 40 mmHg with LVSD → consider valve replacement

TABLE 9.1 (Cont'd)

	Features	Investigations	Management
Mitral regurgitation	**RFs:** degenerative MR, papillary muscle/chordae rupture (acute MI), IE or trauma. **Hx & O/E:** pansystolic murmur over apex → radiates to axilla. Symptoms: reduced exercise tolerance, fatigue, orthopnoea. Signs: decompensating heart failure – pulmonary oedema (commonest PC)	**CXR:** cardiomegaly if heart failure, or may be normal	Asymptomatic and EF > 60% → ACE-i and ß-blocker. Symptomatic or EF < 60% → surgical management, e.g. **Valve replacement + ACE-i and ß-blocker**
Pulmonary stenosis	**RFs:** usually congenital (genetic syndromes, e.g. Noonan's), rare in adults. **Hx & O/E:** ESM, loudest over upper left sternal border→ radiates to left shoulder. Asymptomatic if trivial/mild, if severe: mild exertional dyspnoea. Pulmonic thrill, split S2, systemic venous congestion (hepatomegaly, etc.), CCF		Asymptomatic → Observe. Symptomatic → **balloon or surgical valvuloplasty**
Tricuspid regurgitation	**RFs:** Hx of rheumatic fever/infective endocarditis/left heart failure/IVDU, carcinoid, myxomatous disease. **Hx & O/E:** pansystolic murmur. Symptoms: dyspnoea, abdominal distension, early satiety, dyspepsia. Signs: venous congestion: RUQ pain (hepatomegaly), ↑JVP, peripheral oedema		Treat the underlying cause. Manage any HF: lifestyle changes and medication
Hypertrophic cardiomyopathy	**RFs:** autosomal dominant inherited. **Hx & O/E:** ESM, crescendo-decrescendo. Dyspnoea, syncope/presyncope, angina, early CCF. Split S2, JVP α-wave, double carotid arterial pulse. **FHx:** sudden death/HCM	**ECG:** LVH, deep Q waves, ST waves abnormal. **TTE:** septal hypertrophy-asymmetrical	Reduce exertion. No high-intensity sport. **ICD** will be required if deemed at risk of sudden death
Key Complication Heart failure	More severe disease leads to reduced cardiac output then CHF	↑ BNP. **CXR:** ABCDE, signs of CCF. **Echo.** **TTE:** reduced ejection fraction	ACE-i. ß-blocker. Diuretic for symptomatic relief

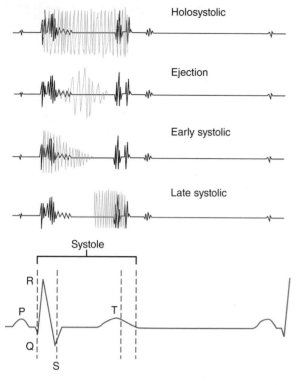

Holosystolic

Ejection

Early systolic

Late systolic

Systole

R

P

T

Q

S

Fig. 9.1 Four classes of systolic heart murmurs. (From Pelech AN. The cardiac murmur. *Pediatr Clin North Am.* 1998;45:107–122.)

In the vignette, ejection systolic murmur (ESM – Fig. 9.1) with dyspnoea (± angina) in an elderly person suggests aortic stenosis (AS), here probably due to valve calcification (senile calcification). She has early signs of failure, due to increased afterload and cardiac remodelling. Reduced exercise tolerance reflects slowly progressive dyspnoea characteristic of AS – would need confirmation via echocardiogram. Mitral regurgitation can be distinguished from AS by the character and location of the murmur. This would be more likely to cause acute heart failure and can be triggered by MI, infective endocarditis, valve prolapse, congenital defects, rheumatic fever or trauma.

REVISION TIPS

- Is a murmur systolic or diastolic? Always feel the pulse when auscultating
- Accentuation to make a murmur easier to hear; *'RILE' Right Inspiration Left Expiration*
- Murmurs are graded 1–6. 1 = very quiet, only heard via careful listening with a stethoscope → 6 = can be heard without stethoscope + cardiac thrill
- Right-sided valvular disease is rare – think IVDU

10

Palpitations

Alice Parker, Alexander Royston, and Viren Ahluwalia

GP CONSULTATION, FEMALE, 50.
FLUTTERING SENSATION IN CHEST

HPC: Started suddenly 1 hour ago, associated with SOB/dizziness. No chest pain. History of previous palpitations – usually terminate in minutes. No identifiable trigger. No previous cardiac history. **PMHx:** HTN, obesity, depression. **DHx:** ramipril, sertraline. **SHx:** non-smoker, drinks 16 units/week.

O/E: CVS: HR 140 (regular), BP: 140/95, HS I+II+0. RS: RR 26, SpO$_2$ 98%, chest clear, equal air entry. Neuro: PEARL, no focal deficit. T 37.3.

1. What is the treatment for suspected supraventricular tachycardia (SVT)?
2. How does it work?
3. What drugs are common causes of this condition?

Answers: 1. Vagal stimuli or adenosine: 6 mg IV, then 12 mg in 1 to 2 minutes if no effect (can repeat), max 30 mg total. 2. Causes AV node blockade, with slowing of ventricular response rate or cessation of atrial tachycardia. Transient. 3. Digoxin, aminophylline, β-agonists, potassium-wasting diuretics, drugs of abuse (cocaine, amphetamine, alcohol).

TABLE 10.1

	Features	Investigations	Management
Cardiac Supraventricular tachycardia (Fig. 10.1)	**RFs:** F>M (75% of cases), CAD, hyperthyroidism. **Hx & O/E:** abrupt onset palpitations, Hx similar episodes, regular pulse. Triggers: alcohol, caffeine, nicotine, stimulants, digoxin, salbutamol	**ECG:** rate >100, narrow QRS, P waves absent/ inverted/ after QRS. AVNRT is commonest SVT. U&Es (↓K), ↑digoxin+ aminophylline levels, TFTs	A→E. Vagal manoeuvres e.g. Valsalva, carotid sinus massage. **Definitive:** IV adenosine 6 mg then 12 mg then 12 mg. DCCV if shocked.
Atrial fibrillation	See *12. DIZZINESS*		

(Continued)

TABLE 10.1 (Cont'd)

	Features	Investigations	Management
Atrial flutter	RFs: as per AF/SVT. Hx & O/E: palpitations, SOB, dizzy. Atrial rate of 300 bpm translates to ventricular rate 150 (2:1 block), 100 (3:1) or 75 (4:1)	ECG: sawtooth appearance of baseline (characteristic in inferior leads)	Treat cause. Rate and rhythm control (as per atrial fibrillation). Anticoagulation
Ventricular tachycardia	RFs: CAD, structural cardiac disease (valvular/hypertrophy), hypoxia, acidaemia, anti-psychotics/anti-arrhythmic drugs. Hx & O/E: palpitations, SOB, dizzy, chest pain, syncope. Regular pulse. Unstable rhythm: high risk of VF → shock (hypotension, pain)	ECG: rate >100, broad QRS. Torsades de pointes: polymorphic VT. U&Es($\downarrow$K), calcium, magnesium, troponin, ABG	A→E. DCCV if shocked. Definitive: Amiodarone IV. Torsades de pointes: MgSO$_4$
Wolff-Parkinson-White syndrome	RFs: most common in young people, FHx (rare). Hx & O/E: tachycardia, palpitations, may trigger SVT, AF, flutter	ECG: short PR interval, delta wave	Unstable: DCCV Stable: radiofrequency ablation of accessory pathway
Extra-cardiac Anxiety	RFs: sex (F>M, 2:1), anxious personality traits, stress, trauma, substance misuse, comorbid depression. Hx & O/E: widespread disproportionate worry, duration ≥6 months. Physical symptoms include chest/abdo pain, palpitations	TFTs, LFTs, CBG. Urine: drug screen. ECG: sinus tachycardia GAD7	Education, lifestyle advice, SSRI. Definitive: psychological therapy (often CBT). β-blockers only if physical symptoms problematic (short-term use)
Thyrotoxicosis	RFs: smoking, other autoimmune disease, FHx of thyroid disease. Hx & O/E: tremor, goitre, weight loss, tachycardia/ palpitations, diarrhoea, oligomenorrhea, sweating, exophthalmos (in Graves'), thyroid acropathy	ECG: sinus tachycardia TFTs: $\downarrow$TSH, $\uparrow$T4, thyroid autoantibodies (Graves'). FBC/CRP: inflammatory markers ($\uparrow$thyroiditis)	Initial: β-blockers – symptom control. Definitive: antithyroid-carbimazole, propyl-thiouracil. Radioactive iodine (uncontrolled Graves'/toxic multinodular goitre). Thyroidectomy
Phaeochro-mocytoma	RFs: FHx, autoimmune/other endocrine disorders, MEN2, von Hippel-Lindau disease, NF1. Hx & O/E: triad; palpitations, labile hypertension, sweating. Weight loss, headaches	Often paroxysmal. Urine: 24 h metanephrines CT: abdomen, pelvis	Alpha-blockers (phentolamine), β-blockers Definitive: surgery – adrenalectomy

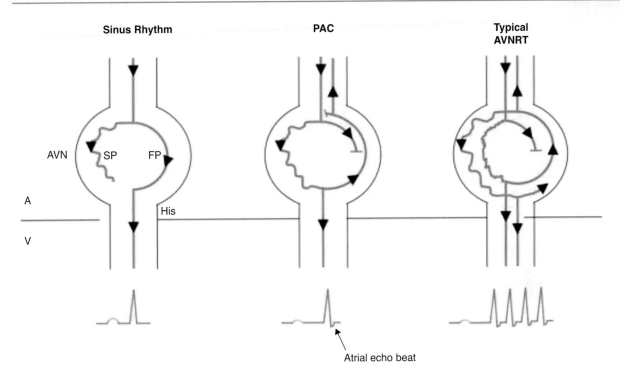

Fig. 10.1 Prototype of dual AV nodal pathways physiology in sinus rhythm, with a premature atrial complex (PAC) which trigger a typical "slow–fast" AVNRT. *SP*, slow pathway; *FP*, fast pathway. (From Carrizo AG, Ballantyne B, Baranchuk A. Atrioventricular node reentrant tachycardia. In: Vasan RS, Sawyer DB, eds. *Encyclopedia of Cardiovascular Research and Medicine*. Elsevier; 2018:224–241.

This patient has risk factors for several conditions that predispose to tachycardia. Her history of mental health illness puts her at risk of anxiety, similarly her age and gender mean she is at heightened risk of autoimmune disease of which hyperthyroidism is a common manifestation (her obesity makes this perhaps less likely). The diagnosis here is SVT, suggested by the speed of onset, the previous palpitations and her being otherwise asymptomatic.

REVISION TIPS

- Causes of palpitations with a regular pulse include SVT, VT, atrial flutter, anxiety, thyrotoxicosis, phaeochromocytoma and WPW
- Causes of palpitations with an irregular pulse include atrial fibrillation, atrial flutter with variable conduction, ectopics

- Management of SVT = IV adenosine, VT = IV amiodarone
- Management of AF: Rate versus Rhythm control:
  - Rate, e.g. bisoprolol, verapamil, diltiazem, digoxin, amiodarone
  - Rhythm (<48 h or post-3-weeks anticoagulation/clear TOE): DCCT, flecainide, amiodarone

11

Chest Pain and Pain on Inspiration

Lucy Andrews and Chetna Kohli

EMERGENCY DEPARTMENT, MALE, 36.
CHEST PAIN

HPC: Two-day history of worsening, stabbing central chest pain. Eased by sitting forward. No sweats, palpitations, nausea. Recent bad cold. **PMHx:** Nil. **SHx:** non-smoker. **FHx:** nil of note.

O/E: RS: No respiratory distress, equal breath sounds. **CVS:** No oedema, DVT or diaphoresis; rubbing noise throughout precordium; regular pulse; CRT <2 sec. **Ix:** ECG: PR depression, widespread ST elevation.

---

1. Chest pain, worse with movement, does not radiate and is reproduced by palpating the chest wall. ECGs, troponins, CXR normal. What is the *most likely* diagnosis?

2. Unilateral chest pain, SOB, productive cough. Reduced air entry and crackles in the right lung base. What is the *most likely* diagnosis?

3. Patient with SOB and chest pain, RR 28. No cardiac RFs, examination unremarkable apart from tachypnoea. ECG, troponin and D-dimer normal. Her blood pH is 7.52. What is the *most likely* diagnosis?

Answers: 1. Musculoskeletal (muscle/tendon strain, myalgia following coughing, soft tissue). 2. Pneumonia. 3. Anxiety/panic attack. Respiratory alkalosis may be evident on a blood gas due to hyperventilation.

TABLE 11.1

	Features	Investigations	Management
ACS; STEMI	**RFs:** age, smoking, diabetes, HTN, obesity, alcohol, dyslipidaemia, FHx, cocaine, SLE. **Hx & O/E:** crushing, central pain, radiation to arm/neck/jaw. Nausea, SOB, palpitations, sweating. **Non-cardiac sounding/atypical pain** especially women/diabetics	**Serial ECG:** dynamic changes, > 1 mm ST elevation in two contiguous leads – more elevation needed in V2-3, possibly LBBB (Sgarbossa criteria). ↑ **Troponin.** **CXR:** to assess for other causes. **Coronary angiography** (as part of PCI).	**(MONA):** Metoclopramide and morphine. Oxygen if <94%. Nitrates (GTN sublingual or nitrates IV). Antiplatelets (aspirin 300 mg + ticagrelor 180 mg/clopidogrel 300 mg). **Secondary prevention (BASH):** Beta-blocker, Aspirin, Statin, HTN (ACE-i). **STEMI:** PCI < 120 min, thrombolysis if no PCI.

TABLE 11.1 (Cont'd)

	Features	Investigations	Management
ACS; NSTEMI	As above	**ECG:** non-specific ST depression or T wave inversion. ↑Troponin. CXR. Coronary angiography.	*As above for MONA + BASH.* **Unstable:** PCI/CABG + anticoagulant + P2Y12 inhibitor. **Stable:** PCI/CABG considered.
ACS; Unstable angina	As above – may present as a new/worse pattern of stable angina or as 'crescendo' angina.	**ECG:** may be normal, or as NSTEMI. **Troponin:** no rise. CXR. **Coronary angiography**	*As above for MONA + BASH.* + P2Y12 inhibitor. Discuss with cardiologist – for early angiography/ revascularisation.
Pericarditis	**RFs:** preceding viral/bacterial illness. **Hx & O/E:** recent MI (Dressler's), eased by leaning forward, precordial rub.	**ECG:** global saddle-shaped ST elevation, PR depression. ↑CRP. May have ↑WCC. **Echocardiogram:** ± effusion. Troponin usually normal, but may not be ↑	Ibuprofen, colchicine, PPI. Rest. Treat underlying cause. Treat tamponade if present.
Aortic dissection	**RFs:** HTN, connective tissue disorder, FHx. **Hx & O/E:** sudden tearing pain through to back, haemodynamically unstable, new aortic regurgitation murmur, BP different between arms; GI ischaemia; neurological.	**CXR:** widened mediastinum, pleural effusion – can be normal. **ECG:** may show ST changes, most commonly inferior leads. **Troponin:** often normal. **Bedside USS:** may see dissection flap. **CT angiogram:** dissection. Crossmatch blood.	Analgesia. **Aggressive BP control:** target SBP 100–120 mmHg and HR 60–80/min. **Urgent cardiothoracic surgery referral**
Pneumothorax	**RFs:** tall, thin younger male smoker. Respiratory disease, connective tissue disorder. **Hx & O/E:** SOB, pleuritic chest pain. Hypoxia, trachea deviated (if tensioning); absent breath sound on affected side, hyper-resonant percussion	**Tension pneumothorax suspected:** clinical diagnosis, investigations should not delay decompression. **Non-tension:** **CXR:** lucency between chest wall and lung. **FAST scan:** absence of lung sliding indicates pneumothorax.	Oxygen. **Tension:** immediate decompression, 14 G or 16 G cannula into 2nd intercostal space, mid-clavicular line then chest drain. **Non-tension:** observe/aspirate/ chest drain.
Pulmonary embolism (PE)	**RFs:** malignancy, immobilisation, FHx, previous VTE, surgery, pregnancy. **Hx & O/E:** pleuritic chest pain, SOB, haemoptysis, signs of DVT, tachycardia, low saturations, collapse	**Wells' score >4:** CTPA, therapeutic dose anticoagulation. **Wells' score ≤4:** if D-dimer positive, do CTPA (interim anticoagulation if any delay). If D-dimer negative, consider alternative diagnosis. Low D-dimer in 'low risk' patient <50 yo rules out PE. Use age-adjusted D-dimer for patients >50 yo (10 × age gives upper limit of normal). **ECG:** see *Revision Tips*	Oxygen (aim 94%–98%). **PE confirmed and haemodynamically stable:** DOAC (provoked: 3 months, unprovoked: 6 months). **PE confirmed and haemodynamically unstable:** Unfractionated heparin + thrombolysis. After thrombolysis, unfractionated heparin can be switched to a DOAC. Thrombectomy or IVC filters may be considered.

(Continued)

TABLE 11.1   (Cont'd)

	Features	Investigations	Management
Pleurisy	**RFs:** parietal pleural inflammation. **Hx & O/E:** chest pain that worsens with coughing, breathing, sneezing – usually sharp or stabbing in nature.	Investigations to rule out dangerous differentials, e.g. ECG, CXR, Wells' scoring, bloods. Isolated rib fractures do not require imaging.	Treat cause - e.g. pneumonia, PE, pneumothorax, viral, lung/pleura malignancy, rib fracture. Analgesia
Gastro-oesophageal reflux disease	See *81. CHRONIC ABDOMINAL PAIN*		
Acute Pancreatitis	**Causes/RFs:** Mnemonic 'I GET SMASHED' (idiopathic, gallstones, ethanol, trauma, steroids, mumps/malignancy, autoimmune, scorpion sting (Tityus), hypercalcaemia/hypertriglyceridaemia, ERCP, drugs). **Hx & O/E:** sudden onset severe abdominal pain, often radiates to back, N&V	Raised inflammatory markers, ↑↑Amylase, might have cholestatic LFTs. **CBG:** ± ↑Glucose (DM) **Erect CXR:** rule out pneumoperitoneum. **Abdominal USS:** look for gallstones. **MRCP:** If USS inconclusive. **CT AP:** may show complications.	Eat and drink as tolerated. IV fluids + analgesia ± oxygen (only if needed). Urinary catheter in elderly patients/AKI/dehydration. No antibiotics unless later imaging shows necrosis. Glasgow-Imrie scoring (involve ICU services if ≥3). Monitor for alcohol withdrawal if causative. **ERCP:** if CBD calculus. Visualises and removes. **Consider cholecystectomy** ('hot lap chole')

Chest pain is a very common, and often high-risk, emergency presentation (Fig. 11.1). In the vignette, the patient has positional chest pain with a preceding illness and ECG changes classically seen in pericarditis – PR depression, widespread ST changes. The history reveals the diagnosis and should not be replaced by merely ordering a troponin and ECG. Approaching with the attitude of 'what is the worst thing this could be' allows you to consider the higher risk differentials early and guards against missing a subtle PE or anticoagulating a dissection. This patient would still have been investigated for acute coronary syndrome given his presentation, as missing myocardial ischaemia in this case is unacceptable.

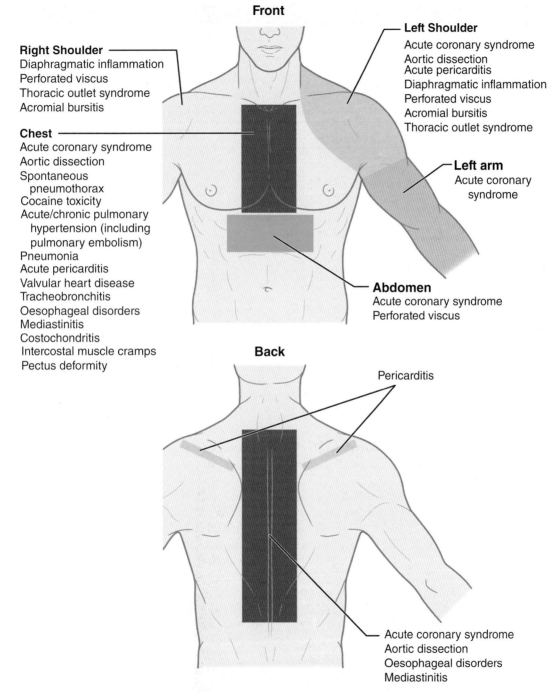

Front

Right Shoulder
Diaphragmatic inflammation
Perforated viscus
Thoracic outlet syndrome
Acromial bursitis

Chest
Acute coronary syndrome
Aortic dissection
Spontaneous
  pneumothorax
Cocaine toxicity
Acute/chronic pulmonary
  hypertension (including
  pulmonary embolism)
Pneumonia
Acute pericarditis
Valvular heart disease
Tracheobronchitis
Oesophageal disorders
Mediastinitis
Costochondritis
Intercostal muscle cramps
Pectus deformity

Left Shoulder
Acute coronary syndrome
Aortic dissection
Acute pericarditis
Diaphragmatic inflammation
Perforated viscus
Acromial bursitis
Thoracic outlet syndrome

Left arm
Acute coronary
  syndrome

Abdomen
Acute coronary syndrome
Perforated viscus

Back

Pericarditis

Acute coronary syndrome
Aortic dissection
Oesophageal disorders
Mediastinitis

Fig. 11.1 Causes of (referred) chest pain. (Reproduced with permission from Fenster BE, Lee-Chiong TL, Gebhart GF, Matthay RA. Chest pain. In: *Murray & Nadel's Textbook of Respiratory Medicine.* 7th ed. Elsevier; 2022:521–531.e2.)

REVISION POINTS

- Women and diabetics with ACS are more likely to present atypically
- Thrombolysis is absolutely contraindicated in: previous ICH; ischaemic stroke within last 3/12; suspected dissection; current bleeding; brain tumour; cerebrovascular lesion; serious head trauma in last 3/12

- All patients with chest pain require ECG, most need troponin and CXR
- ECG in PE – most likely sinus tachycardia, 'S1Q3T3' (prominent S wave in lead I, Q wave and inverted T wave in lead III) rarely seen; R heart strain, p-pulmonale; RAD (normal ECG does not rule out PE)

12

Dizziness

Margarita Fox, Alexander Royston, and Viren Ahluwalia

EMERGENCY DEPARTMENT, FEMALE, 80. DIZZINESS THAT STARTED THIS MORNING, ASSOCIATED WITH PALPITATIONS.

HPC: Palpitations onset within 30 minutes, and ongoing. 'Light-headed', tired, reduced exercise tolerance. No vertiginous symptoms, no loss of consciousness. **PMHx:** Hypothyroidism, IHD, hypertension, aortic stenosis **DHx:** ramipril, levothyroxine, atorvastatin. **SHx:** Alcohol 30 units/week, non-smoker.

 O/E: CVS: HR 120 (irregularly irregular), BP: 149/91, HS I+II+ESM radiating to carotids. RS: RR 18, SpO$_2$ 98% on air clear to auscultation, afebrile. Abdomen soft, non-tender, bowel sounds present. Neuro: nil focal.

1. What is the next step in this lady's management?
2. What are the clinical scoring systems used to assess risk in this condition, and why do we use them?
3. A 57-year-old smoker, 20–30 units/week, T2DM 170/95, high cholesterol; walking 'drunk', dysarthria, dizziness, nausea, diplopia, nystagmus, past-pointing, dysdiadokinesia. What is the key investigation?

Answers: 1. Fast AF, stable, onset <48 hours: heparinise, treat with rhythm (DCCV/amiodarone) or rate control. Lifelong anticoagulation (CHADSVASc >2). Echo to grade AS severity and establish whether dizziness is from arrhythmia or valvular disease. 2. CHADSVASc and HASBLED. Used when assessing risk of stroke and then bleeding (if put on anticoagulation). 3. Posterior stroke. CT head: rule out haemorrhagic stroke.

TABLE 12.1

	Features	Investigations	Management
Cardiovascular Atrial fibrillation (Fig. 12.1)	**RFs:** IHD, hypertension, heart failure, valvular disease, thyroid disease, electrolyte disturbance, caffeine, alcohol, age. **Hx & O/E:** asymptomatic or palpitations, SOB, dizziness, chest pain. Irregularly irregular pulse. **Unstable** hypotension, chest pain, SOB, dizziness, syncope, shock	**ECG:** absent P waves, irregular narrow QRS. U&Es, Mg, Ca, TFTs, troponin	**New onset fast AF:** A-E. **Unstable→ immediate DCCV.** **Stable <48 h:** rate or rhythm control + LMWH. **>48 h:** rate initially, then cardioversion after 3 weeks anticoagulation. *Rate:* bisoprolol, diltiazem, verapamil. *Rhythm:* flecainide or amiodarone. Consider anticoagulation
Aortic stenosis	See *9. HEART MURMUR*		

(Continued)

TABLE 12.1 (Cont'd)

	Features	Investigations	Management
Orthostatic hypotension	RFs: age, antihypertensives dehydration, autonomic neuropathy (diabetes, PD). Hx & O/E: lying standing BP. Postural drop: falls >20 mm Hg systolic/10 diastolic within 3 min of standing-light-headed, collapse.	ECG. Anaemia, CBG (hypoglycaemia). Tilt table testing (rare): autonomic dysfunction	Medication review. Encourage fluid intake. **Fludrocortisone** (monitor U&Es), **midodrine** (avoid supine HTN)
Anaemia	RFs: iron deficiency/diet. Hx & O/E: fatigue, dizzy, palpitations, SOB, pallor, hair loss, koilonychia	FBC: hypochromic microcytic anaemia. Ferritin: low. TIBC/ transferrin high	**PO Ferrous sulphate.** Investigate for cause and treat
Non-cardiovascular: Neurological/ENT			
Posterior circulation stroke	RFs: as for stroke. Hx & O/E: acute vestibular syndrome-sudden onset dizziness, nausea + vomiting, ataxia. Confusion, headache, weakness, diplopia, dysarthria, LoC	CT: r/o haemorrhagic stroke. MRI brain: lesion demonstrating cerebellar infarction/ haemorrhage	Aspirin 300 mg. **Thrombolysis** if eligible (within 4.5 h, no contraindications). Secondary prevention: 75 mg OD clopidogrel
Peripheral vestibular causes (BPPV, Meniere's, labyrinthitis, vestibular neuronitis)	**BPPV** (hours): dizzy turning head. **Meniere's** (weeks/months): tinnitus, hearing loss, vertigo. **Acute vestibular syndrome:** labyrinthitis (hearing loss), vestibular neuronitis (no loss).	**BPPV:** Dix-Hallpike manoeuvre **Meniere's:** pure tone audiogram (PTA)	**BPPV:** Epley manoeuvre. **Meniere's:** betahistine prophylaxis, prochlorperazine (acute attacks). **Vestibular neuronitis/ labyrinthitis:** prochlorperazine
Peripheral neuropathy	RFs: ageing, diabetes, low vitamin B$_{12}$, hypothyroidism, alcohol Hx & O/E: disequilibrium/ unbalanced, unsteady. Sensory: paraesthesia, pain. Motor: weakness. Autonomic: constipation, low BP	FBC, U&Es, LFTs, CRP, vitamin B$_{12}$, folate, TSH, glucose, HbA1C. Nerve conduction studies. Electromyography	Symptomatic management. Pain: Amitriptyline. Hypotension: high salt/fluid diet, compression garments, midodrine/fludrocortisone
Iatrogenic	RFs: polypharmacy; anxiolytics, antidepressants, antipsychotics, aminoglycosides, NSAIDs, antihistamines, anticholinergics	Clinical	Medication review
Acute alcohol intoxication	Dizziness, feeling intoxicated, disorientation, ataxic gait. May have ALD signs: telangiectasias, palmar erythema, muscular atrophy, etc.	LFTs – γGT, ALT	A-E. Correct any electrolyte disturbances (K$^+$ likely). Correct hypoglycaemia. Pabrinex/ thiamine/CIWA

ALD, alcoholic liver disease.

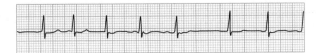

Fig. 12.1 Electrocardiogram (ECG) of atrial fibrillation. Irregularly irregular QRS complexes, saw-tooth baseline of uncoordinated atrial activity, absent P waves. (Reproduced with permission from Slater TA, Waduud MA, Nadeem Ahmed N. *Palpitations, Pocketbook of Differential Diagnosis*. 5th ed. 342–344, Copyright © 2022 by Elsevier, Ltd. All rights reserved.)

Dizziness is a common presenting symptom in older people. It can have cardiovascular, neurological or ENT-based origins. If you suspect pre-syncope with a cardiovascular cause, then assessing haemodynamic stability is priority. AF can produce symptoms (haemodynamic compromise, pre-syncope) and predispose to complications (notably stroke). In the vignette, sudden onset palpitations and irregularly irregular pulse point towards AF. Whilst AS is commonly progressive, sudden deterioration is uncommon. Risk for a thromboembolic event can be estimated with scores such as CHADS-VASc (congestive heart failure, hypertension, age ≥ 75, diabetes, stroke, vascular disease, age 65 to 74 and sex category (female)).

REVISION TIPS

- **Vertigo:** false sense of spinning – suggests vestibular involvement, and makes central causes unlikely
- **Light-headedness:** suggests pre-syncope causing reduced blood/oxygen to brain (cardio-inhibitory: structural/valvular heart disease, arrhythmias; or vaso-depressive: hypotension). Can be hypoglycaemia
- **Disequilibrium:** unsteadiness or imbalance (e.g. musculoskeletal (MSK), impaired proprioception in peripheral neuropathy, visual impairment, ageing)
- **Vague:** 'floating/wooziness/heavy-headedness' (more likely psychogenic)

13

Obesity - Outline

Marcus Drake

Body mass index (BMI) = kg/m² (weight divided by height squared);
- WHO classification: normal weight – BMI 18.5 to 24.9 kg/m²; obese – BMI ≥ 30 kg/m² (Table 13.1).
- For people of Asian descent: normal weight – BMI 18.5 to 22.9 kg/m²; obese – BMI ≥ 27.5 kg/m²
- Consider age, ethnicity, fluid status, muscularity (e.g. waist circumference or waist-hip ratio) to avoid overclassifying someone as overweight or obese

Phenotypes: Abdominal/central ('apple-shaped') or hip-thigh-gluteal ('pear-shaped').

Primary obesity- imbalance in energy intake and expenditure.

Secondary obesity- due to disease or medication;
- Hypothyroidism, growth hormone deficiency, Cushing syndrome, pseudohypoparathyroidism, depression (over-eating/binge eating), eating disorders, neurological (e.g. hypothalamic disease, brain tumour), Prader-Willi or Bardet-Biedl syndromes
- Look for striae (can suggest Cushing syndrome), acanthosis nigricans (insulin resistance), acne/hirsutism polycystic ovary syndrome (PCOS), goitre

- Endocrine evaluation, glucose tolerance test, polysomnography (OSA), ultrasound for non-alcoholic fatty liver disease or PCOS
- Medication can cause weight gain by stimulating appetite, stimulating fat storage, slowing metabolism, fluid retention, reducing exercise tolerance
- Drug classes that may be relevant include; anti-depressants, antipsychotics, diabetes drugs, steroids, anticonvulsants, opioids, beta-blockers, antihistamines, hypnotics

Monogenic obesity: mutation in melanocortin 4 receptor, leptin deficiency/receptor mutation, pro-opiomelanocortin deficiency.

Obesity complications;
- Cardiovascular disease, hypertension, DVT/PE
- Metabolic syndrome, diabetes, dyslipidaemia, gout
- Non-alcoholic fatty liver disease/steatohepatitis
- Osteoarthritis
- OSA/hypoventilation
- Gastroesophageal reflux
- Malignancy (breast, endometrial, colorectal, renal, oesophageal)

Medications to treat obesity can reduce fat absorption (orlistat), or improve appetite/satiety (e.g. liraglutide)

TABLE 13.1

	Features	Investigation	Treatment
Overweight	BMI 25–29.9 kg/m²	Fasting lipid panel, fasting glucose, HbA1C, LFTs. Check BP with appropriate cuff size	Lifestyle modification: reduced calorie diet, physical activity, behavioural therapy. Medication if obesity complications
Obese	BMI ≥30 kg/m² *mild = 30–34.9, moderate = 35–39.9, morbid ≥40*		Lifestyle modification. Medication. Bariatric surgery (Fig. 13.1); BMI ≥40, or ≥35 with obesity complications

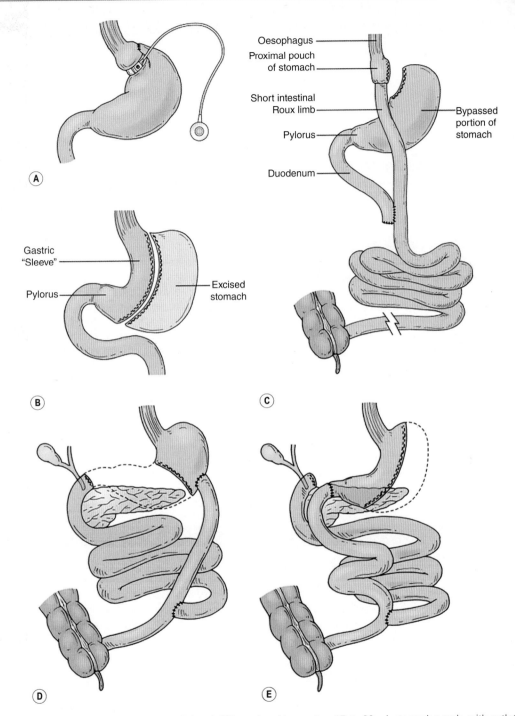

Fig. 13.1 Bariatric Surgery. (A) Adjustable gastric band. Silicone band to create a 15- to 20-mL stomach pouch, with outlet adjusted via a subcutaneous port. (B) Sleeve gastrectomy, stapling vertically and removing the fundus and greater curve. (C) Roux-en-Y gastric bypass (RYGB). A small gastric pouch created by division of the upper stomach, connected to 100 to 150 cm limb of jejunum. (D) Biliopancreatic diversion (BPD). Bypassing most of the small bowel, a short channel absorbs calories and nutrients. Less risk of protein malnutrition than for RYGB. (E) Biliopancreatic diversion with duodenal switch, to avoid dumping syndrome and maintain the pylorus. (Adapted with permission from Ding S-A, McKenzie T, Vernon AH, Goldfine AB. Bariatric surgery. In: Jameson JL, De Groot LJ, de Kretser DM, et al., eds. *Endocrinology: Adult and Pediatric.* 7th ed. Elsevier; 2016:479–490.e4.)

14

Scarring

Katie Turner and Richard Barlow

DERMATOLOGY CLINIC, MALE, 24. LESION ON SHOULDER

HPC: Raised purple lesion, occasionally itchy. Surgery at this site 5 months previously. Bothered by appearance.

O/E: 3 × 1 × 0.5 cm, irregularly shaped, non-tender, hairless purple lesion on the posterior aspect of the right shoulder, shiny smooth surface, firm/rubbery texture. Fitzpatrick type 6 skin.

Answers: 1. Mnemonic DID NOT HEAL – Drugs, infections/ischemia, diabetes, nutritional deficiency, oxygen (hypoxia), toxins, hypothermia/hyperthermia, excessive tension, acidosis, local anaesthetics. 2. Inflammation of the epidermis stimulates melanin production, which can enter the dermis leading to PIH. Patients often misinterpret PIH as scarring, but it gradually resolves with time. Post-inflammatory hypopigmentation is often permanent, after more damaging trauma such as burns. 3. Full-thickness ulcers, burns, surgery. There are also scarring and non-scarring variants of many inflammatory disorders, e.g. lichen planopilaris and discoid lupus.

1. List the factors associated with poor wound healing.
2. What is post-inflammatory hyperpigmentation (PIH)?
3. Give examples of scarring skin disorders.

TABLE 14.1

	Clinical	Investigations	Management
Keloid scar	**RFs:** young adults, dark skin, sternum, shoulder, neck, face **Hx & O/E:** enlarged, raised scar beyond the boundaries of the original wound. Shiny, hairless, smooth, hard, painless, rubbery. Colour ranges from pink to purple. Does not regress with time.	Clinical diagnosis. Skin biopsy if suspicious of malignancy	Intra-lesional/topical/tape preparations of corticosteroids to reduce size and symptoms. Other treatments have varying success: combinations of surgical excision, cryotherapy, laser. May exacerbate the problem
Hypertrophic scar	Raised scar confined to the boundaries of the original wound. May be painful and itchy, can regress with time	Clinical diagnosis. Skin biopsy if suspicious of malignancy	As above

TABLE 14.1   (Cont'd)

	Clinical	Investigations	Management
Atrophic scar	Indented scar, often result of acne or chickenpox. Types; • Boxcar (round/oval craters) • Ice pick (deep, narrow pitted scars) • Rolling (uneven appearance with sloping edge)	Clinical diagnosis	Subcision, disruption of tethered rolling scars often resulting from acne via specialised needles, encourages new collagen deposition to resolve the scar. Other options often not available on NHS: dermabrasion, laser therapy (e.g. pulsed dye laser), needling, radiofrequency
Contractures	Occur after burn injury. Shortened, hypertrophic regions of scars. Wounds crossing joints are at high risk. Restricted movement in affected joint	Clinical diagnosis	Splints. Physiotherapy
Stretch marks (striae)	**RFs:** rapid weight loss, steroids, obesity, pregnancy, bodybuilding. **Hx & O/E:** indented streaks – abdomen, breast, hip, buttock. Red, purple, brown may turn white. Painless	Clinical diagnosis	Moisturisers. Topical retinoid therapy. Chemical peels. Pulsed dye laser therapy. Skin needling

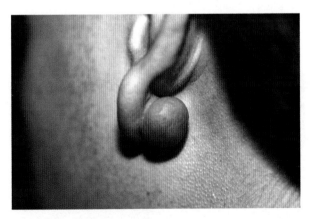

Fig. 14.1 Keloid scar on an earlobe. (From Kliegman RM et al. *Nelson Textbook of Pediatrics*. Philadelphia: Saunders; 2011.)

The vignette is describing a keloid scar (Fig. 14.1). Risk factors include the patient's ethnicity and recent surgery. They often arise behind the earlobes following ear piercings. Keloid scars are difficult to manage and can be exacerbated by conventional treatment methods. Whilst not the case in this scenario, consider self-induced mechanisms of scarring, especially when the pattern or distribution is atypical. Dermatitis artefacta describes skin lesions arising from the patient's own actions and may imply a psychological problem; elicit what may be driving the process without being accusatory.

REVISION TIPS

- Damage to deeper skin increases chances of scarring
- Keloid scars extend beyond the borders of the original wound whilst hypertrophic scars do not
- Keloid and hypertrophic scars can mimic malignancies if the history of surgery or trauma is not forthcoming. They are not at risk of malignant transformation

15

Acute Rash

Katherine Parker, Alexander Royston, Jennifer Powell, and Richard Barlow

HPC: Spread proximally to his trunk over past 2 days. Recent sore throat/fever. **PMHx:** Herpes labialis. **DHx:** valacyclovir for flares. **SHx:** PE teacher/swimming coach.

O/E: Annular lesions of varying sizes on the hands, arms and trunk (eyes and genitals unaffected). Central blisters with surrounding paler skin and darker red borders are noted. A cold sore on the left side of the lower lip is present. He is systemically well.

1. What is the pathophysiology of urticaria?
2. What is chronic urticaria?
3. What type of reaction occurs in Stevens-Johnson syndrome (SJS)/toxic epidermal necrolysis (TEN)?
4. What is erysipelas?

Answers: 1. IgE-mediated degranulation of mast cells/basophils, releasing histamine/vasoactive mediators (bradykinin, leukotriene C4, prostaglandin D2), hence extravasation into the dermis leading to itchy urticarial lesions. 2. Daily itchy weals for more than 6 weeks. 3. Type IV hypersensitivity reaction. 4. Form of cellulitis involving more superficial dermal structures; raised and well-demarcated borders.

TABLE 15.1

	Features	Investigations	Management
Urticaria (Fig. 15.1)	**RFs:** triggers (acute)-food, bites and stings, vaccinations, drugs (NSAIDS), contact dermatitis, infections (viral/bacterial). Chronic: chronic spontaneous urticaria, inducible (pressure, heat/cold etc.). **Hx & O/E:** intensely itchy weals, resolve <24 h. Raised firm plaques/papules: dermal oedema: mm-cm ±targetoid/ erythema	Clinical diagnosis. Investigate if: unidentified trigger, prolonged attacks suggestive of urticarial vasculitis, angioedema. *EXCLUDE ANAPHYLAXIS* airway compromise or shock	Identify/avoid trigger (symptom diary). Urticaria Activity Score (UAS7) or Dermatology Life Quality Index (DLQI) – assess severity. *Mild* Avoidance. *Moderate* Non-sedating antihistamine: <6 weeks (urticarial doses). *Severe* also consider oral corticosteroid <7 days (completion risks rebound flare). **Definitive:** dermatology if; painful/persistent, treatment-resistant severe food/latex allergy, chronic

TABLE 15.1   (Cont'd)

	Features	Investigations	Management
Contact dermatitis	Consider if unusual eczema distribution. **Irritant (80%):** affects anyone, e.g. bleach, detergent. **Allergic (<20%):** delayed type IV hypersensitivity, may exceed area of contact. **Causes:** topical or airborne irritant/ allergen. Occupational: metal work, aerosols, acrylic nail products, cosmetics	Clinical diagnosis. **Patch Testing** to investigate for allergic contact dermatitis	Avoid trigger. Treatment of eczema: emollients/ topical corticosteroids. Typically improves in weeks. **Definitive:** consider dermatology referral-severe/persistent, chronic/ recurring, Occupational
Erythema multiforme	**Causes:** infections (n.b. HSV, *Mycoplasma pneumoniae*), drugs (penicillin, NSAIDs), vaccination. **Hx & O/E:** prodrome/URTI → rash (post-24–48h). Symmetrical. Starts distally→proximally, ± pruritus, target lesion. Mucosal involvement uncommon	Clinical diagnosis. Note: does not progress to SJS/ TEN	Self-limiting (1–5 weeks), may recur. Heals without scarring. Symptomatic: analgesia, mouthwash, topical corticosteroid. **Definitive:** aetiology dependent. HSV: antiviral therapy (recurrent). Withdraw causative drug
Stevens-Johnson syndrome (SJS) and toxic epidermal necrolysis (TEN)	Acute evolving rash 1–14/7 after starting new medication. Antibiotics (most common), allopurinol, anticonvulsants, NSAIDs. **Hx & O/E:** prodrome 2–3/7, with constitutional symptoms. Painful, various morphology: macules, bullae, erythema, targetoid lesions ± mucosal involvement. Nikolsky sign +ve. Systemic compromise	Clinical diagnosis. Urgent frozen section of skin biopsy to exclude other pathology (SSSS). **Biopsy:** keratinocyte necrosis with full thickness epidermal necrosis	**Initial/Definitive:** Burns unit referral. Stop causal medication. Rapid assessment (SCORTEN scale). If >3, admit ICU. Supportive measures for skin/other organ systems (treat opportunistic infection). SCORTEN – predicts morality in SJS/TEN
Staphylococcal scalded skin syndrome (SSSS)	*Staphylococcus aureus* exotoxins target epidermis proteins. **RFs:** child (<5-yo), immunodeficiency, CKD. **Hx & O/E:** fever, sore throat/ conjunctivitis, malaise, erythema and skin tenderness. Tender flaccid bullae coalesce and detach. Nikolsky sign +ve	Clinical diagnosis. **Biopsy:** consider to exclude similar disorders. Intra-epidermal cleavage	**Initial/Definitive:** admission. Acute – supportive care: IVI/ electrolyte balance. Emollient: petroleum jellies (skin fragile). Analgesia, antibiotics. Ongoing management; parenteral nutrition (if NBM). Physiotherapy
Cellulitis	**RFs:** immunocompromise (DM, drugs), compromised skin barrier (previous cellulitis, eczema, ulcers, lymphoedema, oedema, venous insufficiency, obesity). **Hx & O/E:** warm, tender erythema ±ulcer or wound. Usually clearly defined border (mark to monitor progression) ±oedema, bullae and systemic compromise	Clinical diagnosis. **Bloods:** inflammatory markers. Categorise severity (Eron classification). Consider varicose eczema in cases of 'bilateral cellulitis'	Manage in primary care (no systemic toxicity/ uncontrolled comorbidities). Urgent admission – sepsis, necrotising fasciitis, rapidly progressing, extremes of age, immunocompromised, facial cellulitis. High-dose oral/IV Abx, analgesia, oral fluids, elevate affected limb, avoid compression garments. Prophylactic Abx only if recurrent

Other Drug Reactions. Also see; *54. BITES AND STINGS; 96. VIRAL EXANTHEMS; 146. ALLERGIES*

Complications

Necrotising fasciitis	Rapidly progressive infection with extensive necrosis and gangrene. Admit urgently for surgical debridement and antibiotics.
Eczema herpeticum	HSV-infected eczema, vesicular rash, requires admission and IV aciclovir. Typically involves the face; therefore, important to seek ophthalmological input.

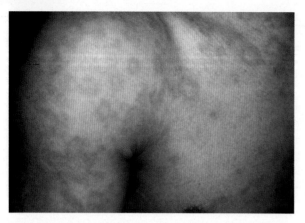

Fig. 15.1 Urticaria. (Reproduced from Elsevier Point of Care. Published June 27, 2016, In Kasparis C, et al: Urticaria and angioedema. In: Lebwohl MG, et al., eds. *Treatment of Skin Disease: Comprehensive Therapeutic Strategies.* 4th ed. London, UK: Elsevier; 2014:777–780.)

Acutely red, itchy rashes are commonplace in dermatology, often due to reactive exanthems (drugs and/or infective processes) and inflammatory dermatoses. The prodromal illness and presence of herpes simplex virus type 1(HSV1) in a person who is systemically well make erythema multiforme the most likely diagnosis in the vignette. Urticaria can feature targetoid lesions; however, intense pruritus would be expected. Chlorine from swimming pools can cause contact dermatitis which is usually irritant in nature and would likely be more widespread. The lack of sheet-like detachment of the epidermis steers away from SSSS and SJS/TEN.

REVISION TIPS

- Erythema multiforme is distinct from SJS and TEN, although all three conditions can have mucosal involvement
- Target lesions resemble a bull's eye: <u>not</u> specific to erythema multiforme

- Single targetoid lesions may represent fixed drug eruptions and often occur at the same site on re-exposure to the offending drug
- Suspect urticarial vasculitis in cases of weals that persist past 24 h or leave bruise-type marks

16

Chronic Rash

Alice Parker, Alexander Royston, Jennifer Powell, and Richard Barlow

---

GP CONSULTATION, FEMALE, 30.
PRURITIC RASH FOR 4 MONTHS

HPC: Associated with pain and swelling of finger joints. **PMHx:** Bipolar affective disorder, gastritis. **DHx:** lithium, emollients, ibuprofen, omeprazole.

O/E: Well-defined erythematous plaques on trunk and limbs inclusive of extensor surfaces, with overlying silvery scale. Pitting of fingernails, distal interphalangeal joint swelling.

---

1. Which bacteria commonly contribute to the inflammatory lesions seen in acne?
2. What factors can exacerbate psoriasis?
3. List the topical steroid treatment ladder in order of potency.

Answers: 1. *Propionibacterium acnes*. 2. Stress, trauma, alcohol, obesity, smoking, beta-blockers, lithium, NSAIDs, ACE-inhibitors, antimalarials. 3. Weakest to strongest: hydrocortisone, clobetasone (Eumovate), betamethasone (Betnovate), clobetasol (Dermovate) = 'Help Every Budding Dermatologist'.

TABLE 16.1

	Features	Investigations	Management
Lupus erythematosus	See *189. MUSCLE PAIN/MYALGIA*		
Chronic plaque psoriasis	**RFs:** FHx, cold environment, smoking, medications: β-blockers, lithium, TNF-α inhibitors, immunosuppression. **Hx & O/E:** erythematous scaly plaques typically on extensor surfaces ± itch. Nail changes: pitting (with psoriatic arthritis), onycholysis	**Clinical diagnosis.** Multisystem disorder: cardiovascular burden and psoriatic arthritis. **X-ray** hands 'pencil in cup' deformity (psoriatic arthritis). Other patterns of joint inflammation can occur	Severity = PASI (Psoriasis Area Severity Index). Phototherapy. Topicals: emollients, corticosteroids, vitamin D analogues and coal tar. **Definitive:** systemic DMARDs-methotrexate, ciclosporin. Biologics: TNF-α inhibitors

(Continued)

TABLE 16.1   (Cont'd)

	Features	Investigations	Management
Seborrhoeic dermatitis	**RFs:** M > F, immuno-compromise, hepatitis C, Down syndrome. **Hx & O/E:** scaly eczematous patches in seborrheic distribution. Dandruff and cradle cap in infants	Scraping to exclude fungal infection	Anti-fungal shampoo, lotion, cream or ointment. **Definitive:** in combination with mild topical corticosteroid
Eczema	**RFs:** atopic eczema associated with asthma and rhinitis, FHx, allergens, stress. **Hx & O/E:** itchy, dry, erythematous eruption. Flexures in children and adults, extensors in infants and children of Asian, Black Caribbean/African origins. Several types, including atopic, seborrheic, varicose, contact	Clinical diagnosis. Consider patch testing in well-demarcated eczema at atypical locations. Severity = EASI (Eczema Area and Severity Index)	**Emollients.** Avoid triggers. ± Phototherapy. **Topical steroid;** *Apply 2+ days after clearance* *Mild* Hydrocortisone. *Moderate* Betamethasone 0.025% (hydrocortisone for face/flexures). *Severe* Betamethasone 0.1% (betamethasone 0.025% face/flexures 5 days max). Topical tacrolimus. Systemics: methotrexate, ciclosporin. Biologics: IL-4/IL-13 inhibitors
Acne	**RFs:** puberty, pregnancy, PCOS, stress. **Hx & O/E:** face, chest, back. *Mild*: open/closed comedones (non-inflammatory). *Moderate*: inflammatory pustules/papules. *Severe*: pustules, papules, nodules, cysts ± scarring	Clinical Diagnosis. Investigations for PCOS (if oligomenorrhoea, hirsutism present). Check axilla/groin (hidradenitis suppurativa)	*Mild* topical benzoyl peroxide or retinoid. *Moderate* Topical Abx (e.g. clindamycin) + benzoyl peroxide/retinoid. Oral Abx (e.g. tetracycline, doxycycline, lymecycline) + topical benzoyl peroxide **OR** COCP/Dianette. *Severe* referral for isotretinoin
Rosacea	**Triggers:** sun, heat, spicy foods, hot drinks, smoking, alcohol, stress, calcium channel blockers. **Hx & O/E:** erythema and telangiectasia with pustules and oedema. Episodic burning, flushing	Clinical diagnosis	Photoprotection, avoid triggers. **Definitive:** refractory erythema-topical brimonidine. Papules and pustules: topical ivermectin, metronidazole or azelaic acid. *Severe* oral tetracycline
Lichen planus	**RFs:** age (30–60 yo), stress, medications. **Hx & O/E:** pruritic, purple, polygonal, papules, plaques. Wickham's striae: white lacy markings (usually oral mucosa). Flexors, scalp, nail, mouth, vulva	Consider hepatitis C screening	Topical corticosteroids. **Definitive:** widespread/severe local disease-systemics

TABLE 16.1 (Cont'd)

	Features	Investigations	Management
Pityriasis versicolor	**RFs:** hot climate, summertime, activity/sweating, age (teens). **Hx & O/E:** hypo- or hyperpigmented patches ± scale. Varied colours (versicolour): pink, red, brown, white. Often on upper trunk	**Skin scrapings-** spaghetti and meatballs sign (*Malassezia* yeast)	Ketoconazole shampoo. Selenium sulphide shampoo. **Definitive** Oral anti-fungal (resistant/recurrent cases)

PCOS, polycystic ovarian syndrome; *TNF-α,* tumour necrosis factor-*α*.

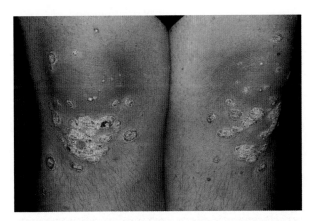

Fig. 16.1 Plaque psoriasis. (Reproduced from Paller AS, Mancini AJ. *Hurwitz Clinical Pediatric Dermatology: A Textbook of Skin Disorders of Childhood and Adolescence.* 5th ed. Philadelphia, PA: Elsevier; 2016.)

The vignette describes an inflammatory pathology, and plaque psoriasis (Fig. 16.1) is suggested by characteristic nail and skin findings in combination with small joint arthritis. Lupus screening would also be appropriate; the subacute cutaneous form may be mistaken for psoriatic plaques in sun-exposed areas and may have joint involvement. Several drugs can trigger psoriasis, including lithium. Medications are also linked with lupus (calcium channel blockers, ACE inhibitors, terbinafine). Seborrhoeic dermatitis can produce scaly eruptions, but usually in seborrhoeic areas (scalp, eyebrows, paranasal region, ears, upper chest).

REVISION TIPS

- Consider alternative causes in treatment-resistant chronic rashes, e.g. mycosis fungoides (cutaneous T-cell lymphoma) can mimic inflammatory skin disease
- **First-line therapy.** For psoriasis, vitamin D + topical corticosteroid; for eczema, emollients + topical corticosteroid for flares; for acne, topical benzoyl peroxide or retinoid

17

Skin Lesion

Katherine Parker, Alexander Royston, and Richard Barlow

GP CONSULTATION, MALE, 60.
SKIN LESION

HPC: 3-month duration on right ear; regularly bleeds and often painful. **PMHx:** Healthy, **SHx:** recently retired from construction work.

O/E: Tender ulceration on the helical rim. Fitzpatrick type II skin, no lymphadenopathy. Numerous hyperkeratotic skin-coloured papules and plaques on the face and dorsa of the hands, with rough sandpaper-like texture.

1. What are the RFs for this condition?
2. What is the gold standard treatment in high-risk basal cell carcinomas (BCCs) amenable to surgery?
3. What is the ABCDE of malignant melanoma?

Answers: 1. Actinic keratosis/Bowen's disease, UV exposure, solid organ transplant, immunosuppression, Fitzpatrick skin types I and II, age (increases), sex (M > F), HPV, smoking, burns. 2. Mohs micrographic surgery. 3. Asymmetry, Border irregularity, multiple Colours, Diameter > 6 mm, Evolving (ugly duckling sign).

TABLE 17.1

	Features	Investigations	Management
Pre-Malignant Lesions			
Bowen's disease	**RFs:** UV, radiotherapy, Fitzpatrick I-II, HPV, immunosuppression. **Hx & O/E:** slow growing lesion, erythematous, hyperkeratotic patch/plaque, bleeds easily, asymmetric distribution, irregular borders (contrast to psoriasis). **Site:** sun-exposed areas	**Dermoscopy:** glomerular vessels ± white circles. **Biopsy:** full-thickness epidermal dysplasia confined to epidermis	Avoid sun, monitor. **Topical:** 5-fluorouracil cream, topical diclofenac, imiquimod, photodynamic therapy, cryotherapy. **Surgical:** curettage, follow-up.
Actinic keratoses	**RFs:** UV, ageing, male, Fitzpatrick I-II, immunosuppression. **Hx & O/E:** slow growing lesion, white/yellow/red/skin-coloured, sandpaper texture ± hyper-keratotic surface. **Site:** H zone of face, top of head, dorsum of hands. Small risk of developing into SCC	**Dermoscopy:** scaly, erythema 'strawberry' pattern often seen on face. **Biopsy:** if unclear diagnosis or concerning features	Avoid sun, monitor, emollient. **Topical:** 5-fluorouracil cream, topical diclofenac, imiquimod, photodynamic therapy, cryotherapy. **Surgical:** curettage, cautery. Follow-up

TABLE 17.1 (Cont'd)

	Features	Investigations	Management
Malignant Lesions			
Basal cell carcinoma (BCC)	RFs: age, UV, x-ray exposure, transplant history, Fitzpatrick I-II. Hx & O/E: lesion grows for months or years, locally invasive. Metastasis rare. *Nodular*: pearly rolled edges ± central ulceration, often face. *Superficial*: scaly, erythematous plaques ± pearly edge. Trunk. *Morphoeic*: poorly defined, scar-like	Dermoscopy: arborising vessels ± pigmentation. Biopsy	Routine referral dermatology, 2WW if large or high risk. Low-risk BCCs can be managed in primary care. *Superficial*: BCC topical treatment (5-fluorouracil cream, cryotherapy), curettage and cautery. *Nodular*: BCC surgical excision ± radiotherapy
Squamous cell carcinoma (SCC)	RFs: UV, age, immunosuppression, radiotherapy, smoking, burns, Fitzpatrick I-II, **actinic keratosis/Bowen's disease**, HPV. Hx & O/E: lesions grow in weeks/ months, hyperkeratotic, crusted nodules, often ulcerate. Tender, indurated ± lymphadenopathy. Can metastasise. Site: sun exposed	Dermoscopy: difficult to diagnose from this alone. Biopsy. USS/CT/MRI	2WW referral. Majority require surgical excision ± radiotherapy (discussion at local MDTs). Newer treatment (immuno-therapy for advanced/ metastatic SCCs) under development.
Malignant melanoma	RFs: FHx/PMHx melanoma, multiple moles, Fitzpatrick I-II, UV, age. Hx & O/E: pigmented lesion (can be amelanotic), ABCDE (see above). Most likely to metastasise	Dermoscopy: ABCDE, blue-white structureless areas. Sentinel lymph node biopsy. ±CT, MRI and PET	2WW referral. 2mm margin excision staging biopsy. Wide local excision of scar; margin guided by **Breslow thickness** ± chemotherapy, immunotherapy or radiotherapy. Photoprotection
Benign Lesions			
Seborrheic keratosis	RFs: >50 yo, Caucasian, FHx. Hx & O/E: well-circumscribed lesion, grey/ brown plaques or papules, waxy, 'stuck on' appearance. May catch on clothing, get irritated	Dermoscopy: keratin plugs, cerebriform surface Biopsy: if unclear diagnosis or concerning features	Usually no intervention required. **Irritated/itching:** emollient, topical corticosteroid or cryotherapy/curettage
Viral wart (HPV)	RFs: children/young adults, immunocompromised, public pools, skin-to-skin contact. Hx & O/E: multiple lesions, rough, skin-coloured papules on hands/feet	Dermoscopy: filiform surface, thrombosed capillaries. Biopsy: if unclear diagnosis or concerning features	Most spontaneously resolve (years). Over-the-counter products usually sufficient. **Symptomatic or obstructing vision:** consider removal (cryotherapy/curettage)
Pyogenic granuloma	RFs: young, trauma to area, COCP/ pregnancy. Hx & O/E: rapidly growing lesions (days/ weeks), vascular, red/purple/yellow polypoid nodule, mm-cm, bleeds easily. Head, neck, fingers	Dermoscopy: vascular structures separated by white lines. Biopsy: if unclear diagnosis or concerning features	Removal (curettage, cautery, shave excision, laser therapy)
Melanocytic naevi (Moles)	Common moles. Follow their own maturation process – junctional, compound and finally intradermal	Dermoscopy: various pigment patterns, e.g. reticular network. Biopsy: if unclear diagnosis or concerning features	No intervention unless clinical concern for malignancy

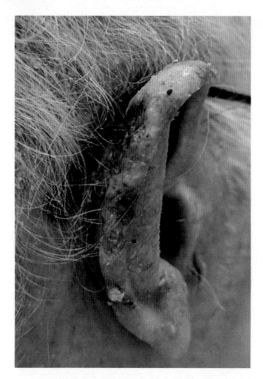

Fig. 17.1 Squamous cell carcinoma (SCC) of the right ear. (Reproduced from Brandt MG, Moore CC. Nonmelanoma skin cancer. *Facial Plast Surg Clin North Am.* 2019;27(1):1–13, Copyright © 2018 Elsevier Inc.)

The most likely diagnosis in the vignette is SCC (Fig. 17.1); tender ulceration in a sun-exposed site. Extensive actinic field change is described on the face and hands from his occupation; a potent RF for subsequent SCC. The temporal aspect is also key: SCCs typically develop over months compared to BCCs, more commonly occurring over years. Unlike solar keratoses, SCCs are tender, often indurated and ulcerated. No hallmarks of melanoma are described, but it must be excluded using dermoscopy.

REVISION TIPS

- Other lumps; acne, epidermal cyst, keloid scars, molluscum contagiosum, folliculitis, keratoacanthoma
- Important benign differentials of tender papules on the ear: chondrodermatitis nodularis helicis
- **S** is for **speedy**, **S**CCs grow faster (weeks to months) than BCCs (many months)
- Actinic keratoses are often easier to feel than see
- Genetic disorders affecting DNA repair can predispose to skin cancers, e.g. xeroderma pigmentosum

18

Skin or Subcutaneous Lump

Alexander Royston and Richard Barlow

GP CONSULTATION, MALE, 47.
SOFT TISSUE SWELLING OF RIGHT UPPER ARM

HPC: Painless mass, 12 months duration, under the skin. Not much changed in size. No trauma or constitutional symptoms, weight stable. PMHx: Fit and well. SHx: Non-smoker.

O/E: Soft, smooth freely mobile, subcutaneous 3 × 4 cm mass, overlying skin unremarkable. No local lymphadenopathy.

---

1. What are the characteristics for liposarcoma compared with lipoma?
2. What condition causes multiple, widespread lipomas which are often tender?
3. What condition causes multiple recurrent epidermoid cysts, with colonic polyps/tumours?

Answers: 1. Liposarcoma: larger than 5 cm at presentation, growing rapidly, deeper and fixed to deep fascia. 2. Dercum disease. 3. Gardner syndrome.

TABLE 18.1

	Features	Investigations	Management
Tumours and Tumour-Like Lesions – Benign			
Lipoma (Fig. 18.1)	Common benign, encapsulated adipose tissue tumour. No malignant risk. RFs: age (40–60 yo), FHx, trauma (debated). Hx & O/E: soft (doughy), mobile, superficial, painless mass. Commonly single, usually subcutaneous (trunk/proximal limbs)- can be in other sites	Clinical diagnosis: imaging/biopsy not indicated unless in doubt	Reassurance. **Definitive:** resection; symptom relief, confirm pathology, cosmetic, if ↑↑size
Epidermoid cyst	RFs: age (20–30 yo), sex (M > F). Hx & O/E: superficial lesion on face/scalp/neck/trunk, tethered to epidermis, rubbery (liquified keratin, foul-smelling contents), central punctum, may leak	Clinical diagnosis	Reassurance. Surgery if recurrent infections

(Continued)

TABLE 18.1   (Cont'd)

	Features	Investigations	Management
Malignant Liposarcoma	**RFs:** age (peak incidence 50 yo), past RTx, trauma, immunocompromise, toxin exposure, genetics (Li-Fraumeni, etc.). Rare, mesenchymal (connective tissue) tumour. Large (most >5 cm), circumscribed mass, ± pain, deep to fascia, recurrence after previous excision	**USS:** urgent direct access scan in adults with unexplained growing lump. **Biopsy.** **CT:** staging	2WW. **Definitive:** surgical excision-stage/histology
Cutaneous metastases	Commonest melanoma, breast (F > M), nasal sinus, lung (M > F). **Hx & O/E:** firm, round/oval, mobile, non-painful nodule (may ulcerate) Can be pigmented or erythematous (cutaneous lymphoma)	Investigate primary	Treat primary- once metastatic, therapy is often palliative
Inflammatory Abscess	**RFs:** smoking, EtOH, DM, obesity, IVDU. **Hx & O/E:** fluctuant lump (beware: late/absent fluctuation), hot erythematous skin, tender, signs of systemic infection. Multiple/recurrent in axilla, groin or perianal may be hidradenitis suppurativa	FBC (↑inflammatory markers). **USS-guided aspiration** (MC&S, treatment)	**Definitive:** incision and drainage, antibiotics Early drainage for patients with DM (risk of necrotising fasciitis)
Tophaceous gout	>10 years after first gout attack. **Hx & O/E:** red, warm, tender tophus near joint. Firm swellings (monosodium urate crystals), chronic can invade soft tissue, joint/bone	As per gout	As per gout (surgery)
Rheumatoid nodule	**RFs:** RA (20%), smokers, extra-articular RA, anti-CCP/RF +ve, methotrexate. **Hx & O/E:** firm, painless (rarely tender) nodules on extensor surfaces of joints	As per rheumatoid arthritis	As per RA. **Definitive:** rituximab. Surgery – will recur
Erythema nodosum	Inflamed fat cells; panniculitis (many other panniculitides). **RFs:** F > M, infection (viral/bacterial/fungal), inflammation (UC, Crohn's, sarcoidosis), pregnancy, medications. Age 20–30. **Hx & O/E:** painful, erythematous, firm, subcutaneous nodules. Anterior lower leg. Associated with arthralgia, pyrexia	Investigate cause	Manage underlying condition. Resolve in 2/3 weeks without scarring

TABLE 18.1 (Cont'd)

	Features	Investigations	Management
Other Causes			
Ganglion (cyst)	Synovial cyst. RFs: young (20's), sex (F > M). Hx & O/E: fluid-filled sac (transluminates), associated with joint, mostly dorsal/volar aspect of wrist, non-tender (maybe wrist pain)	Clinical diagnosis. Size can change, may increase with joint movement	Reassurance. Aspiration of dorsal cysts (therapeutic/diagnostic). Surgery: cosmesis, but can recur
Haematoma (traumatic)	RFs: trauma, coagulopathy (iatrogenic). Hx & O/E: tense, painful collection at trauma site, ± bruising/abscess/nerve compression	Clinical diagnosis (mechanism, ecchymosis). FBC, clotting. USS/CT	Monitor, ice-pack, hold anticoagulation. Drainage (skin necrosis/nerve palsies/infection)

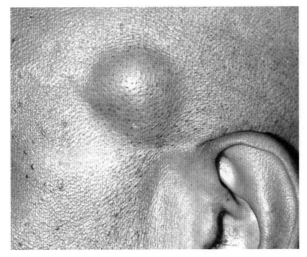

Fig. 18.1 Superficial lipoma. (Reproduced with permission from https://www.clinicalkey.com/?PRODUCT_ID=&PROVIDER_ID=/content/clinical_overview/67-s2.0-516256ec-5b86-45d3-823f-19c6eebd93cb?scrollTo=%2367-s2.0-516256ec-5b86-45d3-823f-19c6eebd93cb-50c440a2-1221-4ffb-ada2-097bac744a6e-annotated)

The vignette describes a lipoma, which is the most common soft tissue tumour. This patient is relatively unconcerned (he is unsure when it first started) and it is growing slowly. Liposarcoma (rare but crucial to identify) typically presents with large size, rapid growth, located deep to the deep fascia; red flag signs include tethering to underlying structures and overlying skin changes. An epidermoid cyst is unlikely (no intermittent foul-smelling discharge, no punctum) and there are no systemic symptoms to implicate an inflammatory cause. The differential diagnosis for a soft tissue swelling is very broad. For example, in the neck: reactive lymphadenopathy, thyroglossal cyst (midline), thyroid adenoma/hyperplastic nodule, multinodular goitre, thyroid cancer, cystic hygroma, branchial cyst, carotid body tumour, lymphoma.

REVISION TIPS

- Benign: typically superficial and <5 cm in size. Masses >5 cm or found deep to the fascia more likely to be malignant. One-third of sarcomas will present as a superficial mass
- Epidermoid cysts: often misnamed as 'sebaceous' (arise from hair follicles, not sebaceous glands)
- Lump O/E: **She Cuts The Fish PERfectly;**
  - Site, size, surface (skin)

- Colour, contour (border), consistency (firm/soft)
- Temperature, tenderness, trans-illuminable
- Fluctuance (fluid-filled), fixity
- Pulsatile (aneurysm)
- Expansile
- Reducible (hernia)

19

Nail Abnormalities – Outline

Katherine Parker, Alexander Royston, and Eleanor Courtney

Nail problems may be primary (Table 19.1) or indicative of wider health aspects (Table 19.2).

TABLE 19.1

	Features	Investigations	Management
Onychomycosis/ Fungal Nail Infection	**RFs:** age, skin infection, psoriasis, DM, Raynaud, PVD, immunocompromise, trauma, use of pools/gyms. **Hx & O/E:** toes greater than fingers. Progressive changes: discolouration, distortion (flaking, onycholysis, subungual keratosis)	**Nail clippings:** fungal MC&S (risk of false negative)	Depends on severity, site, organism. **Self-care** short nails, hygiene. **Topical:** Amorolfine lacquer 6–12 months. **Oral:** dermatophyte – terbinafine 1.5–6 months. Candida/non-dermatophyte-itraconazole 1 month
Acute Paronychia	**RFs:** trauma, artificial nails, finger sucking, immunosuppression, DM, retinoids. **Hx & O/E:** inflammation of skin around nail. Pain, erythema, swollen base ± visible pus	Clinical diagnosis	Warm compress ± antibiotics (topical: fusidic acid, oral: flucloxacillin/clarithromycin). **Definitive:** incision and drainage if collection/abscess formation
Subungual melanoma (subtype of Acral Lentiginous Melanoma)	**RFs:** darker skin tones, not associated with UV. **Hx & O/E:** broad irregular longitudinal bands of pigment underneath the nail, dark brown/black, blurred borders ± Hutchinson's sign (pigmentation of adjacent skin), nail dystrophy	**Biopsy:** nail bed → histology	2WW. **Definitive:** removal of nail apparatus ± amputation of finger/toe. ± Sentinel node biopsy

TABLE 19.2

	Features	Associated Conditions/Aetiology
Leukonychia	Small white patches	**Hypoalbuminaemia** (CKD, malnutrition, nephrotic syndrome), chemotherapy or normal, e.g. post-trauma
Koilonychia	Spoon-shaped nails	**Iron deficiency anaemia**, haemochromatosis, lichen planus, acromegaly, malnutrition, infection, e.g. fungal
Beau's Lines	Transverse furrows	**Temporary growth arrest** during times of stress, e.g. severe infection
Onycholysis	Nail detached from nail bed	Psoriasis, hyperthyroidism, fungal, lichen planus
Mees' Lines	White transverse bands	Poisoning (CO, arsenic), CKD
Nail Pitting	Small pit-like indentations	Psoriasis, alopecia areata, eczema
Clubbing (Fig. 19.1)	Increased curvature, loss of angle between nail and nail fold. Loss of 'Schamroth window'	Many causes. *GI*: IBD, cirrhosis, malabsorption. *CVD*: Cyanotic congenital heart disease, endocarditis, atrial myxoma. *Pulmonary*: TB, CF or other chronic lung suppuration, e.g. empyema, bronchial cancer.
Splinter Haemorrhage	Fine, longitudinal streaks underneath the nail	Microemboli/infarcts. Infective endocarditis, normal (trauma, e.g. gardening), vasculitis
Subungual Hyperkeratosis	Scaling under the nail	Fungal nail infection, psoriasis, crusted scabies
Yellow Nail Syndrome	Nail plate green-yellow. Hard nails, elevated longitudinal curvature ± shedding	Bronchiectasis, lymphoedema, chronic sinusitis

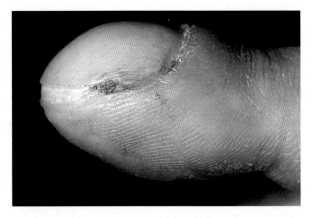

Fig. 19.1 Finger Clubbing. (Reproduced with permission from James GH, Dinulos MD. Nail diseases. In *Habif's Clinical Dermatology*. 1st ed. 2021:961989.e1.)

20

Ear and Nasal Discharge

Christian Aquilina, Alexander Royston, and Shilpa Ojha

**GP CONSULTATION, BOY AGED 9.
1 WEEK OF PAIN IN RIGHT EAR**

HPC: Ear is itchy, hearing is muffled, 2 days of discharge. **PMHx:** Eczema, asthma. **DHx:** salbutamol, hydrocortisone. **SHx:** Enjoys swimming.

O/E: Repeated tugging at right ear, serous discharge from ear canal. Skin is erythematous around external auditory meatus. Otoscopy: red, swollen ear canal containing white debris; tympanic membrane not visible.

1. What is the management of swimmer's ear?
2. What are the RFs for malignant or necrotising otitis externa (OE)?
3. Ototoxic ear drops should be avoided in which patients? Which ones are ototoxic?

Answers: 1. Clean out debris then keep dry, analgesia, topical antibiotic/steroid drops. 2. Diabetes, immunocompromise, often after self-inflicted or iatrogenic EAC trauma. 3. Possible tympanic perforations, including tympanostomy tubes. Those that contain aminoglycosides and alcohol.

TABLE 20.1

	Features	Investigations	Management
Ear Otitis externa	**RFs:** swimming, FBs, burns, blockage(wax, cysts), DM, psoriasis/eczema/seborrhoeic dermatitis, immuno-compromise, OM, stress. **Hx & O/E:** swelling, erythema, discharge, itching, pain (movement of pinna), hearing loss. Bacterial (pseudomonas). Can cause perichondritis (pinna, sparing ear lobule)	Clinical diagnosis. Assess for CN palsies (especially CN7). Immunocompromise: beware necrotising otitis externa (disproportionate pain)	Localised: analgesia, topical antibiotic/steroid drops. Strict water precautions. If diffuse: clean debris in canal (+ above). **Definitive:** oral antibiotics (flucloxacillin) if cellulitis extends past EAC/high-risk patients. D/W ENT on call.
Viral infection	**RFs:** measles or Ramsay Hunt syndrome (herpes zoster oticus). **Hx & O/E:** otalgia, hyperacusis, hearing loss, facial paralysis/paresis, taste disturbance (anterior two-thirds of tongue), decreased lacrimation (affected side), ± rash	Clinical diagnosis. **Otoscopy:** possible erythema and/or vesicles in EAC, auricle, soft palate, lateral border of tongue	Systemic antiviral therapy/steroids (+PPI), analgesia. Eye care: Taping at night, lacrilube, viscotears. Consider ophthalmology review

TABLE 20.1   (Cont'd)

	Features	Investigations	Management
Dermatoses	Eczema (atopic dermatitis), seborrhea (seborrheic dermatitis) Contact (irritant)/allergic dermatitis – depending on exposure	*Eczema:* xerotic scaling, lichenification *Seborrheic:* greasy yellowish scaling	Remove trigger (if possible). Topical steroid
Cholesteatoma	See *21. PAINFUL EAR*		
Acute otitis Media	See *21. PAINFUL EAR*		
Other Foreign body	**RFs:** age (<4 years), learning difficulties **Hx & O/E:** can cause discharge, particularly in children	Examination	Removal by GP if visible. Refer to ENT. Nasal FBs in child must see on-call ENT
Cerebrospinal fluid (CSF) leakage	**RFs:** iatrogenic/idiopathic/skull trauma (dural damage → CSF leakage from nose/ears). **Hx & O/E:** unconscious or headache, visual or hearing changes	CT sinuses/temporal ±MRI head. Beta-2-transferrin to confirm CSF. Halo sign (Fig. 20.2)	Resuscitation as necessary. Neurosurgical referral (as necessary). Skull base defect repair. Tegmen defect with fascial repair (ENT)

CN7, Seventh cranial nerve; *EAC,* external auditory canal; *OM,* otitis media.

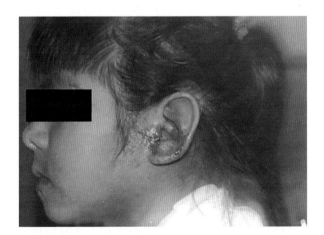

Fig. 20.1 Patient with acute otitis externa, with purulent drainage from the ear canal and mild edema and erythema of the pinna. (From *Feigin and Cherry's Textbook of Pediatric Infectious Diseases.* 8th ed., 2019. ISBN: 978-0-323-37692-1)

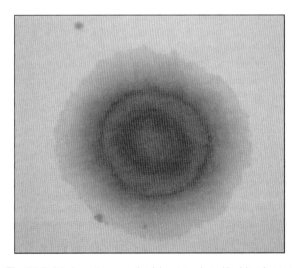

Fig. 20.2 A halo pattern on a bedsheet produced by bloody otorrhea due to basal skull fracture. (Canadian Medical Association Journal, 2013-03-19, Volume 185, Issue 5, Page 416, Copyright © 2013 Canadian Medical Association.)

The vignette describes OE (Fig. 20.1). Cardinal signs present are as follows: otalgia, otorrhoea, abnormal examination of external auditory canal (EAC). Discharge may be serous or purulent. Muffled hearing is caused by oedema in the EAC. This condition is commonly known as swimmer's ear. An important differential is eczematous dermatosis, noting PMHx of eczema and the itch. However, history of swimming and EAC swelling favours OE. A foreign body should be excluded. Otitis media is unlikely due to his age and lack of systemic symptoms.

REVISION TIPS

- Otitis externa: otalgia, otorrhoea, erythematous auditory canal, tenderness to tragus/pinna
- Causative agents: *Staphylococcus, Pseudomonas*. 98% bacterial
- Antibiotics for acute otitis externa only if extending outside ear canal, or specific host factors needing systemic therapy
- Unilateral symptoms in the nose of nasal congestion/epistaxis/polyp are a red flag for cancer

21

Painful Ear

Natalia Hackett, Alexander Royston, and Shilpa Ojha

HPC: Father says crying and off food for 2 days. **PMHx:** uncomplicated birth, croup age 7 months, gastro-oesophageal reflux resolved at 9 months.

O/E: Red bulging left tympanic membrane with 'golden syrup' behind it, temperature 38.5°C, agitated, crying, normal chest auscultation, mild tachycardia.

1. What features in general would suggest a bacterial over viral infection?
2. What are recommended criteria for using ABx? What would you use first-line?
3. What are the criteria recommended by NICE for hospital admission in otitis media?

Answers: 1. Tonsillar exudate, cervical lymphadenopathy, no cough, fever. 2. Systemically very unwell, symptoms and signs of a more serious illness or condition, high risk of complications. Amoxicillin (5–7 days, clarithromycin/erythromycin if allergic). 3. <3 months old with temperature of 38°C, 3–6 months old with temperature of 39°C or complications.

TABLE 21.1

	Features	Investigations	Management
Acute otitis media (AOM)	**RFs:** age (0–4 yo), male, smoking-exposed, bottle-fed, cranio-facial abnormalities. **Hx & O/E:** fever, coryza, otalgia, N&V. Child: irritable, pulling ear. Recurrent: >4 episodes/12 months or >3 episodes/6 months	Clinical diagnosis. Examine CN7, assess mastoid. **Otoscopy:** bulging, erythematous tympanic membrane ± effusion. Loss of light reflex, ± perforation	Analgesia ± Abx. <2 yo: immediate Abx, otherwise delayed script. **Definitive:** admit: fever ≥39°C, systemically unwell/<3 months, concern of mastoiditis/facial nerve palsy. D/W ENT on call
Otitis media with effusion (OME)	**RFs:** age (bimodal: 2, 5 yo), male, smoking-exposed, bottle-fed, cranio-facial abnormalities. **Hx & O/E:** hearing loss ± speech/language delay. May follow AOM, or Eustachian tube dysfunction (young child). Often asymptomatic. Serous otitis media: effusion without signs of infection. Symptoms >3 months = chronic	**Otoscopy:** impaired mobility of TM, bubbles/air-fluid level, opaque TM (Fig. 21.1) **PTA:** CHL	Observe for ≤3 months: resolution is common. **Refer if:** Persistent: >3 months, CHL →significant delay, Foul discharge (cholesteatoma). Trisomy 21/cleft palate.

(Continued)

TABLE 21.1	(Cont'd)		
	Features	**Investigations**	**Management**
Cholesteatoma	**RFs:** chronic infections, Eustachian dysfunction, FHx, Down/Turner syndrome, cleft palate/cranio-facial. **Hx & O/E:** persistent discharge from ear >6 weeks despite antibiotics. Can cause hearing loss/tinnitus/vertigo/facial nerve palsy/taste disturbance	**Otoscopy:** 'pearly' white mass in middle ear/behind intact TM. 'Crust' visible (keratin) in TM/perforation. **PTA:** CHL CT scan temporal bone	Referral to ENT. Elderly/frail patients unsuitable for GA: regular micro-suction of keratin. **Definitive:** surgery – main management
Otitis externa	See *20. EAR AND NASAL DISCHARGE*		
Viral infection	See *20. EAR AND NASAL DISCHARGE*		
Foreign body	See *20. EAR AND NASAL DISCHARGE*		

CHL, Conductive hearing loss; *PTA*, pure tone audiometry; TM, tympanic membrane.

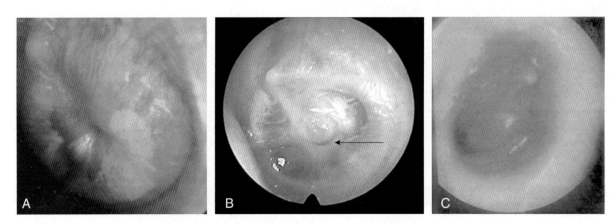

Fig. 21.1 Otitis media. (A) With effusion. (B) Fluid level behind the tympanic membrane (arrow). (C) Acute otitis media. (From Hathorn I. The ear, nose and throat. In: *Macleod's Clinical Examination*. Elsevier; 2018:171–191.)

The vignette describes rapid development of symptoms in an unwell child. Acute otitis media (AOM) is common but may not be obvious, as only two-thirds of children demonstrate ear pain by ear rubbing/ tugging and distress. Instead, there may be non-specific features (fever, fussiness, restless sleep, poor feeding, vomiting, diarrhoea). Symptoms overlap with URTI (when ear symptoms are absent). Otoscopy is key, as the bulging tympanic membrane is pathognomonic for AOM. Otoscopy also excludes cholesteatoma and otitis externa (more common in adults).

REVISION TIPS

- Complications can occur if acute otitis media is not adequately treated, e.g. infection recurrence, hearing loss, tympanic membrane perforation
- Rare but severe complications can include mastoiditis, meningitis, abscess formation

22

Hearing Loss

Natalia Hackett, Alexander Royston, and Shilpa Ojha

GP CONSULTATION, FEMALE, 30.
HEARING LOSS IN BOTH EARS

HPC: associated 'buzzing', recalls her mother having hearing loss at similar age. Currently pregnant, otherwise fit and well. PMHx: coeliac disease, migraines. DHx: COCP before pregnancy.

O/E: otoscopy – red 'blush' on tympanic membrane, external auditory meatus (EAM) clear, Weber's test: no lateralisation, Rinne's test: abnormal (negative) bilaterally.

1. What differential would be most likely if this was a 70-year-old?
2. What is the management of sudden-onset sensorineural hearing loss (SNHL)?
3. What tuning fork is used for tests?
4. What is the commonest viral cause of SNHL?

Answers: 1. Presbycusis. 2. Urgent ENT referral and high-dose steroids. 3. 512 MHz. 4. Cytomegalovirus (CMV).

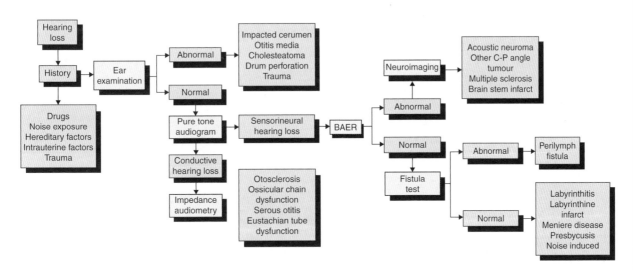

Fig. 22.1 Evaluation of Hearing Loss. *BAER*, Brain stem auditory evoked response; *C-P*, cerebellopontine.

TABLE 22.1

	Features	Investigations	Management
Otosclerosis (Fig. 22.2)	RFs: FHx, sex (F > M), ethnicity (white), age (20–40 yo), viral infection. Hx & O/E: unilateral/bilateral CHL, progression in pregnancy. Schwartze sign: flamingo blush of tympanic membrane (rare)	Otoscopy. Rinne's and Weber's tests. PTA: CHL – Carhart's notch (artefactual dip in bone conduction at 2 kHz)	Routine referral to ENT. Hearing aids (trial). Definitive: surgical assessment for stapedotomy
Cholesteatoma	See *21. PAINFUL EAR*		
Presbycusis	RF: older age (65+). Hx & O/E: may be unaware, gradual, bilateral, no noise exposure/ ototoxic drugs	PTA: bilateral SNHL >2000 Hz. Speech audiogram: ↓perception	Lifestyle changes, hearing rehabilitation
Otitis media with effusion (glue ear)	See *21. PAINFUL EAR*		
Ototoxicity/noise-induced hearing loss	Drugs (aminoglycosides, furosemide, aspirin, antimalarials, cytotoxics, NSAIDs), pesticides, heavy metals, cigarette smoke, noise (occupational). Hx & O/E: bilateral, tinnitus, ± disequilibrium	Comprehensive drug and occupational history. PTA: SNHL	Review medications. Definitive: hearing aids, protection for noise-induced hearing loss (NIHL)
Otitis externa	See *20. EAR AND NASAL DISCHARGE*		
Impacted ear wax (cerumen)	RFs: age (extremes), sex (M > F), learning difficulties, hearing aids, eczema, cotton buds. Hx & O/E: ↓hearing, pain/ itching/fullness, tinnitus, discharge	Otoscopy: wax blocking tympanic membrane	Ear drops (3–5 days). Olive oil ear →sodium bicarbonate. Irrigation/microsuction
Acoustic neuroma	See *23. TINNITUS*		
Meniere disease	See *24. VERTIGO*		

CHL, Conductive hearing loss; *PTA*, pure tone audiogram; *SNHL*, sensorineural hearing loss.

Otosclerosis is the top differential in the vignette, because of the conductive hearing loss (CHL) on tuning fork tests, along with the EAM being clear on otoscopy. Age of onset, FHx and the pregnancy support this – approximately 50% of cases of otosclerosis are inherited. The history does not mention a middle ear infection (pain, fever, bulging TM, younger people) or EAM obstruction (FB, wax, etc.) which are common but rarely occur bilaterally. Overview of assessment is given in Fig. 22.1.

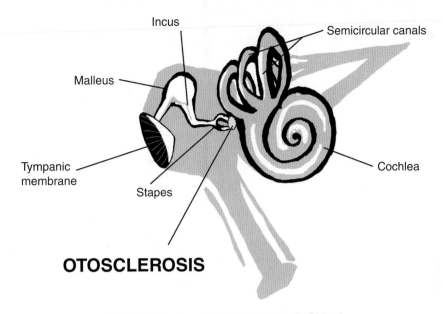

Incus

Semicircular canals

Malleus

Tympanic membrane

Stapes

Cochlea

OTOSCLEROSIS

Fig. 22.2 Otosclerosis. (Picture by Dr Hollie Blaber.)

REVISION TIPS

- Most common causes of hearing loss are ageing and exposure to excessive noise
- Bilateral CHL in younger person with FHx – consider otosclerosis. Begins unilaterally in 60%, progresses to both ears
- Rinne's test: compares air conduction (AC) and mastoid bone conduction (BC). AC > BC is normal. BC > AC – CHL in affected ear
- Weber's test: CHL lateralises to affected ear, SNHL lateralises to unaffected ear
- Otosclerosis shows a distinctive Carhart's notch on PTA (at 2 kHz)
- Consider medications that can cause ototoxicity, e.g. gentamicin

23

Tinnitus

Katherine Parker, Alexander Royston, and Shilpa Ojha

HPC: Constant hissing, 7 months duration. Difficulty hearing in her right ear, intermittent unsteadiness, sometimes walking into things like bannisters. Unsure of timing of onset but never had anything like this before. Mild morning headaches. No other neurological symptoms. No weight loss or fatigue. **PMHx:** Nil.

O/E: Looks well. Obs stable. CNs: reduced hearing on right, Rinne's positive bilaterally, Weber's lateralises to the left side, Fundoscopy NAD. Neck NAD.

1. What are the criteria for immediate referral to secondary care for patients with tinnitus?
2. What are the causes of pulsatile tinnitus?
3. What are the complications of acute otitis media?

Answers: 1. High risk of suicide, sudden onset neurological symptoms, uncontrolled vestibular symptoms e.g. vertigo, suspected stroke, sudden onset pulsatile tinnitus, tinnitus secondary to head trauma. 2. Hyperdynamic states (anaemia, hyperthyroidism), idiopathic intracranial hypertension. 3. Meningitis, mastoiditis, intracranial abscess, sinus thrombosis, facial nerve paralysis.

TABLE 23.1

	Features	Investigations	Management
Unilateral/Bilateral Tinnitus + SNHL			
Acoustic neuroma (vestibular schwannoma) (Figure 23.1)	**RFs:** age (50–55 yo), noise exposure. **Hx & O/E:** gradual/progressive unilateral tinnitus, SNHL ± imbalance/vertigo. Late findings: CN palsies (5, 7, 8), otalgia, ataxia, visual disturbance, nystagmus, persistent headache, ±SOL signs/symptoms. If bilateral: consider neurofibromatosis type II	**PTA:** unilateral, asymmetrical SNHL, progressive. **MRI IAMs:** mass within internal auditory meatus, potentially extending to CPA. Speech audiogram – 'roll-over'	Depends on size/symptoms/progression. Refer skull base MDT. Watch and wait – 60% show no progression. Focused radiation (stereotactic radiosurgery). **Definitive:** surgery (translabyrinthine/retrosigmoid)
Other SOLs (e.g. primary brain tumour)	Morning headache, N&V, seizures, progressive neurological deficits, behavioural abnormalities. Lobe specific symptoms ± papilloedema	CT Head/MRI	Neurosurgical referral. Consider corticosteroids. **Definitive:** surgery, chemo-/radio-therapy
Brain metastasis	Underlying malignancy (esp. breast, lung, melanoma)		

TABLE 23.1	(Cont'd)		
	Features	**Investigations**	**Management**
Intracranial abscess	Immunocompromise, recent infection/trauma/invasive procedure, congenital heart disease. Headache, fever, seizure, N&V, systemically unwell	Raised inflammatory markers. Blood cultures. **CT Head (contrast):** ring enhancing lesion. **MRI.** Pus sample: to guide antibiotic treatment	**Non-operative:** anti-microbial, anti-epileptics (for seizures), treat primary source. **Operative:** abscess excision
Meniere's disease	See *24. HEARING LOSS*		
Drug-induced ototoxicity	Aspirin, NSAIDs, aminoglycosides, loop diuretics, cytotoxic drugs. **Hx & O/E:** bilateral SNHL, tinnitus, dysequilibrium	PTA	Cessation of ototoxic medication. Aspirin SNHL improves on cessation
Noise-induced hearing loss	Occupational/recreational risks. Gradual difficulty understanding speech in loud environments	PTA: SNHL (often bilateral) at 4000 Hz	Counselling, ear protection
Presbycusis	See *22. HEARING LOSS*		
Uni/bilateral Tinnitus + CHL			
Otosclerosis	See *22. HEARING LOSS*		
Impacted ear wax	See *22. HEARING LOSS*		
Otitis media	See *21. PAINFUL EAR*		
Otitis externa	See *20. EAR AND NASAL DISCHARGE*		
Key Complication			
Mental health	Assess with Tinnitus Questionnaire (TQ)/mini-TQ, Insomnia Severity Index. High risk of suicide		

CHL, Conductive hearing loss; *PTA*, Pure tone audiometry, *SNHL*, Sensorineural hearing loss.

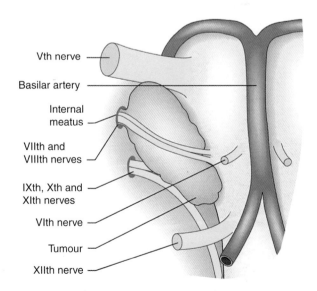

- Vth nerve
- Basilar artery
- Internal meatus
- VIIth and VIIIth nerves
- IXth, Xth and XIth nerves
- VIth nerve
- Tumour
- XIIth nerve

Fig. 23.1 Right acoustic neuroma. (From Myles L, Brennan PM. *Neurosurgery, Principles and Practice of Surgery.* 2018:171–191.)

Tinnitus is a very common presentation; the commonest cause is noise-induced hearing damage. Meniere's disease is also common, particularly in this patient demographic with associated dysequilibrium, but symptoms are more typically fluctuant rather than progressive. Unilateral tinnitus is a red flag symptom for acoustic neuroma and the key diagnostic features in the vignette are the unilateral presentation, progressive nature, and vestibular instability. Some lower facial numbness can be often seen, though headache is less common. Facial nerve paralysis and cerebellar signs are late-stage symptoms and indicate an unstable growth which may need surgical intervention.

REVISION TIPS

- Assessment: onset, quality, duration, and frequency of tinnitus.
  - The features: Uni/bilateral, continuous or episodic? Pulsatile? Associated with hearing loss?
  - Associated symptoms: dizziness, vertigo, facial weakness.
  - Hx of noise exposure, head injury, medications, infections.
- Other presentations which may cause tinnitus but not described here include: MS, head injury.

24

Vertigo

Margarita Fox, Alexander Royston, and Shilpa Ojha

GP CONSULTATION, FEMALE, 42.
5-DAY HISTORY OF INTERMITTENT HEARING LOSS IN HER RIGHT EAR

HPC: She suffers recurrent episodes of 'dizziness', feeling like the room is spinning, and intermittent tinnitus. Feeling of pressure in ear. One previous episode a year ago. **SHx:** never smoked, alcohol: 5 units/week.

O/E: Systemically well. Otoscopy: intact tympanic membrane. Webber's: lateralises to left ear, Rinne's: positive. Romberg test positive, neurological examination is otherwise unremarkable.

1. How do you differentiate central and peripheral causes of sudden persistent vertigo?
2. What are the top differentials:
   a. Elderly lady with 30-second dizzy spells triggered by head turning.
   b. 38-year-old with persistent vertigo and nausea following a 'bad cold'. No hearing loss or tinnitus.
3. What drug-related causes of vertigo can you think of?

Answers: 1. HINTS exam (see Revision tips). 2a. BPPV. 2b. Vestibular neuronitis. 3. Aminoglycosides, salicylates, quinine, metronidazole, co-trimoxazole, furosemide, alcohol intoxication.

TABLE 24.1

	Features	Investigations	Management
Peripheral			
Meniere's disease	**RFs:** age (30–60 yo), autoimmune, migraine, viral infection, trauma. **Hx & O/E:** AAO-HNS criteria (Meniere's disease): two episodes of vertigo lasting 20 minutes to 12 hours, low-frequency sensorineural hearing loss, aural fullness and no other diagnosis. Unilateral -> Bilateral (years)	Clinical diagnosis. **PTA (pure tone audiometry):** fluctuant, low-frequency SNHL, progressive	ENT Referral. Low salt (<2 g/day), avoid caffeine/alcohol/sedatives. Prochlorperazine for acute attacks. Betahistine prophylaxis (poor evidence). Intra-tympanic steroids
Benign paroxysmal positional vertigo (BPPV)	**RFs:** 5th–7th decades, F > M, head trauma/post-labyrinthitis **Hx & O/E:** sudden onset vertigo on turning head position. Brief (20s–30 s), episodic	**Dix-Hallpike manoeuvre** Positive: torsional geotropic nystagmus towards affected side, fatigable.	Epley manoeuvre. Vestibular rehabilitation: Brandt-Daroff exercises. Consider prochlorperazine for acute attacks

(Continued)

TABLE 24.1   (Cont'd)

	Features	Investigations	Management
Vestibular neuronitis	**RFs:** post URTI/viral infection. Episodes can last hours-days. Imbalance may persist. May re-occur several times/year Nausea/vomiting common. No hearing loss/tinnitus	Clinical diagnosis. **Head impulse test** positive – corrective saccade (Fig. 24.1)	Severe vertigo: buccal/IM/PO prochlorperazine/IM cyclizine. Persistent: ENT referral. Vestibular rehabilitation exercises (chronic)
Viral labyrinthitis	**RF:** recent URTI/viral infection. **Hx & O/E:** acute onset vertigo (hours–days), nausea/vomiting, unilateral hearing loss. Can have tinnitus, otalgia, fever. If unsteady gait- falls to affected side	Clinical diagnosis. **Head impulse test** Positive	Often self-limiting. Symptomatic: prochlorperazine/antihistamines (acute attacks)
Acoustic neuroma	See *23. TINNITUS*		
Ramsay Hunt syndrome	Ear pain, vesicular rash ear/soft palate/lateral border of tongue + ipsilateral facial paralysis (severe House-Brackman grade 4+)	Age >60. Clinical diagnosis. **Varicella zoster PCR assay** (consider)	Acyclovir PO 5 days. Oral steroids (prednisolone PO 1 week with PPI cover)
Central			
Vestibular migraine	**RFs:** sleep, stress, weather. **Hx & O/E:** recurrent attacks (mins–hour), headache, aura, photophobia, nausea and vomiting, ataxia	Diagnosis of exclusion. Normal balance. **PTA:** no hearing loss	Acute attacks: NSAIDs/triptans. Vertigo attacks: prochlorperazine Prevention: amitriptyline, propranolol
Vertebrobasilar insufficiency	**RFs:** elderly, neck osteoarthritis. **Hx & O/E:** triggered by neck extension. 3Ns (nystagmus, numbness, nausea). 5Ds (dizziness, diplopia, dysphagia, dysarthria, drop attacks). Ataxia	**CT head:** exclude haemorrhage. **CT angiography/MRA:** atherosclerosis/stenosis in vertebrobasilar arteries	Lifestyle; address RFs. Aspirin, clopidogrel. **Definitive:** surgical repair/endovascular aneurysm repair (EVAR) if severe
Posterior circulation stroke (POCS)	**RFs:** HTN, CVD, smoking, OCP, DM, TIAs, hypercholesterolaemia **Hx & O/E:** sudden onset vertigo, ataxia, unilateral hemiparesis, diplopia, dysarthria, headache, nausea/vomiting, nystagmus	**HINTS HIT:** no corrective saccade. Bidirectional nystagmus. Abnormal test of skew. **CT head** r/o haemorrhagic. **MRI brain**	Aspirin 300 mg. **Definitive:** IV thrombolysis (if <4.5 hours). Secondary prevention: 75 mg OD clopidogrel

EVAR, Endovascular aneurysm repair. *HIT*, Head impulse test.

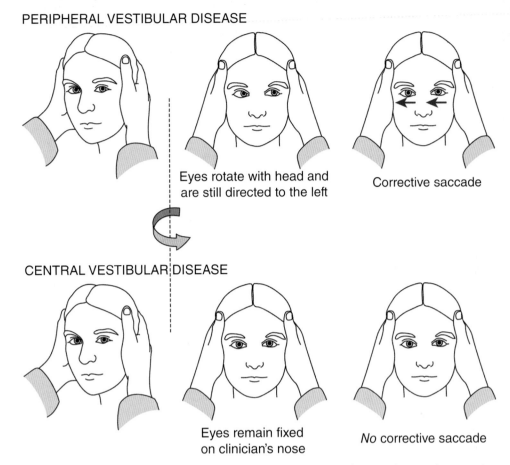

PERIPHERAL VESTIBULAR DISEASE

Eyes rotate with head and are still directed to the left

Corrective saccade

CENTRAL VESTIBULAR DISEASE

Eyes remain fixed on clinician's nose

No corrective saccade

Fig. 24.1 Head-impulse test, evaluates the vestibulo-ocular reflex. If intact: central cause. A corrective saccade suggests CN8 pathology (vestibular neuronitis). (From McGee S. *Evidence-Based Physical Diagnosis*. 2022:611–616. Publisher: Elsevier)

This patient is describing Meniere's disease, which is common in this demographic. The diagnostic challenges in the vignette are mainly around the duration of symptoms. Key to Meniere's is the fluctuating course, with long periods (months) of remission. In this case, there is a 5-day history, with hearing loss/vertigo intermittent within that frame. She has no identified cerebrovascular risk factors and the intermittent symptoms and accompanying hearing loss are both inconsistent with that diagnosis. There are no features of recent upper respiratory tract virus to cause a vestibular neuronitis or viral labyrinthitis.

REVISION TIPS

- Distinguish vertigo from dizziness: 'room spinning around you' versus 'you feel unsteady or lightheaded'
- <u>HINTS</u> for central versus peripheral causes of sudden persistent vertigo; 1. Head impulse test. 2. Nystagmus: (direction-changing nystagmus on lateral gaze = central cause, horizontal nystagmus with a torsional component = peripheral). 3. Test of skew (vertical movement as the eye is uncovered = central cause)
- RFs for CVE: HTN, CVD, DM, smoking, OCP, TIAs, hypercholesterolaemia, sedentary, obesity, arrhythmias, cardiac structural abnormalities
- Timing: prolonged (vestibular neuronitis/labyrinthitis) versus recurrent episodes (Meniere's, BPPV)
- Central: more severe postural instability (even with eyes open), hearing loss/tinnitus is less common

25

Nasal Obstruction

Christian Aquilina, Alexander Royston, and Shilpa Ojha

GP CONSULTATION, MALE, 28.
5-MONTH HISTORY OF BILATERAL NASAL OBSTRUCTION

HPC: Watery discharge, sensation of 'nasal fullness', intermittent loss of taste/smell, snoring. **PMHx:** Asthma. **DHx:** Salbutamol. **SHx:** Non-smoker.

O/E: Systemically well, no nasal deformity. Nasal cavity: bilateral smooth pale growths from mucosa.

1. What would your top differential be if it was unilateral? Or acute onset?
2. What are the adverse effects of using long-term nasal decongestants?
3. What are the side effects of intranasal corticosteroids and how long should they be used continuously before stopping?

Answers: 1. Rule out malignancy. If acute (<12 weeks), more likely URTI or sinusitis. 2. Return of nasal congestion on cessation, mucosal hypertrophy, headache, nausea, irritation, dryness. 3. Nose bleeds, dryness, irritation, sore throat, headache, altered taste/smell. Very potent steroid ≤4 weeks, potent ≤8 weeks.

TABLE 25.1			
	Features	**Investigations**	**Management**
Upper respiratory tract infection	**RFs:** contact with children, asthma/ allergic rhinitis, immunocompromise (CF/ HIV, corticosteroids, transplantation, post-splenectomy), smoking, facial dysmorphia, nasal polyposis. **Hx & O/E:** nasal congestion, discharge, sore throat, sneeze, malaise	Usually viral – rhinovirus. Suspect influenza: fever, more severe malaise. Examine throat/ears to exclude pharyngitis and otitis media	Reassure. Peaks at 2–3 days, resolving by 7 days. Advise rest, simple analgesia, adequate fluids
Allergic rhinitis	See *26. ANOSMIA*		
Sinusitis	See *26. ANOSMIA*		
Deviated septum	**RFs:** adults – idiopathic, traumatic injury/ iatrogenic. Child – injury during birth/ congenital (cleft lip/palate). **Hx & O/E:** visible deformity, unilateral obstruction, noisy/mouth breathing, ↑infections	Clinical examination. **Nasoendoscopy**	Reassurance. **Definitive:** septoplasty

TABLE 25.1   (Cont'd)

	Features	Investigations	Management
Nasal polyps	**RFs:** M>F, aspirin-sensitivity, asthma, allergic rhinitis. **Hx & O/E:** nasal blockage (unilateral/bilateral), discharge, post-nasal drip, taste/smell disturbance, change in voice, widening of nasal bridge	Unilateral; exclude malignancy. Child: exclude CF. **Nasal endoscopy:** soft, pale, painless mucosal outpouching (Fig. 25.1)	EPOS 2020 guidelines. Corticosteroid spray ± prednisolone. Consider macrolide. Surgical: FESS and polypectomy
Foreign body	**RFs:** age (children). Foreign body in the nose or ear can cause discharge	Examination of the ears/nose	Removal by GP/ED. Contact ENT on call
Sino-nasal tumour	**RFs:** smoker, HPV, occupation (wood dust/nickel/leather/chromium), radiotherapy. **Hx & O/E:** blockage, pain, anosmia, epistaxis, mucus, discharge. Eustachian tube obstruction can → unilateral otitis media. Can invade into CN III-VI. Weight loss, ↑fatigue, neck lump/palpable lymph nodes	Nasoendoscopy. EUA. Biopsy. CT±MRI (head and neck). USS neck & FNA (if palpable lymph nodes)	2WW referral to ENT. Surgery, chemotherapy, radiotherapy (often in combination)

FESS, Functional endoscopic sinus surgery

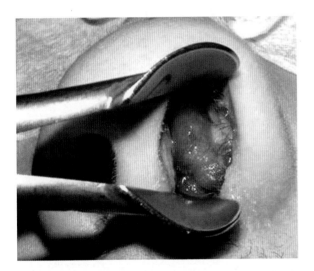

Fig. 25.1 Nasal polyps. (From Insalaco LF. Ferri's Clinical Advisor. 2022:1046.e2–1046.e3; From Swartz MH. *Textbook of Physical Diagnosis, History and Examination,* ed 7. Elsevier; 2014.)

The top differential in the vignette is chronic rhinosinusitis with nasal polyps, a common presentation. 5-months bilateral growing polyps with progressive obstructive symptoms and cough (post-nasal drip) is typical. More common in males and people with asthma, relatively uncommon in children, unless cystic fibrosis is also present (where additional signs are likely). Sino nasal tumours are possible but unlikely with bilateral presentation (assume a unilateral polyp is neoplastic until proven otherwise). Lack of trauma or symptoms of UTRI make other differentials unlikely.

REVISION TIPS

- Very common presentation and usually benign cause (URTI) but must rule out cancer
- Surgery is last resort for nasal polyps – high recurrence rate after polypectomy

26

Anosmia

Mariella Williams and Vincent Cumberworth

RHINOLOGY CLINIC, FEMALE, 60.
REDUCED SENSE OF SMELL (BOTH NOSTRILS)

HPC: 2 years history of difficult nasal breathing, pre-and post-nasal drip. Prolonged use of nasal steroid sprays, oral steroids, antihistamines, saline douching. No trauma or nasal bleeding. No ear or throat symptoms. **PMHx:** Asthma, eczema, hay fever. **DHx:** ventolin, symbicort. **SHx:** non-smoker.

O/E: Increased body habitus, round face, mouth breathing. Flexible nasoendoscopy (FNE): multiple large nasal polyps bilaterally.

1. What is the top differential for the vignette?
2. Anosmia may be an early sign of what group of neurological diseases?

Answers: 1. Chronic rhinosinusitis with bilateral nasal polyps. 2. Neurodegenerative.

TABLE 26.1

	Features	Investigations	Management
Upper respiratory tract infection	See *25. NASAL OBSTRUCTION*		
Allergic rhinitis	**RFs:** allergies, hay fever, atopy (pollen, dust mites, fur, chemicals). **Hx & O/E:** sneezing, rhinorrhoea, nasal itching/ congestion, ± eye irritation/ redness/tearing	Skin prick testing. RAST testing (IgE)	Allergen avoidance. Nasal saline, nasal steroid/oral antihistamine. Immunotherapy (if severe)
Sinusitis	**RFs:** recent URTI, smoking, pollution, allergies/asthma, cocaine, deviated septum, nasal polyps, cleft palate, adenoids. **Hx & O/E:** nasal obstruction, discharge, ±pain/pressure, ±hyposmia. Acute bacterial: >10 days, severe pain, pyrexia, purulent	Clinical diagnosis for uncomplicated sinusitis. **FNE.** **CT scan:** paranasal sinuses if chronic (>12 weeks). *Immunocompromised (DM)* beware invasive fungal sinusitis	Reassure, analgesia. If ≥10 days: saline douching, nasal corticosteroid. Refer to ENT if systemically unwell or chronic refractory

TABLE 26.1 (Cont'd)			
	Features	**Investigations**	**Management**
Nasal polyps	See **25. *NASAL OBSTRUCTION***		
Sino nasal tumour	See **25. *NASAL OBSTRUCTION***		
Foreign body	See **25. *NASAL OBSTRUCTION***		
Deviated nasal septum	See **25. *NASAL OBSTRUCTION***		
Olfactory nerve damage	Base of skull fracture (Fig. 26.1) damages olfactory bulb/ nerves in cribriform plate (ethmoid)	**CT/MRI:** sinuses, skull base, frontal lobes	
Neurodegenerative disease	Anosmia is an early feature of Alzheimer/Parkinson/diffuse Lewy body/multisystem atrophy		
Rheumatological	Sarcoidosis, Churg–Strauss, Wegener's granulomatosis		

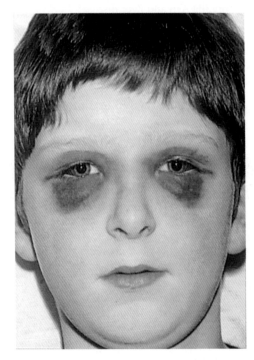

Fig. 26.1 'Raccoon eyes' in basilar skull fracture. (From Mir MA. *Atlas of Clinical Diagnosis*. London: WB Saunders; 1995.)

Anosmia is the inability to perceive smell. Normal ageing reduces cells in the olfactory bulb and olfactory epithelium. Anosmia is a feature of some forms of COVID-19 infection. Drug-induced anosmia may follow chronic nasal steroid use ('rhinitis medicamentosa'), cocaine, and sometimes aspirin, β-blockers, antithyroid drugs, dihydropyridine, ACE inhibitors and intranasal zinc. 70% to 85% are due to nasal/paranasal sinus inflammatory disease, i.e. rhinosinusitis (infection, allergens, drugs, environmental inhalants, hormones, systemic disease). The ARIA initiative (Allergic Rhinitis and Its Impact on Asthma) develops internationally applicable guidelines. A unilateral nasal polyp is a red flag feature requiring ENT referral due to possible underlying neoplasm.

REVISION TIPS

- Unilateral polyp/mass, bloody nasal discharge, crusting may be due to sinonasal tumour
- Diplopia or reduced visual acuity may indicate periorbital/orbital cellulitis
- Focal neurological signs suggest intracranial involvement

27

Epistaxis

Christian Aquilina, Alexander Royston, and Shilpa Ojha

EMERGENCY DEPARTMENT, FEMALE, 79.
3 HOURS OF EPISTAXIS

HPC: Started spontaneously and continued despite compression. Soaked through several tissues and needed insertion of a rapid rhino nasal pack. Feels well in herself, no chest pain, dizziness or confusion. **PMHx:** AF, osteoarthritis, migraine. **DHx:** warfarin.

O/E: Looks well. HS I+II+0, normal observations, pulse: irregularly irregular. Chest clear, abdomen soft non-tender, GCS 15.

1. What is a normal INR and how often should it be checked?
2. What are the clotting factors affected by warfarin, haemophilia A/B and liver disease?
3. Which factors affect PT and APTT values?

Answers: 1. In AF, usual target INR is 2–3, checked ≤12 weekly. 2. Warfarin: vitamin K-dependent factors (II, VII, IX, X, proteins C and S); haemophilia A/B factor VIII/IX, respectively; liver disease: reduced II, V, VII, IX, X, XI, antithrombin, protein C and S, excess VIII and vWF. 3. PT extrinsic pathway, APTT intrinsic pathway.

TABLE 27.1

	Features	Investigations	Management
Trauma	**RFs:** nose picking (children), trauma, recent nasal surgery. Beware of NAI in children and falls/neglect in the elderly	Full observations (rule out shock). FBC (↓Hb). Examine nasal passages.	Sit with head tilted, mouth open, pinch cartilaginous part of nose 10–15 minutes. Nasal cautery/packing. If persists, refer to ENT
Medications	**RFs:** PMHx (AF, DVT and CVD). Anticoagulants/antiplatelets prolong bleeding from minor trauma if over medicated. Topicals (corticosteroids/decongestants) damage the mucosa. Cocaine.	Observations (r/o shock). FBC (↓Hb), Clotting (warfarin: ↑INR)	Resuscitation. Simple measures to stop bleeding. **Definitive:** reversal drugs if severe; andexanet alfa (rivaroxaban/apixaban), vitamin K (warfarin), idarucizumab (dabigatran)
Bleeding disorders	**RFs:** FHx, sex (male). **Hx & O/E:** bruising/prolonged bleeding (may be 1st presentation), heavy menstrual flow. Fatigue, weight loss, splenomegaly, ↑infections, bone pain, may be haematological malignancy	FBC (↓Hb/↓platelets), clotting, blood film. Results depend on underlying condition; haemophilia, von Willebrand, thrombo-cytopenia, leukaemia.	Resuscitation, as required. Refer to haematology

TABLE 27.1	(Cont'd)		
Vascular disorders	*Hereditary haemorrhagic telangiectasia.* Causes telangiectasia (skin/mucosal) → GI bleed/epistaxis. Also pulmonary/cerebral/hepatic AVM risk	Autosomal dominant. Clotting often normal. FBC (↓Hb), ↓haematinics. **Screen for AVMs:** CXR, contrast CT, MRI brain, TTE	Blood/iron transfusion. Specialist treatment ± surgery for AVM. Epistaxis: absorbable adrenaline-soaked packs (not cauterisation). ENT (long-term care)
	Granulomatosis with polyangiitis Hx & O/E: age >65 yo. Fever, arthralgia/myalgia, headache, malaise, ↓appetite, weight loss. Upper respiratory tract first (epistaxis, sinusitis, saddle-shaped nose deformity), then lungs (haemoptysis, cough, dyspnoea) and kidneys (renal failure, proteinuria, haematuria)	Formerly called Wegener's granulomatosis; autoimmune small/medium cell vasculitis. **Urinalysis:** blood, protein cANCA positive, ↑CRP/ESR. **CXR:** (± infiltrates/cavitation lesions). **Renal biopsy**	Refer to secondary care. Immunosuppressants: steroids/cyclophosphamide
Infection	**RFs:** URTI (inflammation mucosal→ bleeding). **Hx & O/E:** febrile, coryza, fatigue, discharge	Clinical diagnosis. Examine nasal passages	Usually self-limiting. Analgesia and rest
Key Complication			
Hypovolaemia	Agitation, pallor, altered consciousness, palpitations, rapid breathing, clamminess	↓BP, ↑HR, ↑CRT, ↑RR, oliguria, ↓GCS. FBC (↓Hb)	A→ E resuscitation. IV fluid bolus, transfusion ±FFP, catheterisation

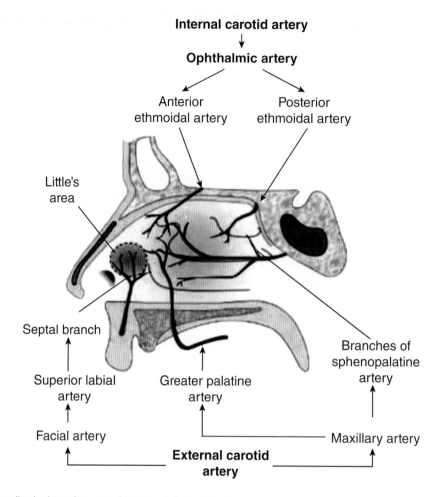

Fig. 27.1 The Kiesselbach plexus is a vascular network from five arteries supplying the nasal septum, the anterior inferior quadrant of which is Little's area. (From Ali T. *Ferri's Clinical Advisor.* 2022:591.e5–591.e6. Elsevier.)

The vignette describes a common occurrence, namely spontaneous epistaxis in someone on anticoagulation therapy. Once trauma is excluded, whilst other causes of coagulopathy are important to consider, the likely cause of bleeding is her use of warfarin for AF. If she had not been on warfarin, then age would make an inherited coagulopathy highly improbable, making thrombocytopaenia in haematological malignancy the next most likely consideration. Reversal of warfarin is sometimes necessary in epistaxis, to restore INR to the target range quickly avoiding subtherapeutic anticoagulation. The commonest location of bleeding is Little's area (Fig. 27.1).

REVISION TIPS

- *'Play Tennis OUTSIDE'*, i.e. PT is EXTRINSIC; *'Play Table Tennis INSIDE'*, i.e. PTT is INTRINSIC
- Haemostasis requires vasoconstriction, platelet plugging and coagulation cascade
- Disorders of platelets or blood vessels cause prolonged bleeding, easy bruising, and mucosal bleeding
- Coagulation defects can cause delayed bleeding into muscle or joints

28

Sore Throat

Leia Alston and Juliet Brown

Leia Alston and Juliet Brown

GP CONSULTATION, FEMALE, 15. SORE THROAT, TWO WEEKS

HPC: Worsening pain on swallowing, radiates to neck and ears. Mild headaches for a week, intermittently hot and sweaty. She has no cough. Self-managing with paracetamol, not improving. Able to drink fluids.

O/E: HR 89 bpm, BP 124/85 mmHg, RR 14, SpO$_2$ 99% (air), T 38.6. Tender, mobile level 2 lymph nodes bilaterally, swollen tonsils bilaterally with exudate.

1. A 2-year-old with sore throat, drooling, and muffled cry. Which differential must be ruled out?
2. Small drop-shaped patches of dry, scaly skin on chest/arms/legs/scalp after sore throat. What is the likely diagnosis?

Answers: 1. Acute epiglottitis, from group A beta-haemolytic *Streptococci* (historically *Haemophilus-b* before Hib vaccine). Do not examine the throat as this may cause airway closure. 2. Guttate psoriasis can occur after *streptococcal* throat infection. On white skin the patches look pink/red and scale looks white. On black/brown skin, the patches can look pink/purple/dark brown, with grey scale.

TABLE 28.1

	Clinical	Investigations	Management
Tonsillitis	**RF:** young age **Hx & O/E:** sore throat, fever, odynophagia, anterior cervical and submandibular lymphadenopathy. Most commonly viral. Bacteria; group A *Strep.* (*Streptococcus pyogenes*), *Streptococcus pneumoniae*, *Haemophilus influenzae*, *Moraxella catarrhalis*, *Staphylococcus aureus*	Clinical diagnosis (Fig. 28.1). **Scores:** FeverPAIN or Centor criteria predict likelihood of streptococcal infection. Consider a throat swab. Bloods: raised inflammatory markers. Monospot test (EBV heterophile antibodies). Consider blood cultures if sepsis signs	Safety net, analgesia, fluids. *No antibiotic* if FeverPAIN 0–1/ Centor 0–2, *back up prescription* if FeverPAIN 2–3, *immediate antibiotic* if FeverPAIN 4–5/Centor 3–4). Phenoxymethylpenicillin or clarithromycin. Difflam mouthwash and analgesia. Admit if very unwell, can't swallow fluids, quinsy, immunocompromise; follow local guidelines for Abx choice (e.g. Benzylpenicillin or clarithromycin). Consider dexamethasone, IV fluids. *Recurrent tonsillitis*: consider tonsillectomy (see revision tips)

(Continued)

TABLE 28.1   (Cont'd)

	Clinical	Investigations	Management
Quinsy (peritonsillar abscess)	RFs: tonsillitis, young age, smoking. Hx & O/E: trismus, 'hot potato voice', tonsillitis-type symptoms (usually unilateral pain), peritonsillar fullness, ± uvula deviation away from affected side. Bacteria; group A *Streptococcus*, *Haemophilus influenzae*, *Staphylococcus aureus*	Clinical diagnosis. Raised inflammatory markers, monospot test (heterophile antibodies). Blood cultures if signs of sepsis.	Aspiration or incision and drainage, antibiotics (local guidelines, e.g. benzylpenicillin and metronidazole). Dexamethasone, difflam mouthwash, analgesia and consider IV fluids. Consider tonsillectomy if previous quinsy
Infectious mononucleosis (glandular fever)	RFs: kissing, sexual, sharing food/cutlery, intrauterine. Hx & O/E: sore throat, fever, posterior cervical lymphadenopathy, splenomegaly (uncommon in adults), malaise. EBV. Complications: hepatitis, thrombocytopenia, GBS, spleen rupture, glomerulonephritis.	Bloods: raised inflammatory markers, LFTs may be deranged. Monospot test (heterophile antibodies) positive (false negative in first two weeks). If less than 12 years old or immunocompromised, test for EBV viral serology. EBV is associated with Burkitt's lymphoma	Treatment as per tonsillitis. Consider steroids. Do not give amoxicillin (macular rash). Avoid alcohol/contact sports for 8 weeks. Admit if stridor, respiratory distress, unable to eat and drink or severe abdominal pain. If deranged LFTs on admission, GP to repeat in community to monitor trend (usually LFTs improve as symptoms improve). See *94. JAUNDICE*

EBV, Epstein-Barr virus; *GBS*, Guillain-Barré syndrome; *LPS*, Liverpool Peritonsillar Abscess Score.

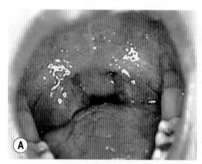 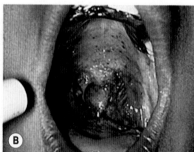 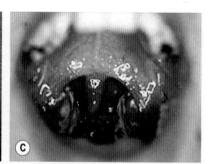

Fig. 28.1 (A) Non-exudative tonsillitis, (B) tonsillitis with petechiae, (C) exudative tonsillitis. (From Marx JA et al. *Rosen's Emergency Medicine*, ed. 8. Philadelphia: Elsevier; 2014.)

In the vignette, she has a FeverPAIN score of 4 – associated with 62%–65% isolation of Streptococcus. She scores a 4 on the Centor criteria. There are no signs of quinsy requiring admission, but immediate prescription for antibiotics is appropriate – she has already attempted self-management and symptoms have lasted longer than the usual course of a sore throat. Due to her age, it would be sensible to test for glandular fever and safety net regarding complications of this.

REVISION TIPS

- Viral sore throat: rhinovirus, coronavirus, parainfluenza, adenovirus, EBV, HSV, influenza
- Non-infectious sore throat: physical irritation (smoking), allergy (hay fever), GORD
- Tonsillectomy in recurrent tonsillitis if: ≥7 bad sore throats in a year OR ≥5 annually for 2 years OR ≥3 annually for 3 years
- Diabetic on insulin and unable to eat/ drink, consider sliding scale

29

Hoarseness and Voice Change

Alice Parker, Alexander Royston, and Shilpa Ojha

GP CONSULTATION, MALE, 54.
PERSISTENT HOARSE VOICE

HPC: Gradually worsened over 2 months, with ody-nophagia and dysphagia. No cough or haemoptysis. Weight loss 4 kg. No recent infections. **SHx:** Smoker 15/day for 20 years. Ex-professional singer.

O/E: HR 74, BP 129/89, RR 15, SpO$_2$ 98%, T 36.5. Hoarse sounding voice, mouth/throat appear normal. No neck lumps or lymphadenopathy.

1. What are the risk factors for laryngeal cancer?
2. What conditions cause hoarseness to get worse throughout the day as the vocal cords fatigue?
3. A patient presents with a hoarse voice. They have recently undergone treatment for persistent hyper-calcaemia. What is the likely underlying cause?

Answers: 1. Smoking, HPV. 2. Myasthenia gravis, Parkinson's disease, muscle tension dysphonia, phonotrauma. 3. Recurrent laryngeal nerve palsy following parathyroidec-tomy operation.

TABLE 29.1

	Features	Investigations	Management
Laryngeal cancer	**RFs:** smoking, prior head/neck cancer, irradiation, occupation (dust/chemical), ↑↑EtOH, GORD, laryngeal dysplasia. **Hx & O/E:** new/persistent hoarseness, odynophagia, dysphagia, otalgia, weight loss. Lump, haemoptysis, stridor	**Nasoendoscopy:** vocal cord paresis, lumps, dysplasia (Fig. 29.1). **CXR.** **Panendoscopy + biopsy.** **CT larynx:** systemic staging for all except T1N0/T2N0 disease (NICE guidance)	2WW referral for suspected laryngeal cancer. **Definitive:** depends on stage. Transoral laser surgery vs radiotherapy. Total laryngectomy (T3/T4)
GORD (reflux laryngitis)	**RFs:** obesity, smoking, alcohol, hernias. **Hx & O/E:** heartburn, odynophagia, acid-brash. Atypical: chronic cough, hoarseness, wheeze	PPI ± antacids (therapeutic trial). **Barium swallow.** **OGD.** **Oesophageal manometry**	Stop smoking, weight loss, reduce caffeine/alcohol/spice/NSAIDs, elevate bed head. PPI. Nissen fundoplication
Vocal cord nodules	**RFs:** phonotrauma (singing/shouting), smoking, alcohol. **Hx & O/E:** husky hoarse voice	**Nasoendoscopy**	Speech therapy. Surgical excision (rare cases)

(Continued)

TABLE 29.1 (Cont'd)

	Features	Investigations	Management
Laryngitis	**RFs:** viral URTI, overuse, smoking, allergies. **Hx & O/E:** hoarseness, odynophagia, dysphagia, fever/coryza	Clinical diagnosis	Supportive. Phenoxymethylpenicillin if secondary bacterial infection
Reinke's oedema	**RFs:** smoking, overuse, hypothyroidism, GORD. **Hx & O/E:** deep hoarse voice	**Nasoendoscopy**	Smoking cessation. SALT. Microlaryngoscopy, biopsy (exclude SCC), lateral cordotomy, drainage
Recurrent laryngeal nerve palsy	**RFs:** recent neck/chest op., intubation, thyroid/lung/oesophagus/larynx cancer, aneurysm, TB, polio, syringomyelia. **Hx & O/E:** weak hoarse voice, cough, SOB	**CXR. CT larynx. USS thyroid** (if thyroid lump)	2WW referral to ENT. Treat underlying cause (may be idiopathic). SALT (voice therapy). Consider medialisation (injection/thyroplasty). Ansa cervicalis nerve reinnervation
Hypothyroidism	**RFs:** PMHx/FHx autoimmune, Turner/Down syndrome, previous head/neck radiation, thyroid surgery, medications. **Hx & O/E:** hoarse, tired, weight gain, cold intolerance, constipation, thin hair, dry skin	TFTs (↑TSH, ↓T4), ↑TPOAb (Hashimoto's)	Levothyroxine
Myasthenia gravis	**RFs:** sex (F > M, 2:1) age (30 F, 50–60 M), other autoimmune disorders, thymoma. **Hx & O/E:** weakness with movement, proximal (face/neck/arms), fatiguability- 'end of the day'. Ocular: ptosis, diplopia, dysphagia (later sign). Hoarse ±myasthenia crisis (acute respiratory failure)	Antibodies: anti-AChR (raised 90%). **Tensilon test:** give edrophonium IV; +ve if power improves in ≤1 minute. **EMG:** decreased response to a train of impulses. **Thymus CT:** likely thymus involvement	Anticholinesterase (pyridostigmine). Prednisolone (relapses – can be combined with azathioprine/methotrexate). **Definitive:** consider thymectomy. See also *30. DIPLOPIA AND PTOSIS*
Muscle tension dysphonia	**RFs:** vocal misuse, personality/psychological, disease. **Hx & O/E:** hoarse voice that tires easily. May have globus symptoms	Functional disorder	Reassurance. Speech therapy

TPOAb, Thyroid peroxidase antibodies.

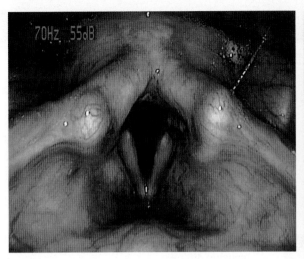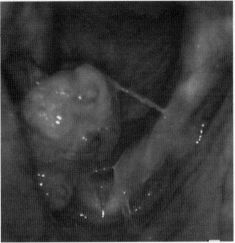

Fig. 29.1 Endoscopic view of the larynx. *Left*, Quiet respiration: vocal folds are moderately abducted. *Right*, Laryngeal squamous cell carcinoma. (Left image: From Standring S. Larynx. In: *Gray's Anatomy*. 2021:717–734.e4. Right image:)

The vignette illustrates basic red flag criteria, even though the individual clinical features may have benign origins. A smoker with progressive hoarseness, significant weight loss and dysphagia requires 2-week wait referral for head and neck cancer. The differential includes GORD, vocal cord nodules and Reinke's oedema, but weight loss and dysphagia are worrying (meriting investigation in their own right). Lack of lymphadenopathy is not reassuring and will likely have been missed on examination. Lifestyles of singers who smoke may stereotypically include consumption of strong dark alcoholic spirits – another carcinogen causing head and neck cancers.

> **REVISION TIPS**
>
> - Red flags for laryngeal cancer include: new and persistent hoarseness of voice that has got worse, odynophagia, otalgia, weight loss, smoker, neck lump, haemoptysis, stridor
> - Recurrent laryngeal nerve palsy causes a hoarse voice and is often caused by cancer

30

Diplopia and Ptosis

Stella Hristova, Mary Xie, and Nick Rees

**GP CONSULTATION, FEMALE, 28.
DOUBLE VISION**

HPC: Right-hand weakness over 3 months, difficulty chopping food. Towards the evening she has difficulty reading novels due to double vision. **PMHx:** Hashimoto's thyroiditis. **DHx:** Levothyroxine. **FHx:** Mother – Type 1 diabetes, stroke at 60 years. **SHx:** Chef, independent, non-smoker, social drinking.
  O/E: Right-hand power 4/5, normal fundoscopy.

1. List red flag signs and symptoms of orbital disease causing diplopia.
2. In CN3 palsy, what does a dilated pupil suggest?

Answers: 1. Proptosis, pain, optic nerve compromise (drop in vision/loss of colour vision/visual field defect/RAPD), resistance to retropulsion, eyelid retraction, periorbital oedema. Any of these indicate orbital imaging. 2. Pupil involvement (dilated) in CN3 palsy could reflect posterior communicating artery aneurysm and needs urgent imaging.

TABLE 30.1

	Features (ptosis + diplopia)	Investigations	Management
Myasthenia gravis	Nicotinic autoantibodies. Peak 30 (F), 50–60 (M). Acquired autoimmune, thymoma. **Hx & O/E:** weakness (face, neck, arms). Fatigue with repetition 'end of the day'. Diplopia/ptosis. Dysphagia (late). Aggravated by pregnancy, thyroid disease, stress	Acetylcholine receptor (anti-AChR), muscle-specific kinase (anti-MUSK) antibodies. EMG, CT or MRI (thymus), edrophonium test. Ice pack test (reduced ptosis)	Anticholinesterase (pyridostigmine), oral corticosteroid, immunomodulators. Thymectomy. See also *29. HOARSENESS AND VOICE CHANGE*
Thyroid eye disease (TED). (Graves' disease 90%; rarely euthyroid/severe Hashimoto's)	Autoimmune response (inflamed/swollen orbital muscles/adipose). **RFs:** F>M, smoking, FHx. **Hx & O/E:** irritated eyes, diplopia (worse in morning), lid retraction, exophthamos, lagophthalmos, periorbital swelling, conjunctival injection/chemosis, restricted movements. Emergency: acute optic neuropathy, exposure keratopathy. Severe- loss of vision. Signs of hyper- or hypothyroidism	TFTs. Anti-TSH receptor/ anti-TPO, anti-thyroglobulin antibodies. Orbital imaging	Endocrinology. Treat thyroid disease. Selenium (mild TED). Corticosteroids based on disease clinical activity score. Immunomodulators. Radiotherapy. Surgical decompression in acute progressive optic neuropathy

TABLE 30.1 (Cont'd)			
Cavernous Sinus Syndrome, including cavernous sinus thrombosis (CST)	**RFs:** facial infection, surgery, pregnancy/early post-partum, clotting disorders, oral contraceptives. **Hx & O/E:** any of ophthalmoplegia (CN3/4/6), Horner syndrome, periorbital reduced sensation (CN5), retro-orbital pain, conjunctival injection, chemosis, proptosis, venous congestion.	Clinical diagnosis. FBC, CRP. ESR/ACE/other immunology if inflammatory cause. CT/MRI of head/orbits. Venogram	Treat according to cause. If CST: Abx, liaise with relevant specialties if infection needing surgical drainage
Ophthalmoplegic migraine	One or more ocular CN palsies (often CN3), headache. Eye pain, loss of peripheral vision, mydriasis, ptosis, N&V, light sensitivity. Usually unilateral. See *99. HEADACHE*	Clinical diagnosis. Imaging to rule out intracranial/orbital pathology	Trigger avoidance, analgesia, antispasmodics, pregabalin, beta-blocker. Botulinum toxin injections
Wernicke encephalopathy	Thiamine-deficiency causing; nystagmus/ophthalmoplegia, ataxia, altered mental status. **RFs:** alcohol excess, anorexia, hyperemesis gravidarum, malabsorption	Clinical diagnosis. Folate and thiamine (low)	Thiamine IV (Pabrinex) with ongoing oral supplement. Alcohol cessation with support. Prompt treatment– signs can be reversed
Features (Ptosis)			
Horner syndrome	Ptosis, miosis, ±facial anhidrosis. **Acquired neuron lesion:** first-order (hypothalamus, brainstem, spinal cord), second-order (lung apex, anterior neck) or third-order (carotid, skull base, cavernous sinus, orbit). Pancoast tumour (apical lung). **Congenital:** affected eye has lighter-coloured iris	Apraclonidine/ cocaine eyedrop tests. MRI/MRA of head, neck, orbits. CT thorax. MRI of brain/upper chest. MRA of the neck	Treatment according to underlying cause

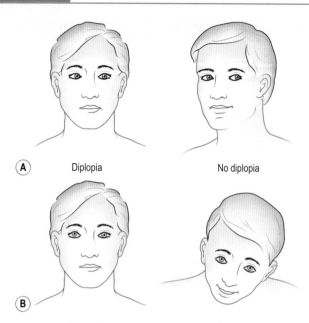

Fig. 30.1 Compensatory head positions for diplopia. (A) Right lateral rectus palsy. A right esotropia is present in primary gaze; however, by turning the head to the right (in the direction of action of the weak right lateral rectus muscle), the patient can move the eyes into left gaze and maintain both eyes on target (orthotropia), thereby achieving binocular single vision. (B) Acute right superior oblique muscle palsy. The right eye extorts (excycloduction) because of the unopposed action of the right inferior oblique muscle. When the patient tilts the head to the left and forward (in the direction of action of the weak muscle), the right eye is passively intorted while the left eye actively intorts to compensate and maintain binocular single vision. The head also tilts forward to compensate for the weak depressor action of the weak right superior oblique. (From Jankovic J et al. *Bradley and Daroff's Neurology in Clinical Practice*, ed 8, Philadelphia: Elsevier; 2022.)

Diplopia is the perception of two images of a single object: it can be monocular (persists when unaffected eye is covered; due to refractive error or cataract) or true binocular diplopia (due to ocular misalignment, resolves when either eye is covered). Elicit its nature (horizontal vs vertical) and any associated features, such as headaches. Look for compensatory head position (Fig. 30.1). Isolated cranial nerve palsies can be caused by; aneurysm, microvascular ischaemia, raised ICP, demyelination, vasculitis, trauma, tumour, etc. Multiple cranial neuropathies can suggest cavernous sinus or brainstem pathology. Orbital causes include: thyroid eye disease, inflammatory or infiltrative disease, as well as trauma (orbital blowout fracture with rectus muscle entrapment). Myasthenia gravis is a disease of the neuromuscular junction, which most commonly presents with ocular symptoms such as ptosis and diplopia. In the vignette, the most likely diagnosis is myasthenia gravis, given the history of fluctuating fatiguability. However, also consider thyroid eye disease (in PMHx).

REVISION TIPS

- Oculomotor palsy (CN3): Vertical and horizonal diplopia, ptosis, large unreactive pupil. Loss of adduction, elevation, and depression; eye remains abducted, depressed and turned in
- Trochlear palsy (CN4): Vertical and/or torsional diplopia. Particularly bad when looking down and inwards. Difficult going downstairs
- Abducens palsy (CN6): Horizontal diplopia. Gets worse looking laterally towards the affected side

31

Squint

Emmanuella Ikem, Alexander Royston, and Denize Atan

GP CONSULTATION, FEMALE, AGED 4. 6-MONTH HISTORY OF INTERMITTENT SQUINT

HPC: Left eye is often turned inwards, worse when tired and when looking at close objects. Well, no recent viral infection/headache/vomiting/double vision. **PMHx:** Low birth weight. **FHx:** Childhood squint (father).

O/E: Left-sided esotropia based on corneal reflections and cover test. Full range of eye movement, normal visual acuity, equal and reactive pupils, no ptosis, no nystagmus.

1. How is the esotropia described in the vignette managed? What is the aim of treatment?
2. What are the causes of paralytic squints (most commonly in adults)?
3. What is a pseudosquint and how does one differentiate?

Answers: 1. Initially corrective lenses, further options are surgery or Botulinum toxin injections. Aim is to prevent the squinting eye from becoming amblyopic or lazy, and to improve cosmesis. 2. Microvascular ischaemia, space-occupying lesion (aneurysm, tumour), congenital, demyelination, meningitis, iatrogenic, idiopathic, trauma, infection (rare). 3. Apparent squint due to facial or eyelid shape in babies (often wide epicanthic folds); differentiated by corneal reflections.

TABLE 31.1			
	Features	**Investigations**	**Management**
Esotropia (Childhood)			
Accommodative esotropia	**RFs:** FHx (squint). **Hx & O/E:** intermittent squint, worse when looking at near objects. Esotropia (Fig. 31.1), normal visual acuity with glasses	Observe corneal reflections. **Prism cover tests:** cover and alternate cover test with prisms, smooth pursuit eye movements	Routine ophthalmology assessment. Corrective glasses for hypermetropia (long-sightedness) with convex lenses
Non-accommodative or partially accommodative esotropia	**RFs:** poor vision in one eye, FHx (squint). **Hx & O/E:** intermittent or constant squint. May have poor vision in squinting eye with or without glasses	Corneal reflections. **Prism cover tests**	Rapid ophthalmology. Corrective glasses if hypermetropia. Occlusion therapy if vision reduced due to amblyopia. Squint surgery

(Continued)

TABLE 31.1 (Cont'd)

	Features	Investigations	Management
6th nerve palsy	**RFs in children:** congenital, tumour (non-localising sign). **Hx & O/E:** esotropia, ipsilateral head turn, features of ↑ICP, limited abduction	Observe corneal reflections. **Prism cover tests.** **CT/MRI:** Tumour	Urgent ophthalmology. Treat cause. Treat esotropia as above
Exotropia (Childhood)			
Exotropia	**RFs:** myopia, poor vision in one eye, neurodevelopmental. **Hx & O/E:** intermittent squint, worse when tired/looking at bright lights. No squint looking at near objects. Exotropia, normal visual acuity with glasses if due to myopia	**Prism cover tests**	Routine ophthalmology. Corrective glasses (concave lenses) if myopia. Occlusion therapy if vision reduced due to amblyopia. Squint surgery to straighten eyes in some cases
Poor Vision in One Eye (Child)			
Amblyopia (lazy eye)	**RFs:** uncorrected refractive error, squint. **Hx & O/E:** child dislikes covering one eye. Impaired visual acuity	Routine referral for ophthalmology assessment	Occlusion therapy (eye patch)
Congenital cataracts	See *32. LOSS OF RED REFLEX*		
Retinoblastoma	See *32. LOSS OF RED REFLEX*		
Adult-Onset Squint—Non-Paralytic			
Exotropia	**RFs:** chronic childhood exotropia or consecutive (after childhood esotropia or squint surgery) or chronic poor vision in one eye	**Prism cover tests**	Routine ophthalmology. Cosmetic squint surgery to straighten eyes in some
Esotropia	**RFs:** can be consecutive (after squint surgery) or chronic poor vision in one eye	**Prism cover tests**	Routine ophthalmology. Cosmetic squint surgery to straighten eyes in some
Adult-Onset Squint—Paralytic			
Cranial Nerve palsies 3/4/6	**RFs:** DM, HTN, injury, infection, tumour, aneurysm, congenital. **Hx & O/E:** CN3 diplopia, ptosis/ mydriasis, pain, proptosis, 'down and out' pupil, fixed dilatation. CN4 vertical diplopia, contra-lateral head tilt, slight upward deviation (cannot look down/in). CN6 horizontal diplopia, ipsilateral head turn, medial inward deviation, ↓lateral movement	Paralytic cause of squint: far more adult-onset. CN6: tumour (falsely localising sign), features of ↑ICP. **CT/CTA:** tumour, aneurysm	Urgent ophthalmology. Acute CN3 palsy emergency (risk of aneurysm). Treatment depends on underlying cause; CN4 vertical prism for diplopia, CN6 base-out prism for esotropia

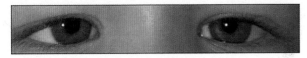

Fig. 31.1 Infantile esotropia. The child is fixing with her left eye; note the temporally decentred light reflex in the right eye. (From Kinori M, Robbins SL. *Ophthalmology.* 2019;11(6):1210–1216. e1. Copyright © 2019 Elsevier Inc. All rights reserved.)

Childhood squints (strabismus) are very common, most often due to refractive error. This child in the vignette had an esotropia associated with hypermetropia (long-sight). Children who are short-sighted (myopia) might present with exotropia (divergent squint). Children with reduced visual acuity may have serious underlying pathology, such as retinoblastoma, so squint requires dilated eye examination. Crucial pointers here are features of the squint (worse examining objects up close), family history, normal visual acuity and normal ocular motility.

REVISION TIPS

- Convergent squints are the commonest type of squint in children, mostly hypermetropia, sometimes idiopathic
- Myopia is rare in childhood
- Paralytic squints; rule out red flags (trauma, symptoms of ↑ICP, sudden onset post-school age)

- Amblyopia means reduced visual acuity in one eye and is treated by occlusion therapy
- Amblyopia can cause squint and vice versa
- Surgery is not a treatment for amblyopia, only for squint

32

Loss of Red Reflex

Margarita Fox, Alexander Royston, and Denize Atan

GP CONSULTATION, FEMALE, 18 MONTHS. RIGHT EYE LOOKS 'DIFFERENT TO THE LEFT'

HPC: Mother also states her daughter looks 'slightly cross-eyed' and is having difficulty seeing. **PMHx:** nil, unremarkable developmental history, NVD at term.
  O/E: Using Cardiff cards; acuity on right 6/18, left 6/12. Red reflex test reveals white reflex in right eye (leukocoria). No cataract.

1. What are management options for retinoblastoma?
2. Name some complications of congenital cataract.
3. What pre-natal infections may result in leukocoria?

Answers: 1. Depends on tumour size, vitreous seeding and metastasis; generally uses plaque radiotherapy to preserve eye. 2. Amblyopia, strabismus, retinal detachment, pupillary abnormalities, cystoid macular oedema, endophthalmitis; glaucoma and posterior capsule opacification (surgical complications). 3. TORCH syndrome (toxoplasmosis, other agents, rubella, CMV, herpes simplex) by causing congenital cataracts and/or retinal scarring.

TABLE 32.1

	Features	Investigations	Management
Paediatric Retinoblastoma	**RFs:** age (<3 years), FHx (10% hereditary: autosomal dominant). **Hx & O/E:** leukocoria (commonest presentation), strabismus, visual problems	**Fundoscopy + EUA.** **OCT:** macula/fovea, tumour growth, subretinal/vitreous seeding. **B-scan USS:** mass, calcification, shadowing. **MRI/CT of orbit:** to check for extraocular extension	2WW referral. Depends on stage; external beam radiation, plaque therapy, chemotherapy, photocoagulation/cryotherapy. Enucleation – if very advanced
Congenital cataracts	**RFs:** birth (polar), trauma, infection (VZV/rubella), genetics. **Hx & O/E:** squint, leukocoria, loss of red reflex, reduced visual acuity	**Fundoscopy:** lens opacification → loss of red reflex	If affecting vision, cataract surgery (phacoemulsification) ± lens implant
Persistent foetal vasculature	Embryologic mesenchymal tissue in vitreous cavity. **RFs:** genetic, syndromic, idiopathic. **Hx & O/E:** leukocoria. Maybe with cataract or microphthalmia (small eye)	**Fundus exam ± EUA:** short axial length. **USS:** r/o detachment and retinoblastoma	Observation. Lensectomy, glaucoma management

TABLE 32.1   (Cont'd)

	Features	Investigations	Management
Retinopathy of prematurity	Ischaemic retinal vasculopathy. RFs: prematurity, low birth weight, Hx of high-dose oxygen. Hx & O/E: strabismus, leukocoria	Fundoscopy: lack normal vascularisation of peripheral retina	Aim: reduce risk of retinal detachment. Argon/diode laser intravitreal anti-VEGF
Coats disease	RFs: M > F, age (~5–6 years). Hx & O/E: strabismus, unilateral. Yellow-eye effect: lipid rich, subretinal exudate, loss of vision	Fundoscopy: more yellow than white. Telangiectasias, aneurysms. OCT/ USS: distinguish from retinoblastoma	Photocoagulation. Cryotherapy. Intravitreal steroid/anti-VEGF injections
Astrocytic hamartoma	RFs: linked to Tuberous Sclerosis (TS). Hx & O/E: creamy-white tumour, TS features (shagreen patch, facial angiofibromas)	Fundoscopy: circumscribed lesion with 'glistening' yellow calcification	Mostly stable: do not require treatment
Retinal detachment (children)	Rare, can be rhegmatogenous, exudative and tractional. RFs: retinitis of prematurity, trauma, cataracts, myopia, vitreoretinopathies, Coat's. Hx & O/E: leukocoria, reduced acuity, peripheral field loss	Ix as for adults – see 33. FLASHES AND FLOATERS IN VISUAL FIELDS. Urgent ophthalmology <24h	Retinopexy (cryotherapy/laser) ± scleral buckles (bands to relieve traction/support tears). Pars plana vitrectomy not often required
Leukocoria in Adults			
Cataracts (age-related)	RFs: acquired: age, T2DM (nuclear). Hx & O/E: blurred/dim vision, loss of night vision, fading of colours, halos around lights	Fundoscopy: lens opacification	Stronger glasses, use brighter lights. **phacoemulsification** + lens implant
Corneal scarring	RFs: contact lenses, trauma, abrasion. Hx & O/E: painful red eye, blurred vision, photophobia. Irritation/ scratching sensation. Complication of keratitis	Slit lamp: Fluorescein eye stain. Corneal scraping	Discontinue contact lenses. Treat keratitis: topical Abx (quinolones). Analgesia: cyclopentolate. Scarring: UV phototherapy. Surgery: corneal transplant
Vitreous haemorrhage	RFs: age (not seen in children), diabetic retinopathy, retinal tear/ detachment, PVD, eye trauma. Hx & O/E: floaters preceding vision loss, may have flashes, blurred vision, shadows, seeing 'red hue'. Not leukocoria	Dilated fundoscopy: diffuse haemorrhage obscures view of retina. Slit lamp: RBCs in anterior vitreous. B-scan ocular USS: exclude retinal tear/detachment	Blood clears from vitreous with time → vision returns. If due to neovascular: anti-VEGF injections/laser photocoagulation. If tear: retinopexy ± scleral buckles
Retinal detachment	See 33. FLASHES AND FLOATERS IN VISUAL FIELDS		

TS, Tuberous sclerosis; OCT, optical coherence tomography; EUA, examination under anaesthesia.

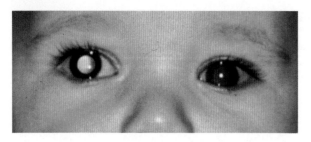

Fig. 32.1 Normal red reflex in the left eye. White reflex in the right eye, later diagnosed with retinoblastoma. (From Martin RJ, Fanaroff AA, Walsch MC, eds. *Fanaroff & Martin's Neonatal-Perinatal Medicine*. 10th ed., Vol 2. Philadelphia: Elsevier/Saunders; 2015: Fig. 103.7, p.1739.)

The commonest cause of leukocoria is cataract, but the likely diagnosis in the vignette is retinoblastoma (example in Fig. 32.1). The key points are onset at 18 months (not congenital) and absence of cataract. Persistent foetal vasculature also presents with leukocoria but is congenital and commonly presents with cataract. Coats disease more commonly affects males and at an older age. This child was born at term (excludes retinopathy of prematurity), with no features of tuberous sclerosis (excludes astrocytic hamartoma).

REVISION TIPS

- Red reflex: should appear red, orange or yellow and symmetrical
- Leukocoria → abnormal white reflection from retina
- Abnormalities require urgent ophthalmology referral
- Loss of red reflex suggests light is not reflecting back → pathology anywhere in retina, vitreous, lens, cornea

33

Flashes and Floaters in Visual Fields

Margarita Fox, Alexander Royston, and Denize Atan

GP CONSULTATION, FEMALE, 69.
SUDDEN ONSET FLASHES IN LEFT EYE

HPC: 'Funny vision' and 'spot-like shadows' which drift on moving her left eye. Denies ocular pain. **PMHx:** Myopia (glasses since age 15), HTN, cataract surgery. **DHx:** Amlodipine.

   O/E: Visual acuity; 6/12 left eye; 6/6 right eye. Visual fields intact. Fundoscopy normal.

---

1. Which of the following is not a symptom of retinal detachment? Flashes, ocular pain, shadow over visual field, reduced acuity.
2. What other non-ocular causes of flashes are important to consider in:
   a. A 77-year-old man with flashes, dizziness and bilateral temporary dimming of vision on standing up?
   b. An elderly lady with bilateral photopsia, vertigo and weakness?

Answers: 1. Ocular pain. Retinal detachment is typically painless. 2. (a) Postural hypotension, (b) Vertebrobasilar insufficiency/TIA of posterior cerebral circulation, specifically if affecting vessels supplying the occipital lobe. Note, vascular insufficiency/TIA affecting the ophthalmic or central retinal artery may cause flashes of light and transient visual loss in one eye only.

TABLE 33.1

	Features	Investigations	Management
Vitreous/Retinal Detachment			
Posterior Vitreous Detachment (PVD)	**RFs:** high myopes. PMHx of intraocular surgery (especially cataracts) or inflammation (uveitis), age (>50 years). **Hx & O/E:** sudden or gradual onset flashes of light in peripheral vision. Floaters. Blurred vision. Painless	**Ophthalmoscopy:** may have Weiss ring (floater from prior attachment around the optic nerve). **Slit lamp:** r/o retinal haemorrhage or tear	Gradual onset floaters: refer ≤1 week. Sudden onset floaters + flashes in one eye: refer ≤24 hours. Symptoms may resolve. May require vitrectomy but risks outweigh benefits

(Continued)

TABLE 33.1	(Cont'd)		
	Features	**Investigations**	**Management**
Retinal detachment	**RFs:** • Rhegmatogenous: as PVD, PMHx retinal tear, myopia, FHx • Tractional: think proliferative diabetic retinopathy • Exudative: rare • Childhood: retinitis of prematurity, trauma **Hx & O/E:** acute flashes/floaters. Painless 'curtain-like' shadow from peripheral to central. Reduced acuity, peripheral field loss. Childhood: squint, leukocoria, loss of red reflex, ↓visual acuity	**Fundoscopy:** leukocoria, abnormal retinal folds. **Visual acuity tests:** central acuity reduced if macula detached. **Slit lamp:** Shafer's sign or 'tobacco dust' = tear in retinal pigment epithelium, resulting in pigment cells in vitreous. **Indirect ophthalmoscopy:** Consider: **B-scan USS** (if opacity, haemorrhage, unable to see retina)	Urgent ophthalmology (<24 hours). Retinopexy (cryotherapy/laser) ± scleral buckles (bands under extraocular rectus relieve traction/support tears) ± pars plana vitrectomy (clear vitreous opacities): less used in children as vitreous has not detached
Other Important Conditions			
Vitreous haemorrhage	See *32. LOSS OF RED REFLEX*		
Migraine (aura)	See *99. HEADACHE*		

PVD, Posterior vitreous detachment.

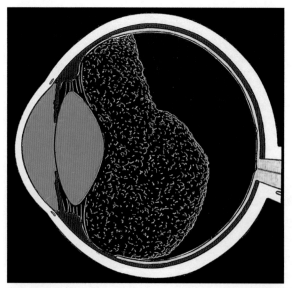

Fig. 33.1 Acute posterior vitreous detachment. (From Kanski JJ., Bowling B. *Synopsis of Clinical Ophthalmology.* © Elsevier; 2013.)

Vitreous detachment is far more common and less serious than retinal detachment, while many risk factors are shared between them. Relevant points for vitreous detachment in the vignette are age, myopia, previous cataract surgery and peripheral onset with no change in visual acuity. The vitreous humour is a gel of aqueous glycosaminoglycans. It peels away from the retina with ageing, which can occur prematurely in high myopes and following ocular trauma or surgery. Retinal detachment is more serious and can affect visual acuity when the macula becomes involved.

REVISION TIPS

- Photopsias are often harmless. Floaters (specks/strings/cobwebs) are vitreous shadows on the retina
- Seek urgent ophthalmology if acute onset flashes floaters with visual field defects → retinal detachment
- Spectrum: PVD → retinal tear → rhegmatogenous detachment

34

Eye Trauma and Foreign Object in Eye

Mary Xie, Mital Patel, and Vidit Singh

EMERGENCY DEPARTMENT, FEMALE, 28. HIT IN THE FACE BY A CRICKET BALL

HPC: Glasses were broken. Left eye; pain, excessive watering, difficulty opening, minimal vision. No loss of consciousness or vomiting. **SHx:** mechanic and welder.
 O/E: GCS 15. Topical LA (tetracaine 1%) to aid the exam. Left eye: periorbital swelling, laceration to upper lid margin, red hue to her vision, restricted up-gaze, chemosis, hyphaema. Visual acuity: PL (perception of light only, no perception of hand movements, finger counting or Snellen letters). Right eye: normal, VA 6/6.

1. Student adding chemical to glass flask which shattered near his face, no eye protection. Bilateral eye pain, redness, watery eyes. What are your differentials?
2. Severe eye pain and progressive vision loss after a punch 7 hours ago. O/E periorbital bruising, ophthalmoplegia, proptosis and reduced pupillary response. What is the diagnosis and management?

Answers: 1. Chemical burns, foreign object, penetrating injury. 2. Retrobulbar haemorrhage, suggested by proptosis. In orbital blowout, the eye tends to be sunken in. Immediate referral for surgical decompression or, in an emergency in the ED, lateral canthotomy.

TABLE 34.1

	Features	Investigations	Management
Corneal abrasion (superficial corneal injury)	RFs: foreign body or scratching eyes. Hx & O/E: tearing, redness, gritty sensation	Slit lamp + fluorescein: increased uptake. Exclude; *microbial keratitis* (white corneal infiltrate, overlying fluorescein), *HSV* (dendritic 'spider-like' uptake)	1. Topical chloramphenicol 2. Lubricant for pain relief 3. Avoid contact lenses 4. Follow up in 24–48 hours If acuity drops ≥2 Snellen lines from baseline refer to ophthalmology

(Continued)

TABLE 34.1   (Cont'd)

	Features	Investigations	Management
Foreign body (FB) in eye	RFs: metal grinding, woodwork, chiselling, etc. Hx & O/E: sensation of FB/grit, watering, irritation, sharp pain, often worse with blinking Superficial (corneal) or intraocular (penetrating/open globe)	Topical LA (tetracaine 1%) – pain from superficial FBs usually resolves in a minute Slit lamp + fluorescein: inspect for penetrating eye injury or globe rupture (positive Seidel sign). Metallic FBs – usually visible, may have 'rust ring' Orbital CT: exclude penetrating/intraocular FB-associated facial fracture	**Urgent ophthalmology in suspected penetrating injury or globe rupture** Check tetanus status Remove FB if no penetrating injury/ globe rupture; 1. Saline to wash out superficial FB or FB in conjunctival fornices 2. Attempt removal with cotton bud/needle/burr 3. Evert lids to look for tarsal FB Topical chloramphenicol, oral analgesia, follow up in 24 hours. If suspect open globe: no topical, no pressure. Eye shield
Penetrating trauma in eye (Open globe injury)	RFs: sharp or high-velocity projectiles, e.g. hammering, chiselling, thorns, lawn mowing Hx & O/E: reduced acuity, irregular pupils, haemorrhagic chemosis subconjunctival haemorrhage. Hyphaema (Fig. 34.1) – red hue/hazy vision, photophobia		
Subconjunctival haemorrhage	See *35. RED EYE*		
Vitreous haemorrhage (post-trauma)	See *32. LOSS OF RED REFLEX*		Urgent ophthalmology
Retrobulbar haemorrhage	RFs: high-impact blunt facial trauma ± antithrombotic medication use Hx & O/E: unilateral painful proptosis, resistance to retropulsion and reduced ocular movements	Inspect for proptosis. Check ocular movement if patient alert/cooperative	**Ophthalmic emergency.** Urgent lateral canthotomy/ cantholysis (prevent CN1 compression); if delay, IV mannitol/ acetazolamide/dexamethasone
Chemical burns	RFs: bleach, concrete, oven cleaner, pepper spray, some plant saps Hx & O/E: reduced acuity, burning sensation, watering, redness	Check eye pH; alkali worse than acid for ocular injury. Inspection (tetracaine 1%). Visual acuities	Topical anaesthesia, irrigation until pH7 (may require >5 L of saline). Urgent ophthalmology: consider antibiotic prophylaxis

FB, Foreign body.

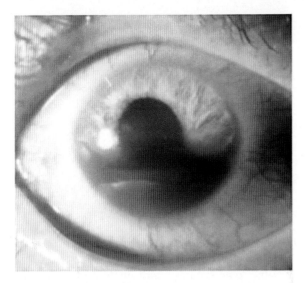

Most eye trauma is managed in the ED and corneal abrasions account for the majority. In high-velocity trauma or suspected penetrating injuries, assess for sight-threatening injuries. Visual acuity is the 'vital sign' of the eye and should be performed in all eye trauma. In the vignette, we are concerned for multiple significant injuries. Her reduced range of eye movement suggests orbital injury and rectus entrapment, while her chemosis, hyphaema and reduced acuity imply globe rupture. These are ophthalmological emergencies and care should be escalated quickly. Also exclude head/cervical spine injury.

Fig. 34.1 Traumatic hyphaema. (From Bowling B. Trauma. *Kanski's Clinical Ophthalmology: A Systematic Approach.* SaundersChina; 2016: 861–885.)

REVISION TIPS

- Painless red eye mostly occurs in subconjunctival haemorrhage. If there is a dull ache/pain consider episcleritis, scleritis or uveitis
- Eye trauma red flags – emergency ophthalmology referral
  1. Metal or organic FB
  2. Suspected penetrating, intraocular, or open globe injury; high speed/high impact/sharp object, irregular pupil(s) ± extruding intraocular contents
  3. Hyphaema or hypopyon
  4. Chemical injury
  5. Significantly reduced visual acuity (two or more Snellen lines)
  6. Deep or large abrasions
  7. Corneal/media opacity with loss of red reflex

35

Red Eye

Emily Warren and Vidit Singh

**OPHTHALMOLOGY CLINIC, FEMALE, 62.
ACUTE ONSET RED EYE**

HPC: Started a day ago, 'stabbing' pain woke her—worse in bright light, struggling to see with it, constantly waters, no unusual discharge. No contact lenses or glasses. **PMHx:** Asthma, eczema, ulcerative colitis, HTN, T2DM. **DHx:** Salbutamol, ramipril, metformin, mesalazine.

  O/E: Obs normal. Right conjunctival injection, watery discharge, unable to open fully. Pupil irregular with hypopyon. Intraocular pressure (IOP) normal. Red reflex seen on fundoscopy.

1. What medications/events can precipitate acute angle closure glaucoma?
2. Name some features which might suggest a benign cause for red eye.
3. Name three extraocular causes of red eye.

Answers: 1. Anything that dilates the eye, e.g. sympathomimetics, atropine, SSRIs. Emotional stimuli, reading/accommodation, dim light. 2. Pupils normal size/reactivity, normal acuity, clear cornea, no proptosis, non-tender eyeball, normal extraocular eye movements, clear anterior chamber. 3. Cluster headache, cavernous sinus thrombosis, orbital cellulitis.

TABLE 35.1

	Features	Investigations	Management
Conjunctivitis	**RFs:** contact with another case (bacterial/viral), atopy (allergic). **Hx & O/E:** eyelid swelling, conjunctival injection, gritty discomfort, itchy eyes. *Bacterial:* mucopurulent discharge, difficult opening eye after sleep. *Viral/allergic:* clear discharge or lacrimation	Clinical diagnosis. Recurrent/persistent: swabs for MC&S, HSV, chlamydia/gonorrhoea and refer to ophthalmology	*Bacterial:* bathe the eyelids, chloramphenicol 0.5%. *Allergic:* reassure, cold compress, anti-histamine drops. *HSV:* acyclovir ointment, refer to ophthalmology. *Chlamydia/gonorrhoea:* treat as for systemic/GU. *Viral:* self-resolves. Consider artificial tears
Subconjunctival haemorrhage	**RFs:** HTN, trauma, straining, anticoagulant, bleeding disorder. **Hx & O/E:** asymptomatic, painless (mild ache or irritation), normal VA	Clinical diagnosis. Check blood pressure	Reassure, cold compress, lubricating drops if severe. Resolves in 5–10 days

TABLE 35.1   (Cont'd)

	Features	Investigations	Management
Acute anterior uveitis	**RFs:** HLA-B27 disorders (IBD, psoriatic/reactive arthritis), sarcoid, SLE, FHx. **Infection:** HIV, TB, toxoplasma – immunosuppression. **Hx & O/E:** acute-subacute pain, watery, reduced acuity, photophobia, conjunctival injection. Likely relapse/chronic	Clinical diagnosis. **Slit lamp:** conjunctival injection, anterior chamber cells ± hypopyon. HLA-B27 serology, toxoplasma/HIV/syphilis. Talbot's test: pain on convergence. Check IOP	Urgent ophthalmology. Tapered topical steroids. Severe: oral steroids, then biologics. Topical cycloplegic (cyclopentolate). <u>Infectious</u>: antibiotics or antivirals (oral steroids can make it worse)
Acute angle closure glaucoma	See *37. ACUTE CHANGE IN OR LOSS OF VISION*		
Keratitis	See *36. EYE PAIN AND DISCOMFORT*		
Episcleritis/ scleritis	See *36. EYE PAIN AND DISCOMFORT*		

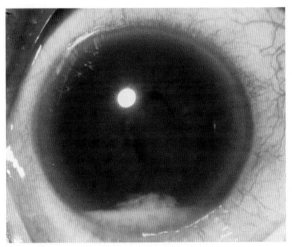

Fig. 35.1 Anterior uveitis with hypopyon and posterior synechiae. (Photo courtesy of Dr. Stephen Orlin.)

Commoner causes of a red eye are usually less serious. While dramatic-appearing, a subconjunctival haemorrhage is often easy to identify and only needs reassurance. Nonetheless, there are potentially sight-threatening emergencies. In the vignette, the patient has IBD, a red eye with blurred vision, photophobia and a hypopyon, making acute anterior uveitis the likely diagnosis. Every patient with an eye complaint should have VA checked ('vital sign' for the eye) and abnormality may warn of significant pathology. An approach to take if struggling with differentials is anatomical; consider causes from the lashes backwards, through the lid, conjunctiva, cornea, sclera, iris to the posterior chamber.

REVISION TIPS

- If someone presents with a red eye and their pupil is dilated, think acute angle closure glaucoma until proven otherwise – it is a sight-threatening emergency
- Background of UC, Crohn's or SLE in vignette? Consider anterior uveitis or scleritis. Background of contact lens wearing/swimming pools? Keratitis

36

Eye Pain and Discomfort

Nicholas Rees, Mary Xie, and Stella Hristova

GP CONSULTATION, FEMALE, 24.
1 DAY PAINFUL RIGHT EYE

HPC: Blurred vision, watering and discomfort looking at bright light, recently been rubbing her eyes. Daily contact lenses – good hygiene practices. No previous episodes of note. **PMHx:** Myopic, ulcerative colitis, hay fever. **DHx:** COCP. **FHx:** NIDDM.

O/E: Right conjunctival injection, hazy patch on cornea.

1. When is same-day ophthalmology assessment indicated in a patient presenting with eye pain?
2. What are your differentials for extra-ocular pain?
3. List the risk factors for all types of keratitis?

Answers: 1. Reduced visual acuity, photophobia, temporal pain, systemic symptoms, trauma, irregular pupil, relative afferent pupillary defect (RAPD), hypopyon, optic disc oedema. 2. Hordeolum, pre-septal cellulitis, giant cell arteritis (GCA). 3. Contact lens use/poor hygiene, trauma, immunosuppression, stress, recent infective contact.

TABLE 36.1

	Features	Investigations	Management
Keratitis	**Viral keratitis** **RFs:** immunosuppression, stress, trauma, recent contact, cold sores. **Hx & O/E:** acute eye pain, reduced acuity, photophobia, conjunctival injection, epiphora. Dendritic corneal ulceration	Clinical diagnosis. Visual acuity (VA), slit lamp, fundoscopy. Fluorescein stain. Swab for viral PCR (HSV-1, herpes zoster)	Same day ophthalmology. Stop contact lenses. Analgesia, topical/PO antivirals (ganciclovir/acyclovir) 10–14 days. Steroids may be indicated – defer if epithelial defect
	Bacterial keratitis **RFs:** trauma, contact lens **Hx & O/E:** aubacute pain, reduced acuity, photophobia, conjunctival injection, corneal opacification, ± hypopyon. Rapid ulceration	Corneal scrape and stain/MC&S.	Same day ophthalmology. Stop contact lenses. Analgesia, topical Abx (e.g. ofloxacin)
	Protozoan **RFs:** unhygienic contact lens use (reusing, tap water, swimming/showering with lenses)	**Hx & O/E:** disproportionate pain. Later, ring-shape infiltrate. **Ix:** corneal scrape, stain/MC&S	Same day ophthalmology. Stop contact lenses. Analgesia, topical anti-parasitic

TABLE 36.1 (Cont'd)

	Features	Investigations	Management
	Fungal keratitis RFs: trauma, topical steroids, immunosuppression. Hx & O/E: red eye, corneal opacities (satellite lesions), ulcers, ± hypopyon. Suspect in corneal ulcer not responding to Abx.	VA, slit lamp, fluorescein stain. Corneal scrape for MC&S (e.g. candida)	Topical anti-fungals as per local guideline
Trauma	RFs: contact lens use, power tool use, windy environments. Hx & O/E: acute eye pain, reduced acuity, photophobia, conjunctival injection, epiphora, foreign body, corneal abrasion	VA, IOP, slit lamp – exclude penetrating injury. Corneal epithelial defect staining with fluorescein	Prevention advice – safety goggles. Foreign body removal at slit lamp/loose epithelium debridement for abrasions. Antibiotics
Uveitis	*Autoimmune uveitis.* RFs: HLA-B27 disorders (IBD, psoriatic/reactive arthritis), sarcoid, Bechet's, FHx. *Infectious uveitis* (e.g. toxoplasma/HSV/syphilis/TB). RF: Immunosuppressed. Hx & O/E: acute-subacute pain, reduced acuity, photophobia, conjunctival injection, ± irregular pupil	VA, IOP, slit lamp, fundoscopy. Blood tests and further investigations based on clinical suspicion, e.g. HLA-B27/ACE/RF/ANA, etc. Toxoplasmosis/syphilis/HIV serology/QuantiFERON.	Urgent ophthalmology. Slowly tapered topical steroids. Severe: oral steroids, then biologics. Topical cycloplegic (cyclopentolate). Infectious: Abx or antivirals (oral steroids can make it worse)
Optic neuritis (typical)	RFs: young to middle-aged, F > M, viral prodrome. May be associated with MS. Hx & O/E: acute-subacute pain worse on eye movement, epiphora, reduced acuity/colour vision, RAPD if unilateral	Clinical diagnosis. Optic disc oedema on fundoscopy. MRI to rule out MS. See also *37. ACUTE CHANGE IN OR LOSS OF VISION*. *Atypical optic neuritis: inflammatory/ infectious/ autoimmune disorder*	Refer to ophthalmology. IV/PO steroid may be indicated, tapered accordingly. In typical cases – good visual acuity recovery. Consider neurology review
Episcleritis	Usually sectoral redness, dull ache, inflammation of episclera	Blanches with topical phenylephrine	Self-limiting, cold compress, lubricants
Scleritis	RFs: systemic autoimmune (50%), especially rheumatoid arthritis. Hx & O/E: deep pain worse on movement (keeps awake at night), blue/purple scleral tinge, photophobia	VA, slit lamp, fundoscopy. Does not blanch with topical phenylephrine. Ophthalmic ultrasound. CRP, ESR, RF, ANCA	Urgent ophthalmology. High-dose NSAIDs with gastroprotection. Steroids. Biologics

TABLE 36.1   (Cont'd)

	Features	Investigations	Management
Hordeolum (stye)	Bacterial (e.g. *S. aureus*) infection of eyelash follicles due to follicle obstruction. RF: blepharitis. Hx & O/E: subacute tender swelling at eyelid margin, ± purulent discharge	Clinical diagnosis	Reassure. Warm compress, eyelid massage, hygiene. Abx + steroid ointment. Pre-septal cellulitis: systemic Abx. Surgical incision and curettage
Other Important Differentials			
GCA/temporal arteritis	Most common vasculitis in adults. Medium-large vessel vasculitis. RFs: female, age > 50 years, polymyalgia rheumatica. Hx & O/E: temporal headache/tender, scalp tenderness, jaw/tongue claudication, ± reduced acuity, ± myalgia, temporal artery beading, ± optic disc oedema. Can get ischaemic optic neuropathy	ESR (raised, can be normal), CRP (very sensitive), ↓ Hb/platelets. **Temporal artery biopsy** (within 2 weeks): demonstrates vasculitis (can be normal). **US of temporal artery:** thick wall, 'halo' sign. **CTA, MRA:** arterial wall thickness/inflammation	**No visual symptoms:** same-day rheumatology. **Visual symptoms:** ophthalmology. 40–60 mg PO **prednisolone** + PPI/bone protection. If visual changes, IV methylprednisolone. Tocilizumab if unresponsive
Angle-closure glaucoma	See *37. ACUTE CHANGE IN OR LOSS OF VISION*		
Endophthalmitis (Fig. 36.1)	**RFs:** recent intravitreal injection/surgery, immuno-suppresion, trauma. **Hx & O/E:** acute subacute reduced acuity, conjunctival injection, pain, hypopyon, poor fundal view	Slit lamp, fundoscopy. USS if no fundal view. Aqueous or vitreous sample for MC&S	Same day ophthalmology. Abx – intravitreal/systemic/topical. Vitrectomy

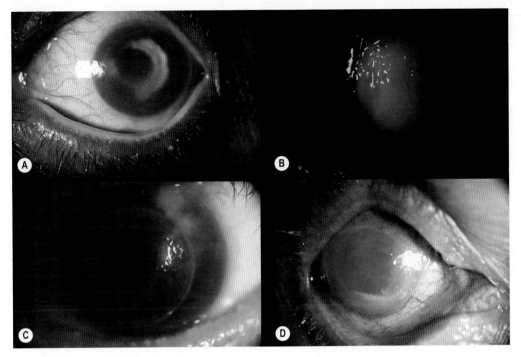

Fig. 36.1 Endophthalmitis after eye surgery. (Reproduced with permission from Robbins CB, Feng HL, Wisely CE, Daluvoy M, Fekrat S. Endophthalmitis after descemet stripping endothelial keratoplasty: microbiological yield and visual outcomes. *Am J Ophthalmol.* 2021;222:34–40.)

For eye pain it is vital to recognise which require immediate ophthalmology assessment. True ocular pain must be distinguished from extra-orbital pain. Key factors which prompt immediate ophthalmology assessment include reduction in visual acuity, marked photophobia, systemic symptoms such as new-onset headache, fever or myalgia and abnormal ophthalmic examination (such as hypopyon, pupillary changes or an abnormal fundus). In the vignette, the history of pain, photophobia and contact lens use, as well as the corneal findings, suggest contact lens-related bacterial keratitis.

REVISION TIPS

1. Eye pain and reduced visual acuity require immediate assessment by ophthalmology
2. Screen for extra-ocular pathology if anterior uveitis is suspected. HLA-B27 disorders mnemonic: PAIR – psoriatic arthritis, anterior uveitis, IBD, reactive arthritis
3. Always consider driving status and onward modes of transport in ophthalmological presentations

37

Acute Change in or Loss of Vision

Lucy Andrews and Vidit Singh

EMERGENCY DEPARTMENT, FEMALE, 66.
LOSS OF VISION, RIGHT EYE

HPC: Gradual onset worsening dull right eye ache, blurry vision, haloes looking at bright lights, nausea and vomiting. Long-sightedness (hypermetropia).
O/E: Diffuse right conjunctival injection, fixed mid-dilated pupil. ↓acuity right eye 6/15 (6/6 left eye).

---

1. A patient with acute eye pain, PMHx ulcerative colitis. O/E there is a hypopyon and an oddly shaped iris. What is the *most likely* diagnosis?
2. A 27-year-old female with blurred 'kaleidoscope' vision, a dull ache behind her left eye and photophobia for 4 hours. Lying down in a quiet space helps. What is the *most likely* cause of the visual disturbance?

Answers: 1. Anterior uveitis. Often HLA B27 haplotype. Associated conditions; ankylosing spondylitis, IBD, reactive arthritis, psoriatic arthropathy. 2. Migraine. Photophobia/ phonophobia, visual disturbance ("zigzags", i.e. visual scotoma). In this case also rule out meningitis.

TABLE 37.1

	Features	Investigations	Management
Painless Loss of Vision			
Retinal detachment	See *33. FLASHES AND FLOATERS IN VISUAL FIELDS*		
Retinal artery occlusion	**RFs:** same as stroke; HTN, smoking, diabetes, etc. **Hx & O/E:** sudden unilateral visual loss ('curtain falling' = amaurosis fugax). Vision loss is complete in central artery occlusion, sectoral in branch occlusion	**CRP/ESR:** r/o atypical (painless) GCA. **Slit lamp:** pale retina, cherry red spot at fovea (Fig. 37.1) ± visible embolus. **Fluorescein angiogram**	Manage underlying RFs. Acute stroke workup. May need injections of VEGF if there is neovascularisation of the retina

TABLE 37.1   (Cont'd)

	Features	Investigations	Management
Painful Loss of Vision			
Optic neuritis	**RFs:** young, female, white. First presentation in 50% of MS cases. Autoimmune conditions (SLE, sarcoid), infection (e.g. Lyme, EBV, syphilis), ethambutol. **Hx & O/E:** acute-subacute pain worse on eye movement, epiphora, reduced acuity/colour vision, relative afferent pupillary defect (RAPD) if unilateral	Optic disc oedema on fundoscopy. Neuro examination. **MRI brain/orbits:** inflamed optic nerve ± demyelination white matter lesions (if MS)	Same day ophthalmology referral if reduced visual acuity. IV/PO steroid, tapered according to response
Acute angle-closure glaucoma	**RFs:** age, hypermetropia, Asian ethnicity, anterior uveitis, FH. **Hx & O/E:** acute pain (nausea, aching), haloes round lights, reduced acuity, conjunctival injection, headache, fixed/dilated pupil, cloudy cornea	**Slit lamp:** cupped disc, shallow anterior chamber, cloudy cornea. **Gonioscopy:** angle closure (Fig. 37.2). IOP (often >40 mmHg, normal 10–21)	Same day ophthalmology. IV acetazolamide, topical beta-blocker (timolol), topical miotic (pilocarpine). Bilateral laser iridotomy
Giant cell arteritis	See *36. EYE PAIN AND DISCOMFORT*		
Acute anterior uveitis	See *35. RED EYE; 36. EYE PAIN AND DISCOMFORT*		

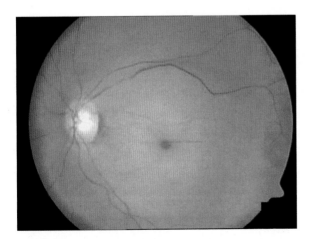

Fig. 37.1 Retinal artery occlusion, with 'cherry red spot' at the macula. (From Fieß A et al. Anterior chamber paracentesis after central retinal artery occlusion: a tenable therapy? *BMC Ophthalmol.* 2014;14:28, Figure 1.)

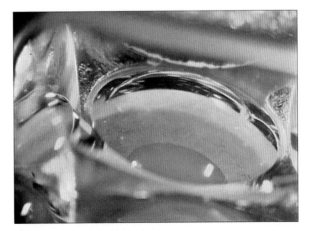

Fig. 37.2 Normal anterior angle on gonioscopy. (Reproduced with permission from Daniel Lee, Edward S. Yung, L. Jay Katz. Clinical Examination of Glaucoma. *Ophthalmology.* Elsevier. 2019.)

The vignette is a classic presentation for acute angle closure glaucoma. She has painful loss of vision, reduced acuity and a fixed, mid-dilated pupil; nausea and vomiting is a common association. Her risk is increased due to her long-sightedness. Further findings included in exam questions are haloes around lights, a hazy cornea, a firm eyeball and symptoms which are worse in the dark. In dim light, the pupil dilates and this worsens the drainage of aqueous humour, thereby worsening symptoms.

REVISION TIPS

- Snellen charts are used to measure visual acuity. Snellen chart measurement of acuity: *numerator* is distance from the chart (6m); *denominator* is distance at which someone with normal vision can read the smallest line the patient can clearly see
- Eye pain and vomiting in an older person – consider acute glaucoma
- Migraine is a contraindication for COCP, which should be stopped/changed accordingly

38

Gradual Loss of Vision

Max Shah, Meijia Xie, and Stella Hristova

OPTOMETRY APPOINTMENT. AFRICAN-AMERICAN, FEMALE, 55. VISION PROGRESSIVELY BLURRIER FOR 12 MONTHS

HPC: Bilateral. No eye redness, discharge or pain. No halos, flashes or floaters. **PMHx:** T2DM, HTN, myopia. **DHx:** Metformin. **FHx:** Sister chronic glaucoma, mother diabetes.

O/E: BP 130/80, CBG 6.8 mmol. Afebrile. Peripheral vision loss in both eyes.

1. What is the key finding on fundoscopy that suggests open-angle glaucoma?
2. What is the definitive treatment for wet age related macular degeneration (AMD)?
3. What is the most common cause of curable blindness in the UK?

Answers: 1. Optic disc cupping. 2. Anti-VEGF drugs (e.g. ranibizumab, bevacizumab and aflibercept). 3. Cataracts.

TABLE 38.1

	Features	Investigations	Management
Primary open-angle glaucoma	**RFs:** ↑IOP, age 40+, FHx, DM, HTN. African American > Hispanic > Caucasian. **Hx & O/E:** detected during routine eye tests. Can cause peripheral vision loss; tunnel vision, even complete loss. Painless optic neuropathy ± ↑IOP.	**Slit lamp, fundoscopy:** optic disc cupping (diagnostic) and pallor. **Tonometry:** ↑IOP (normal 12–22 mmHg). Visual fields assessment. OCT	**Topical:** prostaglandins (latanoprost), β-blockers (timolol), α2-agonists (brimonidine), carbonic anhydrase inhibitors (dorzolamide), miotics (pilocarpine). **Systemic:** CAIs (acetazolamide). **Surgical:** laser trabeculoplasty, trabeculectomy, other glaucoma shunt/drainage
Diabetic retinopathy (Fig. 38.1)	Can be non-proliferative versus proliferative (neovascularisation due to retinal ischaemia); maculopathy (blurred central vision). Sequelae – vitreous haemorrhage, retinal detachment	**Slit lamp, fundoscopy:** microaneurysms, haemorrhages, venous changes, cotton wool spots, exudates, new vessels. Photography, OCT, fluorescein angiography	Optimise glycaemic control and BP. Yearly diabetic eye screening. Depending on disease: pan-retinal laser photocoagulation/anti-VEGF injections/macular laser/retinal surgery

(Continued)

TABLE 38.1   (Cont'd)

	Features	Investigations	Management
Cataracts – *clouding of the natural crystalline lens*	Most common: age-related (other causes, incl. congenital). **RFs:** UV exposure, DM, smoking, trauma, eye surgery. **Hx & O/E:** gradual ↓VA, glare, ↓contrast sensitivity, poorer vision in the dark	**Slit lamp, fundoscopy:** lens opacification (leukocoria/no red reflex in advanced cataract)	Correct refractive error induced by cataracts – glasses/contact lenses. Surgery if affecting QOL, e.g. phacoemulsification (most common in the UK)
Age-related macular degeneration (AMD)	*Dry:* 'wear and tear' drusen deposits. *Wet:* neovascular membrane causing a bleed/ leak. **RFs:** age 70+, Caucasians, smoking, FHx, IHD. *Dry* (90%): slow, milder symptoms. *Wet* (10%): acute/subacute visual decline, straight lines appear wavy	Painless decline in central vision. **Slit lamp, fundoscopy.** *Dry:* drusen, atrophy. *Wet:* haemorrhages. Amsler grid test. OCT, fluorescein angiography	*Dry:* monitoring, zinc with vitamins A, C and E to reduce risk of progression. *Wet:* anti-VEGF injections; surgery (if severe bleed)
Refractive error	Myopia, hypermetropia, astigmatism, presbyopia	Rule out other causes, complete eye exam	Monitor. Corrective glasses and lenses
Neurological	CVE or space-occupying lesion along/near visual pathways, e.g. pituitary adenoma affecting chiasm can lead to bitemporal hemianopia	Complete eye exam. Eye movements (check for diplopia). Formal visual field test. Imaging CT/MRI	Management depending on findings. Stroke or neurosurgical referral. MDT
Other Differentials			
Retinitis pigmentosa	Loss of photoreceptors. Hereditary. Onset childhood to 30s–50 s. Night blindness. Gradual peripheral vision loss, then central	**Slit lamp, fundoscopy:** black or brown pigments, mottling around retina. Tonometry (r/o glaucoma). Electroretinogram	Vision aids. Referral to specialist. Genetic counselling. Manage sequelae
Choroidal melanoma (Fig. 38.2)	Intraocular tumour. **RFs:** fair skin, UV exposure, sunbeds. **Hx & O/E:** often asymptomatic initially; ↓VA, scotomas, flashes. Complications: retinal detachment	**Slit lamp, fundoscopy:** pigmented dome-shaped lesion ± exudative retinal detachment. Ophthalmic USS, OCT, fluorescein angiography	Radiotherapy. Photocoagulation. Surgical – e.g. enucleation. Chemotherapy in metastatic disease

VA, visual acuity.

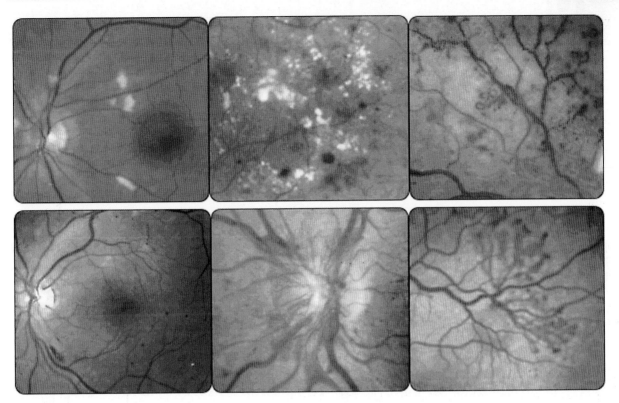

Fig. 38.1 Fundoscopy features of diabetic retinopathy. Top row; cotton wool spots *(left)*, hard exudates *(middle)*, intraretinal arteriovenous shunts *(right)*. Bottom row; microaneurysms *(left)*, disc neovascularisation *(middle)*, neovascularisation elsewhere *(right)*. (Reproduced with permission from https://www.clinicalkey.com/#!/content/clinical_overview/67-s2.0-c5d3a746-a502-42f3-96ac-c0f-5c5edb480?scrollTo=%2367-s2.0-c5d3a746-a502-42f3-96ac-c0f5c5edb480-5bc6267a-87e7-4df8-9ad8-09ba322d7779-annotated).

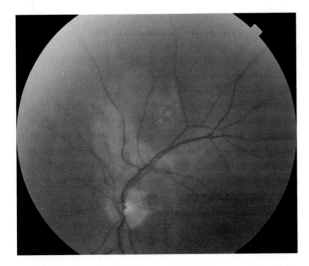

Fig. 38.2 Choroidal melanoma, 7 mm diameter, 2 mm thickness. (Reproduced with permission from Jay S. Duker. Choroidal Melanoma. Atlas of Retinal *OCT: Optical Coherence. Tomography.* Elsevier. 2018.

Driving advice is needed for all vision impairments. The vignette is typical of primary open-angle glaucoma, which leads to painless, insidious peripheral vision loss often picked up at a routine optometrist appointment. Cataracts are common in older people and profoundly affect vision in general, and may cause some drop in contrast sensitivity. Diabetic retinopathy is a crucial differential. AMD is also important, needing urgent ophthalmology due to rapid progression.

REVISION TIPS

- Aide-mémoire for mechanisms of action of glaucoma medications:
  1. The P's 'Pout' = Pilocarpine/Prostaglandin analogoues increase eveoscleral outflow
  2. Drugs reducing aqueous humour hold BAC – Beta-blockers, Alpha-2 agonists, Carbonic anhydrase inhibitors

39

Facial/Periorbital Swelling

Christian Aquilina and Vidit Singh

HPC: 3 days of mild pain and malaise. Mild upper respiratory infection in the preceding week. No change in vision, fevers or rigors.

O/E: Temperature 37°C, HR/RR/BP/saturations normal. Swelling and erythema in both lids of right eye and adjacent tissue, no discharge. No conjunctival redness, pupils normal, normal painless movements of the eye.

1. What is the cause of proptosis in the vignette? Can you name any other causes of proptosis?
2. When are children vaccinated against mumps in the UK?

Answers: 1. The vignette describes periorbital cellulitis. Other causes; orbital cellulitis, Graves' disease, retrobulbar haematoma, tumour (e.g. neuroblastoma), cavernous sinus thrombosis. 2. As part of the MMR vaccine (1st dose at 12 months and 2nd dose pre-school).

TABLE 39.1

	Features	Investigations	Management
Allergic reaction	RFs: recent exposure to new food/drugs/creams, known allergies. Hx & O/E: swelling rapid onset, painful/itchy urticaria, wheals. *Anaphylaxis*: airway swelling (tongue/pharynx/larynx), stridor, difficulty breathing, wheeze, vomiting, circulatory collapse/shock	Clinical diagnosis	Remove trigger. **Allergic reaction:** antihistamine ± oral corticosteroid. **Rapidly developing oedema;** IV/IM hydrocortisone + chlorphenamine. **Anaphylaxis;** establish airway, IM adrenaline 1:1000, O_2, IV chlorphenamine, IV hydrocortisone, nebulised salbutamol
Dental abscess	RFs: poor dental hygiene, previous dental problems, broken teeth. Hx & O/E: throbbing pain (↑ when eating, drinking cold/hot drinks), unpleasant taste, facial swelling, gum swelling/discharge	Usually, clinical diagnosis. Blood cultures/bloods if febrile/septic. OPG x-ray	Analgesia. If systemically unwell, admit under MaxFax. Abx (follow local guidelines, e.g IV co-amoxiclav if not penicillin allergic). May need I&D. F/U with dentist on discharge

TABLE 39.1 (Cont'd)

	Features	Investigations	Management
Preseptal (periorbital) cellulitis	**RFs:** recent local infection (URTI, infected stye, insect bite), age (<10 years old), trauma, sinusitis, eye surgery, dental abscess. **Hx & O/E:** swollen/painful eyelid or periorbital tissues, fever, malaise	Clinical diagnosis, unless worried about orbital cellulitis (see below). No proptosis, normal eye movements and acuity	Same day referral to ophthalmology and ENT. Oral antibiotics (follow local guidelines (e.g. co-amoxiclav if not penicillin allergic)). Admit if systemically unwell. In children admit and treat as orbital cellulitis until proven otherwise. Consider nasal douching and intranasal steroids (ENT input)
Orbital cellulitis	**RFs:** as per preseptal cellulitis. **Hx & O/E:** as above plus; conjunctival injection, chemosis, proptosis, limited/painful eye movement, blurred/double vision, relative afferent pupillary defect (RAPD) progression to involve CNS	Acuity may be impaired. Blood cultures/bloods required. **CT orbit/sinus/brain:** assess location/spread	Same day referral to ophthalmology and ENT IV antibiotics (follow local guidelines. E.g. cefuroxime/ ceftriaxone + metronidazole). ENT/ophthalmology assessment for abscess drainage. Consider nasal douching and intranasal steroids (ENT input)
Mumps	**RFs:** no previous immunisation/ infection. Recent exposure. **Hx & O/E:** non-specific viral prodrome, parotitis (95%) – often bilateral; pain on talking/chewing, fever	Clinical diagnosis. Saliva IgM mumps antibody or PCR. **Complications:** orchitis, oophoritis, aseptic meningitis	Self-limiting (1–2 weeks). Avoid school for at least 5 days from start of swelling. Analgesia and ice packs for pain
Trauma	**RFs:** traumatic injury to the face. **Hx & O/E:** bruising, subconjunctival haemorrhage. Exophthalmos, visual changes, restricted eye movements, focal neurology. Misalignment of teeth/trismus suggests mandible fracture	CT head and facial bones	Referral to ENT/MaxFax for bony facial injuries. Ophthalmology if concerns of rectus entrapment/acute vision loss/globe injury
Ludwig's angina	Sublingual/submaxillary/ submandibular rapidly spreading cellulitis. Dental source common. Fever and systemic toxicity. Airway obstruction; risk of asphyxiation	Priority to **ensure the airway is secure**, potentially by intubation, then for **contrast CT of neck, bloods**	Involve ENT/MaxFax/anaesthetist SpR/consultant quickly. Patient to be placed in resus. Measures to ensure airway patent. Systemic antibiotics and aggressive surgical intervention (untreated mortality 50%)

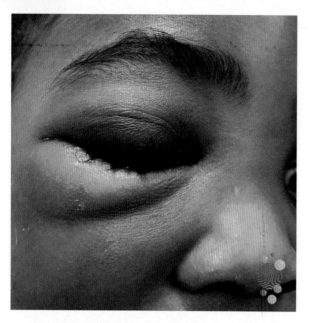

Fig. 39.1 Periorbital cellulitis. (Skin Deep. https://dftbskindeep. com/diagnoses-gallery/#!jig[1]/ML/3644)

Detailed examination differentiates between periorbital and orbital cellulitis; in the vignette, the lack of systemic symptoms and an otherwise normal appearing eye make periorbital cellulitis the likely diagnosis (Fig. 39.1). Generally, the assessment of facial swelling potentially involves several different specialties. Examination needs to be directed to identify the underlying structure and hence form a more accurate differential, as some conditions can be life-threatening.

REVISION TIPS

- If evidence of periorbital infection and ANY change in vision/eye movements, assume orbital cellulitis
- Periorbital is far more common than orbital cellulitis
- Bilateral parotid swelling in child/young adult: consider mumps or bulimia (excessive salivation due to vomiting)

40

Breathlessness

Tejas Netke, Gregory Oxenham, and Rada Ivanov

EMERGENCY DEPARTMENT, MALE, 51. BREATHLESSNESS 36 HOURS

HPC: Presents today as difficult to work (construction worker). Right-sided chest pain, worse on inspiration, relieved with paracetamol. No cough, wheeze, fevers, rash or change in sense of taste/smell. He is generally fit and well. **PMHx:** HTN. **SHx:** Current smoker (15-year pack history). **DHx:** Ramipril.

  O/E: Alert and comfortable at rest, tachypnoeic. Saturations 96%. HR 110, RR 30 and BP 135/80. Chest expansion is equal bilaterally. Hyper-resonance on the right upper zone of the chest, with reduced breath sounds. There is no evidence of a DVT.

1. What is your differential for a patient with chronic breathlessness, haemoptysis and weight loss?
2. What is your differential in chronic breathlessness, crackles at the lung bases and evidence of right heart failure?

Answers: 1. Most likely lung cancer (history of smoking/asbestos exposure) or TB (at-risk group or from endemic area). 2. Pulmonary fibrosis or congestive cardiac failure – distinguishing the velcro crackles of pulmonary fibrosis from wet CHF crackles may be difficult.

TABLE 40.1

	Features	Investigations	Management
Acute Breathlessness			
Acute asthma exacerbation	See *183. WHEEZE*		
Exacerbation of COPD (COPD, See *185. COUGH*)	**RFs:** winter, smoking, severe baseline/long-term O_2 therapy (LTOT), unvaccinated (pneumococcus, flu) genetics (α1AT). **Hx & O/E:** SOB at rest, increased sputum volume/colour change, use of accessory muscles, ↑RR, wheeze; may see fever, cyanosis, also drowsiness in type2 respiratory failure (T2RF). Patients may already have commenced a 'rescue pack' of antibiotics and steroids	Bloods as for asthma, usually no eosinophilia. **VBG/ABG:** assess CO_2 retention. **CXR:** hyperexpanded; assess for pneumothorax/consolidation. **Sputum ± blood cultures:** *Haemophilus influenzae*, *Streptococcus pneumoniae*, *Moraxella catarrhalis*. Frequent exacerbations: prolonged sputum culture (non-TB mycobacteria/*Pseudomonas*). 80% non-infective	O_2 target 88%–92% if known CO retainer; may have severe respiratory. acidosis requiring escalation. **Salbutamol nebulisers ± ipratropium nebulisers ± oral prednisolone/IV hydrocortisone.** **Infection:** Abx, e.g. amoxicillin/clarithromycin. NIV if acute T2RF (senior decision). DECAF score

(Continued)

TABLE 40.1 (Cont'd)

	Features	Investigations	Management
Acute Breathlessness			
Pneumonia	**RFs:** age, COPD, smoking, immunosuppression, cystic fibrosis, bronchiectasis, DM, winter, unvaccinated. **Hx & O/E:** purulent cough, fever, dyspnoea, wheeze, haemoptysis, myalgia, pain (pleurisy). Tachypnoea, localised dull percussion, reduced breath sounds, bronchial breathing. *'Atypical':* dry cough, flu-like, bilateral pneumonia, deranged LFTs/U&Es, immunosuppression	↑WCC/CRP, ± ↑lactate **CXR:** consolidation. Repeat in 6/52 to ensure resolution vs any underlying pathology. Blood/sputum culture. COVID/flu swab: if clinical concern. **Calculate CURB65 score:** 1 point each for; confusion, urea >7 mmol/L, respiratory rate ≥30, BP (DBP ≤60 OR SBP ≤90), Age >65. Legionella/pneumococcal urinary antigens ± respiratory virus screen	CURB65: 0 = PO Abx (e.g. amoxicillin) in community. CURB65: 1–2 = may need hospital admission. CURB65: 3 = admit, may require IV Abx (e.g. co-amoxiclav/clarithromycin) ± HDU/ICU. Also admit if: Abx resistances, young child, frailty, co-morbidities, failure of oral Abx
PE	**RFs:** malignancy, immobilisation, personal/FHx of VTE, surgery, pregnancy, COVID-19. **Hx & O/E:** pleuritic chest pain, SOB, haemoptysis, signs of DVT, tachycardia, low saturations, collapse	**Wells' score:** ≤4 perform a D-dimer, >4 requires CTPA D-dimer <500 in 'low risk' patients <50 years old rules out PE. Older than 50, 10× age is upper limit of normal. D-dimer > upper limit. **CTPA. V/Q scan** (if GFR <30, contrast allergy). **ECG:** sinus tachycardia, *'S1Q3T3'* rarely seen; R heart strain, p-pulmonale; RAD	O_2 (aim 94%–98%) **Stable:** DOAC (provoked: 3 months, unprovoked: 6 months). **Unstable:** UF heparin + thrombolysis. Thrombectomy or IVC filters may be considered.
Pneumothorax	**RFs:** smoker-tall, thin young man. Respiratory (COPD), interstitial lung disease, connective tissue disorder. Altitude. Iatrogenic (ventilation/intervention). **Hx & O/E:** SOB, pleuritic pain. Hypoxia, hyper-resonant, absent breath sounds on affected side, surgical emphysema. Trachea deviated if *tensioning*	Tension suspected clinically, prioritise decompression. **CXR:** lucency between chest wall and lung parenchyma. **FAST scan:** absence of lung sliding. Clotting/FBC before non-urgent drain	**Oxygen.** **Tension:** 14–16 G cannula second inter-costal space, mid-clavicular line, then chest drain. **Non-tension:** observe/aspirate/chest drain. BTS guidelines
Chronic Breathlessness			
Lung cancer	See *185. COUGH*		
Congestive cardiac failure	See *8. PERIPHERAL OEDEMA AND ANKLE SWELLING*		
Bronchiectasis	See *185. COUGH*		

TABLE 40.1 (Cont'd)

	Features	Investigations	Management
Interstitial lung disease	RFs: occupation/environment, connective tissue diseases, drug or radiation injury, sarcoidosis, idiopathic. Hx & O/E: chronic dry cough, exertional dyspnoea. End-expiratory 'Velcro' crackles at lung bases, clubbing, cyanosis	Spirometry: restrictive pattern, reduced transfer factor. CXR: bilateral lower zone fibrosis. High-resolution CT chest: subpleural honeycombing, ground glass, traction bronchiectasis	Smoking cessation, pulmonary rehab., LTOT. Steroids (connective tissue diseases/sarcoid). Anti-fibrotics: Pirfenidone or nintedanib. Lung transplant possible. Often palliative
Other Panic attacks	Sudden, unprovoked – history of anxiety. Tightness, dizzy, tachycardia, hyperventilation ± tingling in peripheries	*Diagnosis of exclusion.* Blood gas = respiratory alkalosis	Reassurance (talking therapy, SSRIs)

PE, Pulmonary embolism.

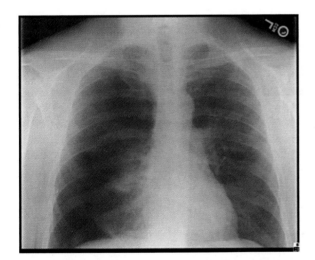

Fig. 40.1 Right-sided pneumothorax. (Reproduced with permission from Fitch RW, Williams J. Evaluation and management of traumatic conditions in the athlete. *Sports Med Clin.* 2019: Figure 9. © 2019 Elsevier Inc.)

In this vignette, acute dyspnoea and hyper-resonance on percussion in combination with reduced air entry indicate pneumothorax. CXR may show linear shadow of visceral pleura with lack of lung markings peripheral to the shadow (Fig. 40.1). Recently practice has moved towards more conservative management of these, with either watchful waiting or needle aspiration. However, a chest drain is likely to be needed for the pneumothorax in Fig. 40.1. Any haemodynamic instability (hypotension, persistent tachycardia, reduced cardiac output, distended JVP, etc.) should prompt immediate decompression; tracheal deviation is a late sign in tension pneumothorax.

REVISION TIPS

- Any patient with breathlessness will eventually need a CXR, **but initial treatment is the higher priority in tension pneumothorax**
- Dry cough, deranged LFT/U&E – think atypical pneumonia
- Normal ECG does not rule out PE

41

Deteriorating Patient – Outline

Harriet Diment, David Roberts, and Alexander Reed

Common causes for becoming acutely unwell in the hospital setting include **sepsis, MI, PE, hypoglycaemia and bleeding**. Critically ill patients are those with physiological derangements that pose an imminent threat to life. Deteriorating patients often (but not always) exhibit progressive physiological derangement, which may progress to cardiorespiratory arrest. Vital signs are key physiological parameters, so basic observations and warning scores are sensitive for deterioration – though not specific for the cause (e.g. tachypnoea occurs in several conditions).

Management (Table 41.1 and Fig. 41.1) follows the principles of:
1. **Supportive care** (the ABCDE approach)
2. **Structured diagnostic approach** to determine the underlying pathology
3. **Specific treatment** directed at the underlying pathology (e.g. the sepsis 6)

The Resuscitation Council UK has produced guidelines on intermediate and advanced life support (ILS/ALS) and all doctors should be familiar with its application (see **43. CARDIORESPIRATORY ARREST**)

TABLE 41.1 A–E Assessment
Danger Ensure personal safety Don protective equipment
Response If a patient responds to voice normally, they have patent airway, are breathing, and have brain perfusion. Lack of response indicates critical illness and/or cardiorespiratory arrest. If the patient looks unwell, call for help immediately.
Airway • Is the airway patent? Check if the patient can breathe, speak and swallow normally. • If not: Can the airway be maintained with positioning or airway manoeuvres? Do so immediately. Suction or remove any FB or secretions that can be done so easily. • Is the airway obstructed or at risk of obstruction? Look for indrawing (supraclavicular, subcostal) or paradoxical movements; look for FBs in the mouth and cyanosis. • Listen to the sound of breathing – calm and quiet versus strained and noisy? Stridor, snoring, gurgling, no sound (complete obstruction)? *Actions: Suction of secretions.* *Airway manoeuvres/adjuncts.* *Administer high-flow oxygen.* *Attach pulse oximetry and measure RR.* *Experts may consider tracheal intubation for a compromised airway. Non-experts should support the airway while ensuring expert assistance is en route*

TABLE 41.1 A–E Assessment (Cont'd)

Breathing

- Assess the adequacy of ventilation. Rapid, shallow breathing pattern versus settled (10–16 bpm) and adequate volume breaths.
- Look for signs of respiratory distress and increased work of breathing. Listen for reduced breath sounds, wheeze, crackles and percussion resonance.
- Is this patient at risk of tiring or struggling to clear their secretion load? If so, escalation of support may be required. Refer early.
- Determine the cause of respiratory difficulty. Is there a lung pathology or is the ventilatory difficulty being driven by another process, e.g. sepsis.

Actions: Administer high-flow oxygen.

Support breathing with a bag-valve mask through an open airway if breathing is inadequate.

Obtain a blood gas and order a portable chest x-ray

Circulation

Life threatening – shock (hypovolaemia/sepsis/anaphylaxis/cardiogenic)

- Clinical assessment of cardiac output and shock:
  Measure HR and BP (noting the MAP).
  Assessment for haemorrhage, e.g. haematemesis, external bleed, melaena.
  Assessment of skin (temperature and CRT).
  Pulses for rate, rhythm and volume (assessing the quality of a pulse requires palpating more central pulses).
  Rapid assessment for other organ dysfunction (neurological dysfunction, renal dysfunction).
- Further assessment for cardiac disease or pathology includes:
  Examination of the heart including auscultation.
  Examination of neck veins for distension.
  12 lead ECG and continuous ECG monitoring.
  Bedside ECHO for tamponade/assessment of global cardiac function.

Actions: HR, BP, ECG and continuous monitoring.

Gain large bore IV access and send bloods for FBC/Coag/G&S/U&Es/troponin/VBG.

Fluid challenge may be indicated (250–1000 mL bolus of crystalloid). Measure urine output, and begin fluid balance chart. Catheterise as necessary.

Vaso-active support: repeated fluid boluses are often an indication for review by a higher level of care, as the underlying issue is not resolving.

Specific treatments for the underlying cause, e.g. cardioversion of malignant dysrhythmias, antibiotics in sepsis, drainage of pericardial effusion in tamponade, reperfusion for myocardial ischaemia

Disability

There are two major things to determine in all patients:

- What is the level of consciousness? Use GCS or AVPU (alert, verbal, pain, unresponsive).
- Are there lateralising signs of focal neurology? Look for pupil size and reactivity. Is there a difference in response to pain between the right and left?

If there is a deficit, think about what the cause could be (e.g. intracranial event: vascular event, trauma, infection, cerebral oedema, endocrine and metabolic derangement, toxins and poisoning). FAST (Facial drooping, Arm weakness, Speech difficulties, Time to call)

Actions: AVPU/GCS.

Glucose – CBG <4 mmol/L requires immediate replacement.

CT head if FAST positive, focal neurology, clinical concern for bleed/stroke.

Consider: LP, MRI, EEG

(Continued)

TABLE 41.1   A–E Assessment (Cont'd)

Exposure
- To examine the patient properly, full exposure of the body may be necessary. Respect the patient's dignity and minimise heat loss.

Actions: Check for trauma, bleeding and rashes.
Check for temperature.
Examine the abdomen – abdominal catastrophes are a common cause of multisystem dysfunction.

Further actions
- Organise investigations.
- Review the notes, drug chart and trends of vital signs.
- Institute specific treatments.
- Consider escalation of care to higher levels (HDU/ICU) for monitoring and organ support.
- Reassess the patient immediately and at regular intervals thereafter

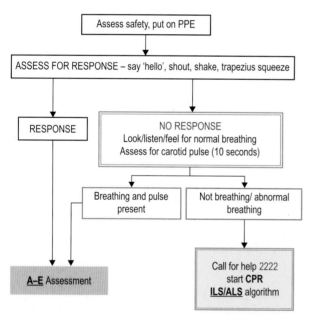

Fig. 41.1 Flow chart of when to use A–E compared to ALS/ILS. (Illustration by Dr Harriet Diment.)

REVISION TIPS

- Some patients may not exhibit vital sign derangements in significant illness, e.g. lack of hypotension in compensating young/fit individuals, absence of tachycardia in elderly/those on β-blockers
- Airway obstruction is a medical emergency; in the majority of cases, simple methods of airway management are all that is required initially
- Reduced level of consciousness (classically taught as GCS 8 or less) may be associated with loss of protective airway reflexes and/or airway obstruction

42

Shock and Low Blood Pressure

Harriet Diment, David Roberts, and Alexander Reed

EMERGENCY DEPARTMENT, MALE, 68. UNCONSCIOUS

HPC: 1-hour history of sudden onset, central, heavy chest pain radiating to both arms and back; associated with nausea, SOB, sweating. Witnessed by wife becoming more breathless and confused before losing consciousness. **PMHx:** HTN, T2DM, hyperlipidaemia, gout, smoker (25 pack-years). **DHx:** atorvastatin, allopurinol, ramipril, amlodipine, bendroflumethiazide.

O/E: SpO_2 90% peripherally (poor intermittent trace), RR 24, HR 115 bpm regular rhythm, cool and clammy, central capillary refill time prolonged >5s, BP 80/45 mmHg (MAP 57 mmHg), E1V1M1 GCS3, HS I+II, dilated neck veins, widespread crackles, abdomen soft.

1. What is the most likely diagnosis in the vignette?
2. What are some important priorities for investigation and management of this case?
3. Name several other causes of low or labile blood pressure not associated with shock?

Answers: 1. Acute MI with profound cardiogenic shock. However, exclude subarachnoid haemorrhage and dissection, as it is unusual for an MI to cause such severe loss of consciousness. 2. Bedside echo may identify if MI is more likely; angiography should then precede CT. If not, immediate CT brain, neck and chest (to exclude SAH/dissection). 3. iatrogenic (medications, e.g. anti-hypertensives), Parkinson's disease/MSA, parasympathetic dysautonomia (DM, alcohol, MS, autoimmune (SLE/Sjogren's))

TABLE 42.1

	Features	Investigations	Management
Hypovolaemic Shock			
Haemorrhagic shock	**Trauma** Major blood loss. **Ruptured AAA:** abdo pain (often radiates to back or flanks), expansile mass. **GI haemorrhage:** haematemesis, melena. **PPH:** 4Ts – Tone (atony); Trauma (laceration, inversion, rupture); Tissue (retained); Thrombin (coagulopathy)	**Urgent bloods:** FBC, U&E, VBG (to define acid-base disturbance, calcium deficiency and other problems), LFTs, **G&S/CM, coagulation tests**	Haemostasis (pressure, surgery), reverse anticoagulants, tranexamic acid. Frugal crystalloids until blood products available; 'like for like' RBCs/platelets/FFP/cryoprecipitate; major haemorrhage protocol. Resuscitation to recover; heart rate, BP, appearance
Fluid losses other than whole blood	**RFs:** very young, very elderly. Burns, diarrhoea, vomiting, polyuria, hyperthermia	U&E, electrolytes, amylase, lipase. Lund and Browder chart for %TBSA burned	IV fluid resuscitation with crystalloid 10–15 mL/kg bolus. Treat underlying cause

(Continued)

TABLE 42.1 (Cont'd)

	Features	Investigations	Management
Cardiogenic Shock			
Acute heart failure with shock	MI. Acute on chronic heart failure. Dysrhythmias (palpitations, light-headedness, syncope). Valvular e.g. endocarditis, MI complication, congenital, degenerative. Congenital heart disease	12-lead **ECG**, cardiac monitoring. Troponins, BNP, U&E. **ABG:** low oxygen levels. CXR. **Echocardiography. Angiography**	Treat underlying cause. Fluid administration (not excessive). Early referral to critical care: inotropic drugs, mechanical assist devices, intra-aortic balloon pump and ECMO to bridge patients to definitive management, e.g. PCI, surgery, transplantation
Obstructive			
Massive PE	RV dysfunction and hypotension; pleuritic chest pain, tachycardia, DVT, hypoxia, PE RFs	**ECG:** often tachycardia **CXR:** wedge shape PE. **Blood gas. Echocardiography:** RV dysfunction/dilation	If haemodynamically unstable – thrombolysis in the absence of contraindications
Cardiac tamponade	**Cardiac Tamponade:** Beck's triad (muffled heart sounds, raised JVP, hypotension), pulsus paradoxus, SOB. Tamponade in trauma is usually due to penetrating injury	**CXR:** globular heart (pericardial effusion). **ECG:** often tachycardia, electrical alternans in pericardial effusion, small volume complexes. **Bedside ECHO:** pericardial fluid, RV diastolic collapse/fixed dilated IVC	Urgent pericardiocentesis (Fig. 42.1) – temporary measure. May need thoracotomy and pericardiotomy. ED thoracotomy – usually in context of penetrating trauma
Tension pneumo-thorax	Respiratory distress, distended neck veins, tracheal deviation, hyper-resonant percussion note, reduced breath sounds		Immediate needle decompression followed by chest tube insertion
Distributive			
Septic shock	**RFs:** very young/old, IVDU, immunosuppressed, indwelling lines, surgery. Chest/abdomen/urine/skin/soft tissues/joints/CNS. **Hx & O/E:** new confusion, febrile, malaise, rash (bacteraemia with septic emboli). Warm, well-perfused, bounding pulse initially, then skin mottling, reduced peripheral pulses.	**SEPSIS 6** – aide memoire *Give 3*: IV broad-spectrum antibiotics, IV fluids, supplemental O_2 (to achieve SpO_2 >94% or 88%–92% in patients at risk of T2RF). *Take 3*: blood cultures (and other microbiology), measure serial serum lactates, monitor urine output. Blood gas, U&E, CRP, FBC, LFT, clotting screen, culture Investigations guided by possible sources, e.g. XR, CT, aspirations, echocardiograph. **Source control:** abscesses and collections must be urgently drained following supportive medical treatment. **Critical care support:** balance of IV fluids and vasoactive support – central venous access, intra-arterial BP monitoring	

TABLE 42.1   (Cont'd)

	Features	Investigations	Management
Anaphylactic shock		See *53. ANAPHYLAXIS*	
Neurogenic shock	**Spinal cord injury:** loss of sympathetic tone. Vasodilation and variably bradycardia if above T1–T4 (due to cardiac accelerator nerve involvement). Potentially respiratory failure (usually above T6). High cervical injuries likely to have neurogenic shock	**Trauma CT** (head, neck, chest, abdomen, pelvis). Later: **MRI spine.** **12-lead ECG** and 3-lead ECG cardiac monitoring	C-spine immobilisation. Critical care input early: IV fluids, positively chronotropic and vasoactive agents should be utilised in vasoplegia and bradycardia to minimise secondary ischaemic injury of the brain and spinal cord. Urgent transfer to specialist spinal centre or spinal surgeons for early spinal cord decompression

PE, pulmonary embolus.

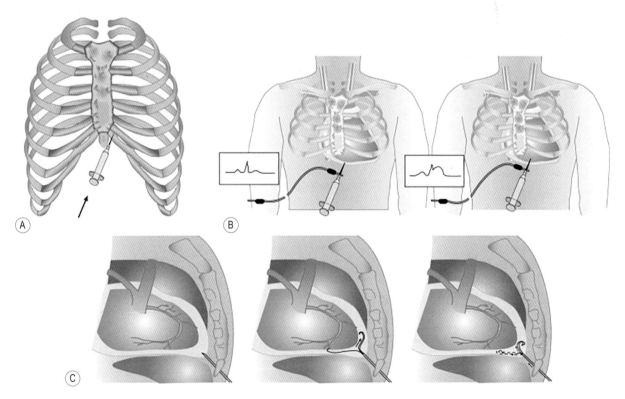

Fig. 42.1 Pericardiocentesis. (A) Subxiphoid approach. (B) A pericardial needle with ECG connection is advanced left lateral to the subxiphoid area aiming towards the left shoulder. ST-segment elevation is seen when the needle touches the epicardium; the needle is then retracted slightly. (C) A guidewire is introduced, the needle is removed, and a catheter is inserted over the guidewire. (Adapted with permission from https://www.clinicalkey.com/#!/content/book/3-s2.0-B9780323446761000066?scrollTo=%233-s2.0-B9780323446761000066-f006-005-9780323446761) Tilak K.R. Pasala, Vladimir Jelnin and Carlos E. Ruiz. Pericardial Tamponade: Clinical Presentation, Diagnosis, and Catheter-Based Therapies Critical Care Medicine: Principles of Diagnosis and Management in the Adult, 6, 72–79.e2.

Shock is circulatory failure associated with inadequate oxygen utilisation by the cells. Hypotension is common and is not always associated with shock state. Causes of shock are categorised into hypovolaemic, cardiogenic, obstructive and distributive. Poor perfusion means skin and extremities are cold and mottled, and neurological state is affected (confused, aggressive, comatose). Palpation of pulses is unreliable for estimating arterial BP. The three components of emergency management are: 1. Supportive care – resuscitation including crystalloids (or blood if indicated) ± vaso-active support. 2. Determine the cause. 3. Specific management of the underlying cause. Excessive fluid therapy in patients without hypovolaemia is likely to lead to harm. As a rule of thumb, after 30 mL/kg of fluid, consider vaso-active support (vasopressor or inotropic medication) in a critical care environment.

REVISION TIPS

- Shock – circulatory failure resulting in inadequate organ perfusion. Defined by systolic BP <90 or MAP <65 with evidence of inadequate organ perfusion, e.g. low urine output, mottling, rising lactate
- Management; supportive care (ABCDE approach) to stabilise, structured diagnostic approach (history, exam, specific investigations for diagnosis) and management of the underlying issue
- IV fluids can harm in large volumes, reassess if you have reached 30 mL/kg

43

Cardiorespiratory Arrest

Lucy Andrews and Chetna Kohli

HPC: Admitted with episode of unstable angina, awaiting angiography ± coronary stenting. **PMHx:** angina, HTN. **DHx:** ramipril, atorvastatin, aspirin, GTN PRN. **SHx:** ex-smoker (10-pack year).

O/E: Unresponsive to voice/pain, no palpable pulse, occasional raspy breath sounds. **Adult cardiac arrest call** is made.

1. What is the most likely cause of a cardiorespiratory arrest following an MI 6/52 ago with recent pleuritic chest pain, increasing SOB and fever?
2. Which metabolic disturbances might lead to cardiorespiratory arrest?

Answers: 1. Dressler's syndrome; inflammatory pericarditis around 6 weeks post-MI, leading to pericardial effusion and potentially cardiac tamponade. Bedside echo shows collapse of the RV during diastole in the presence of a pericardial effusion; treatment is pericardiocentesis (Fig. 42.1). 2. Hypo-/hyperkalaemia, metabolic acidosis (e.g. sepsis, DKA), hypoglycaemia, hypocalcaemia, hypomagnesaemia.

TABLE 43.1

	Features	Investigations	Management
The Ts			
Thrombus – pulmonary	RFs: malignancy/recent surgery, recent DVT, preceding SOB	ECG: sinus tachycardia, RV strain, RAD, widespread ST-segment depression if massive PE, rarely S1Q3T3. CTPA: thrombus in pulmonary arteries ± lung infarct	Thrombolysis (unless contraindicated-see below)
Thrombus – cardiac	Central, crushing chest pain, sweaty, clammy	ECG: ST elevation/depression with reciprocal changes. Angiogram: coronary thrombus	If return of spontaneous circulation (ROSC) → PCI. Consider thrombolysis if PCI is unavailable

(Continued)

TABLE 43.1   (Cont'd)

	Features	Investigations	Management
Tamponade	See *42. SHOCK AND LOW BLOOD PRESSURE*		
Tension pneumothorax	See *40. BREATHLESSNESS*		
Toxins	See *51. POISONING; 52. OVERDOSE*	Administer antidotes promptly, where available. TCAs, CCBs and β-blockers are important in overdose-induced cardiorespiratory arrest. Prolonged CPR often warranted	
The Hs			
Hypovolemia	See *42. SHOCK AND LOW BLOOD PRESSURE*		
Hypokalaemia	RFs: vomiting/diarrhoea, eating disorder, diuretics. Hx & O/E: asymptomatic or may have myalgia, fatigue, weakness	VBG: potassium of <3.5. ECG: U waves, flattened T waves, prolonged PR interval, ST depression, SVT/VT/VF/torsade	IV potassium (diluted in saline)
Hyperkalaemia	See *180. HYPERKALAEMIA*		
Hypoxia	RFs: respiratory failure/asphyxia/drowning. Respiratory arrest is commonest cause in child. Cyanosis, confusion/agitation	↓ SpO_2 ABG: ↓PaO_2; ↑/↓ $PaCO_2$ CXR: may show consolidation, oedema, collapse, effusion, etc.	Oxygen: 15 L/min via non-rebreather. Consider NIV. If low GCS or respiratory effort tiring, consider need for intubation + ventilation – involve seniors/ICU early
Hypothermia	RFs: drowning, exposure, ↓BMI, extremes of age, long lie, cognitive impairment. *32–35°C:* shivering. *30–32°C:* bradycardia, bradypnoea, confusion, ataxia, shivering stops. *<30°C:* coma, fixed dilated pupils, bronchorrhoea	Low-reading thermometer, usually rectal/oesophageal – low temperature. ECG: *30–32°C:* Osborn waves (J waves). *<30°C* sinus bradycardia → AF → VF → asystole. Coagulation screen: hypothermia can cause coagulopathy	Rapid warming: during CPR. Dry the patient, warmed IV fluids, Bair hugger (beware hypotension) Prolonged CPR. Until normothermia

Note: The differentials focused on are the reversible causes of cardiorespiratory arrest, as these are the most important things to rule out initially.

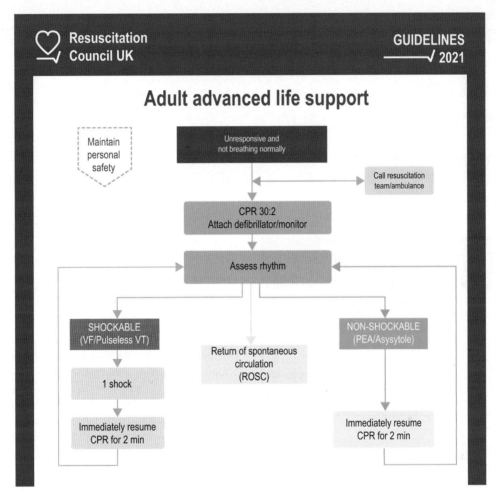

Fig. 43.1 RCUK ALS algorithm 2021. (Reproduced with the kind permission of Resuscitation Council UK.)

Learn the reversible causes of cardiac arrest as they are both easily testable and essential knowledge. The patient in the vignette is likely to have suffered an arrest due to a cardiac aetiology, most likely a coronary thrombosis. Given it occurred in hospital, the initial rhythm may be a VF or a pulseless VT which would prompt immediate defibrillation (Fig. 43.1). If ROSC were achieved, a swift ECG might show widespread ST changes which would confirm the diagnosis, thence proceeding to the cardiac catheter laboratory. Patients with shockable rhythms are more likely to achieve ROSC than non-shockable rhythms. In the modest proportion of patients in whom ROSC is achieved, an ABCDE approach to ongoing resuscitation should be immediately adopted to minimise secondary neurological injury. In Table 43.1, investigations in each case should include FBC, LFT, U&E, VBG & troponin.

REVISION TIPS

- Shockable rhythms: pulseless VT and VF
- Non-shockable rhythms: pulseless electrical activity and asystole

- In the management of hyperkalaemia, calcium gluconate only stabilises the myocardium, it has no effect on serum potassium. Salbutamol and insulin actively reduce serum potassium

44

Trauma and Massive Haemorrhage

Harriet Diment and Chetna Kohli

EMERGENCY DEPARTMENT VIA AIR AMBULANCE, FEMALE, 25.
MOTORBIKE ROAD TRAFFIC COLLISION

HPC: Thrown 5 m, having crashed into a parked car at 60 mph. 1 × 500 mL fluid bolus given at the scene. Sedated and intubated at scene due to reduced GCS.

O/E: HR 125, BP 105/62, RR 14, saturating 100% on FiO$_2$ 0.4, Temp 35.8. Intubated and ventilated. C-spine collar. Equal air entry/chest rise. Obvious deformity of right thigh, pelvic binder in situ. Pupils equal – 4 mm. **Ix:** FAST exam shows free fluid in Morrison pouch.

1. Which blood type can be transfused without cross-matching? What other blood products should be given in a massive transfusion?

2. What differentials should be considered in a 35-year-old female with a stab wound in the left chest, respiratory distress and hypotension?

3. Hypothermia, acidosis and coagulopathy are the 'lethal triad' in trauma; which is she at risk of?

Answers: 1. O negative. O-positive can be considered in an emergency in males. As well as RBCs, FFP, platelets and cryoprecipitate are provided to improve clotting. 2. Haemo-/pneumothorax, but also consider damage to large vessels/spleen, tension pneumothorax and cardiac injury with tamponade. 3. All of them; hypothermia (current low temp, due to exposure and sedation/ventilation), acidosis (poor organ perfusion due to shock state), coagulopathy (blood loss replaced with crystalloid).

TABLE 44.1			
	Features	**Investigations**	**Management**
Trauma With Massive Haemorrhage			
All: (C)ABCDE; G&S/CM; blood products, **major haemorrhage protocol**; tranexamic acid; full-body trauma CT			
External wound/laceration	Deep wound/compound fracture. Arterial bleeding (pulsating, bright red). Venous bleeding (steady blood flow, dark red)	Take down dressings and fully expose; log roll to inspect back	Pre-hospital: direct pressure, packing, haemostatic dressings. Major limb trauma: tourniquet if direct pressure has failed. Early haemostasis with surgery
Long bones	Bony deformity, open fracture, pain, loss of pulses/altered sensation distal to injury, increased CRT	Neurovascular status distal to the injury. Limb radiograph	Haemostasis with splinting. Orthopaedic input, ± surgery

TABLE 44.1   (Cont'd)

	Features	Investigations	Management
Trauma With Massive Haemorrhage			
Chest (haemothorax)	SOB, desaturation, tachypnoea, reduced air entry, chest wall injury or subcutaneous emphysema, asymmetrical chest movement	**Lung USS:** no lung sliding in PTX. Effusion. **CXR:** new effusion, PTX, surgical emphysema, #. **CT thorax**	Finger thoracostomy followed by surgical chest drain. Thoracotomy may be needed
Abdomen (usually organ laceration – e.g. spleen, liver)	RFs: penetrating injury, e.g. stabbing/gunshot. Hx & O/E: blunt – deceleration, direct blow to spleen/liver. Abdo pain, bruising. Splenic rupture: left shoulder tip pain and overlying rib #	**FAST scan:** to assess for free fluid (blood) in abdomen. **CT abdomen ± angiography**	*Depending on extent of injury;* – *Mild/moderate splenic injury* – *angiography/embolisation. Free fluid in abdomen plus shock refractory to initial fluid (blood product);* resuscitate, then laparotomy and abdominal packing ± splenectomy, etc.
Pelvis (fracture)	Leg length discrepancy, unable to straight leg raise, perineal haematoma, PV bleeding, haematuria/urethral bleeding	**Pelvic X-ray:** #	Haemostasis with pelvic binder (Fig. 44.1). Minimise movement. Angioembolisation, surgical repair
Trauma			
Head injury	See *49. HEAD INJURY*		
Airway obstruction	Reduced GCS → loss of protective reflexes. Consider with neck trauma, stridor, altered voice	Clinical diagnosis	Secure the airway, usually intubation. Anaesthetics/ENT involvement
Tension pneumothorax	See *40. BREATHLESSNESS*		
Cardiac tamponade	See *42. SHOCK AND LOW BLOOD PRESSURE*		
Major Haemorrhage			
Ruptured AAA	RFs: male, over 50, vasculopath, FHx, CTDs. Hx & O/E: acute/subacute onset, abdominal/back pain, pulsatile abdominal mass, hypotension ± N&V, clammy	Bedside USS: aorta diameter >5.5 cm. CT aorta: size, location and rupture	Vascular surgery review. Emergency surgical repair (aorta clamping and graft)
Primary post-partum bleeding (major)	RFs: 4 Ts: Tone, Tissue, Trauma, Thrombin. Hx & O/E: >500 mL blood loss from the birth canal within 24 hours of delivery. **Major PPH:** >1000 mL blood loss OR signs of **shock**	FBCs, coagulation profile, CM. **Weigh swabs to estimate blood loss.** May need examination under anaesthetic	Resuscitation with blood products. Catheterise. Uterine compression. Uterotonics e.g. syntometrine/oxytocin. Repair vaginal/cervical tears. Rusch balloon insertion, B-lynch suture, uterine artery ligation, hysterectomy

CM, Cross-match; *PTX*, Pneumothorax.

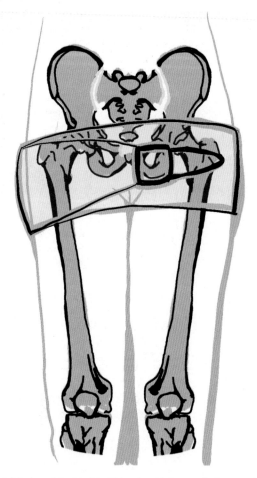

The woman in the vignette has life-threatening injuries following a significant mechanism of injury. She likely has a long bone fracture and an intrabdominal injury (note the free fluid on FAST exam) with haemorrhagic shock. The 'shock index' (HR/SBP) is >1 – essentially if the heart rate is greater than SBP then shock is present. Short-term management includes splinting the fracture and activating the massive transfusion protocol to stabilise her before moving to CT/theatre. Some experienced centres may continue resuscitation with blood products/pressors while transferring to CT and theatre. A thorough primary assessment should look for all life-threatening injuries and aim to reverse or temporise them.

Fig. 44.1 A pelvic binder. This should be applied over the greater trochanters. It can potentially prevent life-threatening bleeding in trauma. (Illustrated by Dr Hollie Blaber.)

REVISION TIPS

- If peripheral IV access fails, move to intraosseous access early
- Bleeding in trauma – *'on the floor and 4 more'*; external (on the floor), long bones, pelvis, abdomen, thorax
- The lethal triad is associated with high mortality rates in trauma – hypothermia, acidosis, coagulopathy. Early correction is key in preventing multi-organ failure

45

Painful Swollen Leg

Damien Mony, Zoe Kay, Omar Amar, Alexander Calthorpe, Christian Aquilina, and Angeliki Kosti

EMERGENCY DEPARTMENT, MALE, 70. ACUTELY SWOLLEN LEG

HPC: Left-sided swelling up to the knee, tender to palpate posteriorly. Weight-bearing but pain on walking. Right leg is unaffected. **PMHx:** Under urology for bladder cancer, TURBT 6 days ago. **SHx:** Ex-smoker, 10 pack years.

O/E: Appears well. T 36.7°C. Examination unremarkable apart from painful swollen left leg, redness extends up to the knee.

1. In which concurrent condition may a DVT lead to stroke?
2. What is post-thrombotic syndrome?

Answers: 1. Patent foramen ovale/atrial septal defects, enabling embolism from the leg to enter the left-sided circulation, and consequently potential for ischaemic stroke. If the foramen ovale has closed, a PE results. 2. Post-thrombotic syndrome follows a DVT or long-standing vascular insufficiency that results in incompetency of the valves in veins. Presents as a change in skin colour/pain/oedema/recurrent venous ulceration.

TABLE 45.1

	Features	Investigations	Management
Deep vein thrombosis (DVT)	Thrombus formation in venous system with embolic potential. **RFs:** immobility, cancer, recent surgery/trauma, personal/FHx of VTE, pregnancy, COCP/HRT. **Hx & O/E:** unilateral limb pain, tenderness, swelling/erythema (Fig. 45.1), ± PE signs. Rarer sites; femoral/arms	2-Level Wells score to stratify risk; a) *Score <2:* DVT unlikely-send D-dimer; • If D-dimer positive request lower limb **duplex USS** • If D-dimer negative, DVT is excluded b) *Score ≥2:* DVT is likely, request duplex USS. NB: D-dimer is sensitive but not specific. If imaging is delayed by >4 hours: give interim anticoagulation	**Thrombus confirmed on USS:** DOAC. (If DOAC is contraindicated give LMWH followed by warfarin). Anticoagulate for 3 (provoked VTE) or 6 months (unprovoked). If anticoagulation is contra-indicated consider IVC filter. Encourage mobilisation and consider graduated compression stockings for distal lower limb. Arrange follow-up

(Continued)

TABLE 45.1 (Cont'd)

	Features	Investigations	Management
Cellulitis	Spreading infection of skin and subcutaneous tissue. Often *Strep. pyogenes*, *Staph. aureus*. **Hx & O/E:** unilateral pain/erythema/swelling, commonly of an extremity, ± systemic signs	**Clinical diagnosis.** Baseline bloods/cultures. Wound swab. Consider imaging (e.g. XR)	Treat sepsis – hospital guidelines for Abx choice. Referral if suspect necrotising fasciitis, septic arthritis, osteomyelitis or orbital cellulitis
Acute limb ischaemia	See *5. COLD, PAINFUL, PALE, PULSELESS LEG/FOOT*		
Compartment syndrome	Pressure in a limb compartment causing neurovascular compromise; bleeding, IVI extravasation, swelling or tight external dressings. **Hx & O/E:** pain out of proportion to clinical signs and on passive stretching. The limb may look swollen	**XR:** to exclude #. **Clinical diagnosis.** However, compartment pressure may be measured (intracompartmental manometry) in confused and unresponsive patients	High index of suspicion and early referral (pulseless, paraesthesia, paralysis are late and serious signs). Urgent referral to Trauma and Orthopaedics. Emergency fasciotomy
Lymphoedema	Protein-rich fluid in interstitial space due to obstruction to lymphatic drainage or surgical removal of nodes; fibrosis. **Hx & O/E:** insidious, painless oedema in an extremity. Initially pitting, later non-pitting. Heavy and/or weak	Often a clinical diagnosis. Lymphoscintigraphy if the diagnosis is unclear	Non-curable. Compression bandaging and massaging. Surgery if significantly impaired function

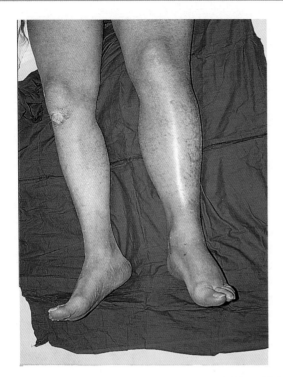

Fig. 45.1 DVT manifesting as an acutely swollen left leg. (Weitz JI, Ginsberg JS. Venous thrombosis and embolism. In: *Goldman-Cecil Medicine*. 2-volume set. Elsevier; 2020. Copyright © 2020 Elsevier Inc. All rights reserved.)

In the vignette, the most likely diagnosis is DVT, suggested by the clinical features and malignancy with recent surgery. The following things should be asked when gathering a history: acute versus chronic presentation, unilateral versus bilateral and painful versus painless. It is also essential to ask about associated symptoms such as fever and potential risk factors.

REVISION TIPS

- If considering cellulitis, rule out serious conditions: necrotising fasciitis, septic arthritis and osteomyelitis
- Red flags: **pain out of proportion** to clinical findings, systemically unwell, unilateral symptoms, SOB, any of the 6 P's
- Remember the 6 P's: Pain, Pallor, Perishingly cold, Pulseless, Paraesthesia, Paralysis

46

Blackouts, Faints and Loss of Consciousness

Louise Mathias and Chetna Kohli

EMERGENCY DEPARTMENT, MALE, 70. COLLAPSE

HPC: Getting up from a chair, went light-headed/sweaty then fell. Wife reports LoC for <1 min with some arm jerks and he passed urine. Quick recovery, no confusion, no injuries from fall. **PMHx:** T2DM, HTN, BPH. **DHx:** amlodipine, metformin, gliclazide, tamsulosin. **SHx:** drives, non-smoker, minimal alcohol, independent.

O/E: Obs; HR 60, RR 16, BP lying 140/85, standing BP 115/80. CVS: Regular HR, HS I+II+0, non-displaced apex. Abdo: Constipated, BO 4 days ago, SNT, BS present. Neuro: no focal neurology, GCS 15, AMT 4. **Ix:** Blood sugar 5.0; ECG: sinus rhythm; bloods: unremarkable.

1. How would your assessment for this patient change if they were on anticoagulants?
2. If the patient was hypoglycaemic, what would be the appropriate management?
3. What cause of collapse should you consider if there was metastatic lung cancer, single leg swelling, a new oxygen requirement and persistent tachycardia?

Answers: 1. No external injury/focal neurology and he can recount the story, with an eye witness, so management would be the same. If head injury can't be excluded (e.g. confused patient, unwitnessed fall) CT head is usually appropriate. 2. Glucose tablets/gel if able to swallow; if unconscious, give glucose 10% or 20% infusion. If IV access not possible, IM glucagon. 3. A PE must be ruled out. Collapse may be the point at which an unwell patient with PE is eventually convinced to attend. With metastatic cancer and high Wells' score, CTPA is required – D-dimer would be non-specific and unnecessary.

TABLE 46.1

	Features	Investigations	Management
Vasovagal syncope (Neurocardiogenic syncope)	**RFs:** stimuli (pain/emotion), dehydration, previous vasovagal. May be situational-e.g. defaecation/micturition/cough/ hot enclosed spaces. Quick onset and recovery. **Hx & O/E:** pre-syncope; nausea, sweating, pale, tunnelled vision, LOC (2–3 minutes) maybe brief muscle jerks	Often a **clinical diagnosis.** **ECG/blood sugar:** key in assessing for alternative diagnoses, especially dysrhythmias and hypoglycaemia	Reassurance and advice on possible triggers

TABLE 46.1   (Cont'd)

	Features	Investigations	Management
Orthostatic hypotension	RFs: *Primary;* autonomic dysfunction. *Secondary:* e.g. diabetic autonomic neuropathy, poor cardiac function, Parkinsonism. *Drug induced;* diuretics, α-blockers, vasodilators, antihypertensives. Dehydration. **Hx & O/E:** dizziness/LOC on standing	Often a clinical diagnosis. **Lying and standing BP.** **ECG.** **Blood sugar.**	Treat cause, hydrate. **Medication review.** Modify behaviours (e.g. get up slowly). Thigh-high compression stockings. Consider oral vasopressors e.g. midodrine
Cardiogenic syncope **Arrhythmias** (tachy or brady) or **Structural** (e.g. aortic stenosis)	RFs: PMHx structural heart disease, FHx of sudden death. **Hx & O/E:** often no prodrome, sudden LOC pre fall, unable to break fall, palpitations, feel 'unwell', spontaneous recovery. LOC during exertion is a red flag	**ECG:** may see heart block (Fig. 46.1), slow AF, WPW, Brugada, conscious VT, hypertrophic CM, arrhythmogenic right ventricular CM. Often normal sinus rhythm. Compare to previous ECG. **Telemetry:** if admitted. **24-hour tape.** **Echo:** structural disease	Depends on arrythmia. β-blockers, anti-arrhythmics. ICD if VT/VF high risk. Pacemaker for ongoing symptomatic bradycardia
Hypoglycaemia	RFs: diabetes medication, e.g. sulphonylureas, insulin. Can occur in sick infants, liver failure, sepsis. **Hx & O/E:** sympathetic; sweating, tremor, anxiety. Neuroglycopaenic; confusion, light-headedness, stupor, seizure	**Blood sugar:** ≤3.9 mmol/L. Recurrent hypoglycaemia can be investigated with a diagnostic fast. **ECG:** symptomatic dysrhythmia and MI can present similarly	**Can swallow:** glucose tablets/sugary drink. **Unconscious:** glucagon IM or glucose 10% or 20% IV. Glucose >4, give long-acting carbohydrate, **review medications/ insulin dose**
Seizure	See *100. FITS/SEIZURES*		
Aortic stenosis	RFs: senile calcification (age >55: ↑prevalence with ↑age), congenital (age <55: bicuspid valve, rheumatic heart disease). **Hx & O/E:** ESM radiates to carotids. Syncope, angina, dyspnoea. Slow rising pulse, narrow pulse pressure	Most common valvular disease. **ECG:** LVH with strain and left atrial enlargement. **Echo:** grade severity	Asymptomatic: observe. Symptomatic: **valve replacement.** Asymptomatic + valve gradient >40 mmHg + LVSD → consider valve replacement
Intracranial bleed	RFs: age, trauma, anticoagulants, heavy alcohol use. **Hx & O/E:** *intraparenchymal bleed/ SAH:* sudden LOC ± focal neurology. *Extradural-*traumatic injury. Raised ICP: pupil asymmetry; bradycardia + HTN. Cushing reflex; irregular breathing, coma, seizures, death	**CTH:** acute blood shows as hyperdense	Acute LOC due to an intracranial bleed often carries poor prognosis. Neurosurgical referral

SAD, Syncope, angina, dyspnoea; *CM,* Cardiomyopathy.

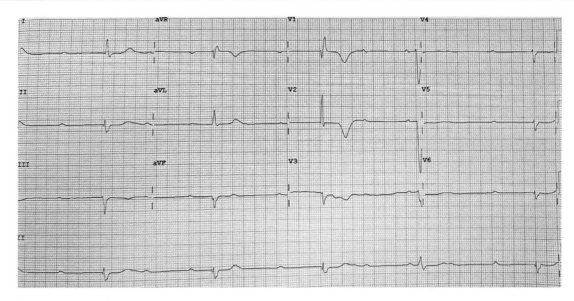

Fig. 46.1 Complete heart block, a cause of syncope. (Reproduced with permission from James Heilman. CC BY-SA 3.0. https://creativecommons.org/licenses/by-sa/3.0, via Wikimedia Commons. https://commons.wikimedia.org/wiki/File:CompleteHeartBlock.jpg. Accessed March 2022.)

The man in this vignette has likely lost consciousness due to multiple factors. His diabetes puts him at a higher risk of autonomic neuropathy while his HTN and antihypertensive medications can cause a labile BP and inappropriate response to position change. These factors, when coupled with LOC on standing, invoke a higher likelihood of orthostatic hypotension as the chief differential. The history is vital here. While jerking of the limbs and incontinence is classically associated with seizure, they are not specific and can be seen in multiple conditions. The key is his quick return to normal consciousness, something which essentially rules out a seizure.

REVISION TIPS

- Consider iatrogenic causes of blackout, especially in the elderly
- Hypoglycaemia can have a broad presentation and sometimes there are few indicators – check blood sugar
- LOC on exertion always requires thorough investigation

Confusion

Margarita Fox and Nicole Lundon

HPC: Woke at 2 am, confused, behaving out of character. Trying to climb out of bed, yelling incomprehensibly, unable to give you a history. Staff report she was her normal self in the evening. **PMHx:** Alzheimer's, T2DM. **DHx:** codeine, paracetamol, morphine, donepezil, metformin.

O/E: Unable to examine as she bats you away. Appears distraught and agitated. Obs: HR 90, BP 110/85, Sats 97% (RA), RR 22, Temp 37.9°C, AMTS 0/4 – not orientated to time, place or person. **Ix:** Blood sugar 6.0 mmol/L.

1. What is the most likely cause for this lady's delirium?
2. What are the non-pharmacological methods of managing delirium?
3. What would you consider if her behaviour posed a danger to themselves/others?

Answers: 1. Multifactorial; post-operative, pain, environmental, opioid use and constipation, anticholinergics, possible infection. NOF repair, advanced age and background of dementia are risk factors. 2. Supportive; consistent staff, reorientation, access to aids (glasses, hearing, walkers). Environmental adaptation: clock, orientate day and time, familiarity (belongings, family). Comfortable noise levels and lighting. Manage day/night reversal. 3. Haloperidol (0.5 mg) – avoid in patients with PD/LBD – consider quetiapine. Lorazepam if required (0.5 mg). Oral route preferable for all medications.

TABLE 47.1

	Features	Investigations	Management
Infection	**RFs:** prolonged admission, recent surgery, indwelling lines/catheters, immunosuppression. **Hx & O/E:** *UTI* (dysuria, frequency, suprapubic tenderness). *Pneumonia* (cough, SOB, pleuritic chest pain, crackles). *Wound* (erythema, pus). *CNS* (acute confusion, headache, fever, neck stiffness, focal neurology)	**Assess for sepsis. Confusion screen:** FBC, blood cultures, CRP, U&Es, bone profile, LFTs, coagulation, TFTs, B12/folate, magnesium, phosphate, glucose, ECG, CXR, urinalysis ± MSU. *Positive dipstick without clinical signs is insufficient to say UTI is causative*	**Treat source.** Refer to local guidelines, e.g. *UTI:* trimethoprim, nitrofurantoin 3–7 days. Send MSU for sensitivities. *Pneumonia:* Amoxicillin, alternative cover required if caught in hospital (HAP)
Post-operative	Multifactorial, e.g. pain, environment change, post-GA, post-op infections, retention	**Confusion screen. Check wound site**	Reorientation, familiarity, diurnal cycle, medication review, analgesia

(Continued)

TABLE 47.1 (Cont'd)

	Features	Investigations	Management
Constipation ± urinary retention	**RFs:** immobility. *Drugs:* opioid, anticholinergics, CCB, NSAIDs, antipsychotic, PPI, iron/calcium, antiparkinsonian. **Hx & O/E:** reduced stool frequency, abdo/bladder distention and discomfort	Confusion screen. Bladder scan. **U&Es:** normal or ↓ Mg, ↓ K, ↓/↑ Ca. Consider AXR	Laxative/stool softener. Remove/replace causative medication. Adequate fluids. Catheter if retention
Electrolyte imbalance	**RFs:** hyperparathyroidism, malignancy, CCF, cirrhosis, renal failure, IV fluids.	Check Na, K, Ca, PO_4, Mg, ECG. See *61. HYPERCALCAEMIA; 179. HYPONATRAEMIA*	
Hypoglycaemia	**RFs:** diabetes medication, e.g. sulphonylureas, insulin. Can occur in sick infants. **Hx & O/E:** sweaty, nauseous, lightheaded, shaky, visual changes	**Blood sugar:** ≤ 3.9 mmol/L. **ECG:** symptomatic dysrhythmia and MI can present similarly	**Can swallow:** glucose tablets/sugary drink. **Unconscious:** glucagon IM or glucose 10%–20% IV. Long-acting carbohydrate and review medications
Polypharmacy	Defined as >4 drugs. Psychoactive (anticonvulsants, antidepressants, benzodiazepines, opioids, sedatives). Dizzy, blurred vision, orthostatic hypotension (anticholinergics, antihistamines, antihypertensives, muscle relaxants)	Clinical diagnosis. **ECG:** ± bradycardia, QT prolongation. Hypotension (postural)	**Medication review.** Stop/reduce/replace where possible. Non-drug treatments, improve environment
Dementia	See *103. MEMORY LOSS*		
Intracranial bleed	**RFs:** HTN, prior bleed, aneurysm, anticoagulant, cerebral atrophy. **Hx & O/E:** stroke-like/chronic subdural type symptoms. Confusion	**Clotting/INR:** in cases of anticoagulant reversal. **CT head**	Blood pressure control. Neurosurgical opinion

The patient in this vignette has hyperactive delirium and is in a state of distress. Patients who come out of delirium may recollect the time when they were confused, and how terrifying it was. Causes are numerous (Tables 47.1 and 47.2). Regardless of cause, it is important to ensure the patient has access to their hearing aids and glasses, is reorientated to time and place, and has family members or familiar items nearby. Diurnal cycle; encourage patients to be awake during the day so they sleep at night. Occasionally simple measures will fail and careful prescription of a sedative or antipsychotic may be required to keep your patient and other patients safe. Medication management of delirium is complex and potentially can prolong a delirium. Delirium is also discussed in **103. MEMORY LOSS** and **104. VISUAL HALLUCINATIONS.**

TABLE 47.2 Mnemonic for causes of delirium

D	Drugs (presence or withdrawal). Dehydration. Discomfort
E	Electrolyte imbalance. Environment
L	Lack of sleep. Lungs (hypoxia)
I	Infection. Infarction (cardiac, cerebral)
R	Restricted mobility/sensory. Renal failure
I	Intracranial (stroke, subdural). Intoxication
U	Urinary/faecal. UTI
M	Myocardial/pulmonary. Metabolic (glucose, thyroid). Metastasis (brain)

REVISION TIPS

- Hyperactive delirium: agitated, restless
- Hypoactive delirium: drowsy, unrousable – do not miss!
- Seek and address underlying causes

Falls

Margarita Fox and Nicole Lundon

HPC: Fell while on the toilet passing urine. Prior to that she felt lightheaded, sweaty, blurry vision. Recovered quickly, thinks she was out briefly. No injury, some pain over left hip. Needs assistance to get up. Describes 'losing her balance' recently, when turning her head. Third fall in 6 months. **PMHx:** cataracts, T2DM with peripheral neuropathy, mild cognitive impairment, HTN, AF, cervical spondylosis. **DHx:** bisoprolol, apixaban, codeine, metformin, gliclazide. **SHx:** lives alone, no stairs, anxious about mobilising, walks with stick. Independent with ADLs. Still driving.

O/E: HR 70, irregularly irregular. BP 170/95 sitting, 145/90 standing. HS I+II+0. Chest clear. Abdomen SNT. Decreased sensation in both feet up to the mid calves, normal power in four limbs. No visible injuries, no head injury. Left hip; not shortened/externally rotated. Mild tenderness over greater trochanter, able to straight leg raise. Can mobilise with stick. **Ix:** blood glucose 5.5 mmol/L, urinalysis + leucocytes, ECG-AF, rate 70. Pelvic x-ray: no fracture.

1. How many factors can you identify which may have led to the fall described in the vignette?
2. An AF patient on digoxin developing falls; what should you consider?

Answers: 1. Frailty; nocturia; orthostatic hypotension – T2DM/HTN/medication; poor vision – cataracts; polypharmacy; impaired gait – cervical spondylosis/mobility aid; peripheral neuropathy; environment – getting up at night/dark; cognitive impairment; possible BPPV; history of previous falls; atrial fibrillation. 2. Digoxin toxicity; GI upset, dizziness, blurred vision, arrythmias, 'yellow-tinged' vision. Toxicity may be precipitated by renal failure or hypokalaemia – vomiting can lead to both.

TABLE 48.1

	Features	Investigations	Management
Mechanical fall	**RFs:** impaired balance or gait, previous falls, peripheral neuropathy, visual impairment, delirium, weakness, frailty, cognitive impairment, urinary frequency/urgency. Poor footwear/lighting, trip hazards. **Hx & O/E:** describes tripping. No LOC or pre-syncope, recalls entire event. O/E likely normal but look for injuries	Gain collateral history. Review of the home environment. Investigations to rule out other causes and injuries (Obs, ECG, Holter, CBG, FBC, U/Es, LFTs, bone profile ± CXR, CT head, echo, MSU, stool chart)	Treat any injuries. **Falls risk assessment:** BP, gait, hearing, vision, drugs, alcohol, urinary, cognition, footwear, environmental hazards. **Physio/OT/social worker/falls prevention programme**

(Continued)

TABLE 48.1 (Cont'd)

	Features	Investigations	Management
Polypharmacy	See *47. CONFUSION*		
Vasovagal syncope	See *46. BLACKOUTS, FAINTS AND LOSS OF CONSCIOUSNESS*		
Orthostatic hypotension	See *46. BLACKOUTS, FAINTS AND LOSS OF CONSCIOUSNESS*		
Balance impairment (e.g. vestibular or proprioceptive dysfunction)	**RFs:** peripheral neuropathy, stroke, neurological disease, Meniere's, BPPV, vestibular neuronitis. *Hx & O/E* (depending on aetiology): sudden onset or persistent vertigo, variable sensory deficit, ataxia, hearing loss, tinnitus	**Balance and gait assessment.** BPPV: Dix-Hallpike manoeuvre. Diabetic: sensory checks, HbA1c. Consider POCS – neuroimaging	See *24. VERTIGO*. Diabetic neuropathy; glycaemic control, gabapentinoids, TCAs, foot checks. Physiotherapy/strength and balance training
TIA/stroke	May present having fallen. See *101. SPEECH AND LANGUAGE PROBLEMS*		
Cardiogenic syncope	See *46. BLACKOUTS, FAINTS AND LOSS OF CONSCIOUSNESS*		
Hypoglycaemia	See *46. BLACKOUTS, FAINTS AND LOSS OF CONSCIOUSNESS* and *47. CONFUSION*		
Key Complications			
Fractures	**RFs:** falls, osteoporosis, frailty, cancer. *Fracture of NOF:* pain, leg shortened/ externally rotated. Pain in groin/thigh may radiate to knee	**X-ray:** AP/lateral hip (Fig. 48.1); visible fracture location/pattern, disrupted Shenton line	**Intracapsular;** hemiarthroplasty. THR if fit, walks independently, not cognitively impaired. **Extracapsular;** DHS/ intramedullary device
Rhabdomyolysis	**RFs:** long duration lie, AKI, compartment syndrome, trauma, prolonged seizures, myositis. **Hx & O/E:** muscle pain (50%), very dark urine (myoglobinuria), AKI	↑CK, ↓Ca, ↑K, ↑PO4, metabolic acidosis. **Urine:** myoglobinuria **ECG:** for ↑K	**Treat cause.** **IV fluids.** Monitoring (risk of overload). Occasionally; renal replacement therapy, alkaline diuresis
Soft tissue and pressure injuries	**RFs:** high Waterlow score, frailty, long lie, immobility	**Physical exam:** wounds, abrasions, pressure injuries	Dressings, monitor for infection. Wound care specialist nursing if pressure injuries

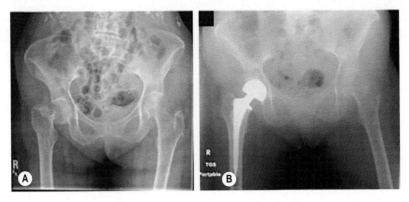

Fig. 48.1 Neck of femur fracture before and after surgery. (Reproduced with permission from Konigsberg BS, Duwelius PJ. Acute femoral neck fracture. In: *Surgery of the Hip*. Elsevier; 2020:Figure: 87.1. Copyright © 2020 Elsevier Inc.)

Beware the phrase 'mechanical fall' – as seen in the vignette, there are usually many reasons in older people. Instead of attributing a fall as 'mechanical', consider describing the cause of the fall instead. The history (including collateral) is crucial. While longer than many of the vignettes in this book, the story is familiar in acute medicine and careful detective work is required in teasing out the nature of a fall. It appears this woman had a multifactorial fall, as is common in the age group. Certain aspects point towards a vasovagal episode (the sensation of pre-syncope when passing urine) but there is also evidence of an orthostatic component.

REVISION TIPS

- Differentiate transient loss of consciousness versus mechanical fall
- If syncope, is it; reflex, orthostatic or cardiac?
- Falls often multifactorial. Keep differentials broad;
  - Environment (stairs, unsuitable walking aids, dark)
  - Medications (psychotropic, antihypertensives)
  - Physiological (impaired hearing/balance, weakness)
- Cardiovascular (vasovagal, postural hypotension, arrythmias, valvular, IHD)
- Acute medical (infection, electrolyte abnormalities, delirium)
- Other (poor vision, incontinence, cognitive impairment, alcohol)

49

Head Injury

Harriet Diment and Chetna Kohli

EMERGENCY DEPARTMENT, MALE, 38. PUNCHED IN THE SIDE OF THE HEAD WITH KNUCKLE DUSTERS

HPC: Witnessed loss of consciousness for 8 minutes, no seizure activity. Dizzy, vomited three times, remains drowsy. Unable to remember the event, reports severe headache.

O/E: GCS 12 (E3 V4 M5). 3 cm laceration on left temporal region, swelling over left eye. Complete left facial nerve palsy with no forehead sparing. Clear fluid dripping from left ear. No boggy deformity over facial bones or cranium.

---

1. How would your differentials change for an 85-year-old male on anticoagulation, who tripped and fell from standing, hitting his head on the floor?

2. Describe differences on head CT between extradural haematoma (EDH) and subdural haematoma (SDH).

3. Your patient develops a right dilated pupil that is unresponsive to light. What has happened?

Answers: 1. Older patients, with brain atrophy, are vulnerable to deceleration forces which shear the bridging veins, causing SDH. Chronic alcohol excess likewise, compounded by thrombocytopenia. Standing height falls can be bad, and older patients may sustain worse injuries compared to those seen in younger counterparts – hence the concept of 'silver trauma'. 2. EDH; biconvex shape, outlining the extradural space. Likely to be high force injury, so high attenuation (bright white). SDH; a crescent shape spanning the entirety of one hemisphere. Likely to be a chronic presentation, so blood is low attenuation (darker than the surrounding brain matter). The attenuation of the bleed can differ by chronicity and CT view. 3. Raised intracranial pressure and compression of the brain stem causing a third cranial nerve (CN3) palsy, often caused by uncal brain herniation – bad prognostic sign.

TABLE 49.1

	Features	Investigations	Management
Concussion/ minor TBI	RFs: young, male, sports, alcohol. Hx & O/E: nausea, dizzy, headache, unsteady, transient visual changes. ≤6 weeks headaches, low mood, fatigue, poor memory/concentration, 'brain fog'	Clinical diagnosis. CT head ± C-spine if meets criteria – *NICE guideline CG 176 (2014)*	Cognitive rest, analgesia, graduated return to exercise. Avoid risk of another TBI. Safety netting regarding worsening symptoms

	Features	Investigations	Management
TABLE 49.1 (Cont'd)			
Subdural haematoma	**RFs:** as for concussion, and; older, anticoagulant, alcohol use disorder. Often seem innocuous mechanism (sliding off bed, fall from sitting). **Hx & O/E:** acute SDH – fluctuating GCS, focal neurological deficit, imbalance. Subacute SDH – as above but slower onset, personality change, sleepy	**CT/MRI head:** bleed/clot ('crescent shaped') ± mass effect, e.g. midline shift, herniation. Age of bleed. Clotting screen (especially if on anticoagulation)	Reverse anticoagulation, e.g. warfarin reversal. Neurosurgical review – surgery dependent on clinical signs, clot size and tempo of accumulation
Base of skull fracture	**RFs:** high-force injury CSF rhinorrhoea/otorrhoea, haemotympanum. **Hx & O/E:** cranial nerve palsies – CN7 (facial paralysis) and CN8 (hearing loss). Periorbital/mastoid ecchymoses (raccoon/panda eyes, battle sign (Fig. 49.1) – presents after 1–2 days)	**CT head:** bone windows show fractures most often in anterior cranial fossa/petrous temporal bone. **CT C-spine:** reduced GCS and significant mechanism. CSF leak, see *20. EAR AND NASAL DISCHARGE*	Regular GCS reassessment. TBI management – initially: avoid secondary neurological injury, secure airway, nurse 30 degrees up, avoid hypoxia/hypovolaemia, normocapnia, C-spine protection. Neurosurgical review
Extradural haematoma	**RFs:** high impact trauma, especially temporal (middle meningeal artery). **Hx & O/E:** lucid period then rapid GCS fall (<50% but common in exams). Confusion, LOC, vomiting, ataxia, seizures, hemiparesis, ipsilateral pupil dilatation. Later, irregular breathing (brainstem compressed), respiratory arrest, death	**CT head:** acute 'lens shaped' bleed ± mass effect. **CT C-spine.** Reduced GCS and significant mechanism	TBI management. Emergency neurosurgical intervention (clot evacuation, ligation of bleeding vessels)
Key Complications			
Subarachnoid bleed	Spontaneous from bleeding aneurysm *or* following trauma. **RFs:** connective tissue disorder, HTN, PKD, FHx, major trauma. **Hx & O/E:** sudden onset 'thunderclap' headache (maximal pain in 5 seconds). Vomiting, seizure, collapse, reduced GCS, focal neurology, meningism. If ruptured berry aneurysms, think PCKD/associated conditions	**CT head:** blood in basal cisterns/subarachnoid, ± intraparenchymal blood, ± hydrocephalus. **Lumbar puncture** – if suspect aneurysmal SAH but normal CT; raised opening pressure, xanthochromia (>12 hours from onset). Angiography (CTA, DSA, MRA). (Multiple grading systems; WFNS grade, Fisher grade)	Neurosurgery; secure the aneurysm – endovascular (coiling, flow-diversion) or surgical (clipping, bypass). Prevent/treat complications; 1. Rebleed (secure the aneurysm), 2. hydrocephalus (CSF diversion), 3. cerebral ischaemia (nimodipine), 4. electrolyte abnormalities (SIADH, cerebral salt wasting), 5. VTE, 6. seizures. Analgesia, antiemetic

TABLE 49.1   (Cont'd)

	Features	Investigations	Management
Facial bone fracture	Swelling/deformity, tender, CN5 sensory deficit, malocclusion of teeth, trismus. Ophthalmoplegia may be rectus muscle entrapment in orbital #	Facial x-rays – lowest radiation but low sensitivity. **CT facial bones** – if suspicion of #	Analgesia. Screen for TBI. Maxillofacial review. Many are managed conservatively

TBI, traumatic brain injury.

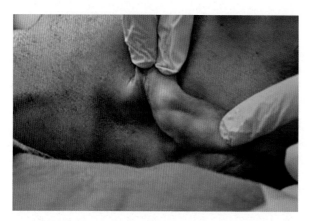

Fig. 49.1 Battle sign. (Reproduced with permission from Krishnan DG. Systematic assessment of the patient with facial trauma. *Oral Maxillofac Surg Clin North Am.* 2013 Nov: Figure 1. Elsevier Inc.)

The vignette describes a situation meeting several requirements for neuroimaging; reduced GCS, evidence of base of skull fracture (CSF otorrhoea and CN7 palsy), vomiting and amnesia. Significant neurological injury is likely – in this case, a fracture through the petrous temporal bone. He would also require a C-spine CT, given his reduced GCS. With head injuries being so common in the ED, an appreciation of the indications for imaging is vital. Minor TBI is the most common presentation, but caution should always apply for intoxicated or confused patients who may conceal significant pathology behind an unclear history.

REVISION TIPS

- For suspected brain bleed, a non-contrast CT head shows blood as bright white in the acute phase
- Head injury patients on anticoagulants should have a CT head within 8 hours of presentation
- The temporal region overlies the middle meningeal artery, hence risk of extradural haematoma

50

Bleeding From Upper GI Tract/Melaena

Meijia Xie, Alexander Calthorpe, and Omar Amar

EMERGENCY DEPARTMENT, MALE, 64. EPIGASTRIC PAIN, HAEMATEMESIS AND MELAENA

HPC: Severe, sudden epigastric pain. Three episodes of dark, foul-smelling stool, several bouts of vomiting blood. No dizziness, no jaundice. Reduced appetite. Weight loss over 2 months. **PMHx:** ulcerative colitis, primary sclerosing cholangitis, cirrhosis. 10 units alcohol/week.

O/E: HR 110, BP 108/75, RR 16, Temp 36.7°C, Sats 98%. Cool peripheries. Tender epigastrium, soft, mild hepatomegaly, bowel sounds present. DRE: no rectal masses, melaena on glove.

1. 92-year-old frail man with epigastric pain/haematemesis for 3 days, elevated CRP. O/E: HR 100, BP 94/60, fine crackles over right mid zone (lung). What is the likely diagnosis and your initial plan?
2. What is the difference between Rockall score and Glasgow-Blatchford score?

Answers: 1. Aspiration pneumonia – a common complication in elderly frail patients. Plan: Sepsis 6, Chest XR. 2. **Glasgow-Blatchford** = risk score **before** OGD (assess if an intervention is needed or patient can be discharged). **Rockall** score = **after** OGD (calculate how severe the GI bleeding was and likelihood of rebleeding).

TABLE 50.1

	Features	Investigations	Specific Management
Peptic ulcer disease	**RFs:** NSAIDs, DOACs, steroids, stress, smoking, alcohol, *Helicobacter pylori*, dyspepsia/reflux. **Hx & O/E:** coffee-ground vomiting, epigastric pain, melaena.	↓ Hb, ↑ Urea. **Erect CXR:** r/o perforation. **Urgent OGD** (diagnostic and therapeutic). *H. pylori* **tests** (often at GP). Urea breath test *or* stool antigen test	Urgent OGD. Offer PPI once endoscopy shows non-variceal upper GI bleed. ↓ smoking, ↓alcohol, stop NSAIDs. Confirmed *H. pylori*: triple therapy. PPI + 2 antibiotics (amoxicillin + clarithromycin/metronidazole)
Oesophageal varices	**RFs:** liver disease, alcohol. Ruptured varices cause copious fresh red haematemesis. **Hx & O/E:** epigastric/retrosternal pain, jaundice, ascites, portal hypertension (spider naevi, hepatomegaly, caput medusa)	↓ Hb, LFTs deranged or normal, ↑ PT/normal. **Urgent OGD**	Resuscitate to stability. **IV Terlipressin, ABx.** **Urgent OGD** for variceal banding. Consider **Sengstaken-Blakemore tube** tamponade (temporary) (Fig. 50.1). **Prophylaxis:** beta-blockers

(Continued)

TABLE 50.1   (Cont'd)

	Features	Investigations	Specific Management
Erosive oesophagitis or gastritis	**RFs:** alcohol, NSAIDs, DOAC, smoking, steroids, hiatus hernia. **Hx & O/E:** reflux, retrosternal pain, worse at night, cough Haematemesis uncommon, no melaena	Clinical diagnosis. **ECG** to r/o cardiac causes. **CXR** to r/o hiatus hernia. If treatment-resistant, endoscopy to r/o malignancy	↓ smoking, antacids, PPI (omeprazole). Stop irritant food/ medication. Treat *H. pylori* if positive
Upper GI malignancy	>55, weight loss, early satiety, N&V, treatment-resistant dyspepsia, anaemia, FHx, mets. *Gastric;* **Virchow's** node. *Oesophagus;* dysphagia (solids then liquids), odynophagia, Barrett's oesophagus	↓Hb, ↑platelets. **OGD + Biopsy.** (2WW referral if new dysphagia, OR age >55 *plus* weight loss and epigastric pain or dyspepsia or reflux). CT CAP ± staging laparoscopy	MDT discussion. *Gastric:* gastrectomy ± adjuvant chemotherapy. *Oesophagus:* stent. Oesophagectomy ± chemo-radiotherapy
Mallory Weiss tear (partial oesophageal tear)	**Minor haematemesis** after violent vomiting, e.g. alcohol, hyperemesis gravidarum, bulimia. Often fresh blood vomited. No melaena	Clinical diagnosis. Baseline bloods to r/o infection and AKI. U&Es may show ↓Cl⁻, ↓K⁺	IV fluids, antiemetics. Often resolve spontaneously
Consider Iron supplements	Ferrous sulphate/fumarate; black stools. Patient otherwise well.	Clinical diagnosis	No further management
Vascular causes of UGI bleed	Examples: angioectasia, Dieulafoy's lesion, AVM, GAVE (gastric antral vascular ectasia). Management: seek senior advice – likely need **endoscopy** for diagnosis and treatment		
Complications Major haemorrhage	E.g. secondary to perforated ulcer, or variceal rupture	**Initial Ix as per UGI bleed.** **Rockall score** = risk of rebleeding after endoscopy	CM 4–6 units RBC (or O neg blood) See *44. TRAUMA AND MASSIVE HAEMORRHAGE*
Oesophageal rupture – Boerhaave syndrome	*Sudden* retrosternal pain + respiratory distress, recent violent retching or vomiting Subcutaneous emphysema, septic	Ix as per UGI bleed. CXR. **CT CAP** with IV and oral contrast: contrast leaks into mediastinum or chest cavity	ABCDE, oxygen, IV fluids, Abx. Urgent endoscopy. Surgical washout of leaked contamination. Consider ITU

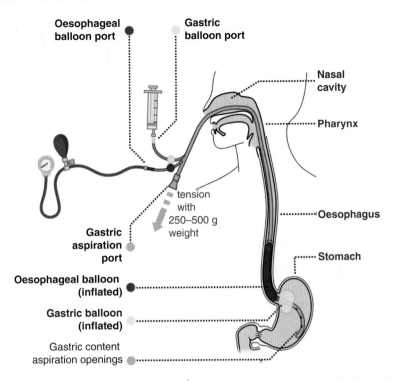

Fig. 50.1 Sengstaken–Blakemore tube in position. (Reproduced with permission from Bridwell RE, Long B, Ramzy M, Gottlieb M. Balloon tamponade for the management of gastrointestinal bleeding. *J Emerg Med.* 2022;62(4):545–558.)

TABLE 50.2	
FOR ALL PATIENTS PRESENTING WITH UGI BLEED/MELAENA	
Baseline Investigations	**Baseline Management**
Bloods: *FBC, CRP, LFT, U&Es, Clotting, Group & Save/CM.* Routine ECG. Calculate *Glasgow-Blatchford bleeding score* (GBBS) to determine urgency/need of endoscopy. Calculate Rockall score post-endoscopy	ABCDE. Two large IV cannulae and IV fluids. Consider blood transfusion (Hb <70). Keep patient NBM. Withhold anticoagulants

Melaena is black tarry sticky stools with a distinctive foul smell. The most likely diagnosis in the vignette is duodenal ulcer. A–E management is essential. Stabilise the patient, ensure all baseline investigations have been carried out (Table 50.2), the initial management has been started, liaise with the specialist team promptly and request an urgent OGD.

REVISION TIPS

- Varices: IV Terlipressin + urgent OGD
- Ulcers: Urgent OGD + PPI once endoscopy shows evidence of recent non-variceal upper GI bleed
- Gastric ulcers WORSE with food; duodenal ulcers relieved by food

51

Poisoning

Lucy Andrews and Chetna Kohli

**EMERGENCY DEPARTMENT, MALE, 37.
REDUCED GCS**

HPC: Found 'passed out' by member of the public, stabilised by paramedics. **PMHx:** Four previous attendances with ↓GCS, metallic mitral valve. **DHx:** Warfarin.
O/E: A – patent; **B** – RR 8, equal breath sounds; **C** – HR 60 regular, HS 'click' + II, BP 110/74; **D** – GCS 12, glucose 4.2, symmetrically constricted pupils; **E** – unkempt, track marks (groin and arms), no trauma, afebrile.

---

1. A patient with PMH of depression presents with shivering, vomiting, anxiety. On examination, hyperreflexia, fever, tachycardia. What is the most likely diagnosis?
2. A patient presents with 1/12 headache, malaise, dizziness, reduced concentration. The headache clears up somewhat when at work. His partner has been feeling more tired lately. Which toxidrome could this represent?
3. An elderly patient presents with confusion. Upon examination, flushed and with dilated pupils. A bladder scan measures 700 mL. Which toxidrome does this represent?

Answers: 1. Serotonin syndrome. Clinical diagnosis. Consider activated charcoal. Cyproheptadine/benzodiazepine to prevent seizure if severe. Provide active cooling and low-stimulus environment. 2. Carbon monoxide. Multiple people from a household with non-specific symptoms that clear up when away from the home. Diagnosed by VBG-↑ carboxyhaemoglobin (COHb) ± ↑lactate. Note smokers have mildly elevated COHb (up to 10%) in the absence of CO poisoning. 3. Anticholinergic syndrome: dilated pupils, flushing, anhidrosis, urinary retention, reduced conscious level/confusion/agitation. Important in older confused patients, especially if polypharmacy.

TABLE 51.1

	Features	Investigations	Management
Opiates	RFs: recent increase in dose, newly prescribed opiate; IVDU – look for track marks (Fig. 51.1). Risk of accumulation in renal failure. O/E: ↓respiratory rate, ↓GCS, pinpoint pupils	Clinical diagnosis. VBG: respiratory acidosis. U&Es: may see renal insufficiency (precipitant cause)	Reversal agent: **naloxone** 100–400 mcg IV, repeated until improvement in clinical status. Short half-life so may need continuous infusion

TABLE 51.1 (Cont'd)

	Features	Investigations	Management
Salicylate/ aspirin	Tinnitus, vomiting, hyperventilation, dehydration, deafness vertigo, sweating. Severe; reduced GCS, seizure, hypotension, heart block, hyperthermia, pulmonary oedema	Salicylate level ↑>500 mg/L (repeat at 2 hours to identify ongoing absorption). Paracetamol level ↔. **VBG:** initial respiratory alkalosis→ metabolic acidosis. Hypoglycaemia, hypokalaemia, AKI	Activated charcoal if ≤1 hour. IV fluids – usually dehydrated. **Sodium bicarbonate** infused over 3 hours if >500 mg/L, metabolic acidosis or symptomatic. Treat hypoglycaemia/hypokalaemia. Haemodialysis for severe poisoning. Consider; gastric lavage, urine alkalinisation. Pulmonary oedema – NIV/intubation
Amphet- amines/ cocaine	**RF:** recreational drug use. **Hx & O/E:** dilated pupils, agitation, tachycardia, HTN, chest pain, seizures. Hyper- thermia predicts mortality	**ECG:** tachycardia, ± ischaemic changes, occasionally SVT. FBC, LFTs, U&Es, CBG-↑/↓. CK (rhabdomyolysis). Troponin (cardiac ischaemia)	**Treat complications:** IVI if depleted, active cooling, ACS treatment if relevant, benzodiazepine for seizures/ agitation
Paracetamol	See *52. OVERDOSE*		

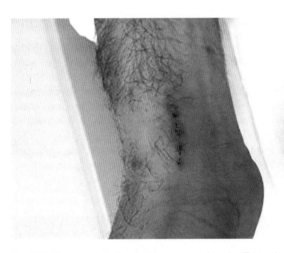

Fig. 51.1 Track marks following the course of a vein. (Reproduced with permission from Cara Hennings MD and Jami Miller MD, Illicit drugs: What dermatologists need to know. *Journal of the American Academy of Dermatology*, 2013,69 (1), 135–142. Copyright © 2012 American Academy of Dermatology, Inc.)

The vignette describes classic signs of opiate toxicity (pinpoint pupils; low RR; reduced GCS) alongside evidence of IVDU. Initial management should be naloxone – this is often administered prior to hospital arrival. His metallic valve is likely a complication of previous endocarditis. The prior attendances suggest this has happened before. Given his reduced GCS and warfarin use, a CTH is needed to assess for intracerebral/cranial bleeding. Caution should be afforded to the patients who are 'just intoxicated' as they may be hiding significant alternative pathology such as subarachnoid haemorrhage or encephalitis.

REVISION TIPS

- Unusual collection of symptoms – think poisoning
- If ingestion <1 hour ago: consider activated charcoal
- Remember safeguarding, especially in children presenting with accidental poisoning
- Someone with alcohol poisoning on a background of chronic alcohol excess, complete a CIWA score and prescribe benzodiazepines to avoid severe withdrawal symptoms

52

Overdose

Harriet Diment and Chetna Kohli

**EMERGENCY DEPARTMENT, FEMALE, 18.
PARACETAMOL OVERDOSE AFTER
ARGUMENT WITH PARENTS**

HPC: 48 tablets ingested 3 hours ago. Nauseated with abdo pain. **PMHx:** Depression. **DHx:** Sertraline, amitriptyline.

O/E: Observations normal, calm, appears well, weight 80 kg, mild abdo tenderness. Normal muscle tone and cranial nerve exam. **Ix:** Pregnancy test and urine dip negative. ECG shows normal sinus rhythm, blood gas is unremarkable.

1. How much paracetamol has she ingested (in mg/kg)? At 4 hours, her blood paracetamol level was 180 mg/L. Use the nomogram (Fig. 52.1) to determine if she requires *N*-acetyl cysteine (NAC).
2. With NAC she develops itching, nausea, urticaria, wheeze, tachycardia. What is this adverse reaction and how is it managed?

Answers: 1. Paracetamol comes in 500 mg tablets. (500 × 48)/80 = **300 mg/kg**. The 4 hour blood paracetamol levels are above the treatment line on the nomogram so NAC is needed. Check which units the paracetamol concentration is given in; using the left-hand side of the nomogram would have led you to underestimate her toxicity. 2. A non-immunoglobulin-E hypersensitivity reaction (anaphylactoid). Stop the infusion, give anti-histamine ± steroid. Once symptoms have settled, restart the NAC at a slower rate. If angioedema, hypotension or bronchospasm – treat as anaphylaxis.

TABLE 52.1

Differentials	Key Words/Features/Hints	Investigations	Management
Paracetamol overdose	Early: asymptomatic, N&V (common). Late: jaundice, coagulopathy, hypoglycaemia, renal failure, encephalopathy. Abdo pain is usually a late feature	Serum paracetamol level: at 4 hours post-ingestion unless overdose is staggered or 'massive' (see Toxbase). LFTs: ↑ALT in liver damage. INR. U&Es: reduced eGFR, ↑creatinine in late OD	Activated charcoal (reduces absorption) if seen in ≤1 hour. Below nomogram treatment threshold at 4 hours: nil. Above threshold/massive/staggered: NAC (SEs: N&V, anaphylactoid-3%; anti-histamine ± steroid, reduce rate of infusion). King's College Transplant Criteria

TABLE 52.1   (Cont'd)

Differentials	Key Words/Features/Hints	Investigations	Management
Sertraline/SSRI overdose	**RFs:** taking multiple serotonergics (SSRIs, MAOIs, TCAs, recreational). Serotonin syndrome; mild (N&V, tremor, agitation), **altered mental state** (confusion, seizures, coma, agitation), **autonomic dysfunction** (tachycardia, hyperthermia, hypotension/HTN, flushing, tachypnoea, dilated pupils), **neuromuscular hyperactivity** (restlessness, hyperreflexia, clonus, ataxia, rigidity, rhabdomyolysis)	**ECG and continuous cardiac monitoring:** QT prolongation, ventricular dysrhythmias possible. CK if prolonged neuromuscular over activity – assess for rhabdomyolysis	Supportive. **For serotonin syndrome:** benzodiazepine (0.1 mg/kg IV lorazepam), cyproheptadine. Avoid further serotonergics. Severe – cooling; intubation, ventilation, neuromuscular paralysis
Tricyclic overdose (amitriptyline, nortriptyline, doxepin, imipramine)	Anti-cholinergic syndrome, also arrhythmias, convulsions, coma, cardiovascular collapse. Features of anti-cholinergic syndrome; tachycardia, confusion, flushing, anhidrosis, mydriasis, urinary retention, dry mouth	**ECG (with multiple repeats):** prolonged PR, QRS, QT intervals. **Cardiac monitoring:** prolonged QRS predicts convulsions/ventricular arrhythmias. Blood gas to assess for acidosis. U&Es, monitor U/O	Consider activated charcoal if within 1 hour of ingestion. Prolonged QRS >100 msec or acidosis – sodium bicarbonate aiming for pH 7.50–7.55. Fluid non-responsive hypotension will need ICU ± vasopressors
Salicylate overdose	See *51. POISONING*		
Anti-psychotic overdose (most commonly quetiapine, risperidone)	Tachycardia, sedation, dystonic. Hypotension, confusion, agitation, respiratory depression, convulsion. Quetiapine: anti-cholinergic syndrome. **Neuroleptic malignant syndrome:** rare life-threatening reaction over 24–72 hours; rigidity, fever, tachypnoea, delirium, autonomic instability (tachycardia, sweating, incontinence and labile BP)	**ECG (with multiple repeats):** assess for QT/QRS prolongation. U&Es with Mg^{2+} and Ca^{2+}: electrolyte derangement. Creatinine kinase ↑↑↑ in rhabdomyolysis	Supportive. Acute dystonic reactions: procyclidine. **For NMS:** stop the drug. Supportive measures, treat rhabdomyolysis, consider bromocriptine

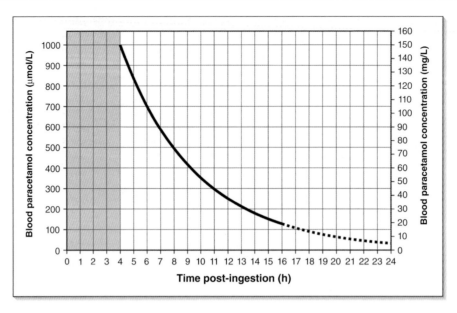

Fig. 52.1 Paracetamol nomogram. (Reproduced with permission from Andis Graudins and Anselm Wong. Paracetamol. *Textbook of Adult Emergency Medicine*, 2020; 25.6, 756–760.)

Overdoses with intent to self-harm always require medical assessment and paracetamol is by far the most common overdose seen in ED. This presentation is consistent with either sertraline or paracetamol overdose. Many patients will say what they have taken. Accessing poison information online provides advice and stepwise management. Essential features to get from the history to treat paracetamol OD are dose of paracetamol, patient weight, timeframe of ingestion and any co-ingested medications. Ingestions of <75 mg/kg usually do not require hospital assessment. The abdominal pain in this case is probably from N&V, as pain is usually a later feature of toxicity – a raised ALT might indicate an earlier ingestion than stated.

REVISION TIPS

- RFs for intentional overdose: previous OD, self-harm behaviour, polysubstance use, psychiatric co-morbidity
- Serotonin syndrome is a risk if two or more serotonergic drugs are used (SSRIs, TCAs, MAOI, St John's Wort)
- Most patients presenting with paracetamol overdose are minimally symptomatic in the early stages
- Get an ECG (with repeats) – many medications cause conduction disturbances in overdose

53

Anaphylaxis

Harriet Diment and Chetna Kohli

EMERGENCY DEPARTMENT, FEMALE, 18. RESPIRATORY DISTRESS SOON AFTER EATING A CHOCOLATE BAR

HPC: Breathing difficulty, new rash, facial swelling. **PMHx:** Eczema, asthma (no previous hospital admissions).

O/E: HR 130, BP 78/50, RR 32, O_2 98% on 15 L non-rebreather, afebrile. Audible wheeze, new widespread rash, swollen lips/tongue.

---

1. What type of sensitivity reaction is this and what mediates it?
2. What is the difference between adrenaline dosing for anaphylaxis versus cardiac arrest?
3. A patient tells you they previously had anaphylaxis to penicillin. Which of the following antibiotics are considered safe: (A) Tazocin. (B) Gentamicin. (C) Ceftriaxone. (D) Co-amoxiclav?

Answers: 1. Severe type 1 hypersensitivity reaction; both anaphylaxis and urticaria are histamine mediated. 2. Anaphylaxis – 0.5 mg IM every 5 minutes (1:1000) versus cardiac arrest – 1 mg IV every 3–5 minutes (1:10,000). 3. (A) Unsafe – contains piperacillin. (B) Considered safe. (C) <10% cross reactivity with cephalosporins – consult infectious diseases team, or use an alternative antibiotic. (D) Unsafe – contains amoxicillin.

TABLE 53.1

	Features	Investigations	Management
Anaphylaxis	**RFs:** allergies, previous anaphylaxis. **Hx & O/E:** rapid onset (minutes); angioedema, urticaria, stridor/wheeze/respiratory distress, circulatory collapse (tachycardia/hypotension = anaphylactic shock – BP >30% below baseline). Diarrhoea/vomiting	Clinical diagnosis. Serum tryptase levels at 1/6/24 hours – false negatives common (poor sensitivity), positively correlated with severity. Formal allergy testing (RAST/CAP/skin prick). *Remove trigger* e.g. bee sting (do not induce vomiting if food trigger).	Call for help. CPR if unresponsive and not breathing normally. <u>IM adrenaline 1:1,000</u> as per age-related guidelines (mid third of thigh/ arm), repeat every 5 mins until response- *max dose 0.5ml/ 0.5mg.* O_2 (mask with reservoir)- target sats. 94–98% (T2RF 88–92%) **Rapid IV fluid** (Hartmann's/ normal saline); adult 500–1000mL, child 10 mL/kg, then IVI. ± Inhaled salbutamol/ ipratropium.
Acute asthma	See *183. WHEEZE*		

(Continued)

TABLE 53.1   (Cont'd)

	Features	Investigations	Management
Other Important Differentials			
Acute urticaria (Fig. 53.1)	**RFs:** idiopathic, triggered by drugs (e.g. penicillins, opiates, NSAIDs), bacterial or viral infection, stings, food, contact allergy (e.g. latex). **Hx & O/E:** pruritic wheals/flares, wide distribution, ± angioedema. Severe allergic urticaria may lead to anaphylaxis	Symptom diary; frequency, duration, severity. Finding cause; withholding medications, patch testing/skin prick testing – contact urticarias. Immunoglobulin E tests for specific allergens	Identify and avoid triggers. Antihistamines (non-sedating) – cetirizine/fexofenadine/loratadine. Prednisolone 40 mg daily 3–7 days. Uncontrolled/recurrent: increase dose/duration of antihistamine, calamine lotion, sedating antihistamine (chlorphenamine). Dermatology/immunology
Panic disorder	**RFs:** anxiety or panic/mood disorder. **Hx & O/E:** usually <30 mins; hyper-ventilation, palpitations, shaking, nausea, hot/cold flushes, dizzy, fear of dying, paraesthesia in fingers/face	VBG: respiratory alkalosis. TFTs: rule out hyperthyroidism	Observation and reassurance. Consider referral for mental health input – talking therapies, CBT, SSRI treatment

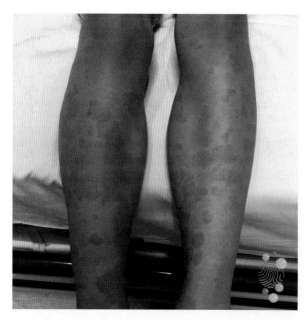

Fig. 53.1 Urticaria. (Reproduced with permission from Skin Deep: https://dftbskindeep.com/diagnoses-gallery/#!jig[1]/ML/3846)

Anaphylaxis needs prompt response; while the patient in the vignette has PMHx of asthma, angioedema, urticaria and shock are vital indicators. The patient is positioned semi-recumbent (if breathing problem), supine ± leg elevation (circulatory), in recovery position (breathing but unconscious), or lying on left side (pregnant); abrupt change in position is dangerous, so take care when transferring. Circulatory collapse (histamine vasodilation/ vascular permeability) is fatal; give IM adrenaline 1:1,000 into the thigh IM (IV adrenaline; 1:10,000 needs specialist setting). Monitor breathing/ wheeze, vital signs (RR, sats, HR, BP, level of consciousness) as indicators of response. Ensure follow up after discharge.

REVISION TIPS

- Anaphylaxis is prime exam material: easy to test and essential to know. Beware biphasic reactions, recurring within 8 hours in 20%- treated in the same way
- Patients can present with anaphylaxis at any age, even in the absence of previous allergy history
- In a life-threatening asthma attack, normal/rising CO_2 levels on ABG indicate impending respiratory failure

54

Bites and Stings

Zoe Kay, Mital Patel, Gregory Oxenham, and Dalilah Restrepo

**GP CONSULTATION, MALE, 19.
ITCHY RED BUMPS ON HIS BACK AND LEG**

HPC: Not painful, no systemic symptoms. He recently returned from a trip to Amsterdam with his friends.

O/E: Multiple small 2 mm red lesions in a vertical pattern along his right flank and right lateral thigh, and two likewise on the forehead. Evidence of excoriation. No abscess/secondary infection.

1. Describe your management of a dog or cat bite.
2. What are the risk factors for developing cellulitis secondary to a bite?
3. What bacteria causes cat scratch disease?

Answers: 1. Assess damage to soft tissue, consider underlying fracture if bitten by a large dog. Assess risk of tetanus (rabies if abroad). Meticulous irrigation (and debride if necessary). Prophylactic antibiotics only if the skin is broken – usually co-amoxiclav. Large/complex wounds from dogs require closure. Small puncture wounds from cats are left open. 2. Diabetes, peripheral arterial disease, unclean wound, leg ulceration or oedema. 3. *Bartonella henselae*.

TABLE 54.1

	Features	Presentation	Management
Wasp/hornet/ bee stings	Painful, itchy. May have a central white area (site of sting). Urticaria. **Complication:** Allergy (Fig. 54.1)		Remove sting if present (more common with bee). Cold compress, avoid scratching. Topical steroid/oral antihistamine for itch
Horsefly bites	Very painful. Red raised lesion. May develop an urticarial rash. **Complication:** Allergy or secondary infection		
Midge bites	Common in UK summer. Itchy and red, look like mosquito bite. **Complication:** Allergy		
Bedbugs	**Complication:** Allergic reaction, secondary bacterial infection. Recurrent exposure as very difficult to remove from mattresses/crevices around bed – professional eradication	Bites occur in straight lines – asymptomatic or itchy: 2–5 mm. Bedbugs feed at night and bite without host noticing	Usually resolve in a week. Topical steroid/oral antihistamine for itchiness/urticaria

(Continued)

TABLE 54.1   (Cont'd)

	Features	Presentation	Management
Mosquito See revision tips below for other diseases	**Malaria:** Groups most at risk: old, young, splenectomy, pregnant. Small red itchy bites on exposed areas. Fever, rigors, headache, GI symptoms, myalgia/arthralgia, hepatosplenomegaly, jaundice. May see a relapsing course due to dormant parasites in liver/blood. Haemolytic anaemia/AKI/haemoglobinuria (blackwater fever) – *P. falciparum*. Cerebral malaria – seizures, coma. Malaria is a **notifiable disease**. See also *98. TRAVELLING ADVICE*	Parasitic disease caused by *Plasmodium* sp. *P. falciparum* is most severe. Presents between 6 days and 1 year from exposure. Symptoms/signs: **Fever and rigors** (cyclical or continuous), malaise, headache, GI symptoms, hepato-splenomegaly, jaundice. **Thick blood film:** detects parasites. **Thin blood film:** identifies species and calculates parasitaemia. Films ×3 with Giemsa stain	Prevention; repellent, net, avoid area with standing water, drug prophylaxis. Uncomplicated *P. falciparum*: artemisinin combination therapy. Quinine (+doxycycline) or atovaquone eproguanil (malarone). IV antimalarial (e.g. artesunate/lumefantrine) if; altered consciousness, acidotic, severe anaemia, AKI, jaundice, severe parasitaemia (>2%)
Tick	*Most tick bites do not transmit disease*, but consider Lyme disease (*Borrelia burgdorferi*). Other tick-borne diseases are rarely seen in the United Kingdom (Rocky Mountain spotted fever, ehrlichiosis, babesiosis). **RFs:** Grassy/woody areas in South England, North England, Scotland Also Eastern Europe, Scandinavia and US Atlantic coast	**Erythema migrans** is pathognomonic of Lyme disease. If present with risk factors, no further investigations required. Other symptoms may include: fever, fatigue, headache, migratory arthritis. Rare cause of Bell's palsy/ heart block	**Prevention:** Long trousers, tick checks, single dose doxycycline (consider if relevant exposure). Enzyme-linked immuno-assay – takes a month Western blot for IgM/IgG. First-line management: oral doxycycline
Scabies (Fig. 54.2)	**RFs:** Poverty/overcrowding, refugee camps, institutional care (rest homes, prisons, hospitals). Immunocompromise; crusted/**Norwegian scabies** – further risk of bacterial infection. **Complication:** Continued infestation without treatment. Impetigo from secondary infection	Transmitted through skin contact. History of itchy household contacts. Intense itching, burrows in the finger webs. Rash weeks later (hyper-sensitivity) – erythematous papules trunk/ limbs, diffuse dermatitis; spares scalp	Dx: dermatoscopy + skin biopsy/microscopy. Treat contacts in past 8 weeks – topical permethrin/ oral ivermectin. Repeat treatment at 8–10 days. Wash all bedding/clothes at >50°C, thorough cleaning/ vacuuming

Other Complications

Anaphylaxis	See *53. ANAPHYLAXIS*
Cellulitis	See *45. PAINFUL SWOLLEN LEG*

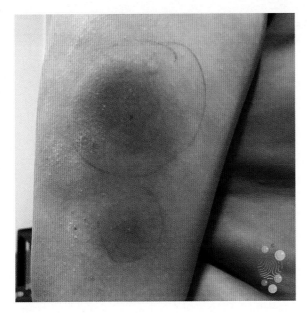

Fig. 54.1 Reaction to a bite with swelling and erythema. (Refer Reaction to a bite: Skin deep: Fig. 2. https://dftbskindeep.com/all-diagnoses/bites/#!jig[1]/ML/3551)

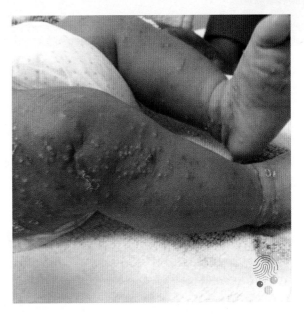

Fig. 54.2 Scabies in an infant. (Refer Scabies in an infant: Skin deep: Fig.1. https://dftbskindeep.com/all-diagnoses/scabies/#!jig[1]/ML/885)

The likely culprit in the vignette is infestation with bedbugs; itchy bites with markings travelling in lines often on parts of the body which make contact with the mattress/pillow. The trip to Amsterdam was likely the source, perhaps from a hostel bedroom. He will need to treat his clothes in a hot wash and vacuum/wash his bag. If he has already spread the bugs to his bed then this will need treating too. If travelling, check under mattresses/sheets for signs of bedbugs (i.e. their faeces) and keep bags off the floor.

REVISION TIPS

- Erythema migrans usually indicates Lyme disease in an exam question
- Exclude petechiae/other skin signs as a cause of rash
- Check travel (internationally and United Kingdom) and vaccination history
- Infection of pet bites: cats > dogs, deep puncturing wound, bitten extremities (hands, feet, face), diabetes mellitus, young/old age
- Mosquitoes transmit malaria, Dengue fever, West Nile virus, Chikungunya, Zika, Japanese encephalitis, Yellow fever. Consider in patients with fever after visit to tropics/subtropics

55

Burns

Katherine Parker and Jajini Susan Varghese

EMERGENCY DEPARTMENT, FEMALE, AGED 3. **HOT COFFEE SCALD**

HPC: Supervised by babysitter, mother says daughter knocked cup of coffee onto her right arm – babysitter applied cold water promptly. She is inquisitive and is often grabbing for things. Babysitter is not present. Mother came straight home and brought patient to ED. **PMHx:** Nil relevant. No allergies. **SHx:** No previous attendances, no involvement with social care, no siblings. Mother and father only cohabitants.

O/E: Patient is distressed. Preferentially using left arm. T 36.8. Right arm – well circumscribed erythema with blistering, sloughing and exudative base. Extends over fingers, back of hand and distal forearm. Torso: 3 × 2 cm area of erythema on right pectoral region.

1. Which aspects of this case mean it is categorised as a 'complex' burn?
2. How would other burns appear?

Answers: 1. Burn is of a critical area (hand) and crosses joints (wrist). 2. Other burns; <u>Superficial epidermal</u>: red and glistening, no blisters, brisk CRT, painful. Heals within 7 days, no scarring. <u>Deep dermal</u> (deep partial thickness): dry, blotchy/mottled and cherry red/stained appearance, blisters may be present, absent capillary refill variable sensation. Possible scarring, may require specialist treatment. <u>Full thickness</u> (previously 3rd degree): dry, leathery, white or black (charred), no blisters, absent capillary refill insensate. Most require surgical intervention.

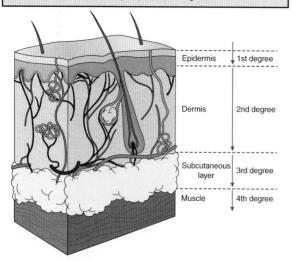

Fig. 55.1 Skin layers and subcutaneous tissue and representative degrees of burn injury based on depth of burn. (From Shiland B. *Mastering Health Care Terminology*. 2nd ed. St. Louis: Elsevier; 2006.)

TABLE 55.1

	Clinical	Investigations	Management
All Burns (Fig. 55.1)	**RFs:** children <5 years, adults >60 years, male, occupational. Erythema, blistering	A–E assessment with full observations. Assess and document time of incident, first aid administrated, location of burns, size, extent and depth. Estimate total body surface area (TBSA) affected (*rule of nines* – adults only, *Lund-Browder chart* – more accurate, used in adults and children, palmar surface). FBC, U&E. **COHb, ABG, CXR** (inhalation injury). ECG (chemical or electrical)	Remove non-adherent clothing and restricting jewellery. Cool the burn (irrigate with tepid water 20 minutes). Analgesia. Tetanus booster if indicated. Consider admission to burns unit
Thermal	**RFs:** alcohol, abuse, epilepsy. Scalds (hot liquid, steam), flames, heated objects. **Inhalation injury:** enclosed space, husky voice, cherry red skin (CO poisoning)		**Non-complex burns:** irrigation (20 minutes), remove loose burned tissue. Dress according to local wound protocol. Review at 10–14 days. **Complex:** admit to burns unit
Chemical	Industrial or household corrosive agents (acids, alkalis, organic products)		Identify chemical, remove affected clothing and brush chemical off skin. Do not try to neutralise. Irrigate with water (1 hour). Admit to burns unit
Electrical	Damage on entry/exit points and internal tissues (including muscle). Extent determined by voltage		Low-voltage source – switch off supply/remove from electrical source using non-conductive material. **Do not irrigate.** Admit to burns unit
NAI	Red flags (implausible/inappropriate explanation, immobile patient, unusual injury)	Full examination. See *156. CHILD ABUSE*	Immediate admission if suspect NAI. Careful documentation of findings Report to safeguarding lead

Key Complications

Early	Respiratory distress, arrhythmias, hypothermia, hypovolaemia, AKI, vascular insufficiency		
Late	Cellulitis, toxic shock syndrome, scarring, psychological complications		
Shock	Hypotension (hypovolaemic shock). Oedema maximal in burn areas after 24 hours. Extravasation of proteins and electrolytes	Hypoproteinaemia and electrolyte imbalance. ECG: arrhythmias. Coagulation: deranged	Parkland formula; 4 mL lactated ringers solution × %TBSA burned × patient's weight in kilograms = total fluid for first 24 hours (half given over 8 hours). Subsequent rate gauged for urine output 30–50 mL/hr

The case in the vignette represents a superficial dermal (superficial partial thickness): red/pale, large blisters, brisk CRT, painful, heals within 14 days, no scarring. Nonetheless, it is a complex burn due to its location affecting a critical area, so should be discussed with the specialist team.

REVISION TIPS

- **Non-complex burns** (previously 'minor') – any partial-thickness thermal burn of ≤15% of TBSA (or 10% in children, or 5% in under 1 year old), that does not cover a critical area
- **Complex burns** (previously 'major') – thermal burn of a critical area (hands, face, feet, perineum, genitalia, across joints or circumferential), thermal burns covering >15% TBSA in adult (>10% in children and >5% in children younger than 1), chemical/electrical, full thickness burns
- Parkland formula – calculate fluid requirements for first 24 hours. Volume of NaCl 0.9% = TBSA of burn (%) × weight × 4, give half fluid in first 8 hours

56

Laceration

*Harriet Diment, Berenice Aguirrezabala Armbruster,
Alexander Calthorpe, and Omar Amar*

**EMERGENCY DEPARTMENT, MALE, 35.
CUT ON ELBOW**

HPC: Fell onto broken glass.
O/E: 6 cm laceration over right elbow, glass shards in the wound. Full range of movement.

---

1. What is the best closure technique for this wound?
2. What would be the best management if this were;
   a. Puncture wound to right index finger, contaminated with soil. No change in sensation, full range of movement

   b. 3 cm head laceration, good edge apposition, clean wound
   c. Pre-tibial laceration with flap

Answers: 1. Interrupted sutures, as the cut is on an area of flexion (steri-strips would not keep the wound edges together). Careful debridement and radiographic confirmation that no glass is left in the wound before closure. 2. (A) Clean and dress wound. Do not close due to risk of infection. Treat with tetanus immunoglobulin. Find out patient's immunisation history to assess whether they need a tetanus booster. (B) Clean and close wound with either steri-strips or glue. (C) Reposition flap and steri-strip in place – do not suture, due to tension which does not allow for swelling.

TABLE 56.1

	Features	Management
Sutures	Use for wounds >5 cm. Wounds subject to tension/flexion (e.g. wounds over joints). Wounds subject to getting wet	Assess damage to tendons, bone, nerves, vessels. Consider XR/CT. Clean wound and remove foreign bodies. LA injection. Suture (see revision tips and Figs. 56.1 and 56.2). Removal of non-absorbable sutures by professional at: 3–5 days for head, 10–14 days for joints, 7–10 days for other sites
Steri-strips	Wounds <5 cm, and NOT subject to tension/flexion/wetting	Don't get wet. Combination with deep absorbable sutures. Self-removal at 3–5 days on head, 7–10 days for other sites.
Glue	Wounds <5 cm. Edges easy to oppose, not subject to tension/flexion or wetting	Take care not to get wet before glue has dried. Glue on top of apposed wound edges – NOT inside wound. Will remove naturally after 7–10 days

(Continued)

TABLE 56.1   (Cont'd)

	Features	Management
Key Complications		
Tetanus	Fever, malaise, trismus, spasms, opisthotonos, dysphagia, arrhythmias, respiratory arrest. **Wounds at risk:** late-presenting wound needing surgery (>6 h), puncture, devitalised tissue, soil/manure, foreign body in wound, compound #, systemic sepsis	**Check immunisation status** (3 primary vaccinations, 2 boosters at 3 and 10 years). **Human tetanus immunoglobulin** (given in tetanus prone wounds regardless of immunisation status). **Booster needed if:** not immunised, status unknown, incomplete primary immunisation, boosters not up to date. **If tetanus develops:** ITU support, tetanus immunoglobulin IM, wound debridement Diazepam for spasms
Complex wounds	**Tendon damage:** reduced movement, deep wound, hand. **Nerve damage:** loss of sensation/movement **Lack of apposition:** complex edge/excess devitalised tissue	Pre-surgical bloods and imaging. Specialist plastics referral – surgery/skin grafts ensuring structure preservation
Infected wound	Contaminated, purulent exudate, delayed presentation, systemically unwell	Clean, pack (prevent apposition) and dress wound. Consider orthoplastics referral for debridement. Abx 5–7 days (e.g. for penicillin non-allergic, flucloxacillin, or co-amoxiclav if soil/faeces/saliva) Review in 3–5 days to assess and decide whether to close wound.

General Suturing Technique

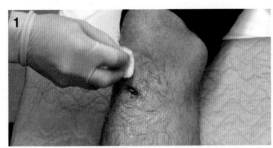

1 Cleanse the skin surrounding the wound with an antiseptic such as chlorhexidine or povidone-iodine. Avoid introducing antiseptic into the wound because it may be toxic to tissue.

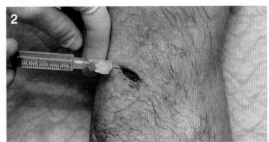

2 Anesthetize the wound prior to exploration and irrigation. Introduce the needle through the wound (as opposed to through the epidermis).

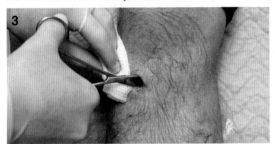

3 Explore the wound to exclude the presence of foreign bodies, gross contamination, or injuries to deep structures. Débride grossly contaminated or devitalized tissue.

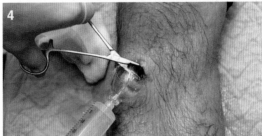

4 Irrigate the wound thoroughly until it is visibly clean. Use of a large syringe with a splash guard is ideal. Retract the wound edges with an instrument to facilitate thorough irrigation.

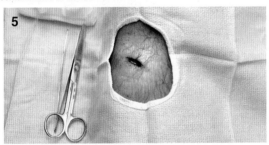

5 Apply a sterile drape, gather the instruments, and ensure that the field is appropriately lit.

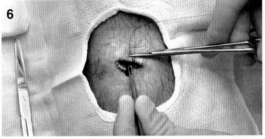

6 Place the first suture at the center of the wound so that it bisects the laceration into two equal segments.

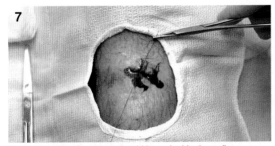

7 Tie the knot. The first throw should be a double throw (ie., surgeon's knot) to prevent it from loosening. Place an additional three (single) throws and then cut the sutures while leaving 1- to 2-cm tails.

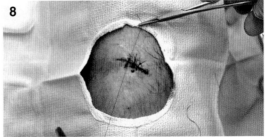

8 Continue to place additional sutures by further bisecting each segment of the laceration. After the last stitch has been placed, cleanse the area and apply an appropriate dressing.

Fig. 56.1 General suturing technique. (From Richard LL, Lovita ES. Methods of wound closure. In: *Roberts and Hedges' Clinical Procedures in Emergency Medicine and Acute Care.* Elsevier; 2019. Copyright © 2019 Elsevier Inc. All rights reserved.)

Instrument Tie

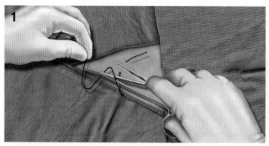

Place the needle driver parallel to the wound and wrap the suture end twice over the needle driver. This forms the surgeon's knot, which prevents the first throw from loosening.

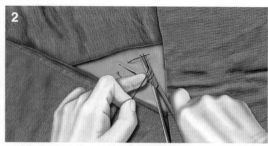

Rotate the needle driver 90 degrees and grasp the short suture end on the opposite side of the laceration.

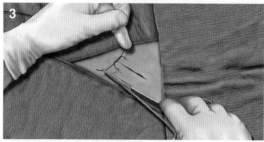

Gently pull the suture ends to the side of the laceration opposite their origin. Tighten only enough to approximate the skin edges; avoid overtightening, which may lead to tissue strangulation.

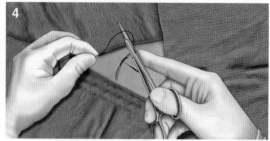

To begin the second throw, again place the needle driver parallel to the laceration. Wrap the long suture end over and around the needle driver once. (Only one wrap is used on throws 2 to 4.)

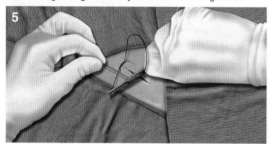

Rotate the needle driver 90 degrees and grasp the short suture end on the opposite side of the laceration.

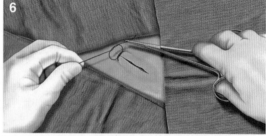

Pull the suture ends to the side of the laceration opposite their origin. On the second and subsequent throws, you can tighten the knot down snugly.

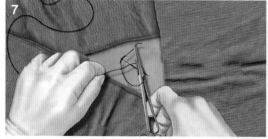

Place an additional two throws (for a total of four), as depicted in *steps 4 through 6*. Remember to place the needle driver parallel to the wound and pull the long suture end over the driver; this will ensure that all knots tied are square knots.

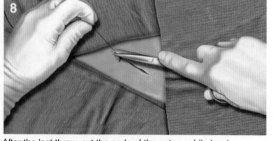

After the last throw, cut the ends of the suture while leaving 1- to 2-cm tails. Avoid cutting the ends too short, which may lead to knot unraveling or difficulty during suture removal.

Fig. 56.2 Instrument tie. (From Custalow C. *Color Atlas of Emergency Department Procedures*. Philadelphia: Elsevier; 2005.)

REVISION TIPS

- When closing wounds – avoid wound edge inversion and skin tension
- LA with adrenaline (vasoconstrictor); reduces LA clearance (enhances effect), less bleeding. Adrenaline CI for digits or appendages (risk of ischaemia). Avoid in severe HTN/ unstable cardiac rhythm

Suture type
- Absorbable sutures: for deep wounds
- Non-absorbable sutures: for superficial wounds

Suture material
- Synthetic: more often used
  - Absorbable synthetic: monocryl, vicryl, PDS
  - Non-absorbable synthetic: Ethilon, Prolene
- Natural: less often used
  - Absorbable natural: collagens
  - Non-absorbable natural: surgical cotton, silk, (steel)

Suture size
- Size 0: Largest suture
- Size 7-0: Smallest suture (the higher the number before the –0, the smaller the suture)

Suture configuration
- Multifilament: easier to handle and tie, higher risk of infection
- Monofilament: more difficult to handle and tie, less risk of infection

57

Snoring

Tejas Netke, Mariella Williams, and Vincent Cumberworth

SETTING: GP. MALE, 56. SNORING

HPC: Worse lying on his back. No breathing difficulty/ gasping. Does not report disturbed sleep or daytime somnolence, occasional morning headache. Systems review: no chest pain, no SOB, no fevers. Increased sweating, intermittent hand tingling (relieved by hanging hand down). **PMHx:** HTN, T2DM. **DHx:** Ramipril, metformin. **SHx:** Non-smoker, low alcohol.

O/E: BMI 26. No nasal polyps, no septal deviation. Prominent supra-orbital ridges, protruding jaw; as you examine his hands, wife says his wedding ring was re-sized recently.

---

1. If a patient presented with snoring/ waking headaches, and had BMI>30, peripheral oedema, hypoxaemia and polycythaemia, then what would be your immediate concern?
2. What are the non-surgical management options for OSA?

Answers: 1. Obesity Hypoventilation Syndrome (OHS)- a specific form of chronic ventilatory failure. 2. Lifestyle modification, mandibular advancement device, CPAP.

TABLE 57.1

	Features	Investigations	Management
OSA	**RFs:** male, excessive snoring, morning headaches, overweight. **Hx & O/E:** unrefreshed sleep, daytime somnolence, irritable, concentration deficit. Pathological airway obstruction	BMI. Epworth sleepiness scale. Polysomnography (PSG); AHI and desaturations. Nasolaryngoscopy: anatomy and obstruction	Weight loss, smoking cessation, physical activity, sleep hygiene. Mandibular advancement device (Fig. 57.1), CPAP. Driving advice. Airway surgery
Pathological airway obstruction	**RFs:** septal deviation, large uvula/turbinates/tonsils, macroglossia, nasal polyps, craniofacial, e.g. retrognathia	Nasolaryngoscopy: assess airway anatomy and level of obstruction	Septoplasty, tonsillectomy, uvulopalatopharyngoplasty, turbinate reduction, tongue base ops., polypectomy, mandibular advancement

TABLE 57.1 (Cont'd)

	Features	Investigations	Management
Simple snoring (diagnosis of exclusion)	RFs: alcohol, sedatives, supine position, smoking, increasing age. Snoring without irregular breathing and hypoxia	Rule out pathological causes	Weight loss, smoking cessation, physical activity, sleep hygiene
Acromegaly (excess growth hormone)	Snoring, morning headaches and bitemporal hemianopia (pituitary adenoma), sweating, carpal tunnel (synovial overgrowth), HTN (visceral hypertrophy), deeper voice (thick vocal cords), dental gaps, weakness, amenorrhoea. T2DM (insulin resistance). Coarsening of facial features and enlargement of hands	Serum IGF-1 (raised if GH is). OGTT (glucose failing to suppress GH). Glucose, phosphate, triglycerides may be raised. Urinary calcium raised. Pituitary MRI: CT may be used to identify ectopic GH/GHRH secretion	Transsphenoidal hypophysectomy. Medical therapy: somatostatin receptor ligands (octreotide), dopamine agonist (e.g. bromocriptine, cabergoline), GH receptor antagonist (pegvisomant)
Hypothyroidism	May contribute to sleep apnoea		

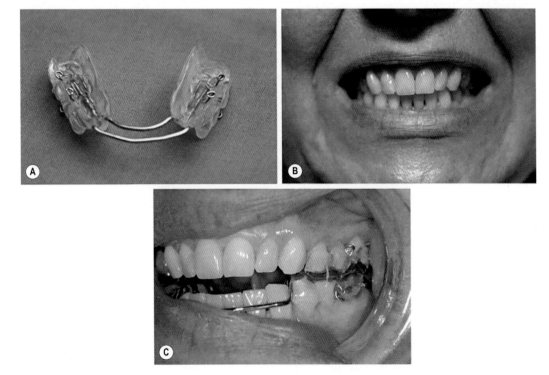

Fig. 57.1 Mandibular advancement device. A) The device. B) Device not in place. C) Device in place. (Reproduced from Park, Si-Myung, Park, Soyeon, Shin, Sangkyun, Lee, Hyeonjong, Ahn, Su-Jin, Kim, Laehyun, Lee, Soo-Hong, Noh, Gunwoo. Designing a mandibular advancement device with topology optimization for a partially edentulous patient. Process of designing mandibular advancement device by topology optimization. 123(6) 850–859. © 2019).

Snoring is noisy breathing due to vibration of relaxed soft tissues of the nose, soft palate or pharynx whilst sleeping or drowsy, and suggests some airway obstruction. In deep sleep, obstruction may prevent breathing (apnoea), leading to lighter sleep to restore airflow. The apnea-hypopnea index (AHI) is the average number of apneas and hypopneas each hour during sleep. Multiple episodes impair daytime functioning, and impair chronic physical/mental health. The vignette suggests acromegaly (sweating, hand tingling, change in ring size), which can cause snoring due to macroglossia. Aims of treatment are to normalise GH/IGF-1 levels and remove the adenoma, while preserving pituitary function. Secondary effects of acromegaly will also need treatment: HTN, DM.

REVISION TIPS

- AHI is categorised as mild at 5–15 episodes per hour, moderate 15–30, severe ≥30
- Oxygen desaturation during OSA; reductions no lower than 90% are mild, dips down to 80%–89% are moderate, <80% are severe

58

Weight Loss

Zoe Kay, Alexander Royston, and Kavita Narula

HPC: Muscle aches and feeling dizzy on standing. No pain or change in bowel habit. No obvious trigger for symptoms, though some stress at work. **PMHx:** nil. **SHx:** Lives with two friends, continues ADLs but feels more tired. Now uses lift instead of stairs due to muscle aches. Non-smoker, 5 units alcohol at weekends.

O/E: Appears pale, wearing loose clothing, otherwise normal. HR 58, BP 100/60, RR 16, SpO_2 99%, Temp 35.8°C.

1. What would blood results show in subclinical hypothyroidism? Is this symptomatic? When do you treat?
2. What are possible complications of thyroidectomy?
3. Which other common condition may thyroid autoantibodies be seen in?

Answers: 1. ↑TSH, T4 normal. This can be symptomatic and if so a trial of levothyroxine is warranted (also if TSH >10). If asymptomatic, treatment is not indicated but TFTs may be monitored. 2. Damage to the recurrent laryngeal nerve and subsequent hoarse voice (airway obstruction if bilateral); parathyroid deficiency, which can ⟶ hypocalcaemia (likely asymptomatic unless all four are removed); compressing haematoma after surgery ⟶ airway compromise; wound infection, pain, scarring. 3. Hashimoto's thyroiditis. Generally hypothyroid but can (rarely) also present with hyperthyroidism. Thyroid peroxidase (TPO) autoantibodies are present in 90% of Hashimoto's thyroiditis, 70% of Graves' (however, TPO autoantibodies can also be found in approximately 10%–15% of normal population).

TABLE 58.1

	Features	Investigations	Management
Endocrine Addison disease	**RFs:** F > M, infection (TB, CMV, fungal), sepsis, ARDS, pneumonia, liver disease. **Hx & O/E:** gum/skin pigmentation (Fig. 58.1), ↓BP/HR, fatigue, weight loss, ↓appetite, syncope, cramps, delayed puberty, amenorrhoea. Co-presents with autoimmune diseases	Lying/ standing BP. U&Es: ↓Na/↑K, ↓9 am cortisol, TFTs (exclude concurrent hypothyroid). **Short Synacthen test:** +ve diagnosis will NOT effectively increase cortisol. Adrenal autoantibodies. CT/MRI: adrenal imaging	Glucocorticoid and mineralocorticoid: hydrocortisone/prednisolone, fludrocortisone. Sick-day rules: ↑dosage with ↑physiological stress (illness/ surgery). MedicAlert bracelet/ necklace/card (see Adrenal crisis below)

(Continued)

TABLE 58.1   (Cont'd)

	Features	Investigations	Management
Hyperthyroidism	**RFs:** smoking, autoimmune disease, FHx. **Hx & O/E:** goitre, tachycardia/palpitations, exophthalmos (Graves'), tremor, acropachy. Red flags: compression (airway noises, dysphagia). Most commonly Graves'. Others: toxic nodular goitre, thyroiditis (de Quervain's), thyroid cancers, drugs (levothyroxine, amiodarone, interferon, PD-1 inhibitors)	**TFTs:** ↓TSH, ↑T4, Thyroid autoantibodies (Graves, disease), FBC/CRP (↑thyroiditis). **USS:** nodules ⟶ FNA (histology)	β-blockers – symptom control **Definitive:** Anti-thyroid: carbimazole, propylthiouracil. Radioactive iodine (for uncontrolled Graves'/toxic multinodular goitre). Thyroidectomy
Malabsorption (and Others)			
Coeliac disease	See *79. FOOD INTOLERANCE*		
Inflammatory bowel disease	See *84. CHANGE IN BOWEL HABIT*		
Malignancy	Increased metabolism, loss of skeletal muscle, fatigue, loss of appetite: cachexia		
Anxiety/depression	**RFs:** PMHx/FHx, life events. **Hx & O/E:** anergia, anhedonia and low mood associated with cognitive or biological symptoms	Diagnosis of exclusion, rule out organic causes	Talking therapies ± antidepressant medications
Key Complications			
Adrenal crisis	Hypovolaemic shock, acute abdo pain, vomiting, diarrhoea, ↓GCS, weakness/cramps. Endocrinological emergency ⟶ immediate hospital management	Never delay treatment for investigations. Addison's patients often carry IM hydrocortisone	If suspected, stat. IV/IM hydrocortisone. Fludrocortisone not needed (weak mineralocorticoid action of hydrocortisone)

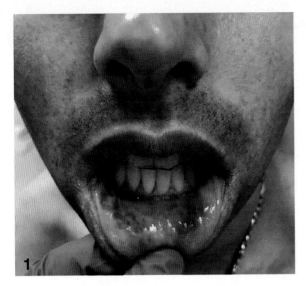

Fig. 58.1 Oral mucosal hyperpigmentation. (From Lee K, Lian C, Vaidya A, Tsibris HC. Oral mucosal hyperpigmentation. *JAAD Case Rep.* 2020 Oct 1;6(10):993–995. Copyright © 2020 American Academy of Dermatology, Inc.)

The vignette describes a vague presentation of fatigue, weight loss and muscle aches – a common presentation in primary care. Postural symptoms, and observations showing hypotension and bradycardia, should prompt

U&Es testing. This would likely show hyponatraemia and hyperkalaemia characteristic of Addison's disease. This patient is female (hence higher risk of autoimmune disease), though she is slightly younger than the typical age of presentation (30–50 yo). Non-organic causes should be considered (including eating disorders), and thyroid disease should be excluded–though this is unlikely with her bradycardia. Malignancy cannot be discounted, although she is young and lacks any convincing risk factors or bowel symptoms suggestive of malignancy.

REVISION TIPS

- Any suspicion of an adrenal crisis, give IV hydrocortisone
- De Quervain's thyroiditis; **painful goitre** + transient hyper- then hypo-thyroidism after a viral URTI
- Acropachy is a dermopathy in Graves disease; soft-tissue swelling of the hands and clubbing
- Hyperpigmentation in Addison's disease is caused by increased cleavage of POMC to produce ACTH, with melanocyte-stimulating hormone as a by-product. Thus, darkened skin indicates a primary rather than a secondary cause of adrenal insufficiency

59

Weight Gain

Katherine Parker, Alexander Royston, and Kavita Narula

GP CONSULTATION, FEMALE, 37.
LOW MOOD AND WEIGHT GAIN

HPC: 6-month history of feeling generally low, poor concentration, 4 kg of unintentional weight gain. No trigger, no change in diet. Fatigues easily looking after 2-year-old daughter. **Systems review:** New constipation, heavy menses. **PMHx:** Vitiligo. **DHx:** COCP, no allergies. **FHx:** Coeliac disease (mother), depression (father).

O/E: Face puffy and pale. Wearing many layers of clothing. Overweight. Visible goitre, thyroid firm and diffusely enlarged. No masses felt. HR 55, BP 125/80. **Ix:** FBC (↓Hb), TFTs (↑TSH, ↓T4).

1. Which test would confirm the likely diagnosis?
2. What are the causes of hypothyroidism?
3. What are the causes of ectopic ACTH secretion?

Answers: 1. Thyroid peroxidase antibodies, when combined with abnormal TFTs, is sufficient to diagnose Hashimoto's. 2. Iodine deficiency (most common worldwide), autoimmune thyroiditis/Hashimoto's (most common in iodine sufficient areas), thyroid damage (surgery, radiotherapy), drugs, iodine excess, transient inflammation (de Quervain's, post-partum), infiltrative (amyloidosis, sarcoidosis, tuberculosis, malignant infiltration, lymphoma, metastasis), congenital. 3. Lung cancer (small cell carcinoma), bronchial carcinoid tumours, phaeochromocytoma, gut carcinoids. Rarer: thymus gland tumours, pancreatic islet cell tumours, thyroid medullary carcinomas.

TABLE 59.1

	Features	Investigations	Management
Primary hypothyroidism	**RFs:** PMHx/FHx autoimmune, Turner's/Down's syndrome, previous head/neck radiation, previous thyroid surgery. Drugs: Lithium, amiodarone, carbimazole, iodine, rifampicin can ⟶ thyroid dysfunction. Preceding thyrotoxicosis (Hashimoto's, de Quervain's) can later ⟶ hypothyroid **Hx & O/E:** ↑weight, fatigue, lethargy, cold intolerance, constipation, weak, menstrual irregularities. Depression, poor memory, dry skin, coarse hair/hair loss (lateral eyebrow), oedema, voice deepening, paraesthesia (carpal tunnel syndrome), oedema, bradycardia, ↓deep tendon reflexes	TFTs (↑TSH, ↓T4), ↑lipids, ↑TPOAb (Hashimoto's). ± screening for autoimmune conditions; FBC (↓Hb, ↑MCV) ↓B12 (pernicious anaemia). ↑HbA1c (T1DM). ↑anti-TTG (coeliac). **ECG:** Bradycardia. **USS Neck:** if palpable thyroid enlargement/focal nodularity. Goitres; Hashimoto's (firm, non-tender)/subacute thyroiditis (de Quervain's: nodular, tender)	Manage in primary care (Levothyroxine). 3-monthly TFTs until two stable results, then annual TFTs. De Quervain's: NSAIDs ± thyroxine (resolves in weeks to months). Endocrinology referral: • subacute thyroiditis • goitre • planning pregnancy • drug-induced hypothyroidism

TABLE 59.1	(Cont'd)		
	Features	**Investigations**	**Management**
Secondary/central hypothyroidism	**RFs:** MEN type 1, head/neck irradiation, PMHx Head injury, post-partum haemorrhage (Sheehan syndrome) **Hx & O/E:** as primary ± hypopituitarism (hypogonadism, secondary adrenal insufficiency). Oligomenorrhoea, atrophic breasts, galactorrhoea	TFTs (↓TSH, ↓T4). ±↑PRL, ↓9 am serum cortisol, ↓testosterone, gonadotropins. **MRI Head:** intracranial mass: headache, papilloedema, bitemporal hemianopia	Levothyroxine. **Definitive:** ± treatment of tumour (medical, surgical, or radiotherapy). + Hydrocortisone (adrenal insufficiency)
Cushing syndrome	**RFs:** long-term corticosteroid use (SLE, RA), adrenal/pituitary tumours, F > M. **Hx & O/E:** weight gain, ↓libido, skin atrophy, purple striae, easy bruising, acne, irregular menses, polydipsia, ↓wound healing, ± pigmentation (ACTH-dependent), mass effect symptoms (pituitary tumour). Hirsutism, facial plethora, hypertension, truncal obesity, buffalo hump, proximal muscle wasting, oedema	↑Serum glucose, U&Es (↓K/↑Na). **Screening tests;** Late night salivary cortisol (↑). 24-hour urinary free cortisol (↑). 1 mg overnight dexamethasone suppression test ⟷ (no suppression). 48-hour low-dose dexamethasone suppression ⟷. **Identify cause;** **Plasma ACTH:** ↓↓/↑↑ ⟶ independent/dependent, **Adrenal CT:** adrenal adenoma/hyperplasia/tumour, OR exogenous steroids **High-dose dexamethasone suppression test.** Suppression ⟶ Cushing disease. Suppression fails ⟶ ectopic ACTH. **Bilateral inferior petrosal sampling:** (↑↑central: peripheral ACTH ratio ⟶ Cushing's). **MRI Head:** pituitary adenoma. **CTCAP:** tumour	Reduce/stop exogenous steroids. Metyrapone/ ketoconazole. **Definitive:** surgery. Adrenal: adrenalectomy/ tumour resection. Cushing's: trans-sphenoidal excision. ± post-surgical corticosteroid replacement therapy. Ectopic ACTH: surgical resection. **DEXA:** osteoporosis
Depression	See *164. LOW MOOD/AFFECTIVE PROBLEMS*		
Medications	Tricyclic antidepressants (amitriptyline), SSRIs, atypical anti-psychotics (clozapine), lithium, carbamazepine, steroids, sulphonylureas (gliclazide), sodium valproate, Depo-Provera		
Key Complications			
Myxoedema coma	Life-threatening complication of severe hypothyroidism: lethargy, bradycardia, hypothermia, seizures, coma – admission to ICU – levothyroxine + hydrocortisone IV		

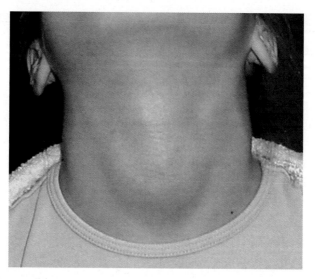

Fig. 59.1 Goitre – Hashimoto thyroiditis. (From Zitelli BJ, McIntire SC, Nowalk AJ. *Atlas of Pediatric Physical Diagnosis*. 6th ed. Philadelphia, PA: Saunders; 2012:369–400.)

The most likely diagnosis in the vignette is primary hypothyroidism caused by Hashimoto's thyroiditis (autoimmune lymphocytic thyroiditis) (Fig. 59.1). Many of her symptoms and risk factors resemble someone with clinical depression: female, young children, fatigue, low mood, poor concentration, and unintentional weight gain; hence that should be considered in the differential diagnosis. However, she has a family and personal history of autoimmune disease, is presenting with cold intolerance, and shows other signs of endocrine dysregulation (bradycardia, menorrhagia, constipation). Her goitre is typical of Hashimoto's and hypothyroidism is confirmed by blood tests. More recently childbirth would make post-partum thyroiditis a strong consideration, which is an immunological 'rebound' from the relative immunosuppression of pregnancy (commonly mistaken for postnatal depression).

REVISION TIPS

- Side effects of glucocorticoids excess 'CUSHINGOID':
- Cataracts
- Ulcers
- Skin (striae, thinning, bruising)
- Hirsutism
- Infections
- Necrosis (AVN)
- Glycosuria/hyperglycaemia
- Osteoporosis
- Immunosuppression
- Diabetes

60

Neck Lump

Margarita Fox, Alexander Royston, and Shilpa Ojha

Margarita Fox, Alexander Royston, and Shilpa Ojha

GP PRESENTATION, FEMALE, 50.
PAINLESS MIDLINE NECK SWELLING

HPC: She reports hoarseness, a sore throat that is not improving and dysphagia, some recent weight loss. Otherwise well. **PMHx:** nil. **SHx:** cigarette smoker: 25 pack years. Alcohol: 20 units/week.

O/E: Obs stable, systemically well, neck examination reveals a firm non-tender midline lump, moving upwards on swallowing.

1. What is the treatment for papillary thyroid carcinoma?
2. 33 yo female, firm lump at bottom of neck with weakness and numbness of her arm on that side. What is the most likely diagnosis?
3. 74 yo man, dysphagia, regurgitation, ongoing cough and halitosis. Examination: midline lump that gurgles on palpation. What is the most likely diagnosis?

Answers: 1. Surgery (usual total thyroidectomy), radio-iodine ablation and levothyroxine. 2. Cervical rib (female adults most commonly, may develop thoracic outlet syndrome). 3. Pharyngeal pouch (older men, usually not visible but if large then see midline lump-gurgles on palpation).

TABLE 60.1

	Features	Investigations	Management
Midline Reactive lymphadenopathy	Benign. Infection (bacterial/viral/ parasitic), sarcoidosis. Symptoms: cause-dependent, systemic/local infective	**USS:** to exclude other causes (if clinical doubt)	Reassurance, treat according to cause
Thyroglossal cyst	**RFs:** Congenital, children/young adults (<20 yo). **Hx & O/E:** painless, smooth, palpable midline mass, elevates with tongue protrusion	**USS:** well-defined cystic lesion (midline internal echoes). **CT/MRI:** if USS ambiguous	Surgical excision of entire thyroglossal tract (Sistrunk procedure). Infection-prone: tender erythematous masses

(Continued)

TABLE 60.1 (Cont'd)

	Features	Investigations	Management
Thyroid adenoma/hyperplastic nodule	**RFs:** F > M age (<20, >70 yo), Iodine deficiency, FHx, genetics. Most are non-functioning (asymptomatic). Midline mass, elevates on swallowing. **Hx & O/E:** retrosternal mass, may compress subclavicular vein → Pemberton's sign (raising arms → facial plethora)	**TFTs:** non-functioning ⟷TSH, toxic ↓TSH. **Iodine[123] scan.** **USS:** solid homogeneous nodules with hypoechoic halo sign, r/o malignancy. **FNA.** **CT (non-contrast)**	Watchful waiting. **Definitive:** subtotal or total thyroidectomy (+ lifelong thyroxine). Radioactive iodine
Multinodular goitre	**RFs:** F > M, age (>70 yo), Iodine-deficiency, FHx, genetics. May be hypo-/eu-/hyper-thyroid **Hx & O/E:** commonly non-toxic and asymptomatic. May be palpable. Compressive; dysphagia, hoarse voice	**TFTs:** non-toxic ⟷TSH, toxic ↓TSH, ↑T3/4. **USS:** multiple nodules, may be solid/cystic. **Iodine[123] scan** uptake in nodules, low in rest of thyroid	
Thyroid cancer	**RFs:** Prior head/neck irradiation, sex (F > M), Hashimoto's, FHx: MEN IIa/IIb syndrome. **Hx & O/E:** often asymptomatic. Painless mass (rapid growth), hoarse/stridor, dysphagia. ↑Risk: nodules >4 cm, firm, fixed, cervical lymphadenopathy, vocal cord paralysis **Papillary:** commonest. Mean diagnosis: 45 yo. Spread cervical LNs (early). Good prognosis. **Follicular:** 10% of thyroid cancers. Spread → haematogenous, often lungs. Mean diagnosis: 50 yo. **Medullary (MTC):** sporadic or part of MENIIa/IIb **Anaplastic:** elderly, rapidly growing solid thyroid mass, hoarseness, dysphagia	⟷TSH (usually), calcitonin (MTC: monitoring). **USS:** hypoechogenic, microcalcifications, absent halo, irregular margins, increased vascularity. **FNA:** cannot differentiate invasive follicular versus benign adenoma (open biopsy required). **CT head and neck.** Genetic screening: MENIIa/IIb syndrome. **Urine:** 24 h VMA/metanephrines	Refer to ENT/thyroid MDT. **Papillary/follicular:** guidelines: >2 cm → total thyroidectomy. Central LNs → level VI selective neck dissection. >4 cm/extrathyroid spread → adjuvant post-op radioactive iodine **MTC:** Total thyroidectomy and level VI neck dissection, consider prophylactic thyroidectomy (children). **Anaplastic:** Poor prognosis. Surgery not indicated. Palliative radiotherapy ± chemotherapy
Also, salivary gland stones/tumours, dermoid cysts, laryngeal swellings			
Lateral (Anterior-Posterior Triangles [Fig. 60.1])			
Branchial cyst	**RFs:** congenital, <20 yo, FHx. **Hx & O/E:** mobile cystic mass, lateral, anterior to sternocleidomastoid (junction of upper ⅔-lower ⅓)	**USS + FNA.** **MRI neck:** (patients 40+ yo consider cystic metastasis from head/neck SCCs	Conservative. Surgical excision. Sclerotherapy

TABLE 60.1 (Cont'd)

	Features	Investigations	Management
Carotid body tumours	Benign paragangliomas (5% malignant). 10% catecholamine-secreting. RFs: chronic hypoxia, genetics. Hx & O/E: pulsatile painless neck lump ± bruit, growing slowly but if large can compress → CN palsies	Doppler USS. MRI/MRA neck/CT neck/ CTA neck. PET-CT. Urine/plasma: 24h metanephrines. MIBG scan if secreting. Angiography: 'Lyre's sign' splaying of external and internal carotid arteries	Conservative: active monitoring/serial imaging. Surgical excision. Radiotherapy (if unresectable)
Further differentials	**Anterior:** Cystic hygroma, thyroid swellings (lobe), pharyngeal pouch, submandibular gland swelling, lymph nodes, parotid swelling. **Posterior:** Cervical rib, lipoma, carotid aneurysm		

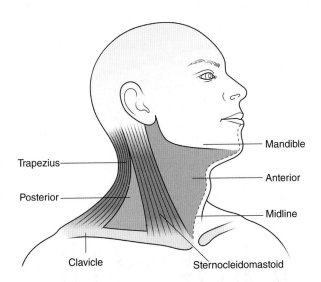

Fig. 60.1 The triangles of the neck. The sternocleidomastoid divides the neck into two triangles. The anterior triangle contains lymph nodes, submandibular gland, tail of the parotid and the carotid bifurcation. The posterior triangle contains lymph nodes and the spinal accessory nerve. (Reproduced with permission from Dhillon RS, East CA. *Head and Neck Neoplasia, Ear, Nose and Throat and Head and Neck Surgery.* 87–117, Copyright © 2013 Elsevier Ltd. All rights reserved.)

The diagnosis of papillary thyroid carcinoma is suspected from the history in the vignette. Whilst a neck lump can have a wide differential and she is slightly older than is typical, this patient reports hoarseness, a persistent sore throat, dysphagia and weight loss against a background of smoking and alcohol. This should trigger a 2-week wait referral to ENT. Papillary carcinomas make up 80% of thyroid malignancies, and this would not be confirmed until a tissue sample is taken. On examination this lump was firm (making it less likely to be benign) and its movement on swallowing is suggestive of fixation (although this does not help differentiate between benign/malignant).

REVISION TIPS

- Lumps (age groups)
  - children – congenital masses: branchial anomalies (branchial cleft cyst/sinus); thyroglossal duct cysts
  - young adults – inflammatory/infectious neck masses (cervical adenitis)
  - older – benign/malignant neoplasms, pharyngeal pouch
- RED FLAGS: if suspicious → USS ± FNA
- Firm, fixed lump
- Dysphagia, stridor, hoarseness
- RFs: smoking, alcohol, PMHx head and neck cancer, irradiation, Hashimoto's thyroiditis. FHx of MEN syndrome
- B symptoms
- CN palsies

61

Hypercalcaemia

Zoe Kay, Alexander Royston, and Kavita Narula

GP CONSULTATION, FEMALE, 54.
NON-SPECIFIC ABDOMINAL PAIN

HPC: Second similar presentation in the last 3 weeks, also back and hip pain unresponsive to ibuprofen. Memory increasingly poor, which she attributes to her depression. **PMHx:** Depression, impacted renal calculus requiring therapy 1/12 ago. **DHx:** Citalopram, macrogol. **SHx:** Never smoked.

  O/E: Sunken eyes and dry lips, no visible JVP at 45 degrees, chest clear, normal heart sounds, abdomen SNT.

1. What condition other than hypercalcaemia is a key cause of an Osborne/J wave on ECG?
2. What is calcium-alkali syndrome?
3. Which lung tumours may secrete parathyroid hormone-related peptide? What are the other paraneoplastic endocrine signs of lung cancer?

Answers: 1. Hypothermia, usually in the context of sinus bradycardia and prolonged QT interval. 2. Excess calcium and alkali ingestion in individuals with renal disease → ↓GFR and further ↓excretion of calcium, ↑water loss and ↓PTH secretions: worsens hypercalcaemia and alkalaemia. 3. Squamous cell lung cancer. See Table 61.2 for lung cancer paraneoplastic endocrine potential.

TABLE 61.1

	Features	Investigations	Management
Primary hyperparathyroidism	**RFs:** FHx, head/neck radiation. Parathyroid hyperplasia/adenoma: → excess PTH (rarely due to underlying cancer). **Hx & O/E:** bones (joint/back pain), abdominal (heartburn, pain, constipation, N&V, ↓appetite), dehydration (headache, thirst, urinary frequency), renal calculi, mental (anxiety, depression, confusion), fatigue, weakness	**ECG:** (Fig. 61.1). ↑PTH, ↑calcium, ↓phosphate, U&Es. **USS** (or CT) of neck. 24 h urinary calcium, kidney imaging, DEXA scan. PTH → ↑bone breakdown, ↑calcium reabsorption in kidneys/absorption in gut, ↑vitamin D production	Hydration (2–3 L water/day). If corrected calcium >2.85 mM: consider cinacalcet (calcimimetic). **Definitive:** parathyroidectomy

TABLE 61.1   (Cont'd)

	Features	Investigations	Management
Multiple myeloma	RFs: age (>50), ethnicity (Afro-Caribbean). CRABI: • Hypercalcaemia • Renal dysfunction (can present as AKI). • Anaemia (+ thrombocytopenia/ bleeding) • Bone (back pain, fractures) • Infections (frequent)	FBC ($\downarrow$Hb, $\downarrow$platelets), U&Es ($\uparrow$urea/creatinine), $\uparrow$calcium, $\uparrow$ESR. **Urine:** Bence Jones proteins. **Serum electrophoresis.** **Serum-free light chain assay:** paraprotein. **Marrow biopsy:** plasma cells. XR: 'punched out' lesions, pepperpot skull, vertebral collapse. **MRI:** whole body	Analgesia, bisphosphonates, transfusions, antibiotics (infections). **Definitive:** chemotherapy. Induction: bortezomib + dexamethasone ± thalidomide. ± stem cell transplant
Hypercalcaemia in malignancy	Late sign of malignancy, suspect in sudden symptomatic rise in calcium. Secondary to bone metastases and osteolytic breakdown (paraneoplastic phenomenon of PTHrP-secretion from tumour)	$\downarrow$/undetectable PTH, $\uparrow\uparrow$calcium. $\uparrow$Inflammatory markers	**Initial:** discuss with patient/NOK if treatment is appropriate. **Definitive:** if symptomatic and for active treatment → admit, IVI and bisphosphonates
Granulomatous diseases	RFs: sarcoidosis, tuberculosis. Granulomas release vitamin D → $\downarrow$renal calcium excretion and $\uparrow$GI absorption	CXR. Sputum culture. Acid-fast Bacilli smear. **Serum ACE**	Steroids to control hypercalcaemia. **Definitive:** treat cause
Drugs	Thiazide diuretics, lithium. Calcium with antacids or vitamin D (calcium-alkali syndrome). Vitamin D or A intoxication. Excess calcium supplements	Medication review. Ix to r/o other causes of hypercalcaemia	Stop medications where possible. Vitamin D is in topicals for psoriasis
Renal disease	RFs: primary glomerular disease, diabetic nephropathy, hypertensive nephropathy, PCKD, chronic interstitial nephritis. **Tertiary hyperparathyroidism:** long-standing $\uparrow$PTH → parathyroid hypertrophy and decoupling of parathyroid activity	**Tertiary:** $\uparrow\uparrow$PTH, $\uparrow$calcium, $\uparrow$phosphate. *Other CKD Ix:* **Bloods** (U&Es), **urine** ACR, **USS.** XR: bony lesions secondary to renal osteodystrophy	Consider treatment for renal condition: eGFR-dependent. **Tertiary:** managed surgically
Immobility	Secondary to excess bone turnover and osteoclast → osteoblast activity	Rule out other causes	Encourage mobilisation. Bisphosphonates
Familial hypocalciuric hypercalcaemia	Benign defect in renal and parathyroid calcium receptors → $\downarrow$renal excretion and $\uparrow$PTH. Rare autosomal dominant. Usually asymptomatic	24 h urinary calcium. U&Es. Ca/Cr clearance ratio <0.01. If inconclusive → genetic testing	No treatment required
Other endocrine diseases	Thyrotoxicosis. Addison disease	Clinical suspicion. Check TFTs/9 am cortisol	Treat underlying cause

(Continued)

TABLE 61.1   (Cont'd)

Key Complications of Primary Hyperparathyroidism

Bone	Osteoporosis
Pancreas	Chronic pancreatitis
Brain	Delirium, psychosis, hallucinations, seizures, neurological signs
Eyes	Corneal calcification
Kidney	Calcium-based kidney stones
Stomach	Peptic ulcers
ECG changes	Variable: shortened QTc, Osborne waves, ST-elevation, T-wave inversions, biphasic T-waves (Fig. 61.1)

TABLE 61.2   Paraneoplastic Features in Lung Cancer

Cancer	Paraneoplastic Features
Small-cell lung cancer	ACTH, SIADH, Lambert-Eaton syndrome, SVC obstruction, carcinoid syndrome
Squamous cell lung cancer	PTH-related peptide (PTHrP), Pancoast tumour/Horner syndrome
Adenocarcinoma	Hypertrophic osteoarthropathy

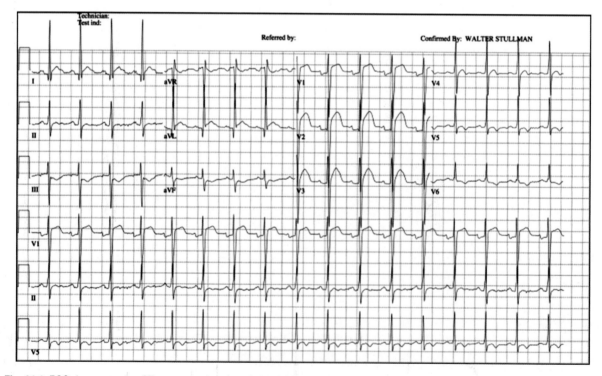

Fig. 61.1 ECG demonstrating ST segment elevations in leads V1 - V4, I, and avL, ST segment depressions in leads III and avF, and biphasic T waves in leads V4 - V6. Serum calcium was 15 mg/dL (~3.74 mmol/l). https://www.sciencedirect.com/science/article/pii/S0735675717300931.

The vignette describes the third commonest endocrine disease which is primary hyperparathyroidism (diabetes and thyroid disease are more common). She has the archetypal presentation of stones, bones, groans and psychic moans. However, many patients present with only dehydration and fatigue. This patient is symptomatic and may need admission for fluid resuscitation if corrected calcium >3.0 mmol/L. ECG changes are not described in the vignette but commonly involve QTc shortening when hypercalcaemia is moderate (and may be variable at higher concentrations). Important differentials to discount are malignancies and myeloma. Although she does report abdominal and bony pain, she has no weight loss, anaemia or fatigue (hypercalcaemia is typically a late-stage complication of cancer). She is also a non-smoker, making lung cancer (and other cancers) marginally less likely.

REVISION TIPS

- Stones, bones, groans and moans – also remember: dehydration (thirst/polydipsia/polyuria/nocturia), fatigue, itch
- Increased PTH is most commonly due to a parathyroid adenoma, less commonly due to parathyroid hyperplasia, and rarely due to parathyroid carcinoma
- A suppressed PTH in context of raised calcium should trigger investigations for malignancy, including CXR to exclude lung cancer or metastases, lymphoma, sarcoidosis or tuberculosis

62

Driving Advice

Natalia Hackett, Alexander Royston, and Jennifer Powell

GP CONSULTATION, FEMALE, 18.
SHE HAS TYPE 1 DIABETES AND WOULD LIKE DRIVING ADVICE

You inform her of the following:
- She needs to inform the DVLA of her condition and that she takes insulin
- She must practise appropriate glucose monitoring, i.e. check her CBG no more than 2 hours before she starts driving and every 2 hours once driving has started
- She should always have a fast-acting carbohydrate on-hand
- She can have no more than one episode of hypoglycaemia requiring assistance before her licence is revoked
- She needs to have hypoglycaemia awareness

1. How would you manage a 30-year-old male with his first unprovoked seizure 1 month ago who is continuing to drive despite being informed previously not to?
2. A patient calls to find out when he can start driving again. He's just had a successful PCI post-NSTEMI. What is your answer?
3. If patient takes lorazepam for anxiety, can he drive? What about if he is a heavy goods vehicle (HGV) driver?

Answers: 1. Inform him that if he continues to drive you will inform the DVLA yourself to revoke his licence. 2. 1 week. 3. Yes, providing his ability to drive is not impaired and his levels are <100 μg/L. Same rules apply for HGV drivers.

TABLE 62.1

	DVLA Restriction (Length of Time Licence Revoked for)
NEUROLOGICAL	
First unprovoked epileptic seizure	6 months
Epilepsy or multiple unprovoked seizures	12 months
Vasovagal episode with provoking factor	No restriction
Unexplained syncope without reliable prodrome	6 months
Solitary loss of consciousness (likely cardiovascular origin, identified and treated cause)	1 month
Sudden unprovoked or unpredictable dizziness	Until symptom control
Parkinson's disease	Determined by disability, case by case
TIA/stroke	1 month

TABLE 62.1 (Cont'd)

	DVLA Restriction (Length of Time Licence Revoked for)
CARDIOVASCULAR	
Angina (if symptoms with rest, emotion or at the wheel)	Until symptoms under control
Post-CABG	1 month
Successful PCI for ACS	1 week
Arrythmias, e.g. atrial flutter/fibrillation, tachycardias, etc.	Until controlled for 4 weeks
Symptomatic aortic stenosis	Disqualified if symptomatic
Pacemaker implantation	1 week
ICD implantation associated with incapacitation	6 months
SUBSTANCE MISUSE	
Alcohol misuse	6 months minimum of abstinence or controlled drinking, normal blood parameters
Alcohol dependence	1 year of abstinence from alcohol
Alcohol-related seizure	6 months
VISUAL	
Reduced visual acuity	Must be at least 6/12 or be able to read a number plate from 20 metres
DIABETES	
Impaired hypoglycaemic awareness	Until GP/consultant confirms adequate awareness
PSYCHIATRY	
Acute psychotic disorder, schizophrenia, stable mania	Until stable for 3 months, treatment adherence, specialist report, free from medication effects that would impair driving
PRESCRIPTION MEDICATIONS <ul><li>Clonazepam</li><li>Diazepam</li><li>Flunitrazepam</li><li>Lorazepam</li><li>Oxazepam</li><li>Temazepam</li><li>Methadone</li><li>Morphine</li></ul>	Covered by the law – and are legal if taken at prescribed doses as limits for the drugs are higher than normally prescribed doses. Patients must not have impaired ability to drive. Threshold levels in blood also apply to recreational drugs that may have been taken by 'accidental exposure'

The guidelines are generally very prescriptive on the management and limitations imposed by medical conditions. In Type 1 diabetes, the assessment of a patient's hypoglycaemic awareness may have a subjective component but clear descriptions are given: severe hypoglycaemia requires the assistance of another person. If necessary, then patients must be advised of the laws and warned of the legal consequences of breaking them.

REVISION TIPS

- Hypoglycaemia symptoms include: hunger, anxiety, irritability, decreased concentration, palpitations, lethargy, decreased vision, confusion
- Whilst doctors have a duty of confidentiality, sometimes public safety risk outweighs risk of breaking confidentiality, but always inform patient before you do so

63

Pubertal Development

Michael Campbell, Alice Parker, and Alex Ridgway

**GP CONSULTATION. MALE, 16.
DELAYED PUBERTY**

HPC: Patient concerned about growth relative to peers and lack of secondary sexual characteristics (enlarging testes, pubic hair). **FHx:** Mother menarche aged 12, father had growth spurt/pubertal development aged 16. **SHx:** Experiences bullying at school.

O/E: Height/weight in 2nd age centile, Tanner 1 pubic hair, Tanner 2 genitals.

1. What may cause gonadal damage that can lead to delayed puberty?
2. When should you actively treat constitutional delay, and what would you treat with?

Answers: 1. Mumps, radiotherapy, chemotherapy, trauma, surgery. 2. Hormone therapy if social/mood problem.

TABLE 63.1

	Features	Investigations	Management
Constitutional delay	Height within mean parental height range, lack of secondary sex characteristics	FHx of late menarche/delayed puberty. ↓FSH/LH, ↓GnRH, ↓Testosterone Hand XR for bone age.	No treatment, generally. If social/mood problems, testosterone 4–6 months
Klinefelter syndrome	Infertility, gynaecomastia, small testes, tall stature, long limbs. Osteoporosis, T2DM, autoimmune	Genetic testing 47XXY. Hypergonadotropic hypogonadism; ↑FSH/LH, ↓testosterone	Testosterone replacement. Surgical breast reduction. Education/behaviour support. Fertility treatment.
Kallmann syndrome	M > F. Delayed start/completion of puberty. **Anosmia**, infertility, small testes, normal height	Genetic testing; 5%–10%. X-linked recessive. Hypogonadotropic hypogonadism; ↓FSH/LH, ↓GnRH ↓testosterone	Sex hormone replacement (testosterone, or oestrogen/progesterone). Fertility treatment
Gonadal damage	Surgery, chemo-/radio-therapy, trauma, mumps	Review patient history. Testicular ultrasound	Depends on cause

TABLE 63.1	(Cont'd)		
	Features	**Investigations**	**Management**
Other Important Differentials			
Malnutrition	Anorexia nervosa: F > M, peak onset 14 years. Self-induced weight loss, distorted body perception. See also *143. INFANT FEEDING PROBLEMS* and *156. CHILD ABUSE*	↓FSH/LH, ↓T3, ↓K⁺. ↓BP, ↓HR. Reduced BMI	Refeeding if life-threatening. Anorexia family therapy. Psychoeducation on nutrition, self-image, support networks
Chronic disease	For example, cystic fibrosis, coeliac disease, Crohn's disease; see relevant cases		
Turner syndrome	See *148. DYSMORPHIC CHILD*		

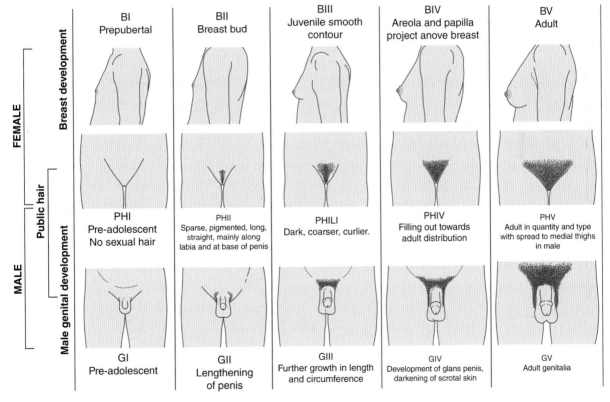

Fig. 63.1 Tanner stages of puberty for breast (B), pubic hair (PH) and genitals (G). (Reproduced with permission from Precocious Puberty. Elsevier Point of Care.)

Pubertal development evaluates breast, pubic hair and genitals (Fig. 63.1). The vignette describes constitutional delay, the commonest cause in males, suggested by FHx and lack of genetic disorder features (e.g. tall stature of Klinefelter's, anosmia in Kallmann syndromes). Eventual height is often normal. Systems review considers underlying chronic disease, psychosocial or significant event (e.g. trauma). Consider Turner syndrome in a female with late breast development or amenorrhea. Rare conditions include complete androgen insensitivity, Noonan syndrome or glycogen storage disorders. Referral to paediatric endocrinology may be needed. Encourage uptake of MMR vaccine in children, since mumps can cause testicular damage through orchitis.

REVISION TIPS

- Male puberty stages: 1. Testis enlargement (>4 mL); 2. Pubic hair; 3. Growth spurt (testis volume >12 mL)
- Precocious if puberty starts <9 years. Delayed if no signs of puberty by 14 years
- Female stages: 1. Breast (8.5–12.5 years); 2. Pubic hair/growth spurt; 3. Menarche (mean 12.7 years)
- Precocious if starts <8 years. Delayed if no periods by 16 years, or no signs of puberty by 14 years

Loss of Libido

Rachel Hawthorne and Anna Ogier

1. What are the physical signs of hypogonadism in a man?
2. What are common pharmacological causes of loss of libido in a woman?
3. What are some contraindications to testosterone replacement?

Answers: 1. Central obesity, reduced testicular size, loss of pubic hair, sarcopenia, more body fat, gynaecomastia, osteoporosis. 2. Hormonal contraception, tamoxifen, aromatase inhibitors, SSRIs, alcohol. 3. Prostate Ca, breast Ca, severe bladder outlet obstruction, OSA, CCF, liver dysfunction, hyperlipidaemia, polycythaemia.

TABLE 64.1

	Features	Investigations	Management
MALE XY Hormonal – hypogonadism (general)	**RFs:** age, obesity, diabetes, CKD, alcohol excess, OSA. **Hx & O/E:** low libido, loss of nocturnal tumescence/erections, fatigue, mood change, hot flushes, infertile. Central obesity, small testes, sarcopenia, increased body fat, gynaecomastia, fracture	LH/FSH, free/total testosterone, prolactin. DEXA scan (osteoporosis). Investigate comorbidities, e.g. T2DM, COPD, CKD, obesity, OSA	Treat cause (e.g. weight loss, lifestyle) and comorbidities. Testosterone replacement (contraindications, see answer to Q3). Monitor: testosterone, LFTs, PSA, lipids, haematocrit
Hormonal – hypogonadism (primary)	Klinefelter's/Noonan's, gonadal dysgenesis, cryptorchidism. *Acquired:* anorchia, orchitis, chemo-/radiotherapy (Leydig cells), alcohol, CRF, idiopathic testicular atrophy, cirrhosis	Early morning serum testosterone ↓, LH n/↑, anti-Müllerian hormone (AMH), inhibin B	If possible treat the cause. Supportive treatment. Testosterone replacement if appropriate. Genetic testing

(Continued)

TABLE 64.1   (Cont'd)

	Features	Investigations	Management
Hormonal – hypogonadism (secondary)	*Congenital:* Prader-Willi, Kallmann, Laurence-Moon. *Acquired:* drugs (opioids, exogenous androgens, LDRH agonists, GnRH antagonists), systemic illness (e.g. COPD, HIV), haemochromatosis	Morning testosterone ↓, LH/FSH ↓, ↓AMH, inhibin B. Exclude cause, e.g. ↑serum ferritin, transferrin saturation	If possible treat the cause. Supportive treatment. Testosterone replacement if appropriate. Genetic testing
FEMALE XX Menopause – primary or secondary	RFs: age, oophorectomy. O/E: vulvar/vaginal atrophy	E2 level, SHBG, total testosterone, calculated free testosterone, prolactin, TSH	Counselling, HRT. See *115. MENOPAUSAL PROBLEMS.* Topical oestrogen
FEMALE/MALE XX/XY Hormonal – hyperprolactinaemia	Pituitary prolactinoma (visual field defects, headaches), CKD, drugs (oestrogen, metoclopramide, imipramine, risperidone, phenothiazine). Hx & O/E: erectile dysfunction, gynaecomastia, galactorrhoea	↑Prolactin, ↓LH, ↓FST, ↓testosterone. **MRI:** brain and pituitary	Treat cause, drug review. Adenoma: dopamine agonist (bromocriptine), radiotherapy, transsphenoidal hypophysectomy
Hormonal – hypothalamo-pituitary axis	Malnutrition, eating disorder, malabsorption, excess exercise, physical/psychological stressors		Treat the cause
Hormonal; hyper-/hypothyroid	Graves' – increased SHBG, reduced testosterone	T3, T4, TSH	Treat the cause
Iatrogenic/pharmacological	See Revision tips. Exclude marijuana, alcohol, narcotics		Risk-benefit assessment of medications
Psychological	Depression, bipolar disorder, stress, insomnia, PTSD	Psychological assessment	Treat the cause
'Sexual aversion'	M: erectile dysfunction. F: vaginismus, dyspareunia, chronic pelvic pain		Treat the cause

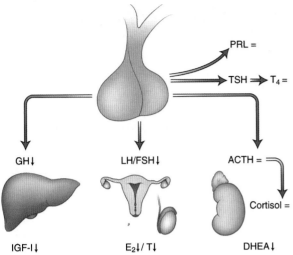

GH↓

LH/FSH↓

ACTH =

PRL =

TSH ⟹ T₄ =

Cortisol =

IGF-I↓

E₂↓/ T↓

DHEA↓

During aging:
Menopause: $E_2\downarrow$
Andropause: $T\downarrow$
Adrenopause: DHEA↓
Somatopause: GH/IGF-I↓

Fig. 64.1 Ageing hormonal changes. Somatopause; reduced insulin-like growth factor 1 (IGF1) due to lower growth hormone (GH). Menopause/andropause; reduced oestradiol (E2)/ testosterone (T) due to lower LH/FSH. On initiation of menopause, LH/FSH increase sharply. Adrenopause; reduced dehydroepiandrosterone (DHEA) without clinically evident changes in ACTH and cortisol secretion. (Adapted with permission from van den Beld and Lamberts, Endocrinology and Aging. In: Williams Textbook of Endocrinology, 14th Edition (Melmed, Koenig, Rosen, Auchus, Goldfine). Elsevier, 2019)

There is a gradual fall in sexual desire with normal ageing (Fig. 64.1). Loss of libido is reduced desire for sexual activity, and can be primary (always absent), secondary (decline) or situational. It is often multifactorial and can signify serious disease. Full history and examination are essential. In the vignette, there are a few possible causes of low libido. Hypogonadism is suggested by T2DM, central obesity, gynaecomastia, small testes and low testosterone. Medications (tamsulosin, finasteride, sertraline), psychological (depression) and smoking/ drinking history need to be considered. Improving general health and rationalising medications should precede testosterone replacement (routes; IM/SC/TD/oral/nasal/buccal).

REVISION TIPS

- Loss of libido is an expected part of ageing, but sometimes there is an important underlying diagnosis, so it should be investigated
- Loss of libido is an adverse effect of medications that either influence hormone levels or psychological processes, or alter drug/hormone metabolism
- Relevant drugs: SSRI, antipsychotic, lithium, α-/β-blocker, 5-α reductase inh., clonidine, ketoconazole, LHRH analogue, spironolactone, antiandrogen, glucocorticoid, hormone contraception, tamoxifen, aromatase inhibitor

65

Gynaecomastia

Lucy Andrews and Natarajan Vaithilingam

BREAST CLINIC, MALE 63.
ENLARGED BREAST TISSUE

HPC: 2/12 painless breast swelling bilaterally. No nipple discharge or nipple/skin changes. No new medications. No anorexia, weight loss or fatigue. T2DM (metformin). 40 units alcohol a week. Ex-smoker.

O/E: Symmetrical enlargement of the breast tissue, no erythema, nipple changes or discharge seen. When palpating, the tissue feels like breast with no discrete lumps. Six spider naevi across the chest.

---

1. How would you expect breast cancer to present in men?

2. A man with symmetrical breast enlargement, no red flags on examination. You notice he recently saw a GP for 'seborrhoeic' dermatitis. PMH alcohol excess. What is the most likely cause of gynaecomastia?

Answers: 1. Unilateral lump/swelling with or without discomfort/nipple changes. Systemic features of fatigue, weight loss or reduced appetite absent unless distant metastases. FHx of breast or ovarian cancers may be present. On examination the breast enlargement is more likely to be unilateral and have concerning features such as firm/hard irregular painless lump with/without fixity to chest wall. Axillary/SCF lymph nodes may be enlarged. 2. Alcoholism with liver dysfunction with/without side effect of medication (it is likely this man was treated with ketoconazole).

TABLE 65.1

	Features	Investigations	Management
INCREASED OESTROGEN			
Physiological	**New-born:** increased oestrogen due to maternal sources. **Pubertal:** oestrogen levels peak before testosterone	Nil required	**Reassure:** new-born/teenage boys should resolve
Alcohol excess	Palmar erythema, Dupuytren's contracture, ascites, >5 spider naevi, hepatomegaly, jaundice	$\uparrow\uparrow$ALT, $\downarrow$albumin, $\uparrow$GGT	Referral for alcohol cessation services
Drugs	Breast development requires oestrogen; medications may have oestrogen-like properties, or they may increase oestrogen availability. Key examples; digitalis, clomiphene, marijuana, spironolactone, anabolic steroids, CCBs, ACEi, neuroleptics, ethanol		Consider modifying dosage/switching the medication/stopping

TABLE 65.1 (Cont'd)

	Features	Investigations	Management
Endocrine	Feminising testicular neoplasm (e.g. Leydig or Sertoli cell), lung/adrenal tumours, thyrotoxicosis (increased peripheral aromatisation), hyperprolactinaemia	Hormonal profile. Imaging for source	Refer to endocrinology

DECREASED TESTOSTERONE

	Features	Investigations	Management
Physiological	Senile gynaecomastia: testosterone decreases with increased age	Nil required if clinically not concerning	Testosterone therapy as appropriate
Testicular	Testicular cancer, mumps/viral orchitis, previous torsion. See *64. LOSS OF LIBIDO; 197. SCROTAL/TESTICULAR PAIN AND/OR LUMP/SWELLING*		
Klinefelter syndrome	Usually presenting at puberty. Tall, small firm testes, infertility, delayed puberty, learning difficulties	**Karyotyping:** XXY. Hypergonadotropic hypogonadism: ↑FSH/LH ↓testosterone	Testosterone replacement therapy
Chronic renal failure	See *177. CHRONIC KIDNEY DISEASE*		
Drugs	Androgens are anti-proliferative for breast tissue; drugs reducing concentration/effect of androgens may cause gynaecomastia. *Key examples*; cyproterone, bicalutamide, cimetidine, finasteride, metronidazole, ketoconazole, phenytoin, psychoactive drugs, metoclopramide		Consider modifying dosage/switching the medication/stopping

OTHER DIFFERENTIALS

	Features	Investigations	Management
Pseudo-gynaecomastia	Global weight gain, increased breast tissue (which feels like adipose tissue). Other RFs absent. See *13. OBESITY*		
Breast cancer	See *1. NIPPLE DISCHARGE*		

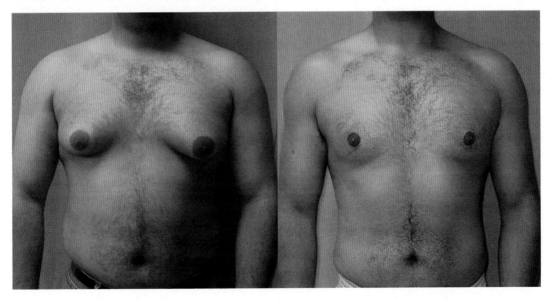

Fig. 65.1 Gynaecomastia. (https://commons.wikimedia.org/wiki/File:GynecomastiaFrontalAsymSevere.jpg) Attribution: JMZ1122 Dr. Mordcai Blau, CC BY-SA 3.0 (https://creativecommons.org/licenses/by-sa/3.0)

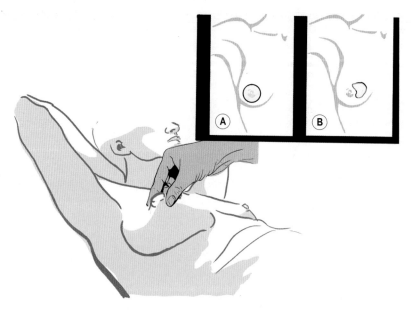

Fig. 65.2 (A) In patients with true gynecomastia, a rubbery or firm mound of tissue concentric with the nipple–areolar complex is felt, whereas in pseudo gynecomastia, no such disc of tissue is found. (B) In patients with malignancy, a hard or firm mass may be felt outside the areola. (Illustrated by Hollie Blaber.)

Gynaecomastia (Fig. 65.1) occurs due to altered balance of active androgen and oestrogen; 35% of men develop it. This can occur due to increased oestrogen or decreased testosterone levels; most are idiopathic. In the vignette, the most likely diagnosis is alcohol excess. However, normal physiological factors may also be contributing (e.g. senile gynaecomastia). This patient has alcohol excess and systemic features of liver damage (>5 spider naevi). On examination (Fig. 65.2) there are no concerning features to point towards malignancy. LFTs would likely show raised ALT, GGT and decreased albumin. Bilirubin is often normal until cirrhosis is advanced. In liver disease there is increased androstenedione from the adrenal glands, increased aromatisation of androstenedione to oestrogen, loss of clearance of adrenal androgens by the liver and a rise in SHBG. He should be offered a referral for alcohol cessation services which can be arranged via his GP.

REVISION TIPS

- Gynaecomastia is a **benign enlargement of male breast tissue**. Malignancy needs to be excluded
- Due to change in the **oestrogen:androgen ratio**, resulting in relative or absolute increase in oestrogen
- If the cause is thought to be physiological/new medication/weight gain further investigation may not be required. **Thorough history and examination, and safety netting advice matter. If there is doubt/suspicion, the cause of the gynaecomastia should be further investigated**
- In absence of identifiable aetiology, **medical therapy** (6-week low dose danazol or 3–6 month tamoxifen 10 mg o.d.) may be trialled in early symptomatic patients. Surgical treatment (**liposuction ± skin excision or sub-cutaneous mastectomy**) may be required

66

Post-Surgical Care and Complications

Harriet Diment and Ben Gibbison

GENERAL SURGICAL WARD, MALE, 45. POST-OPERATIVE PYREXIA

HPC: Exploratory laparotomy 1 day ago for acute abdomen. Adhesions present. No intra-operative bleeding/complications. Inadequate pain relief since operation. No significant PMHx.

O/E: BP 112/65, Temp 38.5°C. SpO_2 96% on 50% FiO_2, RR 26. Midline laparotomy scar – no erythema, no exudate. Reduced breath sounds at right lung base, reduced chest expansion due to pain.

1. What steps are taken to prevent VTE in surgical patients?
2. What would be the diagnosis if:

a. Hoarseness after a thyroidectomy
b. Bradycardia, coma, hypothermia, hypoglycaemia and hyporeflexia after thyroidectomy
c. Shock (hypotension, oliguria) after emergency laparotomy in patient with PMHx of Addison's

Answers: 1. Mobilise early, LMWH enoxaparin 20 mg/40 mg (orthopaedic) SC, graduated compression stockings, intermittent pneumatic compression devices. Stop COCP 4 weeks pre-operatively. 2. (a) Recurrent laryngeal nerve damage during surgery – may be permanent in 0.5% of cases. (b) Myxoedema coma precipitated by thyroidectomy. (c) Addisonian crisis – oral steroids not increased to cover the stress of surgery.

TABLE 66.1			
	Features	**Investigations**	**Management**
Pneumonia	RFs: food/liquid intake, pain, lung disease, stroke. Hx & O/E: crackles, SOB, increased O_2 need, productive cough, purulent sputum	CXR: consolidation (Fig. 66.1). ↑Inflammatory markers. Blood/sputum cultures	If systemically unwell start SEPSIS 6. Fluids, Abx, physiotherapy, CPAP, analgesia
Atelectasis (lung collapse)	RFs: immobility, anaesthesia, underlying lung disease, pain. Hx & O/E: pyrexia, reduced breath sounds at bases, increased O_2 need, reduced expansion	CXR: ↓normal lucency, small volume linear shadows. Note WCC and CRP can be raised by major surgery. Negative blood culture.	Chest physiotherapy. Adequate analgesia to allow normal chest expansion. CPAP

(Continued)

TABLE 66.1   (Cont'd)

	Features	Investigations	Management
Nausea and vomiting	**RFs:** emetic drug use (opiates/anaesthetics). Previous post-op nausea and vomiting. **Hx & O/E:** N&V, dry mucous membranes, low skin turgor ± hypotension	Look for ↑urea/creatinine (dehydration/renal failure) or solute loss (e.g. ↓Na⁺/K⁺)	Treat underlying cause (e.g. change analgesia/exclude bowel obstruction). Anti-emetics. IV fluids
PE	See **11. CHEST PAIN AND PAIN ON INSPIRATION**		
Surgical wound infection	**RFs:** diabetes, non-aseptic technique. **Hx & O/E:** pain, erythema, pus at site, wound dehiscence. Systemic (pyrexia, hypotension, tachycardia)	Baseline bloods (WCC/CRP can be raised by major surgery). **Blood cultures.** **Wound swab:** before Abx **VBG:** raised lactate	If systemically unwell start **SEPSIS 6.** Fluids and Abx (site/culture dependent). Monitor urine output. Surgical exploration; wound closure/drain insertion
Pain	Nociceptive or neuropathic pain	**Baseline bloods:** avoid morphine, use oxycodone if eGFR <30	WHO ladder, PCA, regional analgesia, physical therapy, psychological therapy

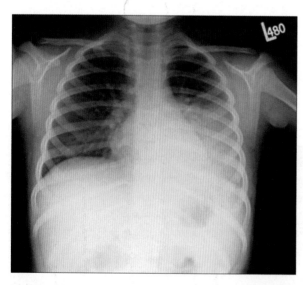

Fig. 66.1 Left lower lobe pneumonia. (Janos C-D, James JG, William BN, Celeste CF, David NH, Derek MC. Treatment of infection in burn patients. In: *Total Burn Care.* Elsevier; 2018. Copyright © 2018 Elsevier Inc. All rights reserved.)

The most likely diagnosis in the vignette is pneumonia. The patient is febrile, with a raised respiratory rate and higher than expected oxygen demand. It can be difficult to delineate between atelectasis and pneumonia after major surgery as the CRP and WCC are raised by the surgery regardless of infection. Consider antibiotics according to local protocol early. If there are signs of sepsis (low blood pressure, high respiratory rate, high lactate) as well, ensure adequate resuscitation with fluid and get early senior help. This problem is common in both exams and real life!

REVISION TIPS

- Consent for procedures must be taken by a clinician that has good knowledge of the procedure and can explain the risk/complications
- Causes of post-operative pyrexia include the 5 Ws:
  - Wind (lungs, e.g. aspiration pneumonia) at 1–2 days
  - Water (genitourinary, e.g. UTI) at 3–5 days
  - Walking (legs, e.g. DVT, PE) at 7–90 days
  - Wound (e.g. surgical site infection, abscess) at 5–7 days
  - Wonder drugs (e.g. transfusion reaction) in hours

67

Acute Abdominal Pain

Emily Warren, Claudia Burton, Berenice Aguirrezabala Armbruster, Shivam Bhanderi, and Rebecca Newhouse

EMERGENCY DEPARTMENT, FEMALE, 28. ACUTE COLICKY ABDOMINAL PAIN

HPC: Started a few hours ago in umbilical region, moved to the RIF, getting worse. Vomited three times, no change in bowel habit. No rectal bleeding, no urinary symptoms, no fever. Non-smoker, minimal alcohol intake.

  O/E: Uncomfortable, holding her abdomen. Guarding, tender RIF, Rovsing's +ve, Murphy's −ve. HS I+II+0, chest clear. **DRE:** No external pathology, no blood, no stools noted.

1. A 35-year-old lady presents with RUQ pain, N&V, no fever, no jaundice/weight loss. O/E: HR 105, BP 117/54, Sats 99% (air), T 37.7°C, abdo soft but tender in RUQ/epigastric region, no organomegaly, active bowel sounds. What are the key differentials?
2. What are the contraindications for NSAID use?
3. What is the Glasgow-Imrie score?
4. Risk factors for an ectopic pregnancy?

Answers: 1. Cholecystitis, pancreatitis, biliary colic, gastritis, gastroenteritis. 2. Asthma, pregnancy, active GI bleeding/ulceration, varicella infection. 3. A score to assess early prognosis of acute pancreatitis based on eight laboratory values. 4. Previous ectopic, pelvic surgery, tubal ligation, IUD/IUS, raised maternal age, assisted reproduction.

TABLE 67.1

	Features	Investigations	Management
GENERAL SURGERY			
Appendicitis	**RFs:** teenage, young adult. **Hx & O/E:** initial dull periumbilical pain then sharper RIF pain, anorexia, worse on movement, ± guarding, mild pyrexia, Rovsing's/psoas/obturator signs	**Urine β-HCG:** r/o ectopic. **Urine dip/MSU:** r/o UTI. **Bloods:** inflammatory markers, G&S, amylase/lipase (r/o pancreatitis). **Abdominal USS or CTAP:** if diagnostic doubt	NBM if for surgery. Analgesia, IV fluids, anti-emetics. IV Abx – follow hospital guidelines. Appendicectomy

(Continued)

TABLE 67.1   (Cont'd)

	Features	Investigations	Management
Acute pancreatitis (chronic pancreatitis, see *81. CHRONIC ABDOMINAL PAIN*)	**Causes:** 'I GET SMASHED' idiopathic, gallstone, alcohol, trauma, steroids, mumps/malignancy, autoimmune, scorpion sting (Tityus), hypercalcaemia/hypertriglyceridemia, ERCP, drugs. **Hx & O/E:** acute central abdo pain radiates to back, tender, fever, tachycardia, N&V	**Bloods:** raised inflammatory markers, ↑↑amylase, ± cholestatic LFTs. **CBG:** ± ↑glucose (DM). **Erect CXR:** rule out pneumoperitoneum. **Abdo USS:** gallstones. **MRCP:** if USS inconclusive. **CT AP:** may show complications	E&D as tolerated (not NBM). Generous IV fluid, analgesia ± O$_2$ (if needed). Urinary catheter (older patient/AKI/dehydration). No antibiotics unless later imaging shows necrosis. Glasgow-Imrie score (ITU services if ≥3). Watch for alcohol withdrawal if causative. **ERCP:** if CBD calculus; see and remove. **Consider laparoscopic cholecystectomy** ('hot lap chole')
Acute cholecystitis	**Causes:** usually a gallstone at gall-bladder neck/cystic duct. **RFs:** 5Fs (female, fat, fertile, forty, fair), 3Ds (diabetes, diet, drugs), Crohn disease. **Hx & O/E:** continuous RUQ pain, radiates to right scapula or epigastrium, fever, Murphy's +ve	**Bloods:** inflammatory markers up, LFTs may be normal, amylase (r/o pancreatitis). **USS:** gallstones in gallbladder, cystic duct, pericholecystic fluid. **CT AP:** inflamed gallbladder, fluid (the gallstones are not always visible). **MRCP:** carried out if stones not detected on USS but stones are still suspected	Clear fluids only orally (if waiting for USS), otherwise E&D as tolerated. Analgesia, IV fluids, antiemetics. **Abx:** hospital guidelines, IV if significant disease. Laparoscopic cholecystectomy (either early or delayed). **Gallstone empyema:** percutaneous cholecystostomy
Biliary colic (symptomatic cholelithiasis)	**RFs:** 5Fs as above. **Hx & O/E:** colicky RUQ pain, radiates to right scapula or epigastrium, can be worse after meals; N&V	**Bloods:** normal or mildly deranged LFTs. **USS:** gallstones. **MRCP:** if USS inconclusive	Analgesia, IV fluids, anti-emetics, reassure. **Gallbladder stone (symptomatic):** elective laparoscopic cholecystectomy. **CBD stone:** if asymptomatic, ERCP or laparoscopic cholecystectomy. If symptomatic, ERCP and lap. cholecystectomy or lap. cholecystectomy + CBD exploration

TABLE 67.1 (Cont'd)

	Features	Investigations	Management
Choledocholithiasis (± ascending cholangitis)	RFs: 5Fs. Hx & O/E: *Charcot's triad*-RUQ pain, fever, jaundice, or *Reynold's pentad*-RUQ pain, fever, jaundice, shock, altered mental status	Bloods: inflammatory, ↑ALT, ↑↑ALP, ↑bilirubin (cholestatic). Blood cultures. USS: gallstones in dilated CBD (>7 mm). MRCP: if dilated CBD and/or deranged LFTs (NICE)	Sepsis pathway: if meets criteria. Analgesia, IV fluids, antiemetics, IV Abx as per hospital guidelines, supportive management. Biliary decompression: ERCP or percutaneous trans-hepatic cholangiography. Lap. choledochotomy/cholecystectomy
Inflammatory bowel disease	See *84. CHANGE IN BOWEL HABIT*		

OBSTETRICS AND GYNAECOLOGY

	Features	Investigations	Management
Ectopic pregnancy	RFs: previous ectopic, pelvic surgery, tubal ligation, IUD/IUS, raised maternal age, assisted reproduction, IVF. Hx & O/E: amenorrhoea or missed period. Abdo/pelvic pain, vaginal bleeding ± clots. GI symptoms. Ruptured ectopic; dizzy, syncope, shoulder tip pain, peritonism	Urine β-HCG: +ve. >1500 highly suggestive. Urine dip/MSU: r/o UTI. Transvaginal/transabdominal USS: no intra-uterine pregnancy, ± ectopic visualised. G&S/Crossmatch	If unstable, two large cannulae, fluids. Medical: if low pain, ectopic <35 mm and β-HCG <1500. IM methotrexate. β-HCG levels decline by >15% at day 4/5. If not, then repeat dose. Surgery: if significant pain, ectopic >35 mm, β-HCG >5000, live ectopic. Lap. salpingectomy or salpingotomy (if damage to contralateral tube). Expectant: if stable, pain free, ectopic <35 mm and β-HCG <1000. NOT FIRST LINE, discuss with senior
Ovarian cyst accident (rupture, haemorrhage or torsion)	Hx & O/E: acute RIF/LIF pain, light vaginal bleeding ± fever/vomiting. Adnexal tenderness ± guarding. Ovarian or adnexal torsion, see *133. PELVIC PAIN*	Urine sample: pregnancy test, MC&S (to r/o UTI). Bloods: pre-op bloods. Transvaginal USS: to assess presentation. CT: consider if suspicious of GI cause or a malignancy	NBM until senior r/v, analgesia, IV fluids. Conservative (analgesia)-cyst rupture in stable patient without significant free fluid. Surgery (laparoscopy/laparotomy) if haemoperitoneum, torsion, acute abdomen, clinically unstable

GENITO-URINARY

Nephrolithiasis	See *197. LOIN PAIN*		
UTI/pyelonephritis	See *200. HAEMATURIA*		

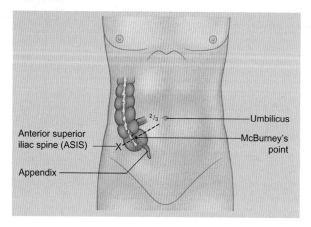

Fig. 67.1 McBurney's point lies two-thirds of the way along a line drawn from the umbilicus to the anterior superior iliac spine. (Steven DW. Chapter 14, Vivian Zhao, a 32-year-old female with right lower quadrant pain. In: *The Chest Wall and Abdomen*. Elsevier; 2023. Copyright © 2023 Elsevier Inc. All rights reserved.)

*The vignette indicates appendicitis. Migrating pain, worse with movement or coughing, N&V, anorexia and malaise. Maximal tenderness at 'McBurney's point' (Fig. 67.1). Peritoneal signs include rebound tenderness, **Rovsing's sign** (left lower quadrant palpation increases right lower quadrant pain), **psoas sign** (right lower quadrant pain when patient is lying on the left and the right thigh is passively extended) and **obturator sign** (pain in the right lower quadrant on passive internal rotation of the flexed right thigh). Be aware of 'stump appendicitis', i.e. inflammation in patients with a previous appendicectomy which did not remove the entire appendix. Atypical presentations; children (non-specific abdominal pain and anorexia), elderly (minimal pain/fever, confusion, shock) and pregnancy (RUQ pain or right flank pain due to displacement of the appendix by the gravid uterus). Variant anatomical position can cause atypical presentations: retrocaecal/retrocolic appendix (right loin pain/tenderness, positive psoas sign, absent muscle rigidity/pain on deep palpation), pre-ileal and post-ileal appendix (vomiting and diarrhoea due to distal ileum irritation), subcaecal and pelvic appendix (suprapubic pain, urinary frequency), long appendix (pain on left lower quadrant).*

REVISION TIPS

- Mnemonic for pancreatitis causes: **I GET SMASHED** (Idiopathic, Gallstones, Ethanol, Trauma, Steroid use, Mumps, Autoimmune, Scorpion Stings, Hypercalcaemia and Hypertriglyceridaemia, ERCP, Drugs). Ethanol and gallstones are the two most common
- **McBurney's point** is the location in the RIF where tenderness is most severe in acute appendicitis
- **Rovsing's sign** is RIF pain elicited by palpation pressure on LIF

68

Abdominal Distension

Tirion Smith, Christian Aquilina, and Angus McNair

HPC: Reduced appetite, nauseous a few days, vomited today. Generalised abdo ache. Recently constipated. **PMHx:** HTN. **DHx:** Ramipril. **SHx:** Alcohol ~90 units/week, ex-IVDU.

O/E: HR 76, BP 118/73, HS I+II+0, RR 14, O_2 sats 99%. Tattooed, cachectic, mild icterus. Palmar aspects of hands are flushed, with palpable thickening. Large, distended abdomen, shifting dullness, fluid thrill. Hard craggy liver edge 1cm below costal margin. Quiet bowel sounds. **Ix:** Deranged LFTs.

1. What blood tests might be included to investigate the cause of liver cirrhosis?
2. List causes of splenomegaly

Answers: 1. LFTs, hepatitis B/C serology, haematinics (ferritin, iron), copper/caeruloplasmin, auto-immune profile (ANA, anti-smooth muscle, AMA, anti-LKM, ANCA), alpha fetoprotein. 2. Haematological malignancy, infective (EBV, malaria, CMV, schistosomiasis, infective endocarditis), portal hypertension, Felty syndrome, sarcoid, amyloidosis.

TABLE 68.1

	Features	Investigations	Management
Ascites	Chronic liver disease (CLD). Hx & O/E: jaundice, bruising, leukonychia, clubbing, palmar erythema, spider naevi, Dupuytren's, caput medusae, hepatosplenomegaly, gynaecomastia	LFTs (↑bilirubin, Alk phos, transaminases, GGT, ↓albumin), clotting (↑PT/INR), hepatitis serology. USS, CT or MRI. Paracentesis: MC&S, cytology, serum – ascites albumin gradient. Screening, e.g. haematinics, auto-anti-bodies. Fibroscan ± biopsy for cirrhosis	Alcohol abstinence (may need chlordiazepoxide, thiamine, vitamin B), nutritional support. Treat clotting abnormalities, encephalopathy, hepatocellular carcinoma, varices. Liver transplantation based on King's College Hospital Criteria
	Malignant – hepatocellular, colorectal, gastric, ovarian, exudative metastases	Imaging (CT/MRI/PET) for diagnosis and staging. Biopsy for histopathology	Referral to relevant specialty/MDT
	Infection – spontaneous bacterial peritonitis	Ascitic paracentesis: MC&S, neutrophils >250/mm³	Urgent admission. IV antibiotics. Ciprofloxacin prophylaxis

(Continued)

TABLE 68.1   (Cont'd)

	Features	Investigations	Management
Obstruction (Fig. 68.1)	**Mechanical** *Small bowel:* adhesions, hernia, stricture, gallstone ileus, intussusception. *Large bowel:* volvulus (Fig. 68.1), diverticulitis, malignancy. **Hx & O/E:** distension, pain, reduced/ tinkling bowel sounds (BS), N&V, obstipation, ±hernia	FBC, U&Es, CRP. Contrast CT abdo/pelvis. ABG: high lactate if tissue ischaemia. Clotting, G&S/CM (surgery).	Limit oral intake/NBM, NG tube. IV fluids, analgesia. Surgery if persists 72 hours. Surgery within 6 hours if ischaemia or strangulation. Treat cause, e.g. tumour resection, stent, hernia repair
	Functional (ileus; no anatomical obstruction) **RFs:** abdo/pelvic surgery, infection, drugs (opioid, anticholinergic, psychotropic), electrolytes (↓K, ↑Ca/Mg), hypothyroid. Signs as above, but less pain and absent BS	AXR or CT: distention of large and small bowel	Limit oral intake. Chewing gum. IV fluids. NGT if vomiting. If possible NBM 7 days, parenteral feeding. When resolving (passing flatus), gradual return to normal diet. Endoscopic decompression of colonic pseudo-obstruction
Perforated viscus	Focal persistent pain, peritonitis (guarding, rebound tender), sepsis	Contrast CT. (Upright CXR; pneumo-peritoneum). Blood cultures	A to E, urgent general surgery. IV antibiotics (amoxicillin, metronidazole, gentamicin ± co-trimoxazole)
Mass	See *70. ABDOMINAL MASS*		
OTHER DIFFERENTIALS			
Faeces	**Constipation/impaction** **RFs:** ageing, sedentary, low fibre diet, dehydration, drugs, post-operative. **Hx & O/E:** indentable mass (left iliac fossa), straining, infrequent hard stools, tenesmus, overflow diarrhoea. DRE	Investigate causes, e.g. TFTs, electrolytes, neurological. AXR or barium enema: faecal loading/cause	Treat the cause, review drugs (e.g. analgesics, anticholinergics, oral iron supplements). Mobilise, dietary fibre, oral fluid. Laxatives; softener (docusate), osmotic (lactulose), stimulant (senna). Enemas/suppositories
	Irritable bowel syndrome (IBS) – functional disorder. Alternating constipation and diarrhoea, distention, pain, PR mucous	Exclude organic and red flag (weight loss, PR bleeding, age >60): colonoscopy. Bloods: exclude thyroid dysfunction, IBD, coeliac. Stool MC&S	Education, reassurance. Symptoms, e.g. antispasmodic, anti-diarrhoeal, laxative. Trial of exclusion diets. Psychological interventions
Retention	See *195. ANURIA AND ACUTE OR CHRONIC URINARY RETENTION*		
Obstetric and gynaecological	*Pregnancy.* *Menstruation* – cyclical lower abdominal bloating. *Fibroids.* *Ovarian:* cancer/cyst	Pregnancy test. Fibroids: TVUS, endometrial biopsy (exclude carcinoma), hysteroscopy or MRI. Ovarian: TVUS, CA-125, doppler, MRI/CT	Obstetric/early pregnancy services, gynaecology. 2WW gynaecological oncology for suspicious ovarian lesions
Obesity	See *13. OBESITY*		

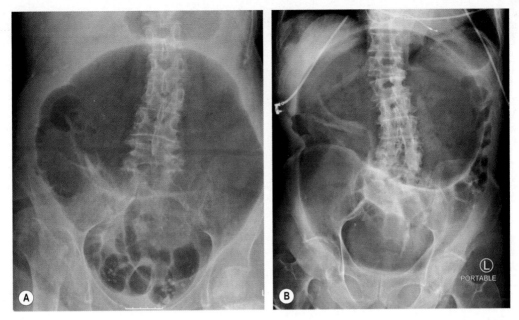

Fig. 68.1 (A) Caecal volvulus. The dilated caecum, which extends to the left of the midline, produces a coffee bean–like appearance with its hilum directed towards the right lower quadrant. (B) Sigmoid volvulus. There is massive distension of the sigmoid colon that extends superiorly to the diaphragm, the so-called northern exposure sign. (From Gore RM, Silvers RI, Thakrar KH, et al. Bowel obstruction. *Radiol Clin North Am.* 2015;53(6):1225–1240, Fig. 5.)

Abdominal distension has multiple potential aetiologies. Look for concurrent red flag symptoms and evaluate these cases fully. CLD has many causes; alcohol, chronic hepatitis, non-alcoholic hepatic steatosis (NASH), other cirrhosis (e.g. auto-immune hepatitis), metabolic (e.g. Wilson disease, haemochromatosis, α-1-antitrypsin deficiency), biliary (PBC, PSC, biliary atresia), vascular (cardiac failure, Budd-Chiari), hepatotoxic drugs. In the vignette, shifting dullness and fluid thrill suggest ascites, and several features of CLD are present. The likely diagnosis is acute-on-chronic decompensation of liver failure, due to alcohol-related cirrhosis. Previous IVDU requires exclusion of hepatitis. Given his cachexia and hard, craggy liver edge, hepatocellular carcinoma should be considered. Treatments for ascites include diuretics (spironolactone ± furosemide), *sodium ± fluid restriction, daily weight monitoring and therapeutic paracentesis, but a serious underlying cause necessitates care with their use.*

REVISION TIPS

- The 'Fs' of some causes of distention: Fluid, Flatus, Faeces, Fat, Foetus, Full bladder, Fibroids
- Serum-ascites albumin gradient: High (>1.1 g/dL) = Transudative. Low (<1.1 g/dL) = Exudative
- 3, 6, 9 rule: normal bowel diameter ≤3 cm for small bowel, ≤6 cm large bowel, ≤9 cm caecum
- Child-Pugh classification of CLD scores encephalopathy, ascites, bilirubin, albumin, prothrombin time

69

Change in Stool Colour

James Chataway and Angus McNair

GP CONSULTATION, MALE, 72. 6-MONTH HISTORY OF VAGUE EPIGASTRIC PAIN

HPC: He has lost weight for 2 months, stools appear pale and are difficult to flush. **DHx:** Amlodipine, atorvastatin. **FHx:** Nil of note. **SHx:** Current smoker (50 pack years). Drinks 14 units a week.

  O/E: Cachectic, jaundiced sclera. **CVS:** HR 110, BP 104/72, HS I+II+0. Abdomen: mild epigastric tenderness but no abdominal masses, normal bowel sounds. **Ix:** raised alk phos and bilirubin. Rest of LFTs normal.

1. What is the classic LFT picture of obstructive cholestasis?
2. What is the tumour marker for pancreatic cancer?
3. How do you treat acute cholangitis with common bile duct stone that is not responding to antibiotics?

Answers: 1. ↑ALP, ↑GGT, ↑bilirubin. 2. CA19-9. 3. ERCP.

TABLE 69.1			
	Features	**Investigations**	**Management**
Pancreatic cancer	**RFs:** FHx, smoking, high BMI, chronic pancreatitis age >65. **Hx & O/E:** vague abdominal pain, fatigue, weight loss, jaundice, pale stools, dark urine, excoriations	**Bloods:** ↑ALP, ↑GGT, ↑bilirubin (obstructive), deranged clotting if liver dysfunction, ↑CA19-9, ↑CEA. **USS:** may show biliary duct dilatation. **CT TAP and pancreas:** staging. **CT PET:** for distant staging. **MRI liver:** for liver metastasis	Analgesia ± coeliac plexus block. Pancreatic enzyme (creon). **Surgical resection:** pancreatico-duodectomy (Whipple procedure) in head of pancreas cancer. Spleno-pancreatectomy for tail. Radical antegrade modular pancreatosplenectomy (RAMPS) procedure for distal/body cancer. Borderline: neoadjuvant chemo-radiotherapy. **Non-resectable (most):** ± chemo-/radio-therapy

TABLE 69.1   (Cont'd)

	Features	Investigations	Management
Cholangiocarcinoma	**RFs:** primary sclerosing cholangitis, bile duct cyst/stone, age >65. **Hx & O/E:** may be asymptomatic initially. Late presentation usually with fatigue, N&V, weight loss, jaundice	↑ALP, ↑GGT, ↑bilirubin, deranged clotting, ↑CA19-9 (in 85%), ↑CA125 (in 65%). **USS:** bile duct dilatation. **CT TAP, triple-phase liver.** **MRCP ± MRI liver:** diagnostic test. **ERCP ± spyglass:** to drain, get histology/cytology	**Resectable** (10%): surgery ± adjuvant chemo/radio-therapy (bile duct removal, partial/extended hepatectomy, Whipple's). **Palliative:** may involve surgery ± chemo-/radio-/immunotherapy (biliary bypass, endoscopic stent, percutaneous transhepatic biliary drainage)
Primary sclerosing cholangitis	**RFs:** ulcerative colitis, young + middle aged men. **Hx & O/E:** vague RUQ/epigastric pain, systemic symptoms (fatigue, weight loss). Cholestatic features can occur	LFTs: obstructive cholestatic, mild-moderate AST/ALT rise. pANCA may be +ve. MRCP/ERCP	No effective medical treatments. Liver transplantation in advanced disease
Primary biliary cholangitis/cirrhosis	**RFs:** female, middle aged, personal/FHx of autoimmune (nb Sjogren sy.). **Hx & O/E:** itching and other cholestatic features. Systemic (fatigue, weight loss)	LFTs: obstructive cholestatic, ALT elevated. M2 anti-mitochondrial antibodies (AMA). Imaging (e.g. US/MRCP) to rule out extrahepatic	Ursodeoxycholic acid. Cholestyramine for pruritus relief. Liver transplantation may be required
Other Important Differentials Gallstone disease causing biliary obstruction (e.g. cholangitis)	**RFs:** history of gallstones. Acute presentation; Charcot's triad (RUQ pain, fever, jaundice), Reynold's pentad: add hypotension, confusion). NB biliary colic + cholecystitis do NOT cause biliary outflow obstruction	Raised inflammatory markers. LFTs: obstructive cholestasis. Abdominal USS. ERCP	Medical emergency. IV fluids and broad-spectrum antibiotics. Early ERCP

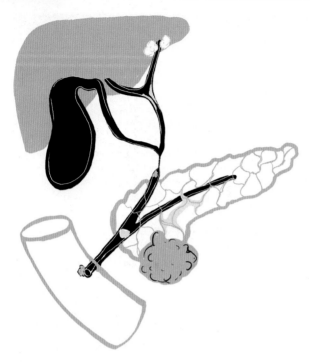

Fig. 69.1 Schematic of where pathology affecting bile can lie. Problems in the liver (malignancy or metastasis), bile ducts (gallstone, atresia, sclerosing cholangitis, tumour) or pancreas (malignancy, pancreatitis). (Picture by Dr Hollie Blaber.)

Pale stools (±dark urine) suggest a cholestatic cause of jaundice (Fig. 69.1). In the vignette, his LFTs (including normal AST/ALT) suggest extra-hepatic (obstructive) is more likely than intra-hepatic (such as hepatitis), but imaging would be needed to confirm this. His chronic presentation with weight loss suggests malignancy. Pancreatic cancer is more likely, since cholangiocarcinoma is rare, and no mention is made of PSC or UC. Other stool colour changes; <u>Yellow</u>; giardiasis. <u>Green</u>; food (e.g. spinach), rapid transit. <u>Chalky</u>; biliary/hepatic. Red; foods (e.g. beets, cranberries, tomato juice), bleeding. <u>Black</u>; liquorice, iron, bismuth (e.g. Pepto-Bismol), melaena. <u>Steatorrhoea</u>; pancreatic, biliary, malabsorption, medication (e.g. orlistat, octreotide). See **50. BLEEDING FROM UPPER GI TRACT/MELAENA, 71. BLEEDING FROM THE LOWER GI TRACT** and **86. DIARRHOEA**.

REVISION TIPS

- Courvoisier's law – if the gallbladder is palpable in a jaundiced patient, it is unlikely to be due to gallstones
- Most common cause of ascending cholangitis is *E. coli*.

Abdominal Mass

Zoe Kay and Shivam Bhanderi

1. Describe the different types of possible stoma and where they tend to be sited on the abdomen.
2. What is carcinoid syndrome and how does it present? What is the significance of it originating in the bowel?
3. What surgical approach is used to resect a low rectal tumour invading the anal sphincter?

Answers: 1. Permanent or temporary (e.g. loop ileostomy). Ileostomy – **spouted** (due to acidic content), normally **right** sided. Colostomy – **flush** with the skin, usually **left** sided, contents are **solid and faecal**. Urostomy – location and appearance like ileostomy, but serves as conduit for the ureters. 2. Carcinoid syndrome is due to carcinoid secreting tumours (**neuroendocrine**), originating in the **bowel** or **lungs**. A colorectal primary gives bowel cancer–type symptoms, and the liver breaks down the carcinoid proteins. Once metastasis to the liver is established, carcinoid gives systemic, **paraneoplastic** features (palpitations, facial flushing, SOB, diarrhoea). 3. Abdominoperineal resection.

TABLE 70.1

	Clinical	Investigations	Management
GENERAL SURGERY			
Colorectal cancer	**RFs:** male, increased age, smoking, red meat/poor diet, FHx. **Hx & O/E:** dark PR bleed, tenesmus, abdo pain, change in bowel habit, weight loss, fatigue. Commonly metastasises to liver due to portal vessels. **Complications** Bowel obstruction, perforation	**Screening:** 60–74 yo FIT (faecal immunochemical test). **DRE:** ± mass, dark blood. **Bloods:** baseline + iron studies. **Colonoscopy, biopsy,** CT colonography. **Staging CT:** 'Apple-core' lesion. **CEA:** carcinoembryonic antigen taken after treatment to identify recurrence	2WW referral. Staging (Fig. 70.1). Neo-adjuvant radiotherapy or chemotherapy. Surgical resection. Consider adjuvant chemotherapy. Symptom control: analgesia, stenting, stoma

(Continued)

TABLE 70.1   (Cont'd)

	Clinical	Investigations	Management
Abdominal wall hernia	**RFx:** obesity, previous pregnancy/surgery. **Hx & O/E:** palpable mass, may be reducible, has **cough impulse**, may be tender, may have overlying inflammatory signs on skin	Baseline bloods, amylase to r/o causes of abdo pain. **AXR:** assess for intestinal obstruction. **CT AP:** clarify anatomy of hernia and ensure no other causes of obstruction if present	If symptomatic or obstructed: for urgent surgery. If no obstruction/reducible: surgery electively, or conservative if causing no problem
GASTROENTEROLOGY			
Constipation	**RFs:** opioid use, stopped laxatives, change in environment or diet. **Hx & O/E:** bowels not opened, overflow diarrhoea. DRE (faecal impaction, r/o anorectal malignancy)	None (in adult functional constipation with no suspected underlying cause)	**Conservative:** increase water, dietary fibre. Trial laxatives ± enemas. **Surgical:** offered in selected cases
Hepato-/splenomegaly	**RFs:** alcohol abuse, right heart failure, primary sclerosing cholangitis, primary biliary cirrhosis, infectious mononucleosis, hepatitis, haematological malignancies. **Hx & O/E:** often accompanied by general health decline. Palpable liver edge on clinical examination. Spleen often significantly enlarged before palpable	Inflammatory markers, viral serology, liver screen, blood film, LDH, tumour markers, renal function (hepatorenal syndrome), Monospot test (for glandular fever). **US liver and portovenous system:** enlargement, abnormal echo-textures, reversed portal flow. **CT TAP:** solid organ malignancy, lymphoma or lymphoproliferative disorder	Manage any decompensated alcoholic liver disease. Stage any malignancies. Ensure co-morbidities optimised. Involve gastroenterology/haematology as needed. Refer to appropriate MDT
VASCULAR SURGERY			
AAA	Asymptomatic abdo mass, expansile aorta. If dissection/rupture, see **44. TRAUMA AND MASSIVE HAEMORRHAGE**	Screen for with abdominal USS. **CT aortogram** to measure width	Smoking cessation, HTN control. Surgical management if the aneurysm is ≥5.5 cm; or >4 cm and has grown >1 cm in 1 year; or symptomatic
OBSTETRICS AND GYNAECOLOGY			
Pregnancy. See **120. NORMAL PREGNANCY AND RISK ASSESSMENT**			

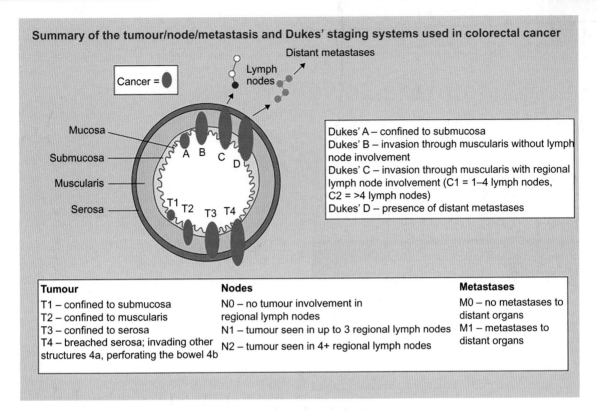

Summary of the tumour/node/metastasis and Dukes' staging systems used in colorectal cancer

Cancer = ●

Distant metastases

Lymph nodes

Mucosa
Submucosa
Muscularis
Serosa

A B C D

T1 T2 T3 T4

Dukes' A – confined to submucosa
Dukes' B – invasion through muscularis without lymph node involvement
Dukes' C – invasion through muscularis with regional lymph node involvement (C1 = 1–4 lymph nodes, C2 = >4 lymph nodes)
Dukes' D – presence of distant metastases

Tumour	Nodes	Metastases
T1 – confined to submucosa	N0 – no tumour involvement in regional lymph nodes	M0 – no metastases to distant organs
T2 – confined to muscularis		
T3 – confined to serosa	N1 – tumour seen in up to 3 regional lymph nodes	M1 – metastases to distant organs
T4 – breached serosa; invading other structures 4a, perforating the bowel 4b	N2 – tumour seen in 4+ regional lymph nodes	

Fig. 70.1 Colorectal cancer staging. (Data from Cancer Research UK. Bowel cancer statistics. Available at: http://www.cancer-researchuk.org/health-professional/cancer-statistics/statistics-by-cancer-type/bowel-cancer. © Cancer Research UK 2023. All rights reserved.)

The most likely diagnosis in the vignette is colorectal cancer. Symptoms suggestive of gastrointestinal malignancy include appetite loss, unexplained weight loss, DVT, abdominal/rectal mass, iron-deficiency anaemia (≥60 years old), iron-deficiency anaemia with rectal bleeding (≥50 years old), unexplained rectal bleeding, abdominal pain with unexplained weight loss (≥40 years old), unexplained abdominal pain with rectal bleeding (<50 years old) and change in bowel habit. In this case, patient is presenting with change in bowel habit, unexplained weight loss and abdominal mass, all of which are suggestive of gastrointestinal malignancy.

REVISION TIPS

- Examine any stoma to check it looks healthy, contents of bag, and exclude parastomal hernia
- Older man with abdominal pain or mass – **always** consider AAA or dissection!
- When suspecting constipation, ask about **absolute constipation**, as this is a red flag for bowel obstruction

71

Bleeding from the Lower Gastrointestinal Tract

Christian Aquilina, Zoe Kay, Shivam Bhanderi, and Jonathan Tyrrell-Price

---

**EMERGENCY DEPARTMENT, MALE, 32.
2-WEEK HISTORY OF RECTAL BLEEDING**

HPC: Bright red blood on the toilet pan after defaecation, itching around anus, occasional pain on defaecation. Systemically well, no other change in bowel habit. No weight loss. No past medical history.

O/E: Normal observations. Small bluish mass on the anal verge. **DRE:** Soft stool, small amount of fresh red blood.

---

1. What does the colour of blood tell you about the point of bleeding?
2. Can you identify the most common age group affected by haemorrhoids?
3. Which parts of the GI tract can be affected by Crohn's disease or ulcerative colitis?
4. Provided the patient is not having a major haemorrhage, what does NICE recommend as the threshold for a blood transfusion?

Answers: 1. Red blood indicates the bleed is from near the anus/rectum. 2. 45–65 years old. 3. Ulcerative colitis only affects the colon, typically ascending proximally from the rectum in a continuous fashion. Crohn's disease can affect any of the GI tract (mouth to anus) and is patchy ('skip lesions'). 4. Hb <70 g/L.

TABLE 71.1			
	Features	**Investigations**	**Management**
General Surgery			
Haemorrhoids	**RFs:** constipation, straining, chronic cough, pregnancy, obesity, increased age. **Hx & O/E:** bright red blood on paper/pan, usually painless but can be painful (e.g. strangulation), ± tenesmus. Rectal pruritis	**DRE:** haemorrhoids. Hb ↓/↔. Consider flexible sigmoidoscopy	Treat constipation. Anal hygiene, topical steroids, simple analgesia. **Surgical:** haemorrhoidectomy (for grade IV haemorrhoids), rubber band ligation (for prolapsing haemorrhoids)
Anal fissure	**RFs:** anorectal trauma (including childbirth), constipation, IBD. **Hx & O/E:** anal pain with defaecation, **mild bright red rectal bleeding**	**DRE** too painful to do. Visible crack in the skin/skin tag	Treat constipation. Anal hygiene, topical steroids, simple analgesia, topical lidocaine, GTN or diltiazem. **Surgical:** EUA to rule out other pathology ± botulinum toxin injection

TABLE 71.1   (Cont'd)

	Features	Investigations	Management
General Surgery			
Colorectal cancer	See *70. ABDOMINAL MASS*		
Diverticular disease. Diverticulitis	**Diverticular haemorrhage:** sudden onset painless severe fresh red PR bleeding, worse if anticoagulated. **Diverticular disease:** intermittent abdo pain (LLQ > RLQ), worse with eating, better with defaecation/flatus, constipation/diarrhoea, bloating, rectal mucus/bleed. **Diverticulitis:** constant abdominal pain, nausea, tachycardia, fever, constipation/ diarrhoea, bloating, mucus/ bleed	**RFs:** increased age, low fibre diet, smoking, medications (steroids, NSAIDs, opioids). Raised inflammatory markers (diverticulitis). **DRE** ± PR bleed. **CT abdomen, pelvis:** diverticula ± inflammation. **Endoscopy:** diverticula ± inflammation	**Diverticular haemorrhage:** free fluids orally, transfuse if indicated, CT angiogram ± embolisation if ongoing bleeding, later endoscopy to exclude cancer. **Diverticular disease:** monitor, diet advice, lifestyle changes, treat constipation. **Diverticulitis:** fluids (IV/PO), antibiotics, analgesia. **Recurrent:** consider surgery
Gastroenterology			
Upper GI bleeding	See *50. BLEEDING FROM UPPER GI TRACT/MELAENA*		
Crohn's disease	See *84. CHANGE IN BOWEL HABIT*		
Ulcerative colitis	See *84. CHANGE IN BOWEL HABIT*		
Inflammatory/ infective/ ischaemic colitis	**RFs:** AF, atherosclerosis, reduced cardiac output, smoking, recent antibiotics, previous *C. diff.* infection. **Hx & O/E:** lower abdo pain with bloody diarrhoea	Raised inflammatory markers. **AXR:** consider toxic megacolon. **CT AP:** extent, assess vessels, r/o perforation. **Stool sample:** exclude infection (e.g. *Salmonella, Shigella, C. diff.*, etc.)	Treat ischaemic colitis with antibiotics, free fluids orally. *C. diff.*; microbiology advice. **Toxic megacolon or perforation;** emergency surgery. Avoid endoscopy in acute phase (risk of perforation)
Key Complication			
Anaemia	Fatigue, dyspnoea, headache, palpitations, pallor	FBC and iron studies. Find cause (imaging, endoscopy)	Iron supplements. Consider blood transfusion

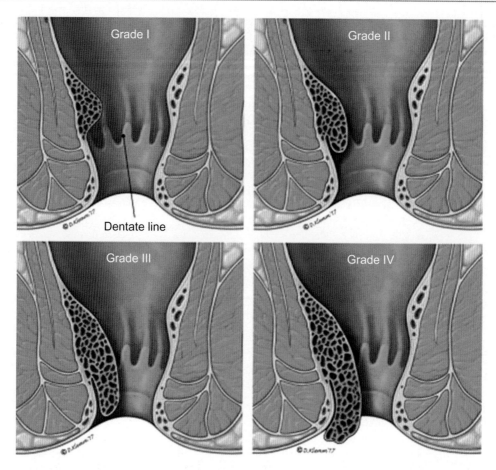

Fig. 71.1 Grading of internal haemorrhoids. Grade I = asymptomatic outgrowth of anal mucosa; grade II = haemorrhoid prolapses but spontaneously reduces; grade III = prolapse must be manually reduced; often with pruritus and soilage; grade IV = haemorrhoid prolapse that cannot be reduced; often with chronic inflammatory changes. (Adapted with permission from https://www.clinicalkey.com/#!/content/undefined/1-s2.0-S0002838X18300224?scrollTo=%23top)

The most likely diagnosis in the vignette is haemorrhoids, which are swollen vascular mucosal cushions in the anal canal. They can be classified as internal (above the dentate line) or external (below the dentate line). Internal haemorrhoids are covered by columnar epithelium and have no pain innervation. External haemorrhoids have modified squamous epithelium (anoderm) and are innervated by pain fibres. Anal pain occurs with prolapsed, strangulated internal haemorrhoids, or thrombosed external haemorrhoids. Internal haemorrhoids are further graded by degree of prolapse (Fig. 71.1).

REVISION TIPS

- Bleeding and evidence of an inflammatory response; consider infection and possible sepsis
- Any cause of bleeding can cause anaemia; resuscitate and possibly transfuse (unwell; think A to E)

72

Lump in Groin

Marie-Louise Lyons, Zoe Kay, and Abraham John

GP CONSULTATION, MALE, 65.
PAINLESS GROIN LUMP

HPC: Present for several weeks, reducible, pops out again on movement or coughing. **PMHx:** Obesity, COPD, appendicectomy. **SHx:** Smoker, non-drinker. Builder.

O/E: An egg-sized lump in the groin, not painful, soft, reducible, disappears on lying down. On coughing, the lump protrudes on the inguinal ligament midway between the pubic tubercle and ASIS. Testes normal. Bowel sounds heard on auscultating the lump. Abdomen soft, non-tender.

1. What is the anatomy of Hesselbach's triangle?
2. What percentage of inguinal hernias strangulate?
3. What are some post-operative complications after hernia repair?

Answers: 1. RIP; Rectus (medial), Inferior epigastric artery (lateral), Poupart's inguinal ligament (inferior). Full anatomy, see (Fig. 72.1). 2. 3%. 3. Urinary retention, groin pain, paraesthesia, haematoma, infection. Long term: recurrence, chronic pain, pelvic adhesions (especially laparoscopic repair), testicular atrophy.

TABLE 72.1

	Features	Investigations	Management
Direct inguinal hernia	**RFs:** male, advanced age, abdo straining, abdo surgery, COPD/smoking, low BMI. Weakness in the posterior wall of the inguinal canal. Lump superomedial to the pubic tubercle, asymptomatic/mild discomfort/dragging sensation on standing/exercise/end of the day	**Clinical diagnosis.** **USS** only if uncertainty – accurate at differentiating types of hernias. **CTAP:** useful in obese patients, Ix of choice in complicated hernias. Herniography and MRI: rarely used	Watchful wait if small and asymptomatic. Analgesia. Truss for non-surgical patients or those who refuse repair. Weight loss (high BMI), smoking cessation. **Surgery: herniorrhaphy or hernioplasty** large or symptomatic hernias. Prophylactic antibiotic not indicated
Indirect inguinal hernia	**RFs:** male, FH, prematurity / low birth weight, connective tissue disorder. Hernia through the deep ring alongside the spermatic cord, may come out through the superficial ring. Hernia does not appear on coughing if deep inguinal ring is occluded digitally		
Femoral hernia	**RFs:** female, obesity, pregnancy. Weakness in the transversalis fascia. Irreducible, mildly painful lump below the inguinal ligament, inferolateral to the pubic tubercle. Higher risk of **strangulation**		Urgent referral. Open or laparoscopic repair ± mesh

(Continued)

TABLE 72.1   (Cont'd)

Other Differentials	Clinical	Investigations	Management
Lymphadenopathy	**RFs:** trauma, malignancy, infection. **Hx & O/E:** firm, non-reducible and tender. Examine lower limb/perianal region for infection/malignancy	FBC, CRP, metabolic panel, CA125, screen for infectious diseases. **USS scan.** **Biopsy:** if suspect malignancy – seek primary (CTAP)	Treat underlying cause
Lipoma	Painless, non-reducible lump, mobile, subcutaneous mass	Clinical diagnosis	Reassure unless infection. Consider surgery
Groin abscess	**RF:** IVDU. **Hx & O/E:** painful lump, systemic signs	Elevated inflammatory markers. **Blood cultures.** **Duplex USS.** **CT angiography:** if suspect pseudoaneurysm	SEPSIS 6 if septic. Abx (hospital guidelines), IV fluids, analgesia. Consider incision and drainage
Femoral aneurysm/ pseudoaneurysm	Pulsating mass, below the inguinal ligament (also above if very large). IVDU is a risk factor for pseudoaneurysm	Peripheral vascular check. **Duplex US.** **CT angiography**	Conservative if <2.5 cm and asymptomatic. Consider femoral aneurysm repair
Saphena varix	Below the inguinal ligament. Soft, non-tender. Disappears on lying down, cough reflex present	Dilated great saphenous vein. **Duplex US**	High saphenous ligation
KEY COMPLICATIONS Bowel obstruction	See **68. ABDOMINAL DISTENSION**	Baseline + pre-operative bloods. **VBG** may show raised lactate. **CT AP:** bowel obstruction. **Erect CXR:** may show perforation	A–E. 'Drip and suck' (NG tube, fluids), analgesia. Urgent surgical referral
Hernia incarceration	**RFs:** age, raised intra-abdominal pressure, previous surgery. Irreducible, painful hernia		A–E. NBM, analgesia. Surgical referral: inguinal hernia repair
Hernia strangulation	**RFs:** same as incarcerated hernia. Severe tenderness, irreducible, erythema, signs of sepsis due to necrosis, disproportionate pain. **Surgical emergency**		A–E. NBM, analgesia. Urgent surgical referral: emergency inguinal hernia repair, resection if bowel ischaemia

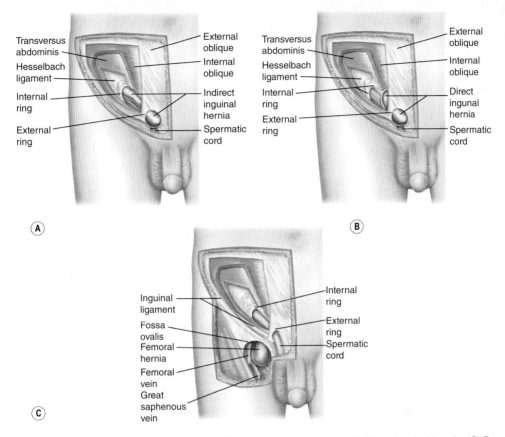

Fig. 72.1 Anatomy of region of common pelvic hernias. (A) Indirect inguinal hernia. (B) Direct inguinal hernia. (C) Femoral hernia. (Monahan FD, et al. *Phipps' Medical-Surgical Nursing*. 8th ed. St Louis: Mosby; 2007.). The Hesselbach ligament, now known as the interfoveolar ligament, reinforces the lateral end of the posterior wall of the inguinal canal.

The top differential in the vignette is a direct inguinal hernia. Despite occlusion of the deep inguinal ring at the midpoint of the inguinal ligament the hernia bulges out on coughing, suggesting that it is unlikely to be an indirect inguinal hernia. His advancing age, smoking, COPD and occupation increase his risk. He has no signs of intestinal obstruction, and it is reducible, painless and non-tender, excluding strangulation.

REVISION TIPS

- Key features to identify when examining a groin lump are its location, cough impulse, whether it is reducible and whether it enters the scrotum
- The anatomical borders and anatomy of the inguinal region will help you differentiate between varying groin lumps
- In an abdominal examination, asking the patient to cough whilst lying flat can demonstrate a hernia

73

Perianal Symptoms

Anya Rutherfurd, Tejas Netke, and Abraham John

**EMERGENCY DEPARTMENT, MALE, 39.
TENDER LUMP AT THE EDGE OF HIS BACK PASSAGE**

HPC: 3 days worsening pain, now constant/throbbing, difficult to sit down. No change in appetite, weight or bowel habit. No blood noticed, no anal trauma. Developed a fever and sweats last night. One regular female sexual partner. **PMHx:** Crohn's disease (diagnosed at 29). **DHx:** 2 mg azathioprine oral OD. NKDA. **SHx:** Current smoker, 11 pack year history, infrequent alcohol.

O/E: Right-hand edge of the anus is red and warm to touch, with very tender obvious swelling; DRE not possible. Abdomen soft non-tender. Temperature is 38.1°C, heart rate is 112 bpm and RR is 14.

1. Give two common causative organisms of anorectal abscesses.
2. Can you explain the grading system for haemorrhoids?
3. Describe Goodsall's rule to predict fistula tracts.

Answers: 1. *E. coli*, *Bacteroides* spp. 2. Grade 1 haemorrhoids remain within the anorectum. Grade 2 prolapse during defaecation and reduce spontaneously. Grade 3 prolapse during defaecation and require manual reduction. Grade 4 prolapse and cannot be reduced. 3. Fistulas with their external opening anterior to the transverse anal line usually form a straight track, whereas posterior fistulas form a curved track.

TABLE 73.1

	Features	Investigations	Management
Anorectal abscess (Fig. 73.1)	**RFs:** male, Crohn's disease. **Hx & O/E:** painful perianal swelling, discharge/ bleeding, malaise, fever, tender fluctuant mass	Raised inflammatory markers. **Blood cultures:** if indicated. **Pelvic MRI**	Sepsis pathway if suspected. Analgesia + Abx. Surgical incision and drainage
Perianal fistula	**RFs:** abscess, Crohn's, trauma, radiation, diabetes. **Hx & O/E:** discharge (mucus, blood, pus, faeces), external opening or fibrous tract felt	May have raised inflammatory markers. **MRI pelvis:** to assess fistula	Surgical options include; fistulotomy or laying open (low fistulae), seton insertion or advancement flap (high/ complex fistulae)

TABLE 73.1 (Cont'd)

	Features	Investigations	Management
Anal carcinoma	See *74. RECTAL PROLAPSE AND ANAL CANCER*		
Anal fissure	**RFs:** hard stool, opiates, rectal cancer, pregnancy. pain on defaecation ± blood on the tissue	Clinical diagnosis	High-fibre diet, adequate fluid intake, laxatives, topical diltiazem/GTN. Botulinum toxin injection. Internal sphincterotomy
Haemorrhoids	**RFs:** chronic constipation. **Hx & O/E:** painless bleeding, anal pruritus/mass, DRE often normal. Pain if strangulated internal/thrombosed external haemorrhoids	Internal haemorrhoids have radial folds. **Anoscopy** (diagnostic) ± colonoscopy or sigmoidoscopy to exclude other pathology	Fibre, fluids, laxatives ± topicals/steroids. Admit for symptom control if strangulated/thrombosed. Rubber band ligation, sclerotherapy or coagulation ± stapled haemorrhoidectomy/haemorrhoidal artery ligation
Pilonidal sinus/abscess	**RFs:** male, age 16–40, family history, previous history of abscess, prolonged sitting. **Hx & O/E:** offensive discharge from natal cleft with emergent hair, pain. Abscess; tender lump, purulent discharge	Clinical diagnosis	None if asymptomatic (advise on skin hygiene) I&D, wide excision and open healing, excision and closure, endoscopic ablation; consider pre-op Abx
Peri-anal hidradenitis suppurativa	**RFs:** female, obesity, smoking, acne vulgaris. **Hx & O/E:** fluctuant, tender lumps, purulent discharge. Open comedones	Clinical diagnosis; chronic inflammatory skin disease of perineum/axilla/groin – recurrent abscesses	**Acute abscess:** incision and drainage with oral Abx. **Ongoing disease:** topical Abx
Sexually transmitted disease	**Secondary syphilis:** condylomata lata (painless warty lesion in oral cavity/perianal), skin rash. See also *135. VULVAL LUMP*	**Serology:** treponemal tests, e.g. EIA, TPHA (IgG and IgM). Non-treponemal e.g. VDRL carbon antigen test, RPR test. High sensitivity in secondary and early latent stages	**Primary/secondary syphilis, early latent:** benzathine penicillin IM single dose (non-allergic). **Late latent, cardiovascular and gummatous syphilis:** benzathine penicillin IM weekly, 3 weeks (non-allergic)
	Anogenital warts: HPV 6 + 11 (most commonly) See *139. GENITAL ULCERS/ WARTS*	Clinical diagnosis; painless. May need proctoscopy	May resolve spontaneously. **Topical:** podophyllotoxin toxin, imiquimod. **Ablation:** excision, cryotherapy
	Anogenital herpes: painful, blistering/ulcerating lesions in mouth/perianal ± tender lymphadenitis	**Swab:** HSV DNA detection via PCR	Antiviral drugs (e.g. oral acyclovir) – within 5 days or if systematically unwell

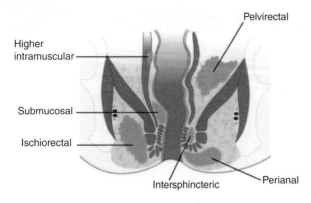

Higher intramuscular

Pelvirectal

Submucosal

Ischiorectal

Intersphincteric

Perianal

Fig. 73.1 Location of common anorectal abscesses. [https://ars.els-cdn.com/content/image/3-s2.0-B9781437735482000410-f041-003-9781437735482.jpg])

The top differential in the vignette is anorectal abscess, noting the history of Crohn's. It is common for perianal abscess to make it difficult to sit down. Perianal fissure or fistula (common in Crohn's) do not present with a warm, erythematous lump and systemic symptoms. Though hidradenitis suppurativa can result in abscesses, they are generally multiple and smaller. A pilonidal abscess would be positioned at the natal cleft.

REVISION TIPS

- Anal fissures usually do not bleed very much and are typically too painful to allow a PR exam
- The most common cause of anal cancer is HPV 16 + 18 (also linked to cervical and penile cancer)
- Chemoradiotherapy is preferred over surgery for anal cancer as it better preserves the anal sphincter

74

Rectal Prolapse and Anal Cancer

Margarita Fox, Berenice Aguirrezabala Armbruster, and Shivam Bhanderi

GP CONSULTATION, MALE, 79.
LUMP ON DEFAECATION

HPC: Pain on passing stools, protruding bulge after opening bowels, constantly feeling need to pass stools. Mucus-like discharge, some blood. Tried bisacodyl, but did not help. History of constipation.

O/E: Obs stable. DRE shows 6 cm protrusion which is red and has concentric folds. Anus appears normal, weakened sphincter.

1. What is the difference between complete and partial rectal prolapse?
2. What features in the vignette overlap with symptoms of rectal cancer and what would prompt a 2WW referral?

Answers: 1. Full-thickness rectal prolapse is when the entire thickness of the wall of the rectum slides out of the anus. Partial (mucosal) prolapse is when the lining (mucosa) of the rectum slides out. 2. Elderly patient, PR bleeding, tenesmus. If there was no prolapse on examination or diagnosis is unclear (e.g. unexplained cause of PR bleeding) further investigations such as sigmoidoscopy/colonoscopy are needed. 2WW: >40 + unexplained weight loss and abdominal pain OR >50 with unexplained rectal bleeding OR >60 with iron deficiency anaemia, change in bowel habit.

TABLE 74.1

	Clinical	Investigations	Management
Rectal prolapse	RFs: intra-abdominal pressure, constipation, straining, heavy lifting, increased age. Hx & O/E: lump at anal verge after defaecation, urge faecal incontinence (unable to reach toilet in time), passive faecal incontinence (leakage), incomplete evacuation, tenesmus ± PR bleed	Partial thickness: only rectal mucosa protrudes Full thickness: rectal wall protrudes. Inspect the visible mucosa for an intussuscepted tumour. If indicated, r/o other causes; proctography, sigmoid/colonoscopy, endoanal ultrasound	Glucogel, ice packs, manual reduction with steady pressure. If chronic, laxatives and avoid excessive straining. Surgery: perineal procedures (Delorme's or Altemeier operation). Abdominal rectopexy

(Continued)

TABLE 74.1   (Cont'd)

	Clinical	Investigations	Management
Haemorrhoids	See *73. PERIANAL SYMPTOMS*		
Anal cancer	**RFs:** HIV +ve, anal trauma, MSM, immunosuppression. **Hx & O/E:** bleeding, hard mass, ulcer, changed bowel habit, pain, palpable inguinal lymph nodes, weight loss. Late presentation (anxiety/assumed haemorrhoids)	**Initial:** anoscopy, followed by EUA + biopsy of tumour. **MRI pelvis/rectum:** For local staging. **CT TAP:** For distant spread Most common type is squamous	Urgent colonoscopy and **2WW colorectal referral** Involve specialist nurses early. MDT assessment. Chemotherapy + radiotherapy. Local excision/abdominoperineal resection

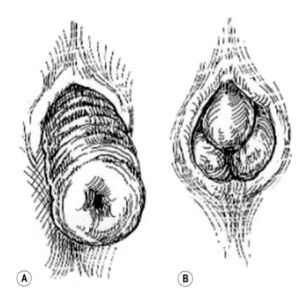

(A)   (B)

Fig. 74.1 (A) Full thickness rectal prolapse, illustrating characteristic concentric folds (internal haemorrhoids have radial folds). (B) Mucosal prolapse. (https://www.ncbi.nlm.nih.gov/pmc/, Public domain, via Wikimedia Commons.)

The most likely diagnosis in the vignette is complete rectal prolapse. Patients present with a lump, initially on defaecation, but later it may occur on coughing or standing. Rectal prolapse differs from haemorrhoids by the presence of symmetrical circumferential folds (Fig. 74.1). It is important to rule out malignancy; ask about constitutional symptoms and arrange appropriate referral.

REVISION TIPS

- Rectal prolapse can be complete (full thickness) or incomplete (only mucosa)
- May present with rectal fullness, sensation of protruding mass, mucus discharge, incontinence or PR bleeding
- Consider referral if rectal/abdominal mass, <50 with rectal bleeding + any one of unexplained: abdominal pain, change in bowel habit, weight loss, iron deficiency anaemia

75

Faecal Incontinence

Margarita Fox, James Chataway, Marcus Drake, and Emma Carrington

---

**EMERGENCY DEPARTMENT, MALE, 90.
BACK PAIN AND RECENT-ONSET FAECAL
AND URINARY INCONTINENCE**

HPC: Ongoing thoracolumbar back pain, weight loss. Weakness and paraesthesia radiating down both legs. **PMHx:** Cognitive impairment, prostate cancer receiving palliative care. **DHx:** Oramorph 5–10 mg PRN, buprenorphine patch 5 μg/h.

O/E: No vertebral tenderness. Afebrile, observations stable. Saddle anaesthesia. Lower limbs; increased tone, brisk reflexes.

1. What are the red flags for lower back pain (which indicate possible spinal cord/cauda equina compression)?
2. What are the three most common causes of metastatic spinal cord compression?
3. What is the innervation of the external anal sphincter?

Answers: 1. Bilateral sciatica, bilateral lower limb neurological deficit, urinary changes (retention or incontinence), faecal incontinence, saddle paraesthesia/anaesthesia, decreased anal tone, lower limb LMN/UMN signs. 2. Breast, lung, prostate. 3. Pudendal nerve (S2–S4).

TABLE 75.1

	Features	Investigations	Management
Chronic constipation/ overflow incontinence	**RFs:** older age, medications (e.g. opioids, sedatives), low fibre diet, immobility	DRE, AXR if suspect faecal impaction	Stool softeners, fluids, high fibre diet, suppositories, enema
Diarrhoea	**Acute:** gastroenteritis (abdo pain, D&V), diverticulitis (LLQ pain, fever, diarrhoea), *Clostridium difficile* (recent hospitalisation/broad-spectrum antibiotics). **Chronic:** e.g. coeliac, diverticular disease, IBS, IBD, lactose intolerance	CRP, FBC, U&Es, LFTs. **Stool culture:** growth if infection. *C. diff* toxin. Further tests as per cause, e.g. colonoscopy, lactose tolerance test	Treatment according to cause. Loperamide. *C. diff*; PO Vancomycin/ metronidazole 10–14 days

(Continued)

TABLE 75.1   (Cont'd)

	Features	Investigations	Management
Medication	Nitrates, calcium channel blockers, β-blockers (alter sphincter tone). Metformin, orlistat, magnesium, digoxin (cause loose stools)		Adjust medication if possible
Rectal prolapse	See *74. RECTAL PROLAPSE AND ANAL CANCER*		
Sphincter damage	During anorectal operations, e.g. haemorrhoidectomy, episiotomy	Endoanal ultrasound, anal manometry	Biofeedback, surgical repair, sacral nerve stimulation
Inflammatory bowel disease	Table 75.2. See *84. CHANGE IN BOWEL HABIT*		
Spinal cord compression	Neoplastic, lumbar stenosis, spinal trauma, disk herniation, abscess. **Hx & O/E:** back pain, worse supine or straining (e.g. coughing, defaecating). Lower limb weakness + numbness (UMN and/or LMN), bilateral sciatica, urinary (retention/ incontinence), faecal incontinence, saddle paraesthesia/anaesthesia, decreased anal tone.	MRI lumbar-sacral spine	**Neoplastic:** high dose dexamethasone + PPI. Urgent oncological assessment for radiotherapy or surgery. **Other causes:** orthopaedic/ neurosurgery
Cauda equina syndrome	See *192. BACK PAIN*		
Neurological (advanced MS, spinal cord injury, stroke, spina bifida, MND)	Increased anal sphincter tone, hence constipation. Areflexic, hence atonic sphincter, reduced peristalsis. Constipation with frequent faecal leaking	Anorectal manometry, EMG. MRI of brain/spinal cord. USS anus	Reflexic; bowel care 1–3 days, rectal suppositories, digital stimulation assist evacuation. Areflexic; daily bowel care, manual evacuation
Dementia	Cognitive decline, immobility, faecal loading		Bowel management programme

TABLE 75.2   Some Key Features of IBD

	UC	Crohn's
Location	Rectum/colon (continuous)	Colon in 2/3, ileum in 2/3, skip lesions
Diarrhoea	+++	+
Rectal bleeding	++	+
Perianal disease	–	++
Gut stricture	–	++
Fistula	–	+
Malignancy	+	++
Ulcers/ cobblestones	–	++

Faecal incontinence (FI) assessment covers type/severity, awareness (urge/passive), timing/frequency, stool characteristics, and associated aspects (e.g. prolapse, urinary/ sexual). History covers obstetric, surgical and medical (DM, stroke, IBD). Examination looks at sphincter (rest/ squeeze/Valsalva), POP, masses, skin irritation, haemorrhoids, fissures and fistulas. Investigations assess sphincter integrity (endoanal ultrasound) and anorectal strength/ reservoir functions (manometry, sensation, volume tolerance, rectal compliance). Dynamic MRI and/or defaecating proctogram may be useful (e.g. if POP). Flexible sigmoidoscopy or colonoscopy may be needed. Symptom scores include Wexner (Cleveland Clinic) or the St. Marks Incontinence Score. MDT participation may include gynaecology, urology and/or neurology. Conservative care (optimise stool consistency, control bowel motility, reduce rectal stool load, perianal skin care, bowel management program, pads/barrier creams, enemas), includes diet advice (foods selection, fluid intake) and medication (treating diarrhoea, constipation or IBS, e.g. amitripty-line). Physiotherapy/biofeedback aim to strengthen and re-coordinate pelvic floor/sphincter in response to rectal distention. Interventional therapies aim to correct structural abnormalities (e.g. haemorrhoids, rectal prolapse, fistulas, deformities), improve sphincter function, or divert the stool (colostomy). In the vignette, lower back pain, neurological signs and incontinence combined with prostate cancer history point towards spinal cord compression, for which urgent spinal MRI and high-dose cortico-steroids/decompression (palliative radiotherapy) are vital.

> ## REVISION TIPS
>
> - In weak sphincter function, dietary fibre requires caution because of increased stool volume or unfavourable stool consistency
> - Extraintestinal manifestations of UC; arthropathies, ocular (episcleritis, uveitis), skin (erythema nodosum, pyoderma gangrenosum), primary sclerosing cholangitis
> - Crohn's may present with joint/back pain (ankylosing spondylitis, sacroiliitis), blurry vision/red eye (uveitis, episcleritis, conjunctivitis), skin lesions (erythema nodosum, pyoderma gangrenosum)

Misplaced Nasogastric Tube and NGT Placement – Outline

Harriet Diment and Angeliki Kosti

1. What are contraindications and relative contraindications to NG tube insertion?
2. What are the indications for NG tube placement?
3. What are the complications of NG tube placement?

Answers: 1. Base of skull fracture, mid-facial trauma, coagulopathies, caustic ingestion, oesophageal stricture/ obstruction, varices. 2. Decompress stomach/GI tract (e.g. ileus, gastric/GI obstruction), gastric lavage (e.g. alcohol excess, drug overdose), feeding/drug administration for people with unsafe swallows or post-operative recovery (e.g. critically ill patients, MND, stroke). 3. Pain, epistaxis, vomiting ± aspiration, tracheal intubation, misplaced through base of skull fracture into anterior cranial fossa, perforation of viscus.

NG Tube Procedure Checklist
Explanation of procedure and verbal consent, include complications. Don PPE – non-sterile gloves and apron
Choose size • Large (e.g. 16–18 Fr) – good for drainage but uncomfortable for patient • Small (e.g. 10–12 Fr) – comfortable for feeding, difficult to aspirate, poor for drainage • Estimate length from nostril to back of throat, and nostril to ~5 cm below xiphoid cartilage
Equipment • NG tube with attachable collecting bag • Lubricant • Bowl with paper towels • Glass of water • pH testing strips • Large syringe (that fits onto NG tube) to aspirate • Xylocaine spray (local anaesthetic) • Tape/NG attachment plaster
Procedure 1. Sit patient upright 2. Insert lubricated tube into nostril, horizontally and with natural curve facing downwards 3. Advance towards the posterior pharynx 4. Encourage the patient to swallow or drink water (using a straw), and continue advancing the tube till you reach the estimated length. Rotation of the tube can assist in insertion when you reach the nasopharynx. Inspect mouth to ensure NGT is not coiling in the oral cavity 5. Confirm position of tube (Figs. 76.1–76.4) 6. Tape the NG tube firmly to the nose; if the patient chokes, gags or struggles to breathe, quickly remove the tube

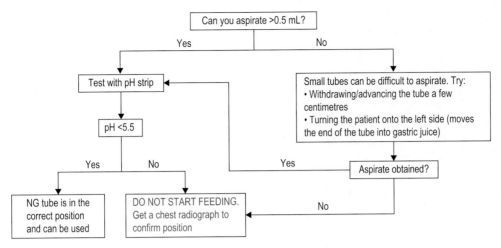

Fig. 76.1 Confirming position of NG tube. Follow local guidelines; most hospitals require a confirmation CXR irrespective of aspirate if the tube is to be used for feeding.

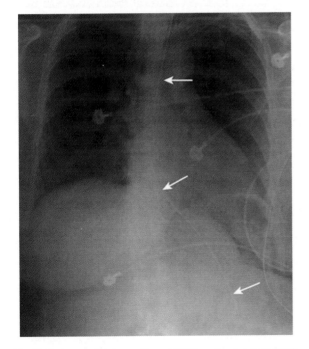

Fig. 76.2 Appropriately positioned NGT on frontal radiograph. Note thin radiopaque curvilinear strip along entire length of NGT (arrows), which extends inferiorly along midline of chest consistent with the oesophagus, with tip overlying expected location of stomach. (Reproduced with permission from Drew A. Torigian and Charles T. Lau . Tubes, Lines, Catheters, and Other Devices. Radiology Secrets Plus, Chapter 22, 189-200. Copyright © 2017 by Elsevier, Inc.)

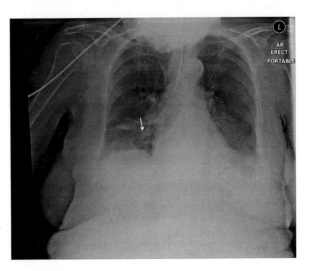

Fig. 76.3 NGT misplacement in the right main bronchus. (Interpreting the chest radiograph. Reproduced with permission from Donna-Marie Rigby and Linda Hacking Anaesthesia and Intensive Care Medicine, Interpreting the chest radiograph. 22(6), 354-358, Copyright © 2021).

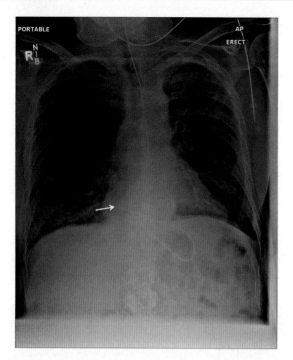

Fig. 76.4 NGT misplacement, coiled in the oesophagus. (Reproduced with permission from Donna-Marie Rigby and Linda Hacking Anaesthesia and Intensive Care Medicine, Interpreting the chest radiograph. 22(6), 354-358, Copyright © 2021).

REVISION TIPS

- PPI or antacid use may make the stomach contents less acidic on pH strip
- NGT needs to be seen crossing the carina, following the midline, and the tip seen under the diaphragm
- Tracheal intubation – feeding through a misplaced NG tube can be fatal and is classed as an NHS never event

77

Swallowing Problems

Emily Warren, Berenice Aguirrezabala Armbruster, Angeliki Kosti, Matthew Boissaud-Cooke, and Harriet Ball

---

EMERGENCY DEPARTMENT, MALE 60. DYSPHAGIA

HPC: Progressive swallowing difficulties, regurgitation, chronic cough and weight loss for a year. Halitosis, no N&V/fever/abdo or chest pain. **PMHx:** Stroke 2 years ago, recurrent aspiration pneumonia. **SHx:** Independent, nil alcohol, non-smoker.

O/E: Observations normal. HS I + II + 0, chest clear, abdomen SNT, CNI-XII intact (able to initiate swallowing motion).

---

1. How is a myasthaenic crisis managed?
2. What are risk factors for carcinoma of the oesophagus?
3. What features help determine if dysphagia is due to a stroke?

Answers: 1. Admit, ITU for ventilatory support, plasmapheresis or IV immunoglobulin. 2. Increasing age, male sex, smoking, increased alcohol, GORD, Barrett's, achalasia, very hot drinks. 3. Sudden onset, alongside other neurological features (e.g. unilateral weakness, speech problems), with new (or newly worsened) dysphagia. Imaging showing ischaemia/haemorrhage in brain region that contributes to swallow control (e.g. brainstem).

TABLE 77.1

	Features	Investigations	Management
NON-MALIGNANT DYSPHAGIA			
Pharyngeal pouch	RFs: elderly. Hx & O/E: dysphagia, regurgitation, halitosis, chronic cough, aspiration, weight loss	Barium swallow	Cricopharyngeal myotomy, endoscopic pouch stapling, diverticulectomy
Achalasia	Progressive dysphagia to solids and liquids, reflux secondary to oesophageal nerve dysfunction	Barium swallow: bird beak appearance. Oesophageal manometry	Nitrates, nifedipine. OGD: for oesophageal dilation or botulinum toxin. Surgery: Heller myotomy

(Continued)

TABLE 77.1   (Cont'd)

	Features	Investigations	Management
Diffuse oesophageal spasm	Odynophagia, intermittent dysphagia for solids and liquids, reflux ± chest pain Rule out ACS	OGD. Barium swallow: corkscrew or rosary bead appearance. Oesophageal manometry. Oesophageal provocation test	Reassure: no significant progression occurs, dietary changes may help. Nitrates, CCB. OGD: dilation (uncommon) Myotomy (uncommon, drastic intervention)
MALIGNANT DYSPHAGIA			
Oesophageal cancer	See *78. DECREASED APPETITE*		
NEUROLOGICAL CAUSES OF DYSPHAGIA			
Myasthenia Gravis	See *102. FACIAL WEAKNESS*		
Stroke	Any of the stroke classifications (TACS, PACS, POCS, LACS) can include dysphagia	The clue that dysphagia is from a stroke comes from the sudden onset, and the other neurological features. See *101. SPEECH AND LANGUAGE PROBLEMS*	

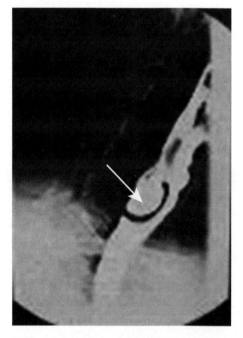

Fig. 77.1 Pharyngeal pouch shown on barium swallow. (Reproduced with permission from Francis Vaz, Nishchay Mehta and Robin D. Hamilton. Ear, nose and throat and eye disease. *Kumar and Clark's Clinical Medicine*, 27, 899-925. © 2021, Elsevier Limited.)

The diagnosis in the vignette is pharyngeal pouch (Zenker's diverticulum), giving rise to dysphagia, regurgitation, aspiration, chronic cough and weight loss. Halitosis may occur due to food decaying in pouch. A barium swallow shows a pharyngeal pouch (Fig. 77.1), and excludes achalasia and diffuse oesophageal spasm. A previous stroke could imply post-stroke complications (but these would only be progressive with repeated events). Myasthenia gravis can affect bulbar muscles and hence swallowing, but extraocular (droopy eyelids, double vision) and proximal limb muscles are most commonly affected. Malignancy should also be considered in progressive dysphagia and weight loss, necessitating 2WW OGD.

REVISION TIPS

- Establish whether they were unable to swallow both liquids and solids from the start or just solids (the latter suggests a physical obstruction)
- 'Bird Beak' = achalasia. 'Corkscrew' = diffuse oesophageal spasms
- Any patient at any age with dysphagia needs a 2WW OGD to investigate for UGI malignancy (as appropriate)

78

Decreased Appetite

Emily Warren and Angeliki Kosti

HPC: Fatigue for a couple of months, previously fit and well. Now unable to undertake usual activities. Denies fevers, SOB, chest pain, or abdo pain. Experiencing reflux and dyspepsia – not unusual for him. Difficulty swallowing solids but not liquids, some vomiting after eating. No change in bowel habit or colour. **PMHx:** Anxiety, GORD. Independent, non-smoker, minimal alcohol intake, very active, healthy diet.

O/E: Normal observations, pale. HS I + II + 0, chest clear, abdomen SNT, epigastric mass felt on palpation, COVID test negative.

1. What are the criteria for an endoscopy in someone presenting with dyspepsia?
2. Name some common side effects of omeprazole.
3. What are your main differentials for (a) melaena, (b) dark red stools, (c) bright red stools, (d) pale stools?

Answers: 1. >55 with ALARM features or if treatment-resistant. ALARM = Anaemia, Loss of weight, Anorexia, Recent progressive dysphagia, Melaena or haematemesis. 2. Abdominal pain, constipation, diarrhoea, dizziness, dry mouth, headache, N&V. 3. (a) Melaena: UGIB, iron supplements. (b) Dark-red stool: proximal colon bleed, e.g. colorectal cancer, IBD, right-sided diverticular bleeds. (c) Fresh-red blood: distal colon bleeding, e.g. sigmoidal diverticular bleeds, colorectal cancer, haemorrhoids, fissure, UGIB with fast transit (high risk haemorrhage). (d) Pale stools: cholangitis, pancreatitis, pancreatic cancer, coeliac disease, cystic fibrosis.

TABLE 78.1

	Clinical	Investigations	Management
Upper Gastrointestinal Malignancy			
Oesophageal cancer (Fig. 78.1)	**RFs:** Barrett's oesophagus (adenocarcinoma), alcohol (squamous cell carcinoma), smoking (both). **Hx & O/E:** progressive dysphagia (solids, then liquids), regurgitation, weight loss, intractable heartburn, dyspepsia	↓Hb ↓MCV ± deranged LFTs if metastasis. **2WW urgent referral** to UGI team for OGD ± biopsy if dysphagia OR >55 with weight loss, upper abdo pain, reflux or dyspepsia. **Endoscopic ultrasound staging.** **CT TAP/PET**	Palliative (most cases). Chemo/radiotherapy, stenting, oesophageal dilation, symptomatic care. **Curative:** oesophagectomy with chemo/radiotherapy Endoscopic mucosal resection for early cancers

(Continued)

TABLE 78.1   (Cont'd)

	Clinical	Investigations	Management
Gastric cancer	**RFs:** *H. pylori*, male, smoking, obesity. **Hx & O/E:** dysphagia, unexplained weight loss, dyspepsia, intractable heartburn, early satiety. Metastasis signs (e.g. Virchow's node, acanthosis nigricans)	Investigations as for oeseophageal cancer	**Surgery (curative):** • Total/subtotal gastrectomy • Endoscopic mucosal resection if early cancer • Chemo/radiotherapy **Palliative:** chemo/radiotherapy, stenting, symptomatic care
NON-MALIGNANT DYSPEPSIA			
Gastritis	See *50. BLEEDING FROM UPPER GI TRACT/MELAENA*		
GORD/PUD	See *81. CHRONIC ABDOMINAL PAIN*		
Barrett's oesophagus	See *81. CHRONIC ABDOMINAL PAIN*		
NON-MALIGNANT DYSPHAGIA			
Achalasia	See *77. SWALLOWING PROBLEMS*		
Diffuse oesophageal spasm	See *77. SWALLOWING PROBLEMS*		
Pharyngeal pouch	See *77. SWALLOWING PROBLEMS*		
OTHER DIFFERENTIALS TO CONSIDER			
Psychological	Depression, anxiety		
Other malignancies	Loss of appetite can be caused by malignancy of various origins		

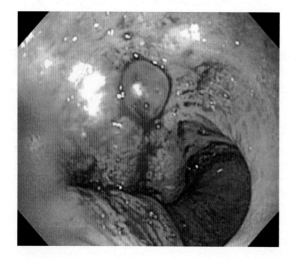

Fig. 78.1 Endoscopic view of T2 oesophageal cancer. (Reproduced with permission from Manu Sancheti and Felix Fernandez . Management of T2 Esophageal Cancer. Surgical Clinics of North America, 92 (5), 1169-1178, Copyright © 2012 Elsevier Inc.)

Anyone with progressive dysphagia, vomiting post-prandially and weight loss has an assumed UGI malignancy until proven otherwise. Important features in the vignette are persisting fatigue, chronic reflux, difficulty swallowing solids with vomiting and epigastric mass. NICE suggests a 2WW OGD in anyone with dysphagia.

REVISION TIPS

• Decreased appetite can result from dysphagia, malignancy, reflux, psychological factors
• Virchow's node is found in the left supraclavicular space between the end of the thoracic duct and left subclavian vein junction. It is often a sign of malignancy
• UGI malignancy is often vague and presents late – know the NICE guidelines for urgent endoscopy referral
• Most cancers are not resectable at presentation

79

Food Intolerance

Lucy Andrews, Alex Carrie, and Matthew Ridd

HPC: Stools looser, no blood or mucus. Lower abdominal pain and bloating in the morning, relieved by defaecation. No weight loss, vomiting or fevers. DHx: None. FHx: Brother has Crohn disease. SHx: Started university 2/12 ago. Drinks 4 cups of coffee daily, 12 units of alcohol weekly.

O/E: Comfortable and orientated. Apyrexial. CVS: HR 70, BP 120/80. Abdomen: Soft, mild tenderness and distention, bowel sounds present.

1. A patient with a symmetrical, intensely itchy and erythematous blistering rash, what is the rash and likely associated condition?
2. What would be your top differential if the patient had presented with sudden onset shortness of breath and wheezing, vomiting and a rash across their torso after a meal, and how would you manage it?

Answers: 1. Dermatitis herpetiformis; commonly associated with Coeliac disease. 2. Anaphylactic reaction; call ambulance, assess A–E, adrenaline, chlorphenamine.

TABLE 79.1

	Features	Investigations	Management
Coeliac disease *Wheat, barley, rye, oats*	**RFs:** F > M, FHx, autoimmune, Turner/Down/Williams syndromes. Due to gluten intolerance. **Hx & O/E:** weight loss, fatigue, abdo pain, pallor, diarrhoea, bloating, failure to thrive, delayed puberty, anaemia. Dermatitis herpetiformis, pyoderma gangrenosum, erythema nodosum	Anti-tTG IgA (tissue transglutaminase; total IgA to rule out IgA deficiency), anti-endomysial IgA – samples taken while on diet containing gluten. OGD and duodenal biopsy. To identify complications; bone profile, Vit D, B12, folate and ferritin TFTs and glucose to r/o associated autoimmune conditions	Gluten-free diet lifelong If non-response, check compliance, repeat OGD. Treat vitamin deficiency. Pneumococcal and flu vaccine due to hyposplenism. Consider genetic testing. Dapsone for dermatitis herpetiformis

(Continued)

TABLE 79.1	(Cont'd)		
	Features	**Investigations**	**Management**
Lactose intolerance *Milk, dairy products*	RFs: recent gastroenteritis, FHx. Less common in white ethnicity groups. Hx & O/E: diarrhoea, abdominal pain, flatulence after consuming dairy products	FBC (check for anaemia). Exclude IBD (faecal calprotectin) and coeliac (anti-tTG, total IgA)	Lactose-free diet. Lactase replacement may be given. Dietician input
Avoidant/ restrictive food intake disorder	Autism spectrum disorder or anxiety. Picky about texture/ temperature/colour of food. Weight loss *in the absence of body dysmorphia*	FBC, ferritin, B12 and folate (check for vitamin deficiency). Reduced BMI	Mental health/eating disorder service. May need nutritional supplementation. CBT/family therapy
Irritable bowel syndrome	See *84. CHANGE IN BOWEL HABIT*		

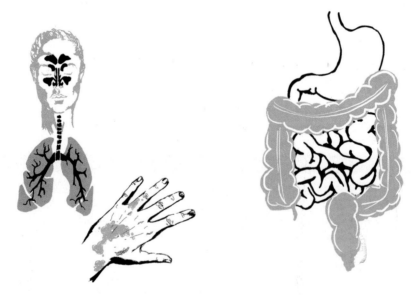

Fig. 79.1 Salicylates (fruits, vegetables, teas, coffee, spices, nuts and honey) and sulphites (preservative in foods, drinks and some medications, naturally in grapes, aged cheeses) can cause wheeze, itch, sinusitis, hives ('WISH'). Diet components, like lactose, gluten and egg, can cause ABCD symptoms of abdo pain, bloating, colitis or diarrhoea.

Key points are symptoms triggered by consumption of a certain food and FH of intolerance. Well-known conditions like coeliac disease or lactose intolerance may spring to mind, but don't forget less well-known contributors (Fig. 79.1). Irritable bowel syndrome (IBS) causes abdominal pain (relieved by passing flatus or stool), bloating, constipation and/or diarrhoea. It is a diagnosis of exclusion – rule out coeliac disease, inflammatory bowel disease (IBD), and colorectal cancer. IBS can be managed by avoiding foods containing FODMAPs (fermentable oligo-, di-, monosaccharides and polyols), notably wheat, apples, pears, peas, sweetcorn, beetroot and cauliflower. Symptomatic care of constipation/diarrhoea, pain and bloating is needed. Coeliac disease is an autoimmune condition where gluten (bread, beer, pasta, sauces (especially soy sauce)) causes small bowel villous atrophy and crypt hyperplasia. Histamine intolerance (fermented foods/ drinks, vinegar, cured meats, dried fruits, citrus, avocados, aged cheeses, vinegar) can result from diamine oxidase or N-methyltransferase deficiency, leading to flushing, headaches, hives, diarrhoea and hypotension.

REVISION TIPS

- Food intolerance does not arise from immune response, unlike food allergy. Intolerance gives milder symptoms after ingestion of the trigger food
- Patients being investigated for coeliac disease must continue to eat gluten whilst awaiting endoscopy to ensure a diagnosis can be made

80

Nausea and Vomiting

Lucy Andrews, Alexander Calthorpe, and Omar Amar

**EMERGENCY DEPARTMENT, FEMALE, 18.
ABDOMINAL PAIN, NAUSEA AND
VOMITING**

HPC: Brought in by mother, concerned she is drowsy, and worried about UTI due to frequent urination recently.
PMHx: Type 1 diabetes mellitus.
  O/E: Chest clear, RR 24, shallow breathing, HS I + II + 0, clinically dry, appears underweight, epigastric pain upon palpation, GCS 13.

1. A patient presents with severe, colicky abdominal pain, bowels not opened for 7 days. Previous appendicectomy. What is the most likely diagnosis?
2. A patient presents with nausea and burning epigastric pain, eased by eating. What is the most likely cause?
3. Which drugs commonly cause nausea and vomiting?

Answers: 1. Bowel obstruction (features are abdo pain, absolute constipation, distension, absent/tinkling bowel sounds, vomiting). 2. Peptic ulcer disease, probably duodenal ulcer (pain that is worse with food is likely gastric). 3. Opiates, NSAIDs, antibiotics, bisphosphonates, chemotherapy.

TABLE 80.1

	Features	Investigations	Management
Diabetic ketoacidosis	**RFs:** T1DM with recent illness, stress, surgery, non-compliance, drug treatment (e.g. steroids). **Hx & O/E:** N&V, abdo pain, Kussmaul breathing, breath smells like pear, fatigue, polyuria, thirst, reduced GCS	**VBG:** acidosis <7.3 or bicarbonate <15 mmol/L. **Ketones:** ketosis >3 mmol/L or +2 on dipstick. **CBG:** hyperglycaemia >11 mmol/L. **Infection screen:** FBC, CRP, CXR, urine dip. **Monitoring:** ECG (hyper/hypokalaemia), **Potassium** – measure every 2 hours via VBG (usually raised, drops with insulin)	**Fluids:** 0.9% NaCl 500 mL bolus if shocked, 1 L over 1 hour if not See also *'revision tips'*. **Potassium** replacement if needed. **Stop short-acting insulin and start FIXED rate infusion** 50 units in 50 mL saline at 0.1 units/kg/hour. Continue long-acting insulin. Start **10% glucose** IV when serum glucose is <14 mmol/L Infusion is continued until ketones <0.3, pH >7.3 and able to eat/drink

	Features	Investigations	Management
Gastroenteritis	N&V, diarrhoea (watery or bloody), epigastric pain. Usually viral	±↑WBC ↑CRP, consider blood cultures. Stool sample MC&S	IV/PO fluids, antiemetics. Consider Abx (rarely used, depending on causative microorganism: salmonella, shigella or campylobacter - usually Quinolone.)
Hypercalcaemia	See *61. HYPERCALCAEMIA*		
Pregnancy	See relevant cases		**Conservative:** ginger, plain foods, avoid triggers. **Antiemetic** (cyclizine) Admit if dehydrated, ketonuria or sustained
Post-surgery (Fig. 80.1)	Long-duration surgery, opiates, inhalation anaesthesia	Monitor pain score, bowels and fluid input/output	Adequate analgesia and fluids. Intra- and post-operative antiemetic (ondansetron)

TABLE 80.1 (Cont'd)

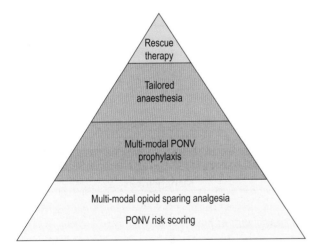

Fig. 80.1 Post-operative N&V prophylaxis/prevention escalating pyramid. (Reproduced with permission from Emma Öbrink, Pether Jildenstål, Eva Oddby and Jan G. Jakobsson. Post-operative nausea and vomiting: Update on predicting the probability and ways to minimize its occurrence, with focus on ambulatory surgery. *International Journal of Surgery*, 15, 100-106. Copyright © 2015)

The most likely diagnosis in the vignette is diabetic keto-acidosis (DKA). This patient is young and her mother reports polyuria. Other features suggesting DKA are: GCS, underweight, Kussmaul breathing, abdominal pain. Finding glucose and ketones in the urine supports the diagnosis.

REVISION TIPS

- Pregnancy testing should be undertaken in women of child-bearing age presenting with N&V
- Dyspepsia + >55 years old OR any ALARM features = 2WW endoscopy. ALARM = Anaemia, Loss of weight, Anorexia, Recent progressive dysphagia, Melaena or haematemesis
- DKA fluid regime: if shocked 500 mL bolus, if not shocked 1 L over 1 hour. Potassium is not added within the first hour of rehydration. Following the first hour: 1 L over 2 hours, 1 L over 2 hours, 1 L over 4 hours, 1 L over 4 hours, 1 L over 8 hours. If serum potassium is 3.5–5.5 then potassium will be added to the 0.9% saline to prevent hypokalaemia as insulin is given
- In DKA, insulin can be changed to sliding scale once ketones <0.6 mmol/L and acidosis has resolved

81

Chronic Abdominal Pain

Berenice Aguirrezabala Armbruster, Emily Warren, Christian Aquilina,
Zoe Kay, Jonathan Tyrrell-Price, and For Tai Lam

GP CONSULTATION, FEMALE, 57. **6-MONTH HISTORY OF EPIGASTRIC AND RUQ PAIN**

HPC: Gradual onset, pain comes and goes, not relieved by simple analgesia, radiates to the back. Worse in the mornings after lying down, not worse after food, oral intake maintained. Nausea, no vomiting. No chest pain/jaundice/change in stool habit/problems passing urine. **PMHx:** NAFLD. Non-smoker, 16 units of alcohol per week.

O/E: Obs normal, comfortable at rest, slightly overweight. HS I + II + 0. Chest clear. Mild epigastric tenderness. No organomegaly or masses felt, bowel sounds present. **Bloods:** Hb 130, WCC 2, Na 137, K 3.6, Amylase 30, LFTs normal.

1. For an *H. pylori* test, for how many weeks prior to testing should PPI and antibiotics be avoided?
2. What is the *H. pylori* triple therapy?

Answers: 1. Avoid PPI for 2 weeks and antibiotics for 4 weeks before the *H. pylori* carbon-13 urea breath test or stool antigen test. 2. Triple therapy for 7 days = PPI + amoxicillin + clarithromycin or metronidazole. If penicillin allergic, PPI + clarithromycin + metronidazole.

TABLE 81.1

	Features	Investigations	Management
CHRONIC ABDOMINAL PAIN – UPPER GASTROINTESTINAL			
Gastritis	See *50. BLEEDING FROM UPPER GI TRACT/MELAENA*		
GORD	**RFs:** alcohol, smoking, obesity, pregnancy, NSAIDs, steroids, bisphosphonates. **Hx & O/E:** dyspepsia, ALARM features (Anaemia, Loss of weight, Anorexia, Recent progressive dysphagia, Melaena or haematemesis)	Assess for ALARM features. **OGD.** **Specialist investigations:** oesophageal manometry and ambulatory 24-hour oesophageal pH monitoring. Barium swallow	Weight loss, smoking cessation, avoid hot drinks/alcohol/caffeine/chocolate/spicy/NSAID/aspirin/eating near bedtime. Raise head of bed/add a pillow. **Proven GORD:** full-dose PPI 8 weeks. **Severe oesophagitis:** full-dose PPI long term. **Refractory/recurrent GORD:** review and adjust medication. Consider add on H2 blocker, refer for specialist investigations and treatment (e.g. laparoscopic Nissen fundoplication)

TABLE 81.1 (Cont'd)

	Features	Investigations	Management
Barrett's oesophagus	Premalignant change due to chronic GORD. Hx: GORD symptoms	OGD: biopsy and sequential longitudinal sampling	Non-dysplastic: PPI, surveillance endoscopy. Low-grade dysplasia: PPI + surveillance OR endoscopic mucosal resection. High-grade: endoscopic resection and ablation (radiofrequency). Oesophagectomy if refractory dysplasia
Peptic ulcer (gastric or duodenal)	RFs: H. pylori, drugs (NSAIDs, steroids, bisphosphonates, SSRIs). Gastric ulcers: pain exacerbated after eating. Duodenal ulcers: pain improves after eating	H. pylori test: carbon-13 urea breath test or stool antigen test. Endoscopy: ulcer identified	Lifestyle changes: e.g. smoking cessation, decrease alcohol. Medication review: avoid NSAIDs. H. pylori treatment if positive
Functional dyspepsia (a.k.a. non-ulcer dyspepsia)	Cause unknown, likely multifactorial. Hx & O/E: dyspepsia symptoms with normal findings on endoscopy	H. pylori test. Endoscopy: normal findings	Lifestyle changes, medication review. Antacids. H. pylori treatment if positive. Low-dose PPI or standard dose histamine receptor antagonist for 1 month
Gastric cancer	See 78. DECREASED APPETITE		

CHRONIC ABDOMINAL PAIN – HEPATOBILIARY

	Features	Investigations	Management
Hepatocellular carcinoma	RFs: male, increasing age, chronic liver conditions. Hx & O/E: may be asymptomatic initially. Later may present with fatigue, anorexia, weight loss, RUQ pain, jaundice, dark urine, pale faeces	Bloods: deranged LFTs, deranged clotting, ↑AFP. Abdominal USS. CT with contrast. MRI with liver contrast	MDT. Treat complications of cirrhosis. Resection and transplantation. Non-surgical; ablative therapies, transarterial chemoembolisation (TACE), targeted cancer drugs. Advanced HCC; sorafenib
Cholangiocarcinoma	See 69. CHANGE IN STOOL COLOUR		
Pancreatic cancer	See 69. CHANGE IN STOOL COLOUR		
Chronic pancreatitis. (Acute pancreatitis, see 67. ACUTE ABDOMINAL PAIN)	RFs: alcohol, gallstones. Hx & O/E: chronic or recurrent epigastric pain which radiates to the back. Relieved by sitting forward or hot water bottle. Exacerbated by fatty food or alcohol. Steatorrhea, weight loss, DM	Raised inflammatory markers, ↑amylase (less than in acute pancreatitis), ↑↑ALP, ↑ALT (cholestatic), ± ↑immunoreactive trypsin (cystic fibrosis). CBG: ± ↑glucose (DM). USS: gallstones. MRCP: if USS inconclusive. CT AP: may show complications	Acute on chronic: IV fluids + analgesia ± oxygen (if needed). ERCP if clear evidence of gallstones. Consider Abx if pancreatic necrosis. Chronic: avoid EtOH, ↓fat, ↑carbohydrates. Creon, ADEK vitamins. DM control. Pancreatic ca monitoring DEXA. scan every 2 years. (Pancreatectomy with islet autotransplantation)
Gallstones	See 67. ACUTE ABDOMINAL PAIN		

(Continued)

TABLE 81.1   (Cont'd)

	Features	Investigations	Management
CHRONIC ABDOMINAL PAIN – LOWER GASTROINTESTINAL			
Irritable bowel syndrome (IBS)	See *84. CHANGE IN BOWEL HABIT*		
Coeliac disease	See *79. FOOD INTOLERANCE*		
Crohn disease	See *84. CHANGE IN BOWEL HABIT*		
Ulcerative colitis	See *84. CHANGE IN BOWEL HABIT*		
Colorectal cancer	See *70. ABDOMINAL MASS*		

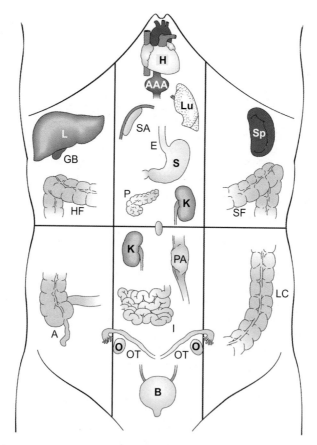

Fig. 81.1 Causes of abdominal pain by location. Key: Right upper quadrant: GB, gallbladder (cholecystitis, steatosis, cholangitis, choledocholithiasis); HF, hepatic flexure (obstruction); L, liver (hepatitis, abscess, perihepatitis). Right lower quadrant: A, appendix (appendicitis,* abscess); O, ovary (torsion, ruptured cyst, carcinoma). Left upper quadrant: Sp, spleen (rupture, infarct, abscess), SF, splenic flexure (obstruction). Left lower quadrant: LC, left colon (diverticulitis, ischemic colitis); O, ovary (torsion, ruptured cyst, carcinoma). Epigastrium: AAA, abdominal aortic aneurysm; E, oesophagus (gastroesophageal reflux disease); H, heart (myocardial infarction, pericarditis, aortic dissection); K, kidney (pyelonephritis, renal colic); Lu, lung (pneumonia, pleurisy); P, pancreas (pancreatitis); S, stomach and duodenum (peptic ulcer); SA, subphrenic abscess. Hypogastrium: B, bladder (cystitis, distended bladder); I, intestine (infection,* obstruction,* inflammatory bowel disease*); K, kidney (renal colic); O, ovary (torsion, ruptured cyst, carcinoma); OT, ovarian tube (ectopic pregnancy, salpingitis, endometriosis); PA, psoas abscess. Generalised abdominal pain: (1) See conditions marked with an asterisk (*), (2) peritonitis (any cause), (3) diabetic ketoacidosis, (4) sickle cell crisis, (5) acute intermittent porphyria and (6) acute adrenocortical insufficiency resulting from steroid withdrawal. (Marshall SA, Ruedy J. Abdominal pain. In: *On Call Principles and Protocols.* Elsevier; 2017. Copyright © 2017 Elsevier Inc. All rights reserved.)

The range of possible causes of abdominal pain is substantial (Fig. 81.1). The most likely diagnosis in the vignette is gastritis, which may present with dyspepsia ± feeling of fullness after eating. Dyspepsia refers to a complex of upper GI symptoms which are typically present for 4 or more weeks, and includes upper abdominal pain or discomfort, heartburn, acid reflux, nausea and/or vomiting. The most common causes of dyspepsia are GORD, peptic ulcer disease (duodenal and gastric ulcers) and functional dyspepsia (a.k.a. non-ulcer dyspepsia). Proven GORD refers to endoscopically determined reflux disease which can be due to oesophagitis or endoscopy-negative reflux disease. Lifestyle factors and medications should be reviewed. Other causes of dyspepsia include Barrett's oesophagus and upper GI malignancy, so it is important to ask about red-flag symptoms (ALARM mnemonic: Anaemia, Loss of weight, Anorexia, Recent progressive dysphagia, Melaena or haematemesis) and arrange endoscopy accordingly.

REVISION TIPS

- When considering causes of abdominal pain consider differentials by location or by system involved
- Crohn's: skip lesions, cobblestone appearance (ulceration + oedema), rose thorn ulcers, string sign of Kantor (narrow terminal ileum)

82

Pruritis

Katherine Parker and Nicole Lundon

GENERAL SURGERY WARD, FEMALE, 75. DEVELOPED INTENSE ITCHING 2 DAYS AFTER CHOLECYSTECTOMY

HPC: Started this morning, no rash, never had this before. Eating and drinking, feels intermittently nauseated and drowsy. Abdo pain 1/10. **PMHx:** CKD2 (recurrent pyelonephritis), impaired fasting glucose. **DHx:** Regular paracetamol and codeine, PRN oral morphine.

O/E: Apyrexial, HR 60 regular, BP 130/85, RR 16, PaO_2 99% (air). Abdo: mildly distended, port sites clean, mild diffuse tenderness, drain 100 mL clear/pink fluid. Skin: excoriation over upper arms and flanks without erythema/scale/dermatitis/abnormal pigmentation. **Ix:** Blood glucose 6.0, WCC 12.5, Urea 22.5 mmol/L (previously 8.5), creatinine 240 umol/L (previously 105)

1. What is tinea incognito?
2. How can discoid eczema be differentiated from tinea corporis on examination?
3. Apart from itching, which other side effects are common with opioids?

Answers: 1. Dermatophyte fungal infection (tinea) which has been misdiagnosed and treated with topical corticosteroids. Typical morphological features have been lost due to inappropriate use of corticosteroids. 2. Tinea is asymmetrical; discoid eczema symmetrical and central clearing less likely. 3. Confusion, dysphoria, constipation, miosis, N&V, urinary retention. High doses – hypotension, respiratory depression.

TABLE 82.1

	Features	Investigations	Management
DERMATOLOGICAL CAUSES			
Atopic dermatitis (eczema)	See *16. CHRONIC RASH*		
Tinea corporis (body)/tinea cruris (groin)	**RFs:** humidity, tight clothes, obesity, hyperhidrosis, immunocompromise, affected contacts. **Hx & O/E:** skin creases or damp areas (toes, groin, scalp). Itchy, erythematous patches, slowly enlarging, central clearing, asymmetrical	Clinical diagnosis. Skin sampling if severe, extensive or uncertain diagnosis	Self-care – loose fitting clothes, hygiene, avoid sharing towels. **Topical antifungal** (mild disease): terbinafine or clotrimazole. **Oral antifungal** (severe): terbinafine, itraconazole

TABLE 82.1   (Cont'd)

	Features	Investigations	Management
Scabies (Figs. 82.1 and 82.2)	**RFs:** overcrowded/institutionalised living, affected contacts. **Hx & O/E:** intense itching, worse at night. Linear burrows (thread-like, whitish-grey)/excoriations between fingers, flexures, umbilicus, genitalia	**Clinical diagnosis. Burrow ink test:** reveals zigzagged line running across and away from the lesion. **Skin scrapings:** for microscopy-mites, eggs or mite faecal material	**Topical permethrin.** Whole body down from chin and ears (old, young, immuno-suppressed: + face and scalp). Repeat after **1 week.** Treat close contacts. Malathion if permethrin contraindicated. Laundry at 60°C. Under 2 months old – paediatric dermatology
Head lice (*Pediculus humanus capitis*)	**RFs:** affected contacts, school outbreak, long hair. **Hx & O/E:** itching of scalp, visible lice	**Wet/dry combing** (live louse found = active infection)	**Topical insecticide + combing.** Dimethicone/malathion – patient and close contacts, repeat after 7 days
Pinworm	**RFs:** young, institutionalised, caring for affected child. **Hx & O/E:** perianal pruritis, worse at night, ± pruritis vulvae. Small white worms, excoriations	**Adhesive tape test + microscopy:** eggs or adult worms	**Hygiene:** hand washing, short nails, change bed linen. **Anti-helminthic:** mebendazole, single dose. Avoid in pregnancy
Dermatitis herpetiformis	**RFs:** coeliac disease, other autoimmune, FHx, HLA-DQ2/DQ8. **Hx & O/E:** rash-symmetrical clusters of itchy blisters, excoriations, hyperpigmentation. Elbows, knees, shoulders, buttocks, sacrum, face	**Bloods:** as for coeliac disease. See *79. FOOD INTOLERANCE.* **Skin biopsy:** to diagnose histologically	Dermatology referral. Dapsone (PO)
SYSTEMIC CAUSES			
Pruritis in chronic kidney disease	Generalised or localised itch, excoriations	See *177. CHRONIC KIDNEY DISEASE*	Emollients, topical/PO analgesia, topical/PO antihistamines, consider gabapentin or pregabalin
Obstetric cholestasis/ other patients with cholestatic/ hepatic disease	**RFs:** >28/40, multiple pregnancy, FHx, Hep C. **Hx & O/E:** itch starts on soles and palms, worse at night. Anorexia, malaise, abdo pain, nausea. Dark urine, pale stools, steatorrhoea. Excoriations, jaundice	Elevated serum bile acids, ± cholestatic LFTs. Viral/autoimmune screening. Urine dipstick (protein). Liver US. CTG. BP	Same day referral to Maternity Unit for bloods/foetal check. Monitor to 2 weeks post delivery. Emollient, cooling measures. Ursodeoxycholic acid. Sedating antihistamines. Vitamin K supplementation
Drugs – allergies or side effects	**RFs:** opioids, allopurinol, amiodarone, statins	**Clinical diagnosis**	Remove offending agent and assess response
KEY COMPLICATIONS			
Eczema herpeticum	HSV-infected eczema (sudden onset eruption of monomorphic vesicles/ erosions with hemorrhagic crusts); admit and give IV aciclovir		
Eczema with bacterial infection	*S. aureus* infection (also *S. pyogenes*) causing increased erythema/oozing. Treat with flucloxacillin (clarithromycin in penicillin allergic, erythromycin if pregnant)		

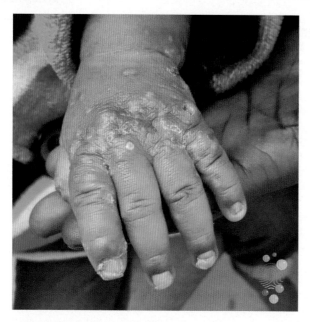

Fig. 82.1 Excoriated lesions on the dorsal hand in scabies (darker skin). (From Skin Deep. https://dftbskindeep.com/all-diagnoses/scabies/#!jig[1]/ML/884)

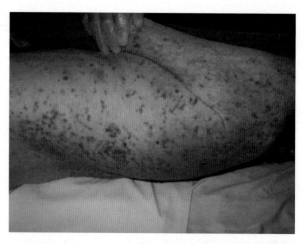

Fig. 82.2 Scabies in a 100-year-old nursing home resident (lighter skin). (Reproduced with permission from Murakonda P, Yazdanbaksh K, Dharmarajan TS. J Am Med Dir Assoc. Jan 2014;15(1):74-5.)

The most likely diagnosis in the vignette is pruritis secondary to opioid use, exacerbated by poor renal function. While it is tempting to assume a dermatological cause in cases of itching, systemic illness can provoke this symptom too and these are the patients you are more likely to see in hospital. Other causes not described in Table 82.1 include:

- *Liver failure*
- *Dermatological – psoriasis, urticaria, pityriasis rosea, lichen planus, lichen sclerosus, prickly heat*
- *Endocrine – hyper-/hypo-thyroidism, hyperparathyroidism*
- *Haematological – polycythaemia rubra vera, iron deficiency anaemia, Hodgkin lymphoma*
- *Psychological – obsessive states, schizophrenia, dermatitis artefacta*

REVISION TIPS

- Help Every Budding Dermatologist; mild – hydrocortisone, moderate – Eumovate, potent – Betnovate, very potent – Dermovate
- Red angry skin in between skin folds in an obese patient – think tinea and provide topical antifungal

83

Ascites

Katie Turner, Berenice Aguirrezabala Armbruster, and Ann Archer

EMERGENCY DEPARTMENT, MALE, 49. ABDOMINAL DISCOMFORT AND DISTENSION

HPC: 6-month history of discomfort and anorexia, with abdominal distension and feeling of fullness for the past week. SOB, especially on stairs. Skin is itchy, shoes feel tight. Drinks 40 units of alcohol a week.

O/E: Jaundice, conjunctival pallor, clubbing, palmar erythema, Dupuytren contracture, koilonychia, several spider naevi on the chest, bilateral pitting oedema of legs. Abdo: distended, shifting dullness, nodular liver palpable 3 cm below costal margin. Bowel sounds present. Temp 37.4°C, BP 110/58 mmHg, HR 75 bpm, RR 22, SpO_2 96 (on air).

1. What can cause non-cirrhotic portal hypertension?
2. What risks should you consent for prior to performing abdominal paracentesis?
3. How would you manage hepatic encephalopathy?

Answers: 1. Schistosomiasis and chronic infection, chronic veno-occlusive disease, idiopathic, PSC, PBC - among others. 2. Pain, failure, infection, bleeding, damage to underlying organs. 3. Lactulose and enemas to establish regular bowel habit aiming for 2–3 soft stools daily. Add rifaximin if recurrent. Education of patient and carers.

TABLE 83.1

	Features	Investigations	Management
Liver cirrhosis	End-stage liver disease: hepato-cellular fibrosis. RFs: alcohol, NAFLD*, viral hepatitis (B & C), metabolic, autoimmune. Hx & O/E: abdominal discomfort, anorexia, breathlessness, fatigue, pruritus. Abdominal distension, shifting dullness, hepatomegaly, splenomegaly, jaundice, peripheral oedema, clubbing, palmar erythema, spider naevi, gynaecomastia, testicular atrophy, cachexia, Dupuytren contracture	**Bloods:** LFTs (↑AST, ↑ALT, ↑ALP, ↑bilirubin, ↓albumin), FBC (↓Hb, low platelets in portal hypertension), prolonged PT, viral hepatitis screen, ferritin, caeruloplasmin, autoimmune panel, immunoglobulins. **USS:** cirrhosis, exclude structural cause, evaluate for HCC. **Transient elastography:** fibrosis. **Liver biopsy:** cause, fibrosis. **± Endoscopy:** exclude varices. **Ascitic tap:** SAAG, r/o spontaneous bacterial peritonitis (SBP)	Alcohol/smoking cessation, dietician review, fluid and salt restriction. Spironolactone, loop diuretics. Ciprofloxacin or norfloxacin to prevent spontaneous bacterial peritonitis. Consider liver transplant. **For tense ascites:** paracentesis, consider TIPS if refractory. *Non-alcoholic fatty liver disease (NAFLD) is now known as metabolic dysfunction-associated steatotic liver disease (MASLD)*

(Continued)

TABLE 83.1 (Cont'd)

	Features	Investigations	Management
Malignancy	Hepatocellular carcinoma, see *81. CHRONIC ABDOMINAL PAIN* Liver metastases from colon, rectum, pancreas, stomach, oesophagus, breast, lung, ovary, etc.		
Budd-Chiari syndrome	Classification: Primary (venous process, e.g. thrombosis or phlebitis); *Secondary* (hepatic vein and/ or IVC constriction by adjacent structure, e.g. tumour). **RFs:** hypercoagulable state (PRV, thrombophilia, pregnancy), female. **Hx & O/E:** severe abdo/RUQ pain, tender hepatomegaly, ascites	Deranged LFTs, deranged U&Es, thrombophilia screen. **USS** with doppler flow studies	Discuss urgently with specialist centre and interventional radiology. **Pharmacological:** anticoagulants, diuretics
Glomerular disease with nephrotic syndrome	Minimal change disease (MCD), focal segmental glomerulosclerosis (FSGS), membranous nephropathy (MN). **Hx & O/E:** generalised oedema, ascites, foamy urine, fatigue, anorexia	**Bloods:** deranged FBC, U&Es, ↓albumin, ↑lipids. **Urinalysis:** protein ++. Daily weights. Consider renal biopsy to identify cause	**MCD/FSGS:** oral prednisolone. **MN:** tacrolimus, cyclophosphamide or rituximab
Heart failure	See *8. PERIPHERAL OEDEMA AND ANKLE SWELLING*		

COMPLICATIONS

	Features	Investigations	Management
Spontaneous bacterial peritonitis	**RFs:** liver cirrhosis, infection, recent endoscopy, GI bleed, previous paracentesis. **Hx & O/E:** ascites, N&V, abdo pain, may show signs of encephalopathy/confusion	**Bloods:** raised inflammatory markers. **Ascitic tap:** cytology, MC&S, neutrophil count >250 cells/mm^3	IV Abx as per local guidelines. Analgesia. Treat decompensated liver disease: consider albumin transfusion; consider re-tap at 48 hours; consider long term prophylactic Abx

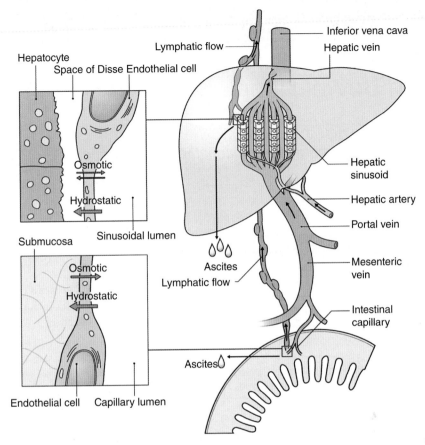

Inferior vena cava

Hepatic vein

Lymphatic flow

Hepatocyte

Space of Disse Endothelial cell

Osmotic

Hydrostatic

Submucosa

Sinusoidal lumen

Hepatic sinusoid

Hepatic artery

Portal vein

Osmotic

Hydrostatic

Ascites

Lymphatic flow

Mesenteric vein

Intestinal capillary

Ascites

Endothelial cell   Capillary lumen

Fig. 83.1 Ascites occurs when the net transfer of fluid from blood vessels to lymphatic vessels exceeds the drainage capacity of the lymphatics; fluid leaks through the hepatic capsule and, to a lesser extent, the intestine. (From Dudley FJ. Pathophysiology of ascites formation. *Gastroenterol Clin North Am.* 1992;21:215–235.)

Ascites is the accumulation of ascitic fluid within the peritoneal cavity (Fig. 83.1), due to portal hypertension (e.g. liver cirrhosis, cardiac failure) or other causes such as peritoneal pathologies (e.g. peritoneal mesothelioma, tuberculous peritonitis, gastrointestinal malignancies). The patient in the vignette has typical features of liver disease and the most likely diagnosis is ascites due to portal hypertension in liver disease. An ascitic tap (diagnostic paracentesis) is a key investigation. Ascitic fluid albumin is used to calculate the SAAG (Serum-Ascites Albumin Gradient); SAAG >11 g/L (high gradient) indicates portal hypertension, SAAG <11 g/L indicates peritoneal pathologies. Management involves treating the cause, dietary salt restriction and spironolactone (add furosemide if needed), with therapeutic paracentesis if large/

symptomatic despite treatment. Consider transjugular intrahepatic portosystemic shunt in refractory ascites that requires frequent paracentesis.

REVISION TIPS

- Child-Pugh classification grades severity of liver cirrhosis; determined by 5 factors including bilirubin, albumin, PT, encephalopathy and ascites
- MELD score is also used to classify severity
- Serum-ascites albumin gradient identifies cause of ascites – SAAG >11 g/L portal hypertension, SAAG <11 g/L indicates another cause (peritoneal)
- Ascites, abdo pain and fever; may be spontaneous bacterial peritonitis, requires antibiotics

84

Change in Bowel Habit

Emily Warren, Christian Aquilina, Zoe Kay,
Berenice Aguirrezabala Armbruster, and Jonathan Tyrrell-Price

GP CONSULTATION, FEMALE, 25. 6-MONTH HISTORY OF INTERMITTENT DIARRHOEA

HPC: Recurrent abdo pain, worse with stress, better after defaecation. Mucus in stool. PR bleed rarely, only on wiping. Colorectal cancer in first-degree relative. Current smoker (2.5 pack years), 10 units of alcohol a week, independent, active lifestyle, dairy-free diet.

O/E: Observations normal. HS I + II + 0. Chest clear. Abdo soft non-tender, no organomegaly, active bowel sounds. DRE: no anal fissures/skin tags/masses/blood.

1. What are the two most common features on biopsy which differ between Crohn disease and ulcerative colitis (UC)?
2. What is the tool used to assess the severity of UC and what are the six variables included?
3. What are the side effects of 5-ASA?

Answers: 1. UC, crypt abscesses; Crohn disease, granulomas. 2. Truelove and Witts criteria; motion/day, rectal bleeding, temperature, resting pulse, haemoglobin and ESR. 3. Rash, haemolysis, hepatitis, pancreatitis and paradoxical worsening of colitis.

TABLE 84.1

	Features	Investigations	Management
Irritable bowel syndrome (IBS)	**RFs:** genetics, infection, inflammation, diet, drugs, stress. **Hx & O/E:** abdo pain relieved by defaecation or associated with altered stool frequency or appearance. Altered stool passage (straining, urgency, tenesmus), bloating, mucus in stools, symptoms worse after eating	Tests to r/o differentials (especially if diarrhoea). **Stool:** MC&S, calprotectin. TFTs, coeliac screen, AXR	Avoid triggers, exercise, low **FODMAP diet**, soluble fibre (↑ in constipation, ↓ in diarrhoea). Laxative (for constipation), loperamide (for diarrhoea), mebeverine (anti-spasmodic). **Consider antidepressant** (TCA, SSRI if TCA not appropriate)
Coeliac disease	See *79. FOOD INTOLERANCE*		

TABLE 84.1 (Cont'd)

	Features	Investigations	Management
Crohn disease	**RFs:** FHx, smoking, psoriasis, infectious gastroenteritis, COCP. **Hx & O/E:** generalised abdo pain, tenesmus, faecal urgency, diarrhoea, vomiting, ± PR bleed, ± mucus in stools. Extra-intestinal manifestations; pauci-articular arthritis, erythema nodosum, aphthous mouth ulcers, episcleritis, bone disease. *Not related to disease activity;* axial or polyarticular arthritis, pyoderma gangrenosum, psoriasis, uveitis, hepatobiliary	**Bloods:** may show ↓Hb, ↑CRP, ↓ferritin, ↓Vit B12, ↓folate, ↓Vit D, ↓albumin. **Stool:** ↑Faecal calprotectin. **Endoscopy + biopsy:** cobblestone appearance, full thickness of intestinal wall. **CT/MRI/barium studies:** to identify complications. (R/o other differentials: coeliac bloods, stool MC&S)	**Inducing remission:** corticosteroid (1st line) or budesonide. **Add-on therapy:** if normal thiopurine methyltransferase (TPMT), offer thiopurine drug, e.g. azathioprine, mercaptopurine. If reduced TPMT activity, offer low dose thiopurine drug. If deficient TPMT offer methotrexate. **Biologicals:** infliximab or adalimumab. **Maintenance of remission** 1. Thiopurine, 2. Methotrexate, 3. Biological agent
Ulcerative colitis	**RFs:** FHx, NSAIDs, non-smoker. **Hx & O/E:** generalised abdo pain, faecal urgency, tenesmus, diarrhoea, PR bleed. Extra-intestinal manifestations like Crohn disease with the addition of VTE	**Bloods:** ↓Hb, ↑CRP, ↓ferritin, ↓Vit B12, ↓folate, ↓Vit D, ↓albumin. **Stool sample:** ↑Faecal calprotectin. **Endoscopy + biopsy:** pseudo polyps, only mucosa affected. **CT/MRI/barium studies** to identify complications. (R/o other differentials: coeliac bloods, stool MC&S)	**Mild–moderate flare:** corticosteroids and/or 5-ASA (e.g. mesalazine, sulphasalazine, pentasa). **Moderate-severe flare:** biologics, Janus kinase inhibitors. IV corticosteroids if severe. **Maintenance:** 5-ASA after mild–moderate flare up. Azathioprine or mercaptopurine after severe flare up/≥2 flare ups in 12 months/ ineffective treatment with 5-ASA alone. Biologics and JAK inhibitors
Colorectal cancer	Fig. 84.1, see *70. ABDOMINAL MASS*		

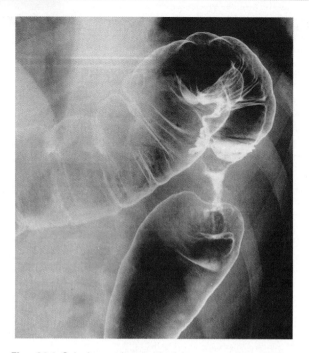

Fig. 84.1 Colonic carcinoma: barium enema examination. Typical 'apple-core' lesion just distal to the splenic flexure. (CLINICAL OVERVIEW: Colorectal cancer. Elsevier Point of Care. Updated April 27, 2022. Copyright Elsevier BV. All rights reserved. From Quick CRG et al. Colorectal polyps and carcinoma. In: Quick CRG et al. *Essential Surgery: Problems, Diagnosis and Management*. 6th ed. Elsevier; 2020:374–386, Fig. 27.5. © 2016 Copyright Elsevier BV. All rights reserved.)

The most likely diagnosis in the vignette is irritable bowel syndrome (IBS), which is classified by the predominant stool type (Rome IV criteria) into diarrhoea predominant (IBS-D), constipation predominant (IBS-C), mixed (IBS-M) and unclassified (IBS-U). Change in bowel habit can be a sign of colorectal cancer. Refer (2WW) the following: (1) Tests showing occult blood in faeces; (2) Age ≥40 with unexplained weight loss and abdo pain; (3) Age ≥50 with unexplained rectal bleeding; (4) Age ≥60 with iron-deficiency anaemia, or change in bowel habit.

REVISION TIPS

- Weight loss and anaemia are red flags for malignancy
- **Refer for suspected colorectal cancer pathway (2WW):** (1) Tests showing occult blood in faeces; (2) age ≥40 with unexplained weight loss and abdominal pain; (3) age ≥50 with unexplained rectal bleeding; (4) age ≥60 with iron-deficiency anaemia, or changes in bowel habit
- **Consider referral for suspected colorectal cancer pathway (2WW):** (1) Adults with a rectal or abdominal mass; (2) age ≥50 with rectal bleeding and unexplained abdominal pain/change in bowel habit/weight loss/iron deficiency anaemia

85

Constipation

Emily Warren and Jennifer Phillips

HPC: Usually, bowels opened every 2 days. Increased fibre and water intake did not help. Recent discharge for THR, prescribed oramorph. Intermittent mild generalised abdo tenderness. No vomiting, passing flatus. **PMHx:** HTN, T2DM, THR. Current smoker (2 pack years), 10 units of alcohol a week.

O/E: Normal obs. Abdomen SNT not distended, BS present. Chest clear, HS I + II + 0. DRE: haemorrhoids, no blood, hard stool.

1. What is the most common cause of small bowel obstruction?
2. An AXR shows the classic coffee bean sign. What type of volvulus causes this?
3. State an example of a bulk-forming laxative
4. State an example of a stimulant laxative.
5. State an example of a softener laxative.
6. State an example of an osmotic laxative.

Answers: 1. Adhesions (80%), followed by hernia. 2. Sigmoid volvulus. 3. Ispaghula husk, sterculia, methylcellulose. 4. Bisacodyl, senna, sodium picosulphate, glycerol suppositories, co-danthramer/co-danthrusate. 5. Methylcellulose, docusate sodium, glycerol suppositories. 6. Lactulose, macrogol.

TABLE 85.1

	Features	Investigations	Management
Constipation secondary to **medication**	Opioids, antimuscarinics, antidepressants, antiepileptics, antihistamines, antispasmodics, diuretics, iron/calcium supplements	Clinical diagnosis. **DRE:** impacted stools, strictures or masses. Check for fissures, fistulae or external haemorrhoids. **AXR:** to r/o obstruction. **Investigations for likely underlying medical condition**, e.g. bloods for calcium, TFTs. Colonoscopy if >50 years with changes in bowel habit or constipation plus ALARM features	Treat cause (e.g. ↑fibre, treat hypercalcaemia). Laxatives (stimulant and softener if opioid-induced constipation). ↑Fluids if poor oral intake. Treat complications (e.g. UTI, urinary retention)
Constipation secondary to **diet**	Poor oral intake, poor fibre intake		
Constipation secondary to **underlying medical condition**	**Endocrine:** hypercalcaemia, hypothyroidism. **Neurological:** MS, stroke Parkinson's disease. **Gastrointestinal:** IBS, IBD. **Malignancy:** colorectal cancer, spinal tumour		
Bowel obstruction	See *68. ABDOMINAL DISTENSION*		

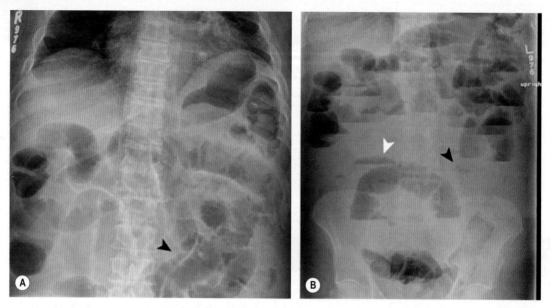

Fig. 85.1 (A) Supine abdominal radiograph showing small bowel obstruction, with distended small bowel loops (*black arrowhead*). (B) Upright radiograph showing gas-fluid levels, giving rise to the 'tortoise-shell' sign (*white arrowhead*), and the 'string-of-pearls' sign (*black arrowhead*). (Reproduced with permission from Stuart E. Mirvis MD, FACR, Wayne S. Kubal MD, Kathirkamanathan Shanmuganathan MD, Jorge A. Soto MD and Joseph S. Yu MD. Nontraumatic Abdominal Emergencies Problem Solving in Emergency Radiology, Chapter 13, 368-466.)

The most likely diagnosis in the vignette is constipation secondary to opioid use. A good history is essential, including reviewing the medication history noting any new drugs. Check if the patient has tried any laxatives previously and if any specific laxatives have worked well. Treat underlying cause and any possible complications associated with constipation. Ensure you rule out bowel obstruction (Fig. 85.1).

REVISION TIPS

- Check which medications the patient is on when considering a diagnosis for constipation
- If someone presents with constipation, anal fissures and skin tags, top differential = Crohn disease

86

Diarrhoea

*Katie Turner, Emily Warren, Berenice Aguirrezabala Armbruster,
and Jennifer Phillips*

**EMERGENCY DEPARTMENT, FEMALE, 24.
DIARRHOEA AND VOMITING**

HPC: Over the past 24 hours, five episodes of loose, non-bloody stools and three episodes of vomiting. Feels tired and weak. Abdo cramps, resolve on opening bowels. Returned from a holiday in Morocco 3 days ago, generally fit and well.

O/E: Dry mucous membranes. CRT 3 seconds. Generalised abdo tenderness. T 38.2°C, BP 89/54 mmHg, HR 95 bpm, RR 18, SpO_2 98% (on air).

---

1. What are the features of haemolytic uraemic syndrome? What bacteria cause it?
2. What clinical features make up the modified Truelove and Witts criteria for the diagnosis of acute severe ulcerative colitis?
3. What findings would be seen on duodenal biopsy in Coeliac disease?
4. What are some of the alarm symptoms that warrant further investigation in a patient presenting with possible IBS?
5. Name some differential diagnoses for villous atrophy.

Answers: 1. AKI + microangiopathic haemolytic anaemia + thrombocytopenia; caused by *E. coli* 0157:H7. Can also be caused by *Shigella*. 2. >6 bloody stools per day and systemic toxicity with at least one of: temperature >38.5°C, pulse >90 bpm, haemoglobin <105 g/L or CRP >30 mg/L. 3. Villous atrophy, crypt hyperplasia, increase in intraepithelial lymphocytes, lamina propria infiltration with lymphocytes. 4. Weight loss, aged >50, short history of symptoms, nocturnal symptoms, FHx colon cancer, anaemic, rectal bleeding. 5. Giardia, lymphoma, Whipple disease, tropical sprue, NSAIDs, hypogammaglobulinaemia.

TABLE 86.1

	Features	Investigations	Management
Gastroenteritis	*E. coli* (most common in travellers), *Giardia*, *Vibrio cholerae*, *Shigella*, *S. aureus*, *Campylobacter jejuni*, *Bacillus cereus*, amoebiasis. **Hx & O/E:** diarrhoea ± cramps, fever, N&V, ± blood in stool	Baseline bloods may show ↑WCC, deranged U&E, ↑CRP. **Consider stool MC&S**	Consider admission, PO/IV fluids, anti-emetics, analgesia. See *98. TRAVELLING ADVICE*
Ulcerative colitis	See *84. CHANGE IN BOWEL HABIT*		

(Continued)

TABLE 86.1   (Cont'd)

	Features	Investigations	Management
Crohn disease	See *84. CHANGE IN BOWEL HABIT*		
Irritable bowel syndrome	See *84. CHANGE IN BOWEL HABIT*		
Coeliac disease	Watery diarrhoea, see *79. FOOD INTOLERANCE*. Steatorrhoea, see below		
Steatorrhoea	Maldigestion; exocrine pancreatic insufficiency (EPI; e.g. chronic pancreatitis) or lack of bile (e.g. advanced PBC). Can be >30g fat/day. Malabsorption; mucosal diseases (e.g. coeliac disease), SIBO. Less severe. Hx & O/E: bulky, pale, foul-smelling oily stools, float in the toilet bowl, difficult to flush away. Chronic diarrhoea, bloating, abdominal discomfort, weight loss	Stool fat quantification: >9.5g/100g suggests pancreatic or biliary cause. Pancreatic enzyme trial. Small bowel imaging. Upper/lower GI endoscopy. Test for fat-soluble vitamin (A, D, E, K) deficiencies	EPI; pancreatic enzyme replacement therapy, with normal to high-fat diet and vitamin supplementation. PBC; ursodeoxycholic acid. PSC; ERCP with stent dilatation. SIBO; trial of Abx, e.g. rifaximin

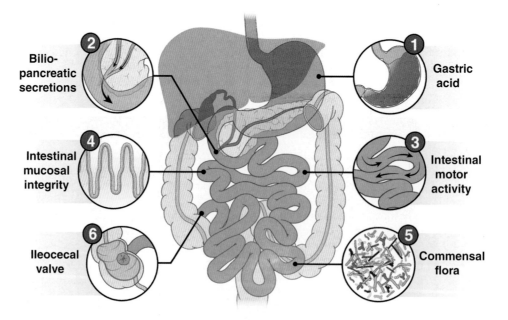

Fig. 86.1 Factors that protect against the development of SIBO in health and that may be susceptible to disruption in disease. (Reproduced with permission from Daniel Bushyhead, Eamonn M.M. Quigley. Small Intestinal Bacterial Overgrowth—Pathophysiology and Its Implications for Definition and Management. *Gastroenterology*. Elsevier. September 2022)

The most likely diagnosis in the vignette is gastroenteritis. The patient is presenting with a short history of diarrhoea and vomiting and reports no previous similar history. Consider admission if unable to maintain oral hydration/intake, raised WCC/CRP or at risk of complications. Chronic diarrhoea lasts ≥4 weeks and is classified by appearance into watery, fatty or inflammatory. Exclude anaemia, dehydration and protein loss. Watery diarrhoea may need stool analysis, small bowel radiography, sigmoidoscopy or colonoscopy with biopsies, bile acid sequestrant trial, and endocrine studies. Sometimes, watery diarrhoea is caused by undisclosed use of laxatives (this can be suspected by looking at the faecal osmotic gap). The most common causes of chronic diarrhoea are coeliac disease, chronic infection, IBS, inflammatory bowel disease, lactose intolerance, endocrine causes, medications and ischaemic colitis. Steatorrhoea reflects maldigestion or malabsorption of fat. Small intestinal bacterial overgrowth (SIBO) reflects maldigestion and malabsorption where colonic microbiota may colonise the small intestine (Fig. 86.1). Availability of breath tests has increased diagnosis, though interpretation needs caution.

REVISION TIPS

- Dysentery is used to describe diarrhoea with blood and mucus – important causes include *Campylobacter, Shigella, Salmonella,* and norovirus
- Diarrhoea is classed as chronic if lasting >14 days
- Steatorrhoea causes: pancreatitis, coeliac disease, chronic liver diseases (PBC, PSC), advanced pancreatic cancer, disease of the distal ileum (e.g. Crohn resection), SIBO, giardiasis
- Traveller's diarrhoea; more than three loose stools a day starting within 24 hours of foreign travel
- The transmural inflammation in Crohn disease can lead to complications such as stricture and fistulae that are not commonly seen in UC
- When considering a diagnosis of IBS, diarrhoea predominance warrants further investigation

87

Pallor

Zoe Kay, Alexander Royston, and Julia Wolf

GP CONSULTATION, MALE, 64.
PALLOR AND FATIGUE

HPC: Symptoms worsening over 3 months. **PMHx:** Crohn disease. **DHx:** Ferrous sulphate. **SHx:** Lives with partner, ex-smoker (10 pack years), no alcohol.

O/E: Appears pale, conjunctival pallor. Obs normal, nil else on examination. Significant negatives: no angular stomatitis, no koilonychia. **Ix:** Hb 103(↓) MCV 106(↑).

---

1. What are the principles of management of B12 deficiency?

2. When would oral iron, IV iron or a packed cell transfusion be prescribed in iron deficiency anaemia?
3. What are the symptoms of anaemia?

Answers: 1. Investigate cause (rule out pernicious anaemia/Ca), dietary advice if necessary. Replace B12 before folate: IM cobalamin loading regime (three times a week for 2 weeks). Maintenance every 2–3 months. 2. Oral iron is the main treatment. Iron infusion in malabsorption, or if poorly tolerated. Packed cell transfusion in severe anaemia: cardiovascular instability. 3. Fatigue, pallor, SOB, tachycardia, palpitations, angina, dizziness and syncope.

TABLE 87.1

	Features	Investigations	Management
MACROCYTIC (MCV >100)			
B12/folate deficiency. Megaloblastic (impaired DNA synthesis)	*B12-deficiency* RFs: pernicious anaemia, Crohn's, dietary insufficiency, bariatric surgery. Hx & O/E: weight loss, fatigue, pallor, altered taste, confusion, Δmood, ataxia, paraesthesia, ↓vision, glossitis. *Folate deficiency* RFs: dietary, ↑excretion, ↑demand (pregnancy), folate antagonists (methotrexate/trimethoprim). Hx & O/E: atrophic glossitis, thrombocytopenia, leucopenia, diarrhoea, fatigue	FBC, reticulocyte count (classically ↓). Serum: ↓folate, ↓B12, LFTs, TSH. Haemolysis screen: (LDH, bilirubin, haptoglobin, reticulocytes, blood film, direct antiglobulin test (DAT). Blood film: hypersegmented neutrophils, oval macrocytes, anisopoikilocytosis	B12 (IM). Folic acid (oral). **Check B12 BEFORE replacing folate (risk subacute combined neurodegeneration)** – see *111. UNSTEADINESS*

TABLE 87.1 (Cont'd)

	Features	Investigations	Management
Non-megaloblastic macrocytic anaemias	• Liver disease (incl alcohol) • Hypothyroidism • Reticulocytosis (immature, large RBCs) • Myelodysplastic syndrome • Drugs (e.g. cytotoxics, antiepileptics)	**Bloods.** As above. Blood film: round macrocytes/macroreticulocytes	Treat underlying cause (hypothyroidism: thyroxine). Investigate haemolysis if present. Discuss with haematology
NORMOCYTIC (MCV 80–100)			
Haemolytic anaemia. (Can be macrocytic due to reticulocytes)	*Immune* Autoimmune haemolytic anaemia (warm/cold). Allo-immune haemolytic anaemia (transfusion/haemolytic disease of foetus and newborn). Drugs. *Non-immune* Microangiopathies, infection, DIC, mechanical haemolysis (heart valves), pregnancy-related. *Hereditary disorders* Haemoglobinopathies (Sickle disease), membrane disorders (hereditary spherocytosis), enzyme deficiencies (G6PD-deficiency)	**Presentation:** pallor, jaundice, dark urine, fever, weak, dizzy, confusion, splenomegaly. **Haemolysis screen:** ↑bilirubin, ↓haptoglobin, ↑reticulocytes, ↑LDH. Blood film: schistocytes/spherocytes/RBC fragments suggest microangiopathic haemolytic anaemia-consider TTP/other causes. **DAT +ve** ⟶immune haemolysis. **USS:** splenomegaly	Treat underlying condition. May require immunosuppression; glucocorticoids, immunosuppressants, plasmapheresis or splenectomy. Blood transfusion if required – severe or life-threatening
Renal anaemia	**RF:** CKD. ↓Erythropoietin	FBC, reticulocytes, U&Es, serum erythropoietin (EPO), iron studies, calcium/PTH. **Urinalysis.** **USS kidneys** ± Renal biopsy	EPO injections ± iron supplementation. **Definitive:** transplantation
Haematological malignancy	**RFs/presentation:** dependent on malignancy. May present with pancytopenia: ↓Hb, ↓WCC, ↓Plts	**Bloods:** incl blood film, LDH, folate, B12. **Bone marrow/LN biopsy:** further investigations	Haematology referral. MDT involvement. Chemo/immunotherapy, ± bone marrow transplant
MICROCYTIC (MCV <80)			
Iron deficiency	**RFs:** rapid growth cycles, heavy menstruation, malabsorption, GI bleed, pregnant, delayed wean, alcohol excess. **Hx & O/E:** fatigue, pallor, fingernail changes, headache, infection, pica, hair loss, SOB, restless legs	FBC (↓Hb/MCV/MCH), ↓ferritin, ↓transferrin saturation, ↑TIBC. Blood film: microcytic, hypochromic (may show poikilocytosis, anisocytosis). **Endoscopy/colonoscopy:** no obvious bleeding site	Iron replacement (oral/IV). Blood transfusion (if symptomatic – risk:benefit). Treat underlying cause

(Continued)

TABLE 87.1 (Cont'd)

	Features	Investigations	Management
Thalassaemia	Autosomal recessive mutations in Hb chains. RFs: certain ethnicities, FHx. Hx & O/E (if severe): signs of anaemia, hepatosplenomegaly, bony deformities, jaundice. Severity varies from life-incompatible ⟶ asymptomatic. Severe forms present early	Screening for all pregnant women. FBC: ($\downarrow$Hb/$\downarrow\downarrow$MCV/$\downarrow$MCH). Serum iron/ferritin ($\uparrow$ if transfusion-dependent). **Genetic testing**	Blood transfusions (according to severity). Aim: suppress extramedullary haematopoiesis (target Hb is often higher >100). Transfusions may cause iron overload (chelation)
Anaemia of chronic disease	RFs: infections (chronic: TB/HIV), autoimmune diseases, cancer, CKD, IBD, CCF, DM. Hepcidin is upregulated causing functional iron deficiency (mechanism to deprive pathogens of free iron). Hx & O/E: anaemia symptoms, malaise	Chronic inflammatory state: $\downarrow$RBC production/survival. FBC ($\leftrightarrow$/$\uparrow$Plts, inflammatory markers may be $\uparrow$, $\uparrow$ferritin, $\leftrightarrow$/$\downarrow$TIBC, $\downarrow$transferrin saturation, $\downarrow$reticulocytes, U&Es (rule out renal cause). Blood film: $\pm$ microcytosis/normocytosis, hypochromic/normochromic	RBC transfusions, erythropoiesis-stimulating agents. Ferritin will be high in inflammation and can mask iron deficiency (consider treating). Treat underlying condition

KEY COMPLICATION

Type 2 MI	MI (Dx with biomarkers) that occurs due to: mismatch in myocardial oxygen supply and demand – absence of CAD. May be secondary to: hypotension (e.g. sepsis), severe anaemia, tachyarrhythmias. Consequent $\downarrow$myocardial oxygenation

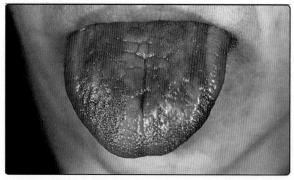

Fig. 87.1 Painful glossitis in pernicious anaemia. (From Howard MR, Hamilton PJ. *Megaloblastic Anaemia, Haematology: An Illustrated Colour Text*. 4th ed. Elsevier; 2013:13, 26–27. © 2013 Elsevier Ltd)

The vignette describes macrocytic anaemia secondary to B12 deficiency, which was itself likely caused by his Crohn disease. A clinical diagnosis without blood tests is not straight forward, but some hints are there even without the characteristic neuropathy. Conjunctival pallor and fatigue are typical for anaemia, but non-specific. The slow onset (3-month) is also non-specific, but the absence of prominent signs of iron deficiency (cheilitis, koilonychia) and iron supplementation suggests a normocytic/macrocytic cause is more likely (despite his RFs for bowel cancer). His main risk factor for B12 deficiency is Crohn disease.

REVISION TIPS

- Coeliac disease is often found when investigating iron deficiency anaemia: check anti-tTG
- **Ferritin** is a measure of the intracellular iron stores: interpretation is impossible in acutely ill patients **(acute phase protein)**
- **TIBC:** measures the amount of transferrin in the blood. Iron travels bound to transferrin. **Transferrin saturation** in combination with TIBC shows the spare capacity there is to bind iron

	Iron deficiency	Anaemia of chronic disease
Ferritin	Low	Normal (or high)
Serum iron	Low	Low
Transferrin saturation	Low	Low
TIBC/ transferrin	High	Low (or normal)

88

Petechial Rash and Purpura

Katherine Parker, Alexander Royston, Katie Wong, and Julia Wolf

GP CONSULTATION, FEMALE, 38.
PETECHIAL RASH ON HER LOWER LEGS

HPC: Rash is 2 days old. Menorrhagia worsening for 3 months, previously light and regular. On questioning reports one episode of epistaxis lasting 15 minutes. Otherwise well. No recent infections, weight loss, night sweats or fevers.
 O/E: Pallor. Bilateral petechial rash on lower legs, examination otherwise normal. Her renal function is normal.

1. Why do both hypersplenism and hyposplenism lead to a low platelet count?
2. Give two examples of dilutional thrombocytopenia.
3. How does bleeding in thrombocytopaenia differ from coagulation disorders?

Answers: 1. Hypersplenism: early destruction of platelets in the spleen. Hyposplenism: reversible pooling of 90% of the total platelet count. 2. Pregnancy and following blood transfusion. 3. Thrombocytopenia; mucocutaneous. Coagulation disorders; delayed visceral, joint, muscles.

TABLE 88.1

	Features	Investigations	Management
NON-THROMBOCYTOPENIC			
Bacterial meningococcal	See *93. NECK PAIN/STIFFNESS*		
Henoch Schönlein purpura (HSP)/ IgA vasculitis	**RFs:** age (3–15 yo), male, recent URTI/gastroenteritis. **Hx & O/E:** palpable purpura (legs/buttocks), abdo pain, bloody diarrhoea, N&V, arthralgia, headache, ±macroscopic haematuria. Low-grade fever, diffuse abdo tenderness ±nephrotic syndrome/renal failure/ hypertension	**Urinalysis:** microscopic haematuria, proteinuria, RBC casts (renal referral). **Urine protein-creatinine ratio** (PCR). **Bloods:**↑Inflammatory markers, U&Es (↑creat), ↑IgA, auto-antibody screen. **USS** (GI): intussusception (5% risk). **Renal biopsy:** mesangial IgA deposition	*Non-blanching rash (child):* immediate paediatric referral. **Supportive:** analgesia (avoid NSAIDs), rehydration, wound care. **Definitive:** cortico-steroids (severe abdo pain, oedema, renal involvement). ACEi (renal involvement)

TABLE 88.1 (Cont'd)

	Features	Investigations	Management
ANCA-associated vasculitides	RFs: unclear (smoking/infection/genetics). Hx & O/E: palpable purpura, systemic (fatigue/weight loss/fever/night sweats/myalgia/polyarthralgia). Haemoptysis, SOB, persistent sinusitis/otitis, ↓hearing, oral ulcers, scleritis, paraesthesia, weakness, mononeuritis multiplex, arthralgia. Saddle-nose deformity (granulomatosis with polyangiitis (GPA)), nail-fold infarctions, splinter haemorrhages, wheeze	Urinalysis: haematuria, proteinuria. Urine PCR. Bloods: U&Es (↑creat), FBC (↓Hb, ↑Plts, ↑Eosinophils), LFTs (↓Alb), ↑ESR, ANCA. CXR: nodular/fibrotic/infiltrative or diffuse alveolar/pulmonary haemorrhage. CT chest: cavitary nodules. ECG. Tissue biopsy (renal/skin). CRP/ANCA(MPO/PR3) titres (monitor disease activity)	Rheumatology/renal referral. Corticosteroids (induce remission). Definitive: cyclophosphamide/rituximab. Methotrexate/azathioprine or rituximab. Corticosteroids. Adjunct: osteoporosis prophylaxis (vit D/calcium).
Drug-induced	Steroids, sulphonamides		

Differentials	Key Words/Features/Hints	Investigations	Management
THROMBOCYTOPENIC			
Haemolytic uraemic syndrome (HUS)	RFs: child (3 yo), recent infective gastroenteritis, farm animal contact, summer months, contaminated food/water. Causes E. coli O157/STEC (Shiga toxin-producing E. coli; 90%), Campylobacter, Shigella, Pneumococcus, HIV, SLE, drugs. Hx & O/E: gastroenteritis (N&V, profuse diarrhoea ⟶ bloody, abdo pain, fever). 3–10 days+: irritability, weakness, lethargy, oliguria, dehydration, pallor, petechiae, HTN	Microangiopathic haemolytic anaemia, thrombocytopenia and kidney injury. Urinalysis: haematuria, proteinuria. Bloods: FBC (↓Hb/↓Plt), blood film (schistocytes), U&Es (AKI), ↑LDH, ↑inflammatory markers. Stool: culture and phage typing (STEC/E. coli O157), Shiga toxin PCR. Urine: MC&S	Rehydration, fluid balance (meticulous). Definitive: ± RBC transfusion, anti-hypertensives. Dialysis. Renal transplant. E. coli O157: avoid Abx, unless septic. Notifiable disease
Thrombotic thrombo-cytopenic purpura (TTP)	RFs: age (30–50 yo), pregnant/post-partum, autoimmune disease with ↓ADAMTS13 enzyme. Hx & O/E: jaundice, pallor, non-palpable purpura. Classic pentad: Microangiopathic haemolytic anaemia (MAHA). Thrombocytopenia. Neurological deficit (confusion/headache/coma/focal deficit/seizure). Fever. Renal dysfunction. All five are rarely present: suspect if MAHA + thrombocytopaenia	Blood film (essential): microangiopathic anaemia + schistocytes/fragments. FBC (↓Hb/↓↓Plts), U&Es (↑Urea/Creat), ↑LDH, ↓haptoglobin, ↑reticulocytes. Direct Coombs (−ve)	MEDICAL EMERGENCY. Urgent haematology discussion and blue light transfer to TTP centre. Definitive: Plasma exchange. Corticosteroids Folic acid. ±Rituximab. ±Caplacizumab. ±Aspirin. Avoid platelet transfusions: (can exacerbate)

(Continued)

TABLE 88.1   (Cont'd)

Differentials	Key Words/Features/Hints	Investigations	Management

Immune thrombo-cytopenia (ITP)	**RFs:** age (<10/>65 yo), autoimmune, viral (CMV/VZV/HCV/HIV), *H. pylori*, lympho-proliferative disorders.
	Children (acute-onset): preceding viral infection/immunisation.
	Adults (insidious-onset): F > M.
	Hx & O/E: thrombocytopenia signs, minor superficial bleeding (life-threatening bleeding rare)
		FBC/blood film (isolated ↓Plts).
		Clotting (PT/aPTT↔).
		HIV/Hep C screen
			Non-blanching rash (child): immediate paediatric referral.
			Observation ± medical management (severity-dependent); corticosteroids, IVIG, platelet transfusion (only if bleeding/↑↑platelet requirement: surgery).
			Definitive:
			    Eltrombopag/rituximab.
			    Other immunosuppression.
			    Splenectomy (rare)

Disseminated intravascular coagulation (DIC)	Always with other conditions; sepsis, trauma, obstetric complications, malignancy, ABO transfusion incompatibility. **Hx & O/E:** petechiae/purpura, ecchymosis, gangrene, disorientation, hypoxia, hypotension, tachycardia	Simultaneous bleeding and microvascular thrombosis (multiple sites). **Bloods:** FBC (↓Plt), clotting (↑PT, ↑APTT, ↑↑D-Dimer, ↓fibrinogen)	Treat underlying disorder. High bleeding risk/active bleeding; platelet transfusion, FFP, cryoprecipitate. LMWH (consider)

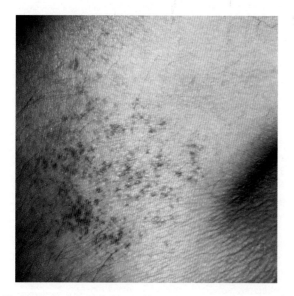

Fig. 88.1 Round to oval petechiae, ≤3mm in diameter. (From Bolognia JL, Schaffer, JV, Duncan, KO, Ko, CJ. Purpura and disorders of microvascular occlusion. In: *Dermatology Essentials.* January 1, 2014:172–181. © 2014.)

The most likely diagnosis in the vignette is ITP, based on petechiae, epistaxis and menorrhagia. She is female (increased risk) and has no red flags for other causes.

The lack of infective symptoms and meningism rules out meningococcal infection, which is the most immediately alarming cause of petechiae. She describes no constitutional symptoms and has normal renal function, which makes ANCA-associated vasculitis unlikely. She reports no gastrointestinal symptoms or fever, which makes HUS less likely. TTP is a rare disease, which should be in your differential- an urgent blood film is the best way to rule this out. Here, the absence of neurological symptoms, fever and renal dysfunction make this less likely. See Fig. 88.1.

REVISION TIPS

- Thrombocytopenia signs: petechiae, bruising, epistaxis, gingival bleeding, haematuria, GI bleeding, menorrhagia, retinal haemorrhage
  - Saddle-nose deformity – think GPA (cANCA) History of asthma – think (eosinophilic) EGPA (pANCA)
- ITP versus TTP:
  - TTP: microangiopathy with fragments 'the terrible pentad' 1. anaemia, 2. ↓platelets, 3. neurological, 4. fever, 5. renal dysfunction: patient UNWELL.
  - ITP: isolated thrombocytopenia without fragments: less likely to be unwell

89

Bruising

Meijia Xie, Max Shah, and Rachael Biggart

Meijia Xie, Max Shah, and Rachael Biggart

GP CONSULTATION, MALE, 2 YEARS OLD. SWOLLEN KNEE

HPC: Stumbled on carpet during play, right knee became swollen and tender. Mother gives collateral history of easy bruising and prolonged nosebleeds. **PMHx, FHx, SHx:** Unremarkable. Normal development.

  O/E: Afebrile, alert. Right knee badly swollen and painful, reduced movement, haematoma above right patella. No evidence of non-accidental injury.

1. A 60-year-old male, septic, bleeding from orifices, jaundice, thrombocytopenia. Blood film: schistocytes. What is the likely diagnosis?
2. A 23-year-old female, mild bruising inner thighs, no history of bleeding after trauma or surgery. No PMHx, DHx or FHx. What is the most likely cause?
3. What is the most common coagulopathy?

Answers: 1. DIC: widespread thrombi with paradoxical bleeding as platelets are consumed – schistocytes not always present on film. 2. Purpura simplex – asymptomatic, idiopathic bruising often in females aged 20 to 40 years. 3. vWD > Haemophilia A > B > C.

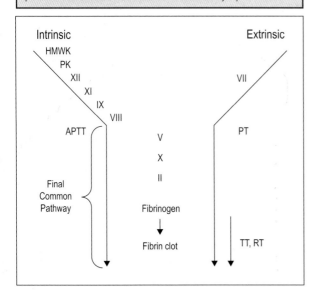

Fig. 89.1 Schematic of the coagulation cascade. Factors II, VII, IX, and X are vitamin K-dependent factors. *APTT*, Activated partial thromboplastin time; *HMWK*, high-molecular-weight kininogen; *PK*, prekallikrein; *PT*, prothrombin time; *RT*, reptilase time; *TT*, thrombin time. Reproduced with permission from Kamal AH, Tefferi A, Pruthi RK. How to interpret and pursue an abnormal prothrombin time, activated partial thromboplastin time, and bleeding time in adults. *Mayo Clin Proc.* 2007;82(7):864–873.

TABLE 89.1

	Features	Investigations	Management
Inherited Coagulation and Bleeding Disorders			
Haemophilias A (factor VIII) B (factor IX; Christmas disease) C (factor XI)	Reduced or absent clotting factors. M > F, child, Caucasian. Acquired (rare) – adult, autoimmune. Hx & O/E: Haemarthrosis (knee, elbow, hip). Thigh, calf haematomas – compartment syndrome. Prolonged bleeding (dental, epistaxis, cuts, spontaneous). Haemophilia C – Ashkenazi Jewish population	**Clotting screen:** normal or prolonged APTT, thrombin/prothrombin/bleeding times. Factor VIII/IX (XI) assay: low or absent. **FBC:** platelets normal. **AST/ALT:** rule out liver cause of prolonged APTT. Joint XR – r/o fracture	Avoid contact sport, IM injection, NSAID/aspirin. Factor concentrate. Haematology review. Genetic counselling (Table 89.2) Acute: ABCDE, clotting factor/FFP, antifibrinolytic, desmopressin
von Willebrand disease (vWD)	Autosomal dominant; von Willebrand factor (vWF) carrier for factor VIII; platelet adhesion Hx & O/E: young/adult female; menorrhagia, easy bruising, mucocutaneous bleeding (dental/epistaxis)	Long bleeding time, mildly prolonged APTT/normal prothrombin time (PT). Platelets normal. vWF antigen level assay and vWF functional assay. Factor VIII may be down	*Mild bleed*: tranexamic acid. Desmopressin. *Severe bleed*: factor VIII concentrate
Hereditary haemorrhagic telangiectasia (HHT) Osler-Weber-Rendu disease	Telangiectasias – lips, mouth, fingers, gastrointestinal (GI), nose (Fig. 89.2). Arteriovenous malformation (AVM) liver, cerebral, pulmonary. Autosomal *dominant* vascular defect. Epistaxis – recurrent	Clinical diagnosis. FBC: potential anaemia. Clotting screen. Blood film: r/o malignancy	Control symptoms. Iron supplements. Embolise AVMs (prevent stroke)
Platelet disorders	ITP, HSP, TTP, DIC. See *88. PETECHIAL RASH AND PURPURA*		
Musculoskeletal			
Ehlers-Danlos syndrome	Young/child, hypermobile, elastic fragile skin, chronic joint/muscle pain, dislocation, bruising (fragile capillaries). Aortic regurgitation, mitral valve prolapse, aortic dissection, SAH	Clinical diagnosis	Symptomatic: physiotherapy/occupational therapy. Analgesia. BP control. Education/ counselling
Inflammatory	In any unilateral joint swelling, consider: • Infection: septic arthritis – febrile, raised WCC, recent trauma/surgery, prosthesis • Rheumatology: crystal arthropathies		
Acquired Causes			
Medication	Drugs increasing bleeding risk: NSAIDs, SSRIs, antiplatelet drugs, warfarin, DOACs (AF, PE/DVT) and certain chemotherapy drugs		
Vitamin K Deficiency	Vitamin K injection to prevent haemorrhagic disease of newborn (signs: bruising (often facial), haematuria, blood in stool). Also seen in adults with cholestatic picture unable to absorb fat-soluble vitamin K.		
Liver Disease	Suggestive history: alcohol excess, craggy liver. Investigation: LFTs (deranged), clotting screen.		

TABLE 89.1 (Cont'd)

	Features	Investigations	Management
Leukaemias: ALL, CLL, AML, CML. Myeloproliferative disorders: CML, MF, PRV, ET			
Shared manifestations: there may be anaemia (breathlessness, fatigue), thrombocytopenia (bruising, epistaxis, dental bleed), neutropenia (recurrent infections, fever), constitutional (fatigue, night sweats, weight loss), hepatosplenomegaly and lymphadenopathy. See *91. LYMPHADENOPATHY* and *92. ORGANOMEGALY* FBC (often shows low Hb, low platelets) and **peripheral blood film**. Definitive test: **bone marrow aspirate and trephine** (BMAT). Flow cytometry, cytogenetics and molecular diagnostics			
Acute Lymphoblastic Leukaemia (ALL)	Mainly children <5 yo, fever, respiratory distress, infection, lethargy, poor feeding, bone pain, hepatosplenomegaly **RFs:** radiation, Down syndrome, EBV	FBC: ↑lymphocytes ±↓Hb, ↓platelets. Blood film: lymphoblasts. BMAT: >20% lymphoblastic	Chemotherapy. Hematopoietic stem cell transplant (HSCT). Chimeric antigen receptor T-cell therapy (CAR-T).
Chronic Lymphocytic Leukaemia (CLL)	Adults >60 yo, often asymptomatic, constitutional symptoms. Signs: lymphadenopathy, splenomegaly. Other assoc: autoimmune haemolytic anaemia, thrombocytopenia (ITP)	FBC: ↑ lymphocyte. Blood film: lymphocytosis, 'smear/smudge' cells. Flow cytometry: clonality. BMAT: often normal	No treatment if uncomplicated. Active monitoring. Tyrosine kinase inhibitor, e.g. ibrutinib. Vaccination, infection prophylaxis
Acute Myeloid Leukaemia (AML)	Mainly adults. **RFs:** myeloproliferative disease, Down syndrome, smoking, obesity, autoimmune. DIC *more common* in AML	Blood film: Auer rods. BMAT: >20% blast cells. Coagulation screen and fibrinogen	Chemotherapy. Allogenic HSCT
Chronic Myeloid Leukaemia (CML)	Mainly adults. Massive splenomegaly. Philadelphia chromosome (BCR ABL1) 95%. CML can transform into AML	Blood film: mature myeloid cells (basophils, eosinophils). BMAT: granulocyte hyperplasia, ↓ myeloid: erythroid ratio. Genetic testing	Chemotherapy: tyrosine kinase inhibitor (imatinib)
Primary Myelofibrosis (PMF)	Massive splenomegaly. 'Dry' tap on bone marrow aspiration	FBC: anaemia. Blood film: 'teardrop' leucoerythroblastic. BMAT: marrow fibrosis	No treatment if asymptomatic. Allogenic HSCT or JAK inhibitor (ruxolitinib). Supportive: transfusions
Primary Polycythaemia (Rubra) Vera (PRV)	Flushed skin; itchy after hot bath, mild/no splenomegaly. Hyperviscosity (e.g. headache), thrombosis (e.g. DVT), leukaemic transformation	Erythropoietin: low. Blood film: ±normal. Genetics: JAK2 (90%)	Venesection, low-dose acetylsalicylic acid. Consider cytoreduction with hydroxycarbamide
Essential Thrombocythaemia (ET)	Persistent thrombocytosis without reactive causes (infection, sepsis, trauma, surgery, chronic inflammation). Rule out iron deficiency	Platelets: ↑ ↑. BMAT: hyperplastic megakaryocytes. Genetics: JAK2 (60%)	Low-dose acetylsalicylic acid. Consider cytoreduction with hydroxycarbamide

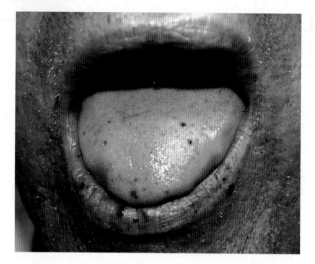

Fig. 89.2 Telangiectases in hereditary haemorrhagic telangiectasia. Reproduced with permission from Pollak JS. Pulmonary Arteriovenous Malformations: Diagnosis and Management. In: Image-Guided Interventions. Expert Radiology Series. 3rd Edition (Author: Thomson; Editors: Mauro, Murphy, Venbrux, Morgan). Elsevier, 2019.

TABLE 89.2   Genetics of von Willebrand Disease, Hereditary Haemorrhagic Telangiectasia and the Three Haemophilias

	X-linked	Autosomal
Dominant		vWD, HHT
Recessive	A, B	C

Coagulation is a complex process (Fig. 89.1), with the liver having a key role through both the hepatocytes (fibrinogen, prothrombin, factors V, VII, IX, X, XI, XII, proteins C/S, antithrombin) and the liver sinusoidal endothelial cells (factor VIII, von Willebrand factor (vWF)). Haematological disease includes myeloproliferative disorders, where there is clonal expansion (lots of the same cells), and myelodysplastic (the cells have altered morphology). In the vignette, lack of hepatosplenomegaly, lymphadenopathy or systemic features (fatigue, night sweats, weight loss) make clonal disorders unlikely. Platelet disorders/von Willebrand disease (vWD) tend to cause mucosal bleeding, such as epistaxis, menorrhagia or easy bruising. Bleeding into joints and within muscles, as in the vignette, occurs in haemophilia – of which type A is more common. Consider imaging to rule out fractures or brain haemorrhage.

REVISION TIPS

- **Inherited** (young patient, historic easy bruising) vs **Acquired** (scrutinise meds and PMHx) vs **Malignancy**
- Massive splenomegaly; CML and PMF. Lymphadenopathy; CLL
- Deranged clotting in a paediatric patient – haemophilia likely
- WCC markedly raised; infection, acute leukaemias (or low; pancytopenia)
- Platelets low and patient unwell; DIC

90

Fever

Lucy Andrews, Alex Carrie, and Sian Maguire

GP CONSULTATION, FEMALE, 18. FATIGUE AND NIGHT SWEATS

HPC: Feeling tired recently, too exhausted to play usual sports. Past 3 weeks waking at night covered in sweat, having to change pyjamas. Weight loss, fevers. **PMHx:** Previous glandular fever. **DHx:** COCP. **FHx:** None.

O/E: BMI 21, general pallor, apyrexial. **CVS:** HR 85, BP 115/20, HS I + II + 0. **Resp:** Chest clear, bilateral cervical lymphadenopathy. **Abdomen:** SNT, bowel sounds present. **Neuro:** No focal neurology.

1. What is the most likely diagnosis for the patient described in the vignette?
2. Describe immediate treatment for a patient who presents with a cough producing white sputum, shortness of breath, HR 110, BP 80/30, sats 88% on air and temperature 38.7°C.
3. What would be the most likely differential if the patient lived in a house share and had a productive cough with haemoptysis and night sweats; how would you treat it?

Answers: 1. Hodgkin lymphoma. 2. Sepsis six = take cultures, lactate, urine output, give fluids, O_2 and broad-spectrum antibiotics. 3. Tuberculosis; 4 months of rifampicin, isoniazid, pyrazinamide and ethambutol, 2 further months of rifampicin and isoniazid.

TABLE 90.1

	Features	Investigations	Management
Infection – general	**RFs:** exposure to infective contacts, immunocompromised. **Hx & O/E:** *Respiratory:* cough, SOB, sputum, coryza. *Urinary:* dysuria, frequency, flank pain. *GI:* change in bowel habit, vomiting, abdominal pain. *CNS:* neck stiffness, rash, headache, confusion, reduced GCS. *Skin:* ulcers, erythema, wounds.	FBC (↑WCC), ↑ CRP. **Blood cultures** to isolate microorganism. **Further investigations** based on focal findings/ suspected source, e.g. urine MC&S, chest x-ray, swabs	Treat according to local antibiotic/anti-infective guidelines. Consider culture sensitivities. Admission; septic (Sepsis 6), haemodynamically unstable, deterioration
Infection – HIV	See *91. LYMPHADENOPATHY*		
Infection – TB	See *95. HAEMOPTYSIS*		

(Continued)

TABLE 90.1 (Cont'd)

	Features	Investigations	Management
Malignancy	**RFs:** FHx, previous cancer, occupational exposures, lifestyle (e.g. smoking). **Hx & O/E:** night sweats, weight loss, fatigue, reduced appetite, lymphadenopathy, localising features, e.g. change in bowel habit	FBC (anaemia, ± deranged white cells if haematological), tumour markers e.g. CA19-9. **Imaging**, e.g. CT TAP to look for mass and metastases. System-specific investigations, e.g. colonoscopy, lymph node biopsy, mammogram	Usually surgery/chemotherapy/radiotherapy with MDT involvement. Potentially active surveillance, or palliation

OTHER CAUSES OF FEVER

		Investigations	Management
Surgery	*Malignant hyperthermia* **RF:** certain anaesthetic agents (suxamethonium, volatile gases), FHx. **Hx & O/E:** muscle stiffness, fever, CO_2 rising	Often no time for investigations. **Lactate ↑, CO_2↑, Sats ↓**	**Dantrolene**, reversal agent needed ASAP, stop triggering agent. Oxygen, IVI
	After surgery – post-op fever **RF:** recent surgery. Wide range of causes, e.g. pneumonia, DVT/PE, wound infection, UTI, transfusion reaction, sinusitis	Low NEWS score. Bloods, imaging, cultures	Anti-pyrexials, e.g. **paracetamol.** Identify and treat cause (Table 90.2)

TABLE 90.2 A Timeline of Typical Causes of Post-operative Pyrexia

Day 0–2	3–5	5–7	Day >7
Physiological, tissue injury response (mild)	Pneumonia	DVT	Abdominal collection
Atelectasis	UTI	Anastomotic leak	DVT
Blood transfusion		Wound infection	

Adapted with permission S Thomasset. Postoperative care and complications. *Principles and Practice of Surgery*, 8 edition, 11, 140–147.

Two main causes of fever are infection and malignancy. Infection is typically more acute and often presents with system-specific symptoms. Use the risk factors, symptoms and examination findings to determine the focus of infection and investigate this system to decide on treatment. Clinically unwell patients (hypotensive, tachycardic) may need admitting for Sepsis 6 initial management. Fever may also be associated with haematological malignancy, as in the vignette. Look out for risk factors; for example, Hodgkin lymphoma typically presents with B-symptoms (weight loss, fever, night sweats – see Revision Tips) in younger patients, and is associated with EBV virus, which also causes glandular fever.

REVISION TIPS

- In the history, ask about travel, infective contacts, exposures/triggers (e.g. meals out)
- Pyridoxine should be prescribed to TB patients taking isoniazid to reduce risk of peripheral neuropathy
- For a child with fever, ask about vaccination history and check the NICE traffic light system
- The Ann Arbor staging of lymphomas includes a number (I–IV) and a letter (A or B). 'A' means absence of systemic symptoms, 'B' indicates their presence

91

Lymphadenopathy

Katherine Parker, Alexander Royston, and Julia Wolf

GP CONSULTATION, FEMALE, 50.
BILATERAL CERVICAL LYMPHADENOPATHY

HPC: She also reports 2 months of increasing fatigue, night sweats and weight loss. Night sweats are drenching and she sometimes feels sweaty during the day. She noticed painless swellings on her neck 10 days ago which are increasing in size. No cough or shortness of breath. Periods regular. **SHx:** No travel abroad.

O/E: Cachectic and pale. Afebrile. Neck: Left-sided 1.5 cm mass, right-sided 3 cm mass consistent with cervical lymphadenopathy. Axillary/inguinal lymphadenopathy. Abdomen: non-tender splenomegaly.

1. What are the management options for Non-Hodgkin lymphoma (NHL)?
2. Which autoimmune diseases can cause lymphadenopathy?

Answers: 1. Active monitoring, chemotherapy, radiotherapy: dependent on sub-type (see Tables 91.1). 2. Sjögren disease, rheumatoid arthritis, Still's disease, SLE, dermatomyositis.

TABLE 91.1

	Features	Investigations	Management
INFECTIOUS			
Reactive lymphadenopathy	See *60. NECK LUMP*		
Tuberculosis	See *95. HAEMOPTYSIS*		
HIV seroconversion illness	**RFs:** IVDU, unprotected sex (receptive anal/vaginal), MSM, needle stick injury, vertical transmission, concurrent STIs.	Pre-test counselling⟶ **HIV antibodies** (ELISA) – 3 months after exposure.	Referral to specialist services. Anti-retroviral therapy.
	Hx & O/E: axillary, cervical, occipital lymphadenopathy. 10 days to 6 weeks following exposure; pharyngitis, fever, maculopapular rash, malaise, arthralgia, myalgia, oral/genital/perianal ulcers	**HIV viral RNA** (serum viral load)/rapid test. Western blot confirmation/repeat test. Sexual health screen. Recurrent/atypical infections, e.g. *Pneumocystis jirovecii* pneumonia, TB	Monitoring; CD4 count/viral load. Education. Prevention; pre- or post-exposure prophylaxis
Epstein Barr virus/glandular fever	See *28. SORE THROAT*		

TABLE 91.1 (Cont'd)

	Features	Investigations	Management
Other infections	CMV, adenovirus, hepatitis, herpes zoster virus; syphilis, lymphogranuloma venereum (*Chlamydia trachomatis*), typhoid; leishmaniasis, Chagas disease, toxoplasmosis, Lyme disease		
HAEMATOLOGICAL Non-Hodgkin lymphoma	**RFs:** ↑Incidence with age, M > F, ethnicity, immunodeficiency (HIV), viral (EBV/HTLV/HCV), bacterial (*H. pylori* ⟶ MALToma). **Hx & O/E:** B symptoms, lymphadenopathy (painless, rubbery), hepato-splenomegaly. Onset dependent on grade (high-rapid, low-slow)	FBC (variable), ↑↑LDH. **LN biopsy** (ideally excisional): diagnostic. **PET CT** staging: Ann Arbor. **CTCAP + neck:** staging	Varies according to subtype; active monitoring, chemotherapy, radiotherapy
Hodgkin lymphoma	**RFs:** age (young adult), EBV. **Hx & O/E:** B symptoms; fevers/ fatigue/night sweats/weight loss. Lymphadenopathy (painless, rubbery, mobile) ± mediastinal mass, hepatosplenomegaly, pruritis. Alcohol-induced LN pain (rare, but characteristic)	FBC (↓Hb, ↑WCC), ↑LDH. **LN biopsy:** Reed-Sternberg cells (Fig. 91.1). **PET CT** staging: Ann Arbor	Combination chemotherapy. ±Radiotherapy (stage-dependent). Consider fertility preservation. High cure rates
Chronic lymphocytic leukaemia	See *89. BRUISING*		
OTHER Non-haematological malignancy	**RFs:** age, PMHx cancer. **Hx & O/E:** weight loss, night sweats, anorexia, fatigue, unilateral progressive swelling of single/ multiple draining LNs (may be matted/firm/fixed)	FBC (↓Hb), markers. **Biopsy:** histology. **Imaging/endoscopy.** Left sided supraclavicular (Virchow's): gastric/lung. Cervical: head/neck. Axillary: breast	Referral to appropriate MDT
Kawasaki disease (mucocutaneous lymph node syndrome)	**Hx & O/E:** fever (>5 days), bilateral non-exudative conjunctivitis, cervical lymphadenopathy, pharyngeal injection, dry lips, strawberry tongue, polymorphous rash, arthralgia, hand/ feet swelling ± skin desquamation	**RFs:** age (1–5 yo). FBC (↑platelets), ↑ESR, ↑CRP, ↑ α1-antitrypsin. **Echocardiogram.** **MR angio** (coronary artery aneurysms)	Aspirin + IV Ig. **Definitive:** ±further Ig/ prednisolone (if ineffective)

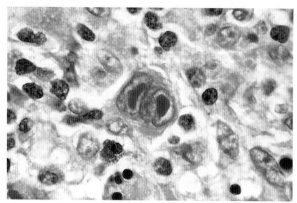

Fig. 91.1 Classic binucleate Reed-Sternberg cell. Each nucleus contains a prominent nucleolus surrounded by a halo. (From Schnitzer B. Hodgkin lymphoma. *Hematol/Oncol Clin N Am.* 2009;23(4):747–768. Copyright © 2009 Elsevier Inc.)

The most likely diagnosis in the vignette is high-grade lymphoma, implied by fatigue, extensive painless cervical lymphadenopathy (which has progressed relatively rapidly) and her night sweats. TB should be in the differential diagnosis, but she lacks a convincing exposure, she is not reporting respiratory symptoms, and lymphadenopathy would typically be slower growing. She also displays non-tender splenomegaly, which can point towards haematological malignancy. Blood results may show anaemia, lymphocytosis or leucopenia (all poor prognostic markers) and will classically demonstrate raised LDH. The diagnostic test is an excisional lymph node biopsy.

92

Organomegaly

Tejas Netke, Alexander Royston, and Julia Wolf

GP CONSULTATION, MALE, 79. FATIGUE, EARLY SATIETY AND REDUCED APPETITE

HPC: Weight loss. Changing his clothes and bedsheets due to sweats, feels feverish on waking. **PMHx:** Type 2 diabetes, hypertension, GORD. **SHx:** Never smoked; occasional alcohol.

O/E: Comfortable, stable obs. Conjunctival pallor. Abdomen soft non-tender, obvious splenomegaly.

1. What is the management of CML? Prognosis?
2. What is the translocation involved in CML?
3. Auer rods are characteristic of which condition?

Answers: 1. Tyrosine kinase inhibitors (Imatinib). If optimum response is achieved, patients have a similar life expectancy to the general population. 2. Philadelphia chromosome: reciprocal translocation of BCR-ABL genetic material between chromosomes 9/22. 3. Auer rods are accumulations of granules seen inside blasts in AML.

TABLE 92.1

		Features	Investigations	Management
HAEMATOLOGICAL				
Acute leukaemia	Acute myeloid leukaemia	Bone marrow failure: anaemia (pallor/SOB/dizziness), thrombocytopaenia, recurrent infections/fevers. Gum infiltration (subtype-specific), leukostasis symptoms (if ↑↑WCC: dyspnoea/hypoxia). ± hepatosplenomegaly, ± lymphadenopathy	**RFs:** age, smoking, benzene, chemotherapy, radiation, genetics, Down's syndrome, FHx, PMHx: PRV/ET/myelofibrosis. **Bloods:** ↓Hb/Plts, ↑↑WCC), LFTs, U+Es, clotting (incl fibrinogen), LDH. **Blood film:** immature granular myeloblasts (Auer rods). **Bone marrow biopsy:** >20% blasts: definitive	Combination chemotherapy. Supportive: transfusions/antibiotics as required. **Definitive:** allogenic stem cell transplant (if required)
	Acute lympho-blastic leukaemia	**RFs:** age (<5 yo, older patients), Down syndrome, PMHx of malignancy, radiation exposure, smoking. Presentation as per AML	FBC (↓Hb/Plts, ↑↑WCC: leucocytosis but neutropenia), LFTs, U+Es, clotting, LDH. **Blood film:** lymphoblasts. **Bone marrow biopsy:** >20% blasts	Combination chemotherapy. **Definitive:** add tyrosine kinase inhibitor (Philadelphia chromosome positive). Consider stem cell transplant/CAR-T

(Continued)

TABLE 92.1 (Cont'd)

		Features	Investigations	Management
Chronic leukaemia	Chronic myeloid leukaemia	**RFs:** age (median 57 yo), radiation, sex (M > F). **Hx & O/E:** massive splenomegaly, constitutional symptoms (weight loss, ↓appetite, night sweats), bone marrow failure (pallor, bruising). 50% incidental diagnosis	↓Hb, ↑Plts/WCC, LFTs, U&Es, clotting, LDH. **Blood film:** mature myeloid cells/basophils/ eosinophils. **Bone marrow biopsy:** disease phase/degree of fibrosis. **Cytogenetics:** Philadelphia chromosome t(9,22)-BCR-ABL fusion gene	Tyrosine kinase inhibitors, imatinib (oral OD)
	Chronic lymphocytic leukaemia	See *89. BRUISING*		
Lymphoma	Hodgkin's	See *91. LYMPHADENOPATHY*		
	Non-Hodgkin's	Fig. 92.1. See *91. LYMPHADENOPATHY*		
Myelofibrosis		Chronic progressive myeloproliferative disorder. **RFs:** age, genetics (JAK2/CALR/MPL), haematological disorders, chemicals, radiation. **Hx & O/E:** constitutional symptoms (weight loss/↓appetite/night sweats/recurrent fevers), massive splenomegaly	FBC (cytopaenias), LFTs, U&Es, clotting, LDH. **Blood film:** tear drop shaped RBCs. **Bone marrow aspirate:** definitive. Often 'dry tap' (fibrosis). **Cytogenetics:** risk scores, JAK2 +ve (60%)	Risk score guides management: (D)IPSS = (Diagnostic) International Prognostic Scoring System. Supportive measures. Transfusions. Ruxolitinib (JAK2 inhibitor). Allogeneic stem cell transplant (potentially curative: high risk)

INFECTION

Malaria		See *54. BITES AND STINGS* and *98. TRAVELLING ADVICE*		
Glandular fever/EBV		See *28. SORE THROAT*		

COMMON, NON-HAEMATOLOGICAL

Liver cirrhosis		See *83. ASCITES*		
Heart failure		See *8. PERIPHERAL OEDEMA AND ANKLE SWELLING*		

AUTOIMMUNE

Felty's syndrome		Rheumatoid arthritis + splenomegaly + neutropenia	↓Neutrophils <2 × 10^9/L. Blood film: exclude haematological causes of neutropenia	1st line: methotrexate (+ folic acid). 2nd line: rituximab

OTHER

Haemolytic anaemias; hereditary spherocytosis, sickle cell anaemia (splenomegaly: childhood only), thalassaemia.
Solid neoplasms and cysts.
Connective tissue disorders; SLE, RA.
Infiltrative disorders; amyloidosis, sarcoidosis.
Gaucher disease

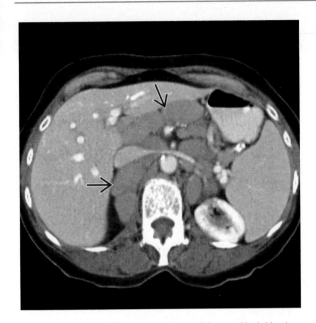

Fig. 92.1 Axial CECT in a patient with non-Hodgkin lymphoma shows splenomegaly and extensive lymphadenopathy (→). (Reproduced with permission from Federle MP, Lau JN. Splenomegaly and hypersplenism. In: *Imaging in Abdominal Surgery*. 316–317. Copyright © 2018 Elsevier Inc. All rights reserved.)

It is unusual to present directly with splenomegaly (or complaints related to it), and additional symptoms are likely to depend on the underlying cause. Mild splenomegaly can be caused by portal hypertension, autoimmune causes and some infections but, as the patient in the vignette is symptomatic, he likely has massive splenomegaly. A cardinal symptom of splenomegaly is early satiety, as the stomach is physically compressed. Massive splenomegaly is caused by myeloproliferative neoplasm (such as CML or primary myelofibrosis), tropical infections (malaria or leishmaniasis), or Gaucher's disease (Glycogen storage disorder). Considering this patient's other symptoms, a haematological malignancy is most likely. A specific diagnosis can only be made after further investigation with blood film and bone marrow biopsy.

REVISION TIPS

- Myelofibrosis: teardrop-shaped RBCs
- Fibrosis can develop secondary to polycythaemia rubra vera (PRV): can also be associated with infection, autoimmune disorder, chronic inflammatory disorder
- CML: typically, triphasic course – progresses from a chronic phase to accelerated phase to blast crisis. Usually diagnosed in chronic phase

93

Neck Pain/Stiffness

Meijia Xie, Alexander Royston, and Eleanor Courtney

HPC: Started feeling unwell the previous night. Intense, widespread headache, vomited several times. Starting to develop a stiff neck with myalgia/arthralgia and occasional rigors. **PMHx:** Physically fit.

O/E: HR 92 bpm, BP 110/76, T 38.9°C. Appears unwell: irritable, subconjunctival haemorrhage, dislikes light on pupillary testing; Brudzinski's/Kernig's sign inconclusive. Patient notes a new rash on upper limb; non-blanching, petechial.

1. What are the likely CSF findings for this case?
2. What is Waterhouse-Friderichsen syndrome?
3. 50-year-old male with sudden, severe headache, neck stiffness, photophobia and vomiting. PMH: CKD stage 4, PCKD. What is the appropriate investigation and expected result?
4. 25-year-old female with trismus, neck stiffness, headache and fever. Her back is arched with neck extended back. What is the likely diagnosis?

Answers: 1. Raised opening pressure, turbid appearance, >1g/L protein (high), <2.2mmol/L glucose (low), glucose serum: CSF ratio <0.4 (low), WCC >500 (high), Gram stain 60%–90% bacteria, 90% PMNs. 2. Adrenal infarction: complication of bacterial meningitis, leading to adrenal insufficiency. 3. SAH, likely due to berry aneurysm (RF: PCKD). Ix: CT head (non-contrast): acute bleed (bright). If CT is negative but history suggests SAH, consider LP at 12 hours (xanthochromia). 4. Tetanus: *Clostridium tetani* from soil-contaminated wound (puncture wounds in the garden, farming tools) – patient might not notice the wound. Management is supportive (wound care, analgesia, muscle relaxants, antibiotics).

TABLE 93.1

	Features	Investigations	Management
Infection			
Bacterial meningococcal meningitis ± septicaemia	**RFs:** close living, infectious contact, travel, birth defects, head trauma, immunocompromise, unvaccinated, hyposplenism, cochlear implant. **Hx & O/E:** fever, non-blanching rash (Fig. 93.1), (petechial→purpuric), N&V, septic shock. Meningism; neck stiffness, photophobia, headache, seizures/focal neurology. Kernig's sign: when leg/knee straightened→neck bends. Brudzinski's sign: passive neck flexion →knees bend. Infants: lethargy, irritation, bulging fontanelle	**Bloods:** FBC, ↑CRP, clotting, CBG, VBG (↑lactate). Blood cultures (BUT DO NOT DELAY Abx). **Lumbar puncture:** cloudy/purulent CSF, ↑↑WCC/neutrophils, ↑Protein, ↓Glucose. Contraindications to LP: any signs of ↑ICP, focal neurology, DIC	Initial (in community) IM benzylpenicillin/ cefotaxime. **Definitive:** sepsis 6, A→E, IV antibiotics (ceftriaxone). IVI: treat shock. Dexamethasone (if age >3 months: strong suspicion). **Notifiable:** contact prophylaxis. Complications; seizures, paralysis, hearing loss

TABLE 93.1 (Cont'd)

	Features	Investigations	Management
Viral meningitis	More common, less severe than bacterial. **RFs**: age (extremes <5, elderly), immunocompromised, enterovirus/VZV/mumps/CMV/HIV. **Presentation** (c/w bacterial): headache, less severe meningism. Can present with seizures	**Lumbar puncture**: ↑WCC/lymphocyte predominant. Mildly ↑protein, ↔Glucose, viral PCR	Do NOT delay IV Abx (for bacterial meningitis) if waiting for LP. Once LP confirms viral, supportive (self-limiting ≤2 weeks). Encephalitis suspected: (focal neurology, altered behaviour, ↓GCS, confusion) → IV acyclovir
Non-infective Torticollis	**RFs** (Acute): age 15–30, idiopathic, genetic, trauma. Also; antipsychotic extrapyramidal side effects. **Hx & O/E**: neck spasm, stiffness, sudden pain (on waking up), unable to move head, flexed away from pain	Clinical diagnosis, avoid cervical imaging	Conservative: heat, analgesia. Muscle relaxant, benzodiazepine. **Definitive**: botulinum, surgery, deep brain stimulation
Acute neck trauma 'Whiplash'	Abrupt flexion/hyper-extension on deceleration/rear-end impact. Neck pain, stiffness, spasm		Encourage early mobilisation. Resting carries worse prognosis → disuse syndrome
Cervical spondylosis ± disc prolapse Myelopathy	Age-related degeneration of cervical vertebrae; pain, stiffness. Postero-lateral disc protrusion: pain radiates→arm, muscle weakness, ↓fine motor/balance. Myelopathy: UMN signs (hyper-reflexia), imbalance, numbness, loss of dexterity, falls ± incontinence	**MRI neck**: suspicion of prolapse/myelopathy	Analgesia, physiotherapy, neck collar. **Definitive**: myelopathy→ surgical decompression
Subarachnoid haemorrhage	See *049. HEAD INJURY*		

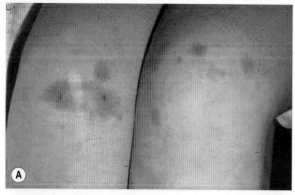

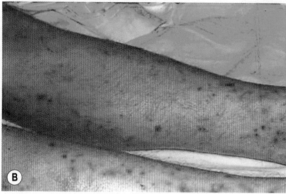

Fig. 93.1 Macular (A) and petechial (B) rashes of meningococcal bacteraemia. (Reproduced with permission from Stephens, DS. Neisseria Meningitidis Infections. In: *Goldman-Cecil Medicine*, 26th ed. Copyright © 2020 by Elsevier, Inc. All rights reserved.)

The vignette describes a relatively clear presentation of bacterial meningitis: starting with non-specific symptoms (fever/headache), progressing to features suggestive of bacterial meningitis. Key bacteria; strep. pneumoniae (gram +ve (G+) cocci), Haemophilus influenzae/ E. coli (gram -ve (G-) rods), N. meningitidis (G- cocci), Listeria monocytogenes (G+ rods-neonates), Strep. agalactiae (G+ cocci- neonates). TB (Acid-fast or fluorescent antibody stain). Note that the meningism was a relatively subtle and late sign, only becoming evident once the peripheral signs of septicaemia were established. Muscular aches are common in those that do frequent exercise, and a normal fitness-related bradycardia can mask some cardiovascular signs from the systemic inflammatory response. A severe headache in this age group prompts thoughts of SAH, but the character of the headache and petechial rash make meningococcal disease more likely. In younger children it may initially resemble acute otitis media, but in this older age group that is far less likely. The differential is narrow in this case, but early recognition is important and prompt treatment with immediate benzylpenicillin and admission is critical.

REVISION TIPS

- Classic meningitis triad: fever, neck stiffness, and altered mental status only present in 27% of meningococcal meningitis cases. More common (58%) in pneumococcal meningitis
- Non-specific complaints common to many self-limiting viral illnesses may be the earliest clinical symptoms (fever, headache, loss of appetite, nausea, vomiting, sore throat and coryza)
- Leg pain is a worrying sign and may be the herald to sepsis, before cold extremities/skin mottling

94

Jaundice

Emily Warren, Dylan Thiarya, and Ann Archer

EMERGENCY DEPARTMENT, MALE 14. 1-DAY HISTORY OF JAUNDICE

HPC: Sent home from school with jaundice and upper abdo pain. Feeling unwell for a few days with a sore throat, headache, fatigue. No regular medications, otherwise healthy.

O/E: Jaundice of eyes and skin. Abdomen is soft, tender RUQ, hepatosplenomegaly. BP 105/82, HR 94, RR 18, temperature 37.6°C. **Ix:** Hb 11.8, WCC 13.1, Platelets 84, Total bilirubin 64, ALP 201, AST 460, ALT 525.

1. What is the difference between jaundice and hyperbilirubinaemia?
2. At what concentration does hyperbilirubinaemia present as jaundice?
3. How might a patient with hepatic encephalopathy present?

Answers: 1. Jaundice is the clinical manifestation of hyperbilirubinaemia, causing yellowing of skin and sclera. Hyperbilirubinaemia is a high concentration of circulating bilirubin. 2. Once bilirubin levels reach >35 µmol/L jaundice may become evident. 3. Mood changes, confusion, mental state changes and sleep disturbance. On examination one may elicit asterixis, clonus or hyperreflexia; along with stigmata of liver disease.

TABLE 94.1

	Features	Investigations	Management
PRE-HEPATIC			
Haemolytic anaemias	See *87. PALLOR*		
HEPATIC			
Paracetamol overdose	See *52. OVERDOSE*		
EBV	See *28. SORE THROAT*		
Hepatitis A	Faecal-oral transmission. Hx & O/E: fever, abdo pain, malaise, jaundice. Adults often symptomatic, child usually asymptomatic	IgM anti-Hep A serology. Elevated LFTs. NOT usually associated with chronic liver disease	Prevention; careful food/water hygiene and immunisation; 2 injections (20 years protection). Treatment: supportive care

(Continued)

TABLE 94.1 (Cont'd)

	Features	Investigations	Management
Hepatitis B	Most common liver infection worldwide. **RFs:** endemic exposure, IVDU, high-risk sexual encounters. Can result in cirrhosis and hepatocellular carcinoma	LFTs raised (low albumin). Surface antigen (HBsAg) and antibody (HBsAb). Core antigen; IgM anti-HBc in acute infection. IgG in chronic infection	Prevention; hepatitis B can be a combined vaccine with hepatitis A. Supportive, anti-virals. Liver transplant may be needed in decompensated cirrhosis
Hepatitis C	Contact with infected blood. Half become chronic. No effective vaccine or postexposure prophylaxis	Serum anti-HCV; a single reactive test does not distinguish acute from chronic or resolved infection. Also test for HBV/HIV	Antivirals; note HBV reactivation may occur. HCV-negative but recently exposed (e.g. needlestick) should be reassessed at 4–6 weeks (HCV-RNA), or 4–6 months (anti-HCV, ALT)
Budd-Chiari syndrome	See *83. ASCITES*		
POST-HEPATIC Cholangitis	See *67. ACUTE ABDOMINAL PAIN*		
Choledocholithiasis	See *67. ACUTE ABDOMINAL PAIN*		

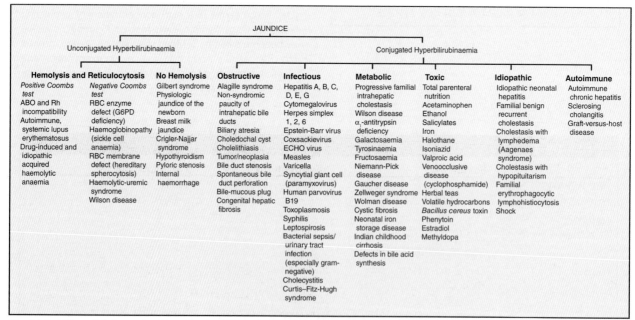

Fig. 94.1 Differential diagnosis of jaundice in childhood. (Marcdante KJ, Robert MK, Abigail MS. Liver disease. In: *Nelson Essentials of Pediatrics.* Elsevier; 2023. Copyright © 2023 Elsevier Inc. All rights reserved.)

The vignette is a case of jaundice secondary to EBV. Usually presenting in young people with general malaise and upper respiratory tract infection symptoms – including a sore throat and fever. Hepatic involvement in EBV infection can elevate alkaline phosphatase/ AST/ bilirubin, peaking 5–14 days after onset, and mostly normal within 3 months. GGT peaks at 1–3 weeks and can be mildly elevated for up to a year. EBV can cause an acute hepatitis with splenomegaly leading to thrombocytopenia and abdominal pain. An atypical/reactive lymphocytosis may be seen on the FBC/blood film. Figure 94.1 describes causes of jaundice in childhood.

REVISION TIPS

- Liver dysfunction contributes to bleeding due to lower platelets and defective clotting factor synthesis
- Painless jaundice is an ominous presenting complaint – see *69. CHANGE IN STOOL COLOUR*
- Jaundice may first be seen in the sclera; always check
- Other important causes of jaundice include: HELLP syndrome, alcoholic liver disease and viral hepatitis
- Minimising blood-borne hepatitis virus transmission; avoid high-risk behaviour, precautions by health care workers, sterilisation of medical equipment

95

Haemoptysis

Tejas Netke, Gregory Oxenham, and Aldoph Nanguzgambo

GP CONSULTATION, FEMALE, 33.
PRODUCTIVE COUGH FOR 6 WEEKS, WITH SPECKS OF BLOOD

HPC: Constant fatigue, worsening dyspnoea, recurrent fevers and night sweats. She has gone down two dress sizes, reduced appetite. No chest pain, wheeze or rashes. **SHx:** Lives with partner, works for the Red Cross, recently returned from a refugee camp in Turkey. Non-smoker. **PMHx/DHx:** nil.

O/E: Pale, cachexic. Slightly tachypnoeic at rest, sats 94–95%. Equal chest expansion, chest clear on auscultation. Cervical lymph nodes non-tender, slightly enlarged bilaterally. **Ix:** Hb 105 g/dL, WCC 30 × 10⁹/L, CRP 27 mg/L and platelets 300 × 10⁹/L. Urine dip negative for RBCs.

1. Why do intravenous drug users (IVDU) have a higher risk of lung abscesses?
2. What are the main side effects of the RIPE drugs?

Answers: 1. Repeated non-sterile IV injection risks bacteraemia and consequent seeding of infection; right-sided endocarditis delivers septic emboli directly to the lung. 2. Rifampicin – <u>R</u>ed/orange urine; Isoniazid – peripheral neuropathy; Pyrazinamide – hyperuricaemia (gout); Ethambutol – <u>E</u>yes (decreased visual acuity).

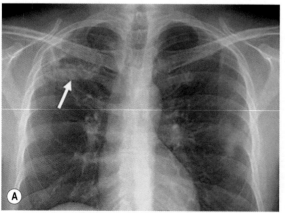
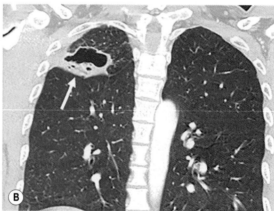

Fig. 95.1 CXR and coronal CT images showing cavitation in a patient with active TB. A) CXR, B) CT. (Reproduced with permission from Restrepo CS, Katre R, Mumbower A. *Radiol Clin N Am.* May 2016; Fig. 9. Elsevier. © 2016 Elsevier Inc. All rights reserved.)

TABLE 95.1

	Features	Investigations	Management
RESPIRATORY			
Lung cancer	See *185. COUGH*		
Pneumonia	See *40. BREATHLESSNESS*		
Active pulmonary TB	**RFs:** environmental exposure, crowded accommodation, travel to area with endemic TB, immunosuppression, HIV, DM, ESRF, solid organ transplant, malignancy. **Hx & O/E:** cough (>4 weeks), fever/weight loss/anorexia/malaise. Extrapulmonary/miliary TB: lymph-adenopathy, bone/joint pain, spinal TB (Pott's disease), abdo/pelvic pain, sterile pyuria (renal TB), meningism, skin lesions (erythema nodosum, lupus vulgaris)	**CXR:** (Fig. 95.1) Primary: Ghon focus/hilar lymphadenopathy. Secondary: reactivated apical lesion. Miliary: 'bird seed'. **Sputum culture:** (gold standard): 4–8 weeks to grow. Ziehl-Neelsen stain (× 3). **Sputum smear of three samples:** stain for acid-fast bacilli or NAAT (can also identify rifampicin resistance). **USS:** LN/FNAC (culture positive). Screening: Mantoux test. Interferon-Gamma Release Assay (QuantiFERON®-TB)	Notifiable disease. Contact tracing. Direct observed therapy: primary antibiotic regimen = RIPE. All 4 drugs for 2 months, then rifampicin/isoniazid 4 months more. Pyridoxine (Vit B6) for those on isoniazid with high risk for neuropathy. Multi-drug-resistant TB: 18–24 months treatment with at least six drugs
Pulmonary Embolism	See *11. CHEST PAIN AND PAIN ON INSPIRATION*		
Bronchiectasis	See *185. COUGH*		
Lung abscess	**RFs:** necrotising pneumonia (*S. aureus*)/tumours, alcohol, aspiration, endocarditis, IVDU, immunosuppressed. **Hx & O/E:** weeks of swinging fever, foul purulent sputum, cough, pleuritic pain, haemoptysis, tachypnoea, clubbing, ± cachectic, poor dentition/infection, ± signs of endocarditis	↑WCC/CRP, ± ↑lactate. **Blood/sputum/BAL cultures.** **CXR:** cavity ± fluid level, may show consolidation/empyema. **Chest CT:** micro-emboli or obstructing bronchial mass. **Bronchoscopy**	**IV Abx:** (2–3 weeks). Can be discharged when stable for home IV Abx (supervised), followed by oral (4–8 weeks). Pulmonary physiotherapy. Treatment failure: bronchoscopic/CT guided drainage or surgical excision (high morbidity)
Fungal disease (Cavitatory pulmonary aspergillosis, Aspergilloma)	**RFs:** immunocompromised, post-TB. **Hx & O/E:** haemoptysis, chest pain, fever, weight loss	**CXR:** infiltrates. **CT:** upper lobe predominance, cavitation with mass inside. Bronchial arteriogram if significant haemoptysis	Embolisation of relevant bronchial artery in ongoing haemoptysis. Antifungal therapy. Surgical resection
CARDIOVASCULAR Mitral stenosis	**RFs:** Rheumatic fever (commonest), age, cardiovascular RFs. **Hx & O/E:** gradual (years) dyspnoea, fatigue, chest pain, haemoptysis, often AF ± embolic events. Mid-diastolic murmur with opening click heard loudest at the apex. Malar flush	**ECG:** may show AF, RAD and bifid P wave if in sinus. **Echo:** reduced valve size, increased pressure gradient, enlarged LA	**AF requires anticoagulation.** Asymptomatic; no treatment. Symptomatic; diuretics, digoxin, beta-blocker, CCB. Surgical valve replacement or balloon commissurotomy

(Continued)

TABLE 95.1   (Cont'd)

	Features	Investigations	Management
Anticoagulation/ antiplatelets	RFs: excessive cough, lung ca. Exclude bleeding from elsewhere, e.g. gum, nose, haematemesis	INR/clotting, FBC, urea, G&S/CM	If no other cause found for haemoptysis, consider stopping causative drug ± reversal agent
AUTOIMMUNE			
Anti-glomerular basement membrane disease (Goodpasture's)	Autoantibodies against Type 4 collagen – basement membrane in kidney/lung. Hx & O/E: SOB, cough, fatigue, change in urine output. Glomerulonephritis and haemoptysis/anaemia	**Urinalysis:** haematuria, proteinuria, RBC casts. **Renal function:** AKI. **CXR:** diffuse alveolar haemorrhage. **Renal biopsy:** For glomerular basement membrane ABs	Plasma exchange. Immunosuppression. Kidney transplantation
Vasculitis (e.g. granulomatosis with polyangiitis, microscopic polyangiitis)	Hx & O/E: haemoptysis, fever, fatigue, joint pain, VTE, renal impairment, skin lesions, nasal symptoms with crusting (including epistaxis), and other upper respiratory tract/ ear. Saddle-nose deformity	**Autoimmune blood screen. Renal function:** Impaired **Urine:** haematuria or proteinuria. **CXR/CT chest:** Patchy or diffuse ground glass opacities or granulomas. **Renal biopsy:** Necrotising glomerulonephritis. Skin/lung/ nasal biopsy	Cyclophosphamide, rituximab, steroids. Large pulmonary haemorrhage: ABCD May need intubation, ICU and bronchoscopy when stable. Consider plasma exchange

In the vignette there are haemoptysis, systemic symptoms (weight loss, loss of appetite, fevers, night sweats), long duration (>6 weeks) and recent relevant travel, so pulmonary TB is high on the differential. Her 'B-symptoms' and cervical lymphadenopathy should also make us consider lymphoma. Cases of TB tend to occur in bigger cities and in more economically deprived groups. More common causes for haemoptysis are lung cancer and pneumonia, but her young age and non-smoking history make primary lung cancer unlikely, and the duration of symptoms makes acute bacterial pneumonia unlikely. TB, once confirmed, is a notifiable disease and contact tracing should be done. Sputum for AFB analysis is the investigation of choice, but with lymphoma being a differential, a biopsy of the cervical lymph nodes would be more informative, with samples sent for both microbiological and histological analysis.

REVISION TIPS

- Questions asking you to diagnose TB will likely include patient contact with high-risk groups – be aware of where TB is prevalent
- All RIPE drugs affect LFTs. Other side effects include; *Rifampicin*: thrombocytopaenia, yellow-orange colour (skin, saliva, urine, sweat, tears- soft contact lenses). Induces hepatic enzymes- affects metabolism of other drugs *Isoniazid*; N&V, peripheral neuropathy *Pyrazinamide*; arthralgia, dysuria, photosensitivity, sideroblastic anaemia *Ethambutol*; hyperuricaemia, optic neuritis, tubulo-interstitial nephritis, peripheral neuropathy

96

Viral Exanthems

Oliver Whitehurst and Matthew Ridd

GP CONSULTATION, FEMALE, AGE 6 YEARS. 2-DAY HISTORY OF RASH

HPC: 6 days of coryzal symptoms, fever, conjunctivitis. Rash began on face, then on body. Not itchy, no photophobia. **PMHx:** Nil. **DHx:** Nil. **FHx:** Nil. Parents did not engage with vaccination program. **SHx:** Lives at home, no pets.

O/E: Bilateral conjunctivitis, watery discharge. Erythematous macular rash on face, chest, back, abdomen, upper arms. Bright red spots with a bluish-white speck on buccal mucosa. Temperature: 38 degrees. **CVS:** HR 87, BP 110/70. **Abdomen:** Soft, non-tender. **Respiratory:** Rate 13 breaths/min, no added sounds.

1. Which of the viral exanthems are unlikely in a vaccinated child?
2. A child is febrile for 3 to 5 days, then suddenly becomes afebrile simultaneously developing a maculopapular rash; which of the viral exanthems is the most likely cause?

Answers: 1. Measles, rubella. 2. Roseola infantum.

TABLE 96.1

	Features	Investigations	Management
Measles (Rubeola) (Figs. 96.1 and 96.2)	**RF:** exposure with incomplete or no prior immunisation **Hx & O/E:** fever and conjunctivitis. Rash on face (starting behind the ears), then body, Koplik spots (buccal white spots). Complications (pregnancy, age <1, immune compromise); pneumonia, encephalitis, sepsis	Diagnosis: salivary swab or serum sample (IgM and IgG)	Self-limiting (resolves <1 week); analgesia, hydration. Immediately notify local health protection team. Self-Isolation: till at least 4 days after initial rash onset. Advise to seek support if complications (short of breath, severe fever, convulsions)
German measles (Rubella) (Fig. 96.3)	**RF:** exposure with incomplete or no prior immunisation. **Hx & O/E:** low-grade fever, maculopapular rash (face, then body), lymphadenopathy	Diagnosis: Rubella serology (IgM). FBC: occasionally thrombocytopenia	Non-pregnant: symptomatic management. Pregnant: referral (risk of foetal infection), intramuscular immunoglobulin

(Continued)

TABLE 96.1 (Cont'd)

	Features	Investigations	Management
Parvovirus B-19 (fifth disease, erythema infectiosum) (Fig. 96.4)	Low-grade fever. Hx & O/E: hot, firm rosy cheeks (2–5 days), then reticular rash on trunk, arms, and legs. Can be a trigger of aplastic anaemia in people with sickle cell anaemia, spherocytosis, or leukaemia	Clinical diagnosis: 'slapped cheek syndrome'. Consider parvovirus B-19 serology (IgM)	Non-pregnant: symptomatic, settles 1–2 weeks. Pregnant: referral (risk of miscarriage and hydrops foetalis)
Streptococci, including scarlet fever	Sandpaper rash: blotchy, rough macular rash, starts on trunk and spreads outwards. Strawberry tongue, sore throat, lymphadenopathy. *Streptococcus pyogenes*, so risk of glomerulonephritis or acute rheumatic fever	Diagnosis: clinical. Consider throat swab for group A streptococcus	Phenoxymethylpenicillin for 10 days. Immediately notify public health. Off school until 24 hours on antibiotics
Herpes virus type 6 (Roseola infantum or sixth disease)	Sudden high fever for 3–5 days, suddenly disappears. Can trigger febrile convulsions. Macular rash on arms, legs, trunk and face. Nagayama spots; blanching raised red lesions on soft palate/uvula	Diagnosis: clinical. Consider enzyme immunoassay or PCR	Symptomatic; analgesia, hydration No time off school needed
IMPORTANT DIFFERENTIALS			
Meningococcal meningitis	See *93. NECK PAIN/STIFFNESS*		
Mumps	Prodromal fever/malaise/headache, then parotid swelling and tenderness. Orchitis, oophoritis, deafness, meningitis, pancreatitis	Clinical diagnosis. Paramyxovirus RT-PCR or viral culture from saliva, urine or CSF	Symptomatic; analgesia, hydration
Kawasaki disease	See *91. LYMPHADENOPATHY*		

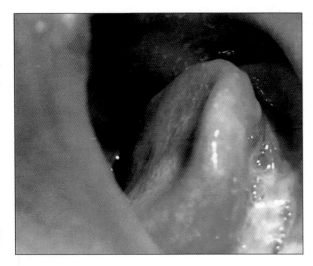

Fig. 96.1 Koplik spots. (Reproduced with permission from Xavier S, Forgie SED. Koplik spots revisited. *CMAJ*. 2015;187:600).

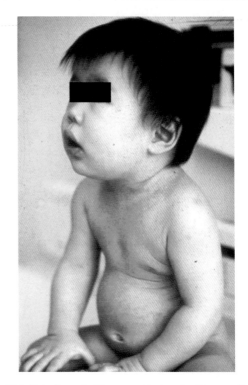

Fig. 96.3 Rubella rash. (Courtesy Centers for Disease Control and Prevention Public Health Image Library.)

Fig. 96.2 Measles rash. (From Ferri FF. *Ferri's Clinical Advisor*. 1st ed. St. Louis: Elsevier; 2019.)

Fig. 96.4 Slapped cheek syndrome (Parvovirus). (Reproduced with permission from Young NS. Parvovirus. In: Goldman L, Schafer AI, eds. *Goldman-Cecil Medicine*. 26th ed. Elsevier; 2019).

Viral exanthems describe rashes associated with a viral infection, generally preceded by a fever. Underlying pathology can range from fairly trivial to life-threatening. In exam questions there will often be key clues, such as poor compliance with the vaccination schedule. In the vignette, the history is typical for a virus, and the spots on the buccal mucosa are likely to be Koplik spots (Fig. 96.1), pathognomonic for measles. Despite being historically described as one of the viral exanthems, scarlet fever is caused by group A strep (Streptococcus pyogenes), so can be treated with antibiotics. 'Strawberry tongue' can be caused by Scarlet fever or Kawasaki disease, but also consider food allergy, glossitis, B12/folate deficiency or Staphylococcal toxic shock syndrome.

REVISION TIPS

- Pay close attention to the vaccination status of the patient
- Koplik spots on the buccal mucosa are unique to measles
- Kawasaki disease, think CRASH and Burn; Conjunctivitis, Rash, Adenopathy, Strawberry tongue, Hands (erythematous hands/feet which later peel), Burn (fever ≥5 days)

Vaccination – Outline

Max Shah, Alice Parker, and Peta Nixon

CHILDREN

TABLE 97.1

	Vaccination Given
8 weeks	6-in-1 (thigh): Diphtheria, tetanus, pertussis, polio, haemophilus influenza B (HiB), hepatitis B Meningococcal B (left thigh) Rotavirus (mouth)
12 weeks	6-in-1 (thigh) Rotavirus (thigh) Pneumococcal conjugate vaccine (PCV – 13 strains) (mouth)
16 weeks	6-in-1 (thigh) Meningococcal B (left thigh)
1 year	HiB/Men C (upper arm/thigh) PCV (mouth) Meningococcal B (left thigh) Measles, mumps and rubella (MMR) (upper arm/thigh)
Primary school age	Live attenuated influenza vaccine (nostrils)
3 years 4 months	4-in-1: Diphtheria, tetanus, pertussis and polio (upper arm) MMR (upper arm)
12–13 years (school year 8)	Human papillomavirus (HPV), 2 doses 6–24 months apart (upper arm)
14 years (school year 9)	3-in-1 booster: tetanus, diphtheria, polio (upper arm) Meningococcal ACWY (upper arm)

HPV vaccination Gardasil (HPV 6, 11, 16, 18) and Gardasil 9 (HPV types 6, 11, 16, 18, 31, 33, 45, 52 and 58) to protect against precancerous lesions/cancers in the cervix, vulva or vagina or anus; genital warts.

ADULTS

TABLE 97.2

	Vaccination Given
65 years	Pneumococcal polysaccharide vaccine (PPV – 23 strains) (upper arm)
65 years (then annually)	Inactivated influenza (upper arm)
70 years	Shingles (varicella-zoster) (upper arm)

Extra vaccinations for people with chronic medical conditions; annual influenza and PPV.

PREGNANT WOMEN

TABLE 97.3

	Vaccination Given
During flu season	Influenza
From 16 weeks pregnant	Whooping cough (pertussis)

Live Attenuated Vaccines

Part of normal schedule: Oral rotavirus, MMR, inhaled/intranasal influenza, Shingles (Zostavax)

Not part of normal schedule: BCG, yellow fever, oral typhoid, varicella/chickenpox

Live attenuated vaccines should not routinely be given to people who are clinically immunosuppressed (either due to drug treatment or underlying illness)

Travelling Advice

Mary Xie, Lucy Harrison, and Jon Dallimore

HPC: She asks for advice regarding malaria and general travel. Routine (UK) vaccinations are up-to-date. **PMHx:** Asthma, depression. **DHx:** Sertraline, COCP. **SHx:** Non-smoker, social drinker (10 units p/w).

1. What may you expect the total white cell count to be in a patient with typhoid? High/low/normal?
2. When would IgM anti-HbC be positive?
3. When should malaria prophylaxis be started and stopped?

Answers: 1. Hb, WCC and platelets low or normal. 2. In an acute infection. 3. Mefloquine should be given 2–3 weeks before until 4 weeks after travel. Doxycycline and Malarone started a few days before travel, and Malarone can be stopped after 1 week.

TABLE 98.1

	Features	Investigations	Management
Diarrhoea	Often bacteria in food/water, can be viral or parasites. Hx & O/E: diarrhoea, abdominal cramps. Self-limiting, usually 3–5 days	Travellers usually self-treat, seeking medical assistance if severe. 1st line Ix: stool culture and sensitivity	Hydration and symptom relief – Loperamide (up to 2 days). Abx only in severe cases. Chronically ill/immunocompromised, consider prophylaxis (rifaximin)
Malaria	Transmitted by bite of infected female Anopheles mosquito. Consider in patients with non-specific symptoms after travel. Hx & O/E: malaise, headache, backache, fever, rigors. Complications: hepatosplenomegaly, jaundice, anaemia, coma	**Serial thin and thick blood films.** Low Hb/platelets, prolonged PT. Lactate raised – severe. 6 days min. incubation. *Plasmodium falciparum* most common	Prophylaxis: start before travel, continue well after return. Treatment: consult latest UK malaria guidelines 2016; artemether/lumefantrine or Malarone. Quinine and doxycycline in severe cases. See also *54. BITES AND STINGS*

TABLE 98.1	(Cont'd)		
	Features	**Investigations**	**Management**
Typhoid	**Hx & O/E:** fever, abdominal pain, headache, anorexia, cough, diarrhoea/constipation. Fever with bradycardia (Faget sign)	Blood/stool culture or bone marrow biopsy. LFTs: mild derangement, transaminase 2–3x normal	Prevention: vaccine – protection lasts 3 years, only effective against one strain. Treatment: ceftriaxone OR cefixime AND azithromycin
Dengue fever	RNA virus, via mosquito bite, can be mild to life-threatening (dengue haemorrhagic fever). **Hx & O/E:** fever, rash, myalgia ('breakbone fever'), headache, arthralgia, pleuritic pain, bruising, hepatomegaly	Leukopenia, thrombocytopenia, elevated haematocrit (due to dehydration). LFTs raised. Serology and PCR positive for dengue virus	Prevention: bite avoidance (e.g. DEET) in endemic regions. Treatment: oral fluids, monitoring, symptom relief Severe: IV fluids, monitor blood parameters for severe haemorrhage, transfusion if necessary. *Notifiable disease*
Schistosomiasis	Trematode via skin exposure (e.g. lake with infected snails, commonly Lake Malawi). **Hx & O/E:** acute schistosomiasis/Katayama fever. Abdominal pain, haematuria, fever, hepato-splenomegaly, 'swimmer's itch' (Fig. 98.1)	Stool/urine microscopy: visualisation of eggs. Urinalysis: haematuria (acute or chronic). Normocytic, normochromic anaemia, eosinophilia (in acute infection). Antibody detection, PCR	Acute = corticosteroid + praziquantel. Chronic = praziquantel. Chronic infection, risk of bladder squamous cell carcinoma
Yellow fever	Infected mosquito bite. **Hx & O/E:** from mild febrile illness to haemorrhagic fever. Fever, Faget sign, jaundice	PCR and serology	Prevention: vaccine available. Now single lifetime vaccination. Treatment: supportive. *Notifiable disease*
Hepatitis A and B	See *94. JAUNDICE*		

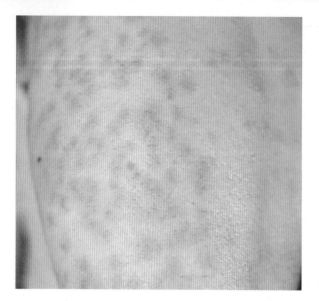

Fig. 98.1 Swimmer's itch – a rash developing soon after exposure to schistosomes. (From James, William D, Elston, Dirk M., Treat, James R., Rosenbach, Misha A., Neuhaus, Isaac M., Andrews' Diseases of the Skin. Published December 31, 2019. © 2020.

You should know which conditions can be immunised against, prevention methods (food hygiene, safe food/drink sources, e.g. checking bottle seals/using water purifying tablets, bite avoidance) and how each is spread. Faecal-oral transmission necessitates caution with ice,

shellfish/seafood, uncooked fruit and vegetables/salads unless washed with clean water. Hepatitis is not uncommon in the United Kingdom, and knowledge of the different types is often tested. Katayama fever may occur 2–12 weeks after non-immune individuals are exposed to Schistosoma or get heavy reinfection. The long incubation means there is risk of misdiagnosis. Symptoms are due to migrating schistosomula and egg deposition, leading to nocturnal fever, cough, myalgia, headache, and abdominal tenderness. E. coli tends to be the cause of bacterial diarrhoea (but diarrhoea will often be viral). Shigella and Campylobacter are the usual causes of bloody diarrhoea (dysentery). Loperamide may make the illness last longer and is contraindicated if there is bloody diarrhoea.

REVISION TIPS

- Vaccines to be considered; typhoid, hepatitis A/B, yellow fever, rabies, meningococcal meningitis, tetanus
- Prolonged febrile illness but normal WCC -> think typhoid
- Hepatitis surface antigen; HbSAg in acute infection, HbSAb in resolved infection or vaccinated
- Hepatitis core antigen; IgM anti-HbC in acute infection. IgG anti-HbC in chronic infection
- Low platelets are seen in malaria and dengue, but haemorrhagic complications are more common in dengue

99

Headache

Louise Mathias, Gregory Oxenham, Dafydd Morgan, and Hamish Morrison

GP CONSULTATION, FEMALE, 27. LEFT-SIDED HEADACHE

HPC: Her third gradual onset, unilateral, throbbing headache – one ED visit. 6-hour duration, with nausea, averse to light – she goes to lie down. Unaffected by position/coughing. No vomiting, no visual disturbance, no obvious trigger. Not relieved by analgesia taken regularly for back pain. Denies any fevers/weakness/sensation change/vision change. **PMHx:** Lower back pain. **DHx:** COCP, co-codamol, ibuprofen. **SHx:** Non-smoker, 18 units alcohol/week, unemployed.

O/E: Afebrile, BMI 35. No rashes, appears well. **Neuro:** CNs normal, no focal neurology, no neck stiffness, no papilloedema, no photo/phonophobia at present.

1. What considerations should be given regarding contraception in this woman?
2. Which migraine prophylaxis medication should be avoided in women of childbearing age?
3. What diagnosis should always be considered in patients presenting with headache aged >50?

Answers: 1. COCP is contraindicated in patients with migraine with aura due to risk of stroke. It is a relative contraindication in migraine without aura. POP and non-hormonal methods are safe to use. 2. Topiramate causes an increased risk of congenital malformations, especially in the first trimester. 3. Always consider temporal arteritis in people over 50 newly presenting with headache especially, in females.

TABLE 99.1

	Features	Investigations	Management
Tension type headache	**RFs:** stress, dehydration, disturbed sleep. Mild/moderate pain, 'band-like', lasts 30 minutes to 7 days	Clinical diagnosis. Normal neurological exam	Simple analgesia. Sleep hygiene, hydration, identify provoking factors
Migraine	CHOCOLATES Chocolate, Cheese, Hormones (COCP), Caffeine, alcohOL, Anxiety, Travel, Exercise, Sleep disturbance. **Hx & O/E:** pulsating, unilateral nature, generally consistent side. Aura – visual (flashes, scintillating scotomas – acuity normal), somatosensory, motor or speech. Photophobia	**Clinical diagnosis** Headache diary. **Diagnostic criteria for migraine without aura:** five headaches lasting between 4 and 72 hours with at least 2 of pulsating, unilateral, moderate or severe pain, aggravated by normal activities. Plus one of photophobia or N&V during attack	**Identification/avoidance of triggers** **Acute:** Simple analgesia, Aspirin 900 mg or Triptan (Sumatriptan 50–100 mg) **Prophylaxis** Propranolol, amitriptyline, topiramate (not if childbearing age) Withhold COCP in migraine with aura

(Continued)

TABLE 99.1   (Cont'd)

	Features	Investigations	Management
Medication overuse headache	Chronic painful conditions/ migraines. Mixed analgesia, especially with codeine	Clinical diagnosis	Withdraw analgesia to ≤6 days/month
Idiopathic intracranial hypertension	See *113. RAISED INTRACRANIAL PRESSURE*		
Cerebral venous sinus thrombosis	See *113. RAISED INTRACRANIAL PRESSURE*		
Meningo-encephalitis	See *93. NECK PAIN/STIFFNESS, 145. THE SICK CHILD*		
Trigeminal autonomic cephalgias (TAC); cluster headache, hemicrania continua, paroxysmal hemicrania and SUNCT/SUNA	**RFs:** FHx, male, 20–50 yo, smoking. Cluster headache by far most common **Hx & O/E:** intense periorbital pain with ipsilateral autonomic symptoms, ptosis, miosis. Occurs in clusters of weeks or months with periods of remission. Not triggered by innocuous stimuli (unlike trigeminal neuralgia)	Classified mainly on duration of symptoms. **Clinical diagnosis. MRI head** to exclude structural cause. (SUNCT or SUNA – Short-lasting, Unilateral, Neuralgiform headaches with Conjunctival injection and Tearing OR cranial Autonomic symptoms)	Dependant on specific TAC. **Cluster headache:** responds to high-dose oxygen, injectable triptans, May require verapamil for prevention. Hemicrania continua: indomethacin
Intracranial space occupying lesion	Headache worse first thing in morning. Early morning vomiting. Focal neurology: unexplained weakness or paraesthesia, progressive. Papilloedema, seizures, confusion, decreased consciousness (Table 99.2)	Neuroimaging, initially plain **CT head**	Neurosurgical referral. Dexamethasone to reduce oedema (liaise with neurosurgery)
OTHER IMPORTANT DIFFERENTIALS			
SAH	See *49. HEAD INJURY and Revision Tips*		
Giant cell arteritis	See *36. EYE PAIN & DISCOMFORT*		
Acute angle closure glaucoma	See *37. ACUTE CHANGE IN OR LOSS OF VISION*		

TABLE 99.2   Headache Red Flags

Headache Red Flags; SSNOOP4	S – Systemic Sx: fever/weight loss S – Secondary RFs (HIV, PKD, metastatic Ca) N – Neurology: confusion, papilloedema, focal deficits, neck stiffness, dysphasia O – Onset: sudden, 'thunderclap' O – Old age >50 yo (consider GCA) P – Previous headache history (new headache or worsening/changing pattern) P – Papilloedema, pulsatile tinnitus, precipitated by exercise P – Precipitated by Valsalva P – Postural aggravation

The most likely cause of the presentation in the vignette is migraine without aura. Characteristics features are recurrent headaches, lasting 4–72 hours, which are aggravated by activities, with associated nausea and/or vomiting, and photophobia and/or phonophobia. For a diagnosis of migraine without aura, five attacks are required with associated features. The lack of exacerbation by positional changes or Valsalva manoeuvres makes a space-occupying lesion unlikely, especially without focal neurological signs. Although she has risk factors for IIH (young, female, overweight), the absence of papilloedema would go against this diagnosis. Cluster headaches can present similarly to migraine, but the patient's attempts to sit still in a quiet room make the latter more likely. Cluster headaches are excruciating and patients tend to become restless during an attack.

REVISION TIPS

- Learn the red flag symptoms of headache – they are easily tested
- Consider all the structures in the head that could cause headache – pressure inside the skull, meninges, sinuses, eyes, blood vessels, muscles, skin, etc.
- *Ottawa SAH rule*; age $\geq$40, neck pain/stiffness, witnessed LOC, onset during exertion, thunderclap headache, limited neck flexion. If any apply, CT is indicated.

100

Fits/Seizures

Margarita Fox, Gregory Oxenham, and Matthew Smith

RECENTLY COME ROUND FROM LOSING CONSCIOUSNESS

HPC: Well, then suddenly 'must have passed out' – unable to provide further history. A friend witnessed him stiffen and fall backwards, hitting his head on the floor, then jerking for 2–3 minutes with incontinence. Slowly came around, disorientated initially, now coherent. Feels tired with a sore head. No vomiting, headache or fevers. **PMHx:** Depression, anxiety. **DHx:** NKDA. Nil regular. **SHx:** His friend reports the patient drinks 2 L cider most days but recently stopped drinking altogether.

O/E: Drowsy. Dishevelled. Temp 37.5°C, HR 92, RR 16, sats 94%, BP 132/91. GCS 13/15 (mild confusion, eyes open to voice). Laceration on tongue, left side. No visible head injury or evidence of skull fracture. No focal neurology. **Ix:** Glucose 5.5 mmol/L, blood gas pH 7.21, lactate 9.0, K 4.0, Na 131, PCO_2 3.7.

1. A boy presents following a seizure starting 35 minutes prior, still fitting despite 2× doses IV lorazepam. What's the most appropriate next step in management?
2. What elements in the vignette point towards a seizure, as opposed to other causes of LOC?
3. List some other causes of seizures to consider in children.

Answers: 1. IV phenytoin or levetiracetam, urgent call to ITU and likely general anaesthesia. 2. Focal prodrome, tongue biting, incontinence, post-ictal period. 3. Febrile convulsions (3 months to 5 years, high fevers), infantile spasms, Lennox-Gastaut syndrome, juvenile myoclonic epilepsy.

TABLE 100.1

	Features	Investigations	Management
Psychogenic non-epileptic seizure (PNES)	**RFs/comorbidities:** childhood trauma, acute stress, head injury, PTSD, dissociative disorder, co-morbid epilepsy. **Hx & O/E:** atypical appearance for seizure (e.g. asynchronous arm movements rapidly changing features). Resistance to eye opening. Immediate recovery	Investigations for seizure, dependent on how confident diagnosis is of PNES	Common – approx. 10% seizure referrals. Acknowledgement of condition and genuine problems it causes. Treatment of underlying mental disorder if present. Psychological therapies

TABLE 100.1 (Cont'd)

	Features	Investigations	Management
Seizure	Temporary dysfunction of brain tissue – twitching, loss of consciousness (ictal phase). Generalised seizure: tonic-clonic movements, head turning to one side/unusual posturing, tongue-biting, urinary or bowel incontinence. Period of disorientation and drowsiness (post-ictal phase). **Epilepsy** means repeated seizures, due to structural abnormality (hippocampal sclerosis, brain tumour, gliosis following a head injury) or idiopathic	**RFs:** epilepsy, alcohol withdrawal, structural brain lesion including SAH, CNS infection, hypoglycaemia, hyponatraemia. **'Provoked' seizures;** due to transient insult (e.g. alcohol withdrawal, acute head injury). **ECG/blood sugar.** **CT head** If first seizure. **EEG** To look for epileptiform activity. Investigation for cause, e.g. septic screen/U&Es	Conservative if seizure has stopped. **Anti-convulsants:** usually where more than one seizure or ongoing risk (e.g. brain tumour). **Safety advice:** driving, bathing/swimming, working at height. Treatment of any specific cause
Cardiogenic syncope	See *46. BLACKOUTS, FAINTS AND LOSS OF CONSCIOUSNESS*		
KEY COMPLICATIONS Status epilepticus	Seizure lasting >5 minutes or ≥2 seizures within 5 minutes without returning to normal between	As for seizure	A–E: airway adjuncts, oxygen, check glucose. IV lorazepam or diazepam. **2nd line:** phenytoin or levetiracetam loading dose. If refractory (30 minutes): general anaesthesia
TOP DIFFERENTIALS: PROVOKED SEIZURES Acute alcohol withdrawal	See *169. ADDICTION*		
Metabolic derangement	**Hypoglycaemia:** palpitations, sweaty, dizzy, shaking, irritable, confusion, seizures, coma. **Hyponatraemia:** N&V, confusion, drowsiness, irritable, muscle cramps, seizures, coma	Bloods as above. Hyponatraemia: –Na$^+$ <135 mmol/L –Seizures likely if Na$^+$ <115	**Treat underlying cause.** IV benzodiazepines for seizure. Seizures with low Na – give hypertonic saline (in HDU/ITU)
Structural CNS lesion (e.g. brain tumour/ stroke/head injury/ hippocampal sclerosis/ SAH)	Lesion location determines seizure e.g. temporal lobe - may get focal seizures with déjà vu sensations and automatisms. Tendency to focal seizures likely to 'secondary generalise' into tonic-clonic seizures	**CT head ± contrast, MRI.** First seizure in adults requires a CT head to rule out a structural lesion	Treat underlying cause/ injury. Symptomatic treatment of epilepsy
Meningoencephalitis	See *93. NECK PAIN/STIFFNESS*		
PRIMARY EPILEPSY SYNDROMES Childhood absence epilepsy, juvenile myoclonic epilepsy, Lennox-Gastaut syndrome	Seizures. Intellectual disability in some cases. Neurophysiological/genetic cause usually implicated	Initial workup to rule out structural causes as above	Anti-convulsants. Vagal nerve stimulator. Ketogenic diet. Epilepsy surgery in refractory focal cases

TABLE 100.2 Overview of Different Seizure Types

Type and Presentation	Investigations	Management
SEIZURE TYPES		
Generalised tonic-clonic: Sudden LOC, tonic stiff limb phase, then clonic jerking. Incontinence, tongue biting, irregular breathing, prolonged post-ictal confusion, myalgia, drowsiness	EEG: bisynchronous epileptiform activity during event in both hemispheres	Levetiracetam. Valproate. Lamotrigine. Topiramate
Generalised myoclonic: involuntary brief jerks **Atonic:** 'drop attacks' **Tonic:** all muscles rigid	As for above Check antiepileptic drug levels for underdosing/non-compliance	Levetiracetam. Valproate. Avoid sodium channel blockers (e.g. lamotrigine, carbamazepine)
Absence; children, suddenly 'stare into space' for 5–10 seconds multiple times/day	EEG: bilateral, symmetrical 3 Hz spike and wave pattern	Ethosuximide. Valproate
Focal: 1. Focal aware (simple), 2. Focal impaired awareness (complex). <u>Location determines activity:</u> Temporal (lip smacking, chewing, déjà vu). Frontal (motor dysfunction). Parietal (sensory disturbances). Occipital (visual/flashes/floaters)	EEG: local discharge. Most often affects temporal lobe	1st line: carbamazepine. 2nd line: valproate or levetiracetam

NB: Valproate is contraindicated in women and girls of childbearing age – teratogenic.

The vignette presents a convincing history of a seizure. A patient will not recollect (if tonic-clonic, although not the case with focal seizures (Table 100.2)) and the witness account is vital. Once stabilised, the key question is whether the event was truly a seizure or another issue, such as syncope. If established as a seizure, any underlying cause needs to be sought. In this case the sudden cessation of alcohol was the culprit and this would be classed as a provoked seizure. Where no clear ongoing cause (e.g. brain tumour) has been uncovered, a single seizure does not usually lead to the patient starting anti-convulsants. Once a second unprovoked seizure has occurred, or there is an ongoing risk, medication is started. For any seizure, informing the patient about driving rules (stopping driving and informing DVLA – see **62. DRIVING ADVICE**) and general safety advice is important.

REVISION TIPS

- Epilepsy: **recurrent** seizures. ≥2 unprovoked seizures >24 hours apart or linked to epilepsy syndrome
- Seziures are common post-stroke and thresholds generally get lower into old age (with brain atrophy)
- Anti-convulsants usually started after second seizure or ongoing risk of seizure (e.g. structural lesion)

101

Speech and Language Problems

Margarita Fox and Matthew Smith

EMERGENCY DEPARTMENT, FEMALE, 75. COLLAPSED

HPC: Well until 45 minutes ago, then sudden weakness, slumped on the sofa. Her daughter tells you that her mum isn't making any sense but appears to understand what she hears. She struggles to make a sentence. **PMHx:** Hypercholesterolaemia, HTN, IHD. **DHx:** Ramipril, atorvastatin. **SHx:** Smoker 40 pack years, nil alcohol.

O/E: BP 165/100, HR 70, afebrile. Neurological: Slow, halted speech. Severe expressive dysphasia. Able to comprehend instructions. Weakness of right CN7 with forehead sparing, right-sided homonymous hemianopia to the right when tested with bilateral stimuli, no dysarthria. Power Left UL: 5/5, right UL: 2/5, Left LL: 5/5, right LL: 3/5. Reduced sensation on right upper and lower limb examination in all modalities. **Ix:** ECG shows atrial fibrillation (new), CT head normal.

1. Which artery is likely affected in the case in the vignette and contributing to her aphasia?
2. What would be your top differential if a patient presented with gradual onset progressive aphasia? What investigations would you order?

Answers: 1. MCA stroke: contralateral hemiparesis, upper extremity may be affected more than lower extremity, contralateral homonymous hemianopia, and dysphasia. Superior division of left MCA supplies inferior frontal gyrus, where Broca's area deficit causes expressive dysphasia. 2. Primary progressive aphasia (frontal dementia spectrum), Alzheimer disease, SOL. Often a clinical diagnosis, including neuropsychological assessment. In primary progressive aphasia, neuroimaging may demonstrate frontal or temporal lobe atrophy and rule out other causes.

TABLE 101.1		
Features	**Investigations**	**Management**
DIFFERENTIALS FOR SUDDEN ONSET DYSPHASIA/APHASIA		
Intracerebral haemorrhage	**RFs:** uncontrolled HTN, anticoagulation, trauma, aneurysm, AVM, and as per ischaemic stroke. Less common than ischaemic strokes. **Hx & O/E:** similar to ischemic stroke, but also headache, nausea, seizures, reduced GCS, LOC	NIHSS score. **CT head:** hyperdense lesion. Possibly underlying vascular malformation/tumour. **Glucose:** normal/raised. **Clotting/INR**	Intensive **BP control** (aim systolic <140). Reverse anticoagulation. Manage raised ICP (extra-ventricular drainage, craniectomy)/seizures (anticonvulsants). Rehabilitation

(Continued)

TABLE 101.1   (Cont'd)

	Features	Investigations	Management
Total anterior circulation stroke (TACS)	**RFs:** HTN, DM, AF, smoking, dyslipidaemia, CVD, carotid artery atheroma, age, gender (M>F), prev TIA, OSA, CKD, migraine, OCP, inherited thrombophilias/acquired prothrombotic or hypercoagulable states. **Hx & O/E:** large stroke of MCA/ACA; all three of 1. Hemiparesis (±sensory deficit) of face, arm, leg 2. Homonymous hemianopia 3. Higher cerebral dysfunction; aphasia, visuospatial	**NIHSS score:** to establish deficits. **Glucose:** normal/raised. **CT head:** rule out haemorrhage – may be normal initially even in large ischaemic stroke. **MRI:** more sensitive than CT. **CT Angio/MRA:** circle of Willis/neck vessels – vital for thrombectomy. **Find cause:** ECG (AF in 50% of strokes, carotid doppler/angiogram to assess for stenosis, TTE to assess for cardiac thrombus, dissection on angiogram	(1) **Reperfusion:** thrombectomy/ thrombolysis (time sensitive, eligibility dependent) (2) **Aspirin** 300 mg PO for 2 weeks **Further management:** control BP/glucose. Swallow assessment ± placement of NGT. VTE prophylaxis. Secondary prevention: vascular factors, clopidogrel 75 mg lifelong (if AF, start DOAC at 2 weeks instead), statin. Consider carotid endarterectomy. Rehabilitation
Partial anterior circulation stroke (PACS)	Two of the three features mentioned above		
Lacunar stroke (LACS)	**RFs:** small vessel disease – HTN, smoking, DM. **Hx & O/E:** pure motor and/or sensory loss or ataxic hemiparesis. No higher cortical dysfunction		
Posterior circulation stroke (POCS)	Cerebellar dysfunction (incl gait/truncal ataxia), isolated homonymous quadrantanopia, acute vertigo and nystagmus, conjugate gaze palsy, motor/sensory deficit. *Posterior inferior cerebellar artery (PICA) stroke;* vertigo, vomiting, headache, tinnitus, dysarthria, diplopia, gait disturbances, ipsilateral horizontal nystagmus		

TYPES OF APHASIA

Receptive aphasia	Inferior division of left MCA, n.b. left superior temporal gyrus -> Wernicke's area (Fig. 101.1). Comprehension is impaired. Speech fluent but non-sensical	Clinical diagnosis supported by stroke syndrome and imaging (dysphasia and aphasia can also be seen occurring progressively in neurodegenerative conditions)	Treat as above for stroke if cause, or other underlying cause
Expressive aphasia	Superior division left MCA, n.b. left inferior frontal gyrus Broca's area. Comprehension intact but speech is disrupted, non-fluent, effortful		
Global aphasia	Lesion impacting all areas (Broca's, Wernicke's, arcuate fasciculus); severe expressive + receptive aphasia. Only able to produce and comprehend few words or greetings/automatic language		

TABLE 101.2 Stroke Summary

TACS (3/3) and PACS (2/3) of	POCS (one out of the following)	LACS (one out of the following)
1. Motor/sensory weakness 2. Homonymous hemianopia 3. Higher cerebellar dysfunction	1. Sensory/motor weakness (contralateral or bilateral) 2. Homonymous hemianopia 3. Cranial nerve dysfunction 4. Cerebellar dysfunction	1. Pure sensory/motor loss 2. Ataxic hemiparesis

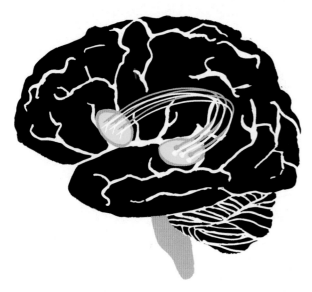

Fig. 101.1 Broca's area (motor speech area in the inferior frontal gyrus) and Wernicke's area (speech comprehension; upper part of the left temporal lobe). (Illustrated by Dr Hollie Blaber.)

disabling deficit such as severe aphasia) who do not have any contraindications and who present within 4.5 hours of onset. Thrombolysis patients should be warned about the approximately 6% chance of haemorrhagic transformation, which may result in even worse deficits. Thrombectomy involves the mechanical retrieval of an intra-arterial thrombus via the distal arteries by interventional radiology, where located in a large vessel such as the proximal MCA. Thrombectomy can be carried out immediately after thrombolysis and has a realistic time window of 12 hours, but is dependent on the extent of penumbra (ischaemic but not irreversibly damaged brain) demonstrated on imaging (often a 'CT perfusion' scan technique). Ischaemic stroke is common, due to atherosclerosis (hypercholesterolaemia, DM, smoking, HTN) and cardioembolic causes (AF, valvular heart disease, previous MI, endocarditis, patent foramen ovale), along with rarer causes: SLE, anti-phospholipid syndrome, DIC, sickle cell disease and dissection.

The woman in the vignette fulfils all criteria required to diagnose a TACS (Table 101.2), NIHSS score at least 12. Assessing for reperfusion therapy is first priority: time is brain. Thrombolysis is usually considered for those with a score >5 (or in those with an isolated and

REVISION TIPS

- Hypoglycaemia is a rare but treatable stroke mimic – check a blood glucose
- Reperfusion treatment is key – effective treatment within a strict time window (time is brain)

102

Facial Weakness

Louise Mathias and Matthew Smith

EMERGENCY DEPARTMENT, MALE, 40. RIGHT-SIDED FACIAL DROOP

HPC: On waking, noted right side of face was sagging, unable to close his right eye fully or smile properly. Previous night felt some pulling in his right cheek. No weakness, sensory changes, problems with walking/balance, visual symptoms. No head trauma. **PMHx:** Type 2 diabetes. **SHx:** Non-smoker, 14 units/week.

O/E: Afebrile, GCS 15, no rashes, normal ear exam. Neuro: R facial droop, unable to raise R eyebrow/close R eye, full range of eye movements, no visual field defects, facial sensation normal, no tongue or uvula deviation. Power, tone, sensation, reflexes and co-ordination normal in all limbs. No aphasia or neglect.

1. If the patient can wrinkle their forehead, does this indicate a UMN or LMN lesion?
2. If the facial palsy was bilateral, what diagnoses would you consider?
3. What differential is likely if the facial weakness is worse at the end of the day, with double vision and difficulty swallowing?

Answers: 1. Ability to wrinkle the forehead implies a UMN lesion. 2. Sarcoidosis, Guillain-Barré (Miller-Fisher), botulism, Lyme disease. 3. Myasthenia gravis.

TABLE 102.1

	Features	Investigations	Management
Bell's palsy	**Hx & O/E:** quick onset CN7 palsy, unilateral sagging of mouth, failure to close eye, decreased taste/lacrimation, hyperacusis. Bell's phenomenon: upwards deviation of eyeball when closing eyelid. Normal finding, but more noticeable in CN7 palsy. **No neurology** aside from LMN facial palsy (involving forehead)	**RFs** idiopathic. Diabetes, pregnancy, secondary. **Clinical diagnosis.** Other investigations (e.g. CT/MRI) if cannot rule out a central cause, or other aetiology. **FBC in children.** Bell's can be the presenting feature of childhood leukaemia	**Prednisolone** 50mg daily for 10 days, or 60mg daily for 5 days followed by a daily reduction of 10mg (total duration 10 days). Artificial tears. Tape over eye at night to protect cornea
Ramsay Hunt syndrome	**RFs:** >60, immunocompromised. **Hx & O/E:** as for Bell's, and pain in the ear/face followed by vesicles in the auditory canal ± on the tongue	Reactivated VZV in CN7 geniculate ganglion. **Clinical diagnosis.** Examine ear canal in all Bell's palsy cases (Fig. 102.1)	As above with oral **acyclovir**

TABLE 102.1   (Cont'd)

	Features	Investigations	Management
Ischaemic stroke	See *101. SPEECH AND LANGUAGE PROBLEMS*		
OTHER IMPORTANT DIFFERENTIALS			
Myasthenia Gravis	**RFs:** autoimmune esp. thymic hyperplasia/tumour, RA, SLE. Commoner in F <50, men >50. **Hx & O/E:** fatigue, facial drooping, ptosis, diplopia, difficulty swallowing. Variability – improves with rest, worse at the end of the day. The weakness shows fatiguability. Myasthenic crisis: weakness of respiratory muscles needing respiratory support	**Antibodies:** raised anti-AChR antibodies, and raised muscle-specific tyrosine kinase. **Repetitive nerve stimulation.** Shows fatiguability – train of impulses on EMG. **Respiratory function:** forced vital capacity. **Thymus CT,** As likely involvement	**Anticholinesterases** e.g. pyridostigmine/neostigmine. **Immunosuppression** e.g. corticosteroids (consider osteoporosis protection) or azathioprine – disease control and treat relapses. IV immunoglobulin or plasma exchange for myasthenic crisis ± ICU Thymectomy
Space occupying lesion	See *99. HEADACHE*		
Parotid tumours/ surgery	Facial nerve runs through parotid gland. Parotid tumour or complication of mastoid/parotid surgery can cause CN7 palsy		
Botulism	Rare, easily missed. Toxin from *Clostridium botulinum* infection (dirty wounds, e.g. IVDU, gardening). Descending paralysis associated with early facial weakness **(bilateral)**, ptosis, pupillary abnormalities and eventual respiratory compromise		
Miller-Fisher syndrome	Similar to botulism – **bilateral** descending paralysis. On spectrum of Guillain-Barré syndrome – parainfectious/immune-mediated peripheral nerve demyelination		

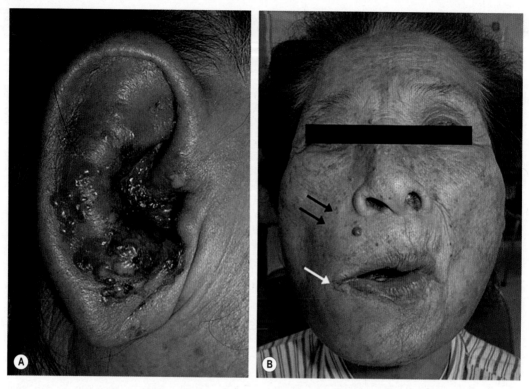

Fig. 102.1 Ramsey-Hunt syndrome, vesicular lesions in the ear (A), flattened nasolabial fold (*black arrows*) and drooping of the angle of the mouth (*white arrow*) (B). (Taguchi T, Ueda S, Kudo T, et al. Ramsey-Hunt syndrome. *J Infect.* Feb. 2011;62(2):Fig.1. Copyright © 2010 The British Infection Association. Published by Elsevier Ltd. All rights reserved.)

A key issue for acute facial paralysis is deciding a central or peripheral cause, i.e. stroke or TIA versus Bell's palsy. Patients presenting with an isolated facial droop might be found to have field defects or speech problems when examined more carefully, suggesting a central cause. In the vignette, the absence of any neurological findings aside from an LMN weakness in CN7, along with the absence of a vesicular rash (Fig. 102.1), indicates Bell's palsy. His history of diabetes puts him at higher risk of both Bell's palsy and stroke. The rare presentation of bilateral facial palsy has few recognised causes and they can be easily tested in exams.

REVISION TIPS

- Facial nerve palsy can be due to central and peripheral causes
- Bell's palsy is 3× more likely in diabetics and 2× more likely in pregnancy
- Facial nerve (CN7) supplies 'face, ear, taste and tear'

103

Memory Loss

Margarita Fox, Gregory Oxenham, and Dafydd Morgan

HPC: Difficulty making decisions and remembering words. Brought in by his daughter, after an episode where he got lost shopping in town. **PMHx:** HTN, ischaemic heart disease, Type 2 DM. **SHx:** Current smoker (45 pack years).

O/E: MMSE 19/30. **Ix:** A confusion screen done by his GP (FBC, CRP, U&Es, bone profile, glucose, LFTs, TFTs, B12/folate, magnesium, phosphate, glucose, MSU) was normal. CT head shows general volume loss with periventricular hypodensities and small vessel disease.

1. What are some of the ameliorable causes of dementia?
2. What type of dementia is most likely in a 68-year-old man with worsening memory and tremor, and he keeps thinking there is a cat in the bedroom?
3. Which drugs may worsen dementia?

Answers: 1. Hypothyroidism, B12/folate deficiency, Wernicke's encephalopathy/alcohol abuse, depression, subdural haematoma, NPH, some cerebral neoplasms, neurosyphilis, HIV-related cognitive impairment. They are not necessarily reversible, but treatment can reduce deterioration. 2. Dementia with Lewy bodies – memory loss, tremor, visual hallucinations. 3. Avoid drugs which impair cognition, e.g. neuroleptics, sedatives, opiates, TCAs, anticholinergics, H2 antagonists. Minimise polypharmacy, 'Start low and go slow'.

TABLE 103.1

	Features	Investigations	Management
Alzheimer's disease	**RFs:** FHx, advancing age, learning disability, depression, heavy alcohol use, low social engagement, rarely genetic. **Hx & O/E:** amnesia, apraxia, agnosia, aphasia. Gradual decline. Later, frontal release signs	**Confusion screen:** assess for reversible causes/delirium. **ACE III:** (attention, memory, fluency, language and visuospatial domains). **MRI:** general atrophy with temporal lobe predilection. Enlarged ventricles, wide sulci. Genetic testing	Education (patient and family). *Mild-to-moderate:* AChE inhibitor (donepezil, galantamine, rivastigmine) ± memantine. *Moderate-to-severe:* memantine
Vascular dementia	**RFs:** as per Ischaemic stroke. See *101. SPEECH AND LANGUAGE PROBLEMS.* **Hx & O/E:** stepwise cognitive deterioration, apathy, disinhibition, short stepping gait, problem-solving issues	**Confusion screen:** assess for reversible causes/delirium **CT head:** small vessel disease, diffuse hypodensities **MRI head** (more sensitive): microhaemorrhages	Address RFs. AChE inhibitor ONLY if co-morbid Alzheimer's, dementia with Lewy bodies or Parkinson disease

(Continued)

TABLE 103.1   (Cont'd)

	Features	Investigations	Management
Dementia with Lewy bodies (LBD)	**RFs:** older age, male, FHx. **Hx & O/E:** visual hallucinations (e.g. small children), fluctuating cognitive impairment, falls, REM sleep behaviour disorder (RBD). ± *Parkinsonism* (suspect LBD if dementia prior to or within 1 year of Parkinsonism)	**Confusion screen:** assess for reversible causes/delirium. **DaT scan:** lateralised reduced dopamine uptake in basal ganglia.	**AChE inhibitors** 1st line: Donepezil/Rivastigmine, 2nd line: Galantamine. Memantine if AChE inhibitors CI (e.g. bradycardia, heart block, unexplained syncope). **Parkinsonism:** Levodopa/carbidopa. **RBD:** Clonazepam or melatonin
Frontotemporal dementia (FTD)	**RFs:** poorly understood but likely FHx. **Hx & O/E:** behaviour/personality, aphasia, younger onset (<65). Pick disease (behaviour variant FTD); social conduct problems, hyperorality, disinhibition, OCD	**MRI head:** frontal and temporal lobe atrophy. 'Knife-blade appearance' indicative of focal gyral atrophy in Pick disease	Non-pharmacological therapies 1st line. Acute agitation/distress: benzodiazepines. Depression/anxiety/sleep disturbance: SSRIs
OTHER IMPORTANT DIFFERENTIALS			
Depression	Suggests *depression over dementia*; onset weeks to months, progressive, biological symptoms, variable Mini-Mental Test, memory loss not restricted to recent memories	Investigations are not routine. Consider confusion screen. Screening questionnaire PHQ-9 (primary care)	Usually reversible. Depends on severity; self-help, group therapy, CBT, SSRIs
Delirium	Suggests *delirium over dementia*; acute onset, fluctuating, inattention, altered consciousness, psychomotor changes/agitation, abnormal perceptions, delusions. See *47. CONFUSION*	4AT, CAMs. Confusion screen: FBC, CRP, U&Es, bone profile, glucose, TFTs, B12/folate, Mg, phosphate. Consider: blood cultures, CXR, ECG, Troponin, LFTs, urinalysis ± MSU	Reversible, treat cause. Orientate/environment modification. 1st line sedative: 0.5 mg haloperidol (or olanzapine). Lorazepam alternative if antipsychotic contra-indicated, e.g. LBD/Parkinson's
Chronic subdural haematoma	See *49. HEAD INJURY*		
Normal pressure hydrocephalus	**RFs:** underlying brain injury/tumour/infection, idiopathic. TRIAD: • Cognitive impairment • Urinary Incontinence • Gait apraxia Personality/mood disturbed	**CT/MRI head:** dilated ventricles, normal sulci. LP: normal opening pressure. **CSF flow studies:** large volume CSF removal can improve symptoms	Ventriculoperitoneal shunt

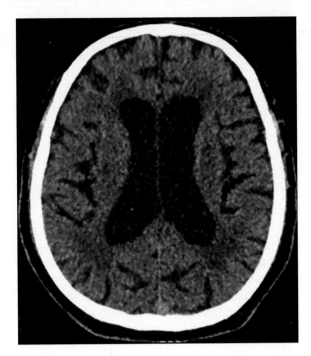

Fig. 103.1 CTH in vascular dementia – periventricular hypodensities and volume loss. (Etherton-Beer CD. *Maturitas*. Oct 2014: Fig. 1. Elsevier Copyright © 2014 Elsevier Ireland Ltd. All rights reserved.)

The vignette describes features of dementia. His cardiovascular risk factors, a relatively rapid 'stepwise' deterioration, coupled with supportive changes on neuroimaging (Fig. 103.1), make vascular dementia most likely. Vascular dementia is also suggested by executive dysfunction, impaired recall and poor attention. Patients with advanced vascular dementia may develop a shuffling gait with a wide base. This patient does not have visual hallucinations or other features of Parkinsonism to suggest Lewy body dementia. Patients with Alzheimer's develop episodic memory loss and can develop executive dysfunction, but they commonly also show signs of parietal cortical dysfunction. Clinicians should screen for depression too, as these entities can co-exist and easily be mistaken for one another. Collecting a collateral history is essential and elaborates how this person lives on a day-to-day basis.

REVISION TIPS

- Dementia leads to a progressive decline in cognition and/or behaviour, which interferes with the individual's activity
- Diagnosis is based on history and examination, timeline of progression, psychometric testing and neuroimaging
- 'Confusion screens' exist to help identify reversible causes of cognitive impairment, not to supplant the role of the history. They are not the same as screening for treatable causes of *dementia*

104

Visual Hallucinations

Alice Parker, Francesca Blest, Dafydd Morgan, and Alice Pitt

GP CONSULTATION, MALE, 75. 2-MONTH HISTORY OF 'SEEING THINGS'

HPC: Seeing people in bedroom at night and furniture moving around the room. Struggling with balance, dizziness on standing. Wife has concerns about his memory and describes increasingly 'vivid dreams' – thrashes about in bed, tries to get up while asleep. **PMHx:** Glaucoma, HTN. **DHx:** Amlodipine, bimatoprost, timolol. **SHx:** 1 bottle of whisky/week.

O/E: Afebrile, obs unremarkable, appears frail, able to hold a conversation and explain many of his symptoms. His memory is better than expected. Neuro: bilateral upper limb rigidity, shuffling gait, appears unsteady.

1. What symptoms are associated with the following seizure types: (a) temporal lobe, (b) frontal, (c) parietal, (d) occipital?
2. What Parkinson-plus syndromes are associated with: (a) autonomic dysfunction, (b) vertical gaze paresis, (c) alien limb phenomenon?

Answers: 1. (a) Temporal lobe = 'HEAD', i.e. hallucinations, emotional/epigastric, automatisms, déjà vu/dysphasia, (b) frontal lobe = motor symptoms, post-ictal Todd's palsy, Jacksonian march, (c) parietal lobe = sensory symptoms, e.g. paraesthesia, motor symptoms, (d) occipital lobe = visual symptoms, e.g. flashers and floaters. 2. (a) autonomic dysfunction = multiple system atrophy, (b) vertical gaze paresis = progressive supranuclear palsy, (c) alien limb phenomenon = corticobasal degeneration.

TABLE 104.1

	Features	Investigations	Management
Delirium	See *103. MEMORY LOSS*		
Alcohol or drug withdrawal	See *169. ADDICTION*		
Dementia with Lewy bodies (LBD)	See *103. MEMORY LOSS*		
Parkinson disease	Visual hallucinations can occur (generally less frequent and less severe than LBD) See *105. TREMOR*		
Charles Bonnet syndrome	Complex visual hallucinations in people with visual impairment (e.g. glaucoma), insight usually preserved Never auditory hallucinations	**RFs:** visual impaired, sudden sight decline, social isolation, old age. **Clinical diagnosis**	No specific treatment, reassurance

TABLE 104.1 (Cont'd)

	Features	Investigations	Management
OTHER DIFFERENTIALS FEATURING VISUAL HALLUCINATIONS			
Schizophrenia	Visual hallucinations are much less common than auditory. See *166. AUDITORY HALLUCINATIONS*		
Migraine with aura	Visual hallucinations/scotoma (Fig. 104.1), zig-zags/flashing lights, then headache	Clinical diagnosis.	See *99. HEADACHE* Extremely unlikely to present as new diagnosis in a 75 year old
Epilepsy	Can cause complex visual hallucinations, especially in occipital cortex		See *100. FITS/SEIZURES*

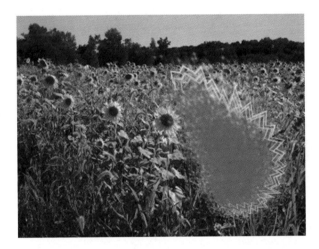

Fig. 104.1 Scotoma, a visual hallucination occasionally seen as part of a migraine aura.

Visual hallucinations alongside fluctuant cognitive impairment are highly suggestive of Lewy Body dementia. In addition, Parkinsonism (bradykinesia, resting tremor and rigidity) and autonomic dysfunction are hallmarks of

the disease. In Lewy body dementia cognitive impairment often precedes symptoms of Parkinson's, but can occur up to 1 year following symptoms of Parkinsonism. In idiopathic Parkinson's this is the reverse. In this vignette, the wife gives a history of REM sleep disorder – something which can precede any cognitive impairment in LBD. Alcohol withdrawal is an important differential to consider here, as delirium tremens is a medical emergency, with hallucinations typically occurring 48 to 72 hours after cessation of drinking. He does have a background of heavy alcohol use, but delirium tremens usually presents more acutely with physical withdrawal symptoms reported and on examination. Migraine with aura is extremely unlikely to present as a new diagnosis in a 75 year old.

REVISION TIPS

- Visual hallucinations are less common in psychosis (which more commonly involves auditory hallucinations)
- In LBD, cognitive impairment often precedes the symptoms of Parkinson's, in idiopathic Parkinson disease it is the reverse

105

Tremor

Margarita Fox and Matthew Smith

**GP CONSULTATION, FEMALE, 65.
TREMOR IN BOTH HANDS**

HPC: Tremor exacerbated by focused tasks, e.g. trying to pour coffee, present >3 years. Feels safe walking/going upstairs, no dizziness. **FHx:** Mother had tremors in older age. **SHx:** Feeling anxious at work recently-aggravates her tremor. It improves with alcohol.

O/E: Tremor is not seen at rest, more noticeable when stretches out her arms. Neurological examination is otherwise unremarkable, gait is normal.

1. How would the diagnosis differ if this were a 74 year old presenting with a unilateral resting tremor and increasing difficulty walking?
2. List some drug/toxin-induced causes of tremor.

Answers: 1. Idiopathic Parkinson disease, or Parkinson plus syndrome (diagnosis often follows, when more symptoms occur). 2. Drugs: lithium, valproate, amiodarone, beta-agonists, theophylline, neuroleptics, SSRIs, TCAs, amphetamines, tacrolimus. Toxins, e.g. alcohol, lead, mercury.

TABLE 105.1

	Features	Investigations	Management
Essential tremor	**RFs:** strong FHx, exacerbated by anxiety/adrenergic stimulation. **Hx & O/E:** usually bilateral – hands and arms affected. Spectrum with 'dystonic tremor' (head and neck). 6–12 Hz, variable amplitude. Can improve with alcohol	**Clinical diagnosis.** DaT scan if atypical features suggest Parkinson disease	1st line: propranolol and/or primidone. 2nd line: gabapentin, topiramate and nimodipine. Deep brain stimulation (DBS) in severe cases
Parkinson disease (PD)	**RFs:** male, age. **Hx & O/E:** resting 'pill rolling' tremor, initially unilateral. Bradykinesia, rigidity, shuffling gait, postural instability, falls, freezing. Flexed, stooped posture (Fig. 105.1). 'Mask-like' face (hypomimia). Cogwheeling. Non-motor symptoms; autonomic, neuropsychiatric, cognitive. Highly sensitive to neuroleptics (e.g. haloperidol, chlorpromazine)	**DaT scan:** reduced dopamine uptake in basal ganglia	**Levodopa** 1st line for bradykinesia/rigidity/tremor. Incomplete response: **dopamine agonist, MAOB inhibitor.** Motor fluctuations ('on' and 'off' in later PD): **COMT inhibitor, amantadine. DBS.** Treatment has little effect on non-motor symptoms, except low mood/anxiety. Consider falls prevention and mitigation (bone protection)

TABLE 105.1   (Cont'd)

	Features	Investigations	Management
Other *parkinsonism* causes	Umbrella term for bradykinesia, tremor, rigidity, postural instability 1. Drug induced (neuroleptics, prochlorperazine, metoclopramide) 2. Toxins (MPTP, copper) 3. Cerebrovascular disease 4. Parkinson plus syndromes (PSP, MSA, CBD, LBD) – tremor is less common than with idiopathic PD	Clinical diagnosis. DaT scan/MRI brain – if unsure of cause	**Withdrawal of neuroleptics** if relevant – long term they cause **tardive dyskinesia.** Anticholinergics, e.g. **procyclidine.** Parkinson plus syndromes are treated with levodopa, but poor response is a diagnostic criterion
Physiological tremor	High frequency (8–12 Hz), low amplitude (present in most people, barely detectable). Secondary causes; hypoglycaemia, hypocalcaemia, hyperthyroidism, alcohol/opioid withdrawal, medications (salbutamol, SSRIs, TCAs, amphetamines)	Worse with caffeine, anxiety. Action tremor. Glucose, U&Es, TFTs, toxicology. Medication review	**Treat underlying cause** (if present). Reassurance usually sufficient – not disabling
Cerebellar dysfunction	**Causes:** toxins (e.g. chronic alcohol, lithium, phenytoin), ischaemic (e.g. stroke), infectious, neoplastic, demyelinating (e.g. MS), genetic (e.g. Friedrich's ataxia). Cerebellar: dysdiadochokinesis, past-pointing, nystagmus, ataxia, slurred speech	Intention tremor, low-frequency 3–4 Hz. MRI brain for underlying cause. Drugs review, alcohol screening	**Treat underlying cause:** tremor poorly responsive to medication. See also *111. UNSTEADINESS*
OTHER IMPORTANT DIFFERENTIALS			
Thyrotoxicosis	See *10. PALPITATIONS*		
Psychogenic	**RFs:** mental health co-morbidities. Varying characteristics (location, frequency). Disappears with distraction, worse with stress	R/o organic causes – see other differentials	Conservative. Psychological therapy. SSRIs 1st line if anxiety
Wilson disease	**RF:** FHx. Copper accumulation in liver, brain, cornea. Young, new tremor (arm/head). Can get asterixis, chorea, parkinsonism, liver disease, dysarthria, psychiatric symptoms		

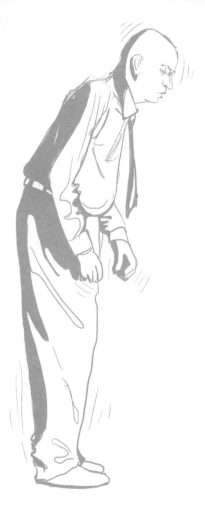

The FHx, worsening on movement and bilateral symptoms, suggest essential tremor as the diagnosis in the vignette. This is the commonest movement disorder, and can be disabling (no longer called 'benign'). Exclude other diagnoses such as chronic alcohol excess and thyrotoxicosis, as well as any offending medications. While idiopathic Parkinson disease may present with tremor, the largely normal neurological exam (including gait), bilateral tremor, and the fact it is postural and on action only (not at rest) favour essential tremor.

Fig. 105.1 Parkinson disease features. (Illustrated by Dr Hollie Blaber.)

REVISION TIPS

Resting tremor: Parkinson disease (often begins unilaterally)

Postural: Holding a position against gravity, e.g. essential tremor

Action: Executing voluntary movement (intention tremor occurs when moving towards a specific target), e.g. cerebellar damage, essential tremor

106

Abnormal Involuntary Movements

Margarita Fox, Gregory Oxenham, and Dafydd Morgan

HPC: Younger brother brings him; initially low in mood, irritable, then had difficulty with tasks–concentration became poor, prone to emotional outbursts–had to leave his job. Increasingly unstable, developing involuntary movements of limbs, and abnormal facial movements.
PMHx: Depression. **FHx:** Adopted. **DHx:** Sertraline.

O/E: Fidgety, easily distracted. Whole body writhing movements, difficulty balancing when asked to stand. Reflexes increased bilaterally, with increased tone throughout. MOCA 23/30.

1. What is the likely diagnosis for a 65 year old with abnormal involuntary movements of the mouth and face, 3 years taking metoclopramide for nausea and constipation; 1 year ago developed repetitive movements of the tongue and jaw which are worsening.
2. A patient describes tremor of both of their hands when performing tasks but which resolve at rest. Provide differentials for postural tremor.

Answers: 1. Tardive dyskinesia; mainly oral-buccal-lingual muscles 2. Physiological tremor, essential tremor, drug-induced tremor, psychogenic tremor. Recent onset postural tremor can also be caused by thyrotoxicosis. Rarer: Wilson's, fragile X-associated tremor/ataxia. Parkinson's classically presents with resting tremor although postural elements are sometimes seen.

TABLE 106.1

	Features	Investigations	Management
Huntington disease	**RF:** FHx autosomal dominant. Insidious progression. Mean onset 40 years. **Hx & O/E:** chorea: irregular 'dance-like' movements. Athetosis: slower writhing movements. Dementia, personality changes, depression, poor coordination, dystonia. Juvenile Huntington disease: may have no chorea	**Genetic testing:** 40+ CAG repeats in Huntington gene (chromosome 4). Cognitive, balance, gait assessments. **MRI:** loss of striatal volume, enlarged lateral ventricles, caudate head atrophy (normal in early disease)	**Chorea:** tetrabenazine, **Depression:** SSRIs, mirtazapine, venlafaxine, **Psychosis:** typical and atypical antipsychotics. **MDT input:** see Fig. 106.1

(Continued)

TABLE 106.1   (Cont'd)

	Features	Investigations	Management
Other causes of chorea	*Hereditary:* benign hereditary chorea, Wilson's *Autoimmune:* MS, SLE, Sydenham chorea (post-streptococcal) *Toxic:* alcohol, CO, post-anoxia *Metabolic:* hyperthyroid, hypo/hyperglycaemia, chorea gravidarum, thiamine deficient *Vascular:* lacunar infarcts affecting basal ganglia *Drugs:* stimulants, neuroleptics, anticholinergics, anticonvulsants		

OTHER HYPERKINETIC MOVEMENTS

	Features	Investigations	Management
Tics	Simple: occur at same site. In children typically self-resolve. Complex (e.g. Tourette's); vocal/motor tics. Associated with OCD, ADHD	Abrupt, repetitive, coordinated movements; may be suppressed. **Clinical diagnosis**	Treat if ADLs affected. Olanzapine, risperidone, clonidine. OCD: SSRIs, CBT
Tardive dyskinesia	Movements; orobuccolingual (e.g. chewing, grimacing), truncal, choreiform. Appears/continues even after drugs stopped	RF: drug-induced; long-term typical antipsychotic / some antiemetics. **Clinical diagnosis.** Abnormal Involuntary Movement Scale (AIMS)	**Gradually withdraw antipsychotics.** If still present at 3–6 months, consider tetrabenazine
Dystonia	*Focal:* blepharospasm, torticollis, writer's cramp. *Generalised:* e.g. primary idiopathic generalised dystonia. Childhood onset, unilateral dystonia in leg, then spreads. Secondary: Huntington disease, PD, Wilson's, anoxia, stroke, drug induced. **Acute dystonia:** cyclizine, metoclopramide, antipsychotic. Oculogyric crisis, trismus, torticollis	Prolonged or intermittent muscle contractions – twisting/abnormal postures. **Clinical diagnosis.** Consider: EMG, EEG, MRI brain, toxicology, genetic testing if primary idiopathic suspected	**Early onset dystonia:** without alternative diagnosis, trial levodopa. **Focal:** botulinum toxin. **Acute dystonia:** procyclidine and stop offending agent
Myoclonus	Sudden 'shock-like' jerks arising from brief muscle contraction, frequently repetitive. Differentials: benign essential myoclonus, physiological, post-stroke, infectious, epileptic. Negative myoclonus – asterixis (hepatic encephalopathy, CO_2 retention)	Depends on suspected cause; EEG, MRI brain, U&Es, toxicology, LFTs	Anticonvulsants (e.g. valproate, levetiracetam, piracetam) effective in cortical myoclonus. Clonazepam may be helpful for all types of myoclonus

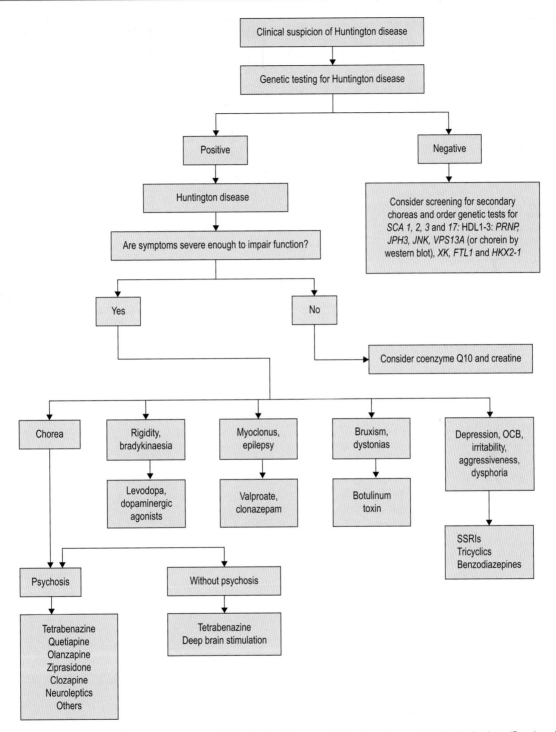

Fig. 106.1 Therapeutic approaches for treatment of Huntington disease. *OCB: obsessive compulsive behaviour.* (Reprinted with permission from Article title is "Treatment of hyperkinetic movement disorders" *Lancet Neurology* 2009;8(9):844–856. Copyright © 2009 Elsevier Ltd.)

In the vignette, insidious symptoms leading to cognitive impairment, personality change and choreiform movements suggest Huntington disease. The patient was adopted; new diagnoses of autosomal dominant Huntington disease are commonly expected in families that carry the gene, so it should be established whether this younger brother is related genetically – genetic counselling would then be relevant. Huntington disease is a neuro-degenerative disorder with no disease-modifying therapies currently available. Death occurs 15–25 years after disease onset.

REVISION TIPS

C: copper deposition (Wilson's), chorea gravidarum, CNS stimulants
H: Huntington's
O: oestrogens, oral contraceptives
R: rheumatic fever (infective causes)
E: endocrine (hyperthyroid, hyperglycaemia, hypoglycaemia)
A: autoimmune (SLE, antiphospholipid), anticholinergics, antihistamines, anticonvulsants, antidopaminergics

107

Facial Pain

Louise Mathias, Felix Miller-Molloy, and Hamish Morrison

HPC: Sudden onset facial pain, comes on while eating, lasts 1–2 seconds, severe and stabbing across R cheek – scrunching her face, makes her eyes water. Sometimes arises when touching her right lower molars. No visual changes. Prone to headaches across her forehead – simple analgesia. Denies fevers/trismus. **PMHx:** Hypothyroidism. **DHx:** Levothyroxine. **SHx:** Lives alone, works as solicitor, EtOH 18 units/week, non-smoker.

  O/E: Appears well, no rashes, good dentition. No pain on palpation of muscles of mastication or temporal area. **Neuro:** Cranial nerves (CNs) normal, visual acuity 6/6 both eyes, no focal findings

1. What is the management for trigeminal neuralgia?
2. What chronic condition is associated with temporal arteritis?
3. How long are shingles lesions contagious?

Answers: 1. Carbamazepine. Secondary medications include oxcarbazepine, lamotrigine, gabapentin, pregabalin and baclofen- microvascular decompression if refractory. 2. PMR – pain and stiffness in the proximal muscles (not weakness), more common in older females. 3. From the time the blisters start oozing to when the lesions scab over – infectivity refers to transmission of VZV, so someone getting the infection would develop chickenpox.

TABLE 107.1			
	Features	**Investigations**	**Management**
Trigeminal neuralgia (TGN)	**RFs:** F >50 years, Asian populations. TGN is a rare presentation of MS. Sometimes due to nerve root compression. **Hx & O/E:** unilateral, short (seconds), sharp stabbing pain, typically mandibular or maxillary branch. Triggers: washing, shaving, eating, cold air	**MRI head:** including trigeminal sequences to look for neurovascular conflict and exclude underlying, e.g. MS. Ensure no dental caries causing similar pain	**Carbamazepine** (first line); effective in 90%, may not be sustained. Oxcarbazepine, lamotrigine, gabapentin, pregabalin, baclofen. Refractory: microvascular decompression

(Continued)

TABLE 107.1   (Cont'd)

	Features	Investigations	Management
Dental abscess	**RFs:** poor dental hygiene, smoking, previous infection, diabetes, medication causing gum hypertrophy (phenytoin, valproate, phenobarbitone)/ dryness. **Hx & O/E:** pain in tooth/jaw, malaise. Severe: trismus, high fever, sepsis, submandibular abscess	Clinical diagnosis. **Orthopantomogram:** caries/abscess. Exclude Ludwig's angina (*39. FACIAL/ PERIORBITAL SWELLING*)	Refer to dentist. Otherwise, oral clindamycin or appropriate alternative
Giant cell arteritis	See *36. EYE PAIN & DISCOMFORT*		
Sinusitis (acute)	See *26. ANOSMIA*		
Temporomandibular disorders	**RFs:** RA, trauma. **Hx & O/E:** pain in temporomandibular joint ± masseter/temporalis. Worse on palpation, chewing or opening/closing the mouth Jaw clicking/locking/dislocation, headache, otalgia	Clinical diagnosis.	Self-management, e.g. soft diet, jaw rest, relaxation techniques, sleep hygiene. Analgesia, ice/heat pads. Referral if: symptoms >3 months, worsening, diagnosis uncertain
Shingles (herpes zoster infection)	**RFs:** elderly, immunocompromised. **Hx & O/E:** burning or stabbing pain (often prior to rash) in dermatomal distribution, followed by vesicular rash which does not cross midline. Vesicles erupt then crust over. Post-herpetic neuralgia – can be chronic	Clinical diagnosis. Slit lamp: corneal epithelial defect on fluorescein if ophthalmic. Hutchinson's sign: lesions on tip of nose mean nasociliary nerve (from the ophthalmic division of CN5) – high risk of ocular involvement	**Refer to ophthalmology if ocular involvement.** Analgesia. Anti-viral therapy within 72 hours if ocular involvement, facial rash, significant pain, immunocompromised
Salivary gland infection/stone can also cause facial pain			

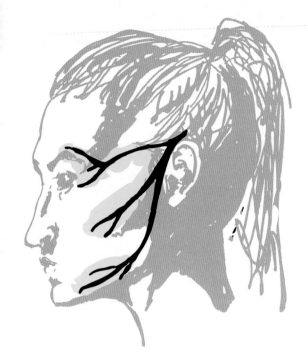

Trigeminal neuralgia (TN) may be subclassified into classical, secondary or idiopathic. Classical TN accounts for 75% of cases and is due to neurovascular compression ipsilateral to the side of pain (Fig. 107.1). Secondary TN accounts for 15% of cases and is attributable to another underlying neurological disease, e.g. MS. No cause is found in 10% of cases (idiopathic). The pain of TN is unilateral, experienced repeatedly over seconds to minutes and often described as a 'lightning-bolt'. TN may be mistaken for toothache, which can lead to inappropriate extractions before diagnosis. Whilst the case in the vignette is most likely to be TN, it is crucial to consider other causes of facial pain such as trigeminal autonomic cephalalgias (in particular cluster headache), GCA and shingles-which have serious visual sequelae. Consider the possibility of atopy in this patient from her hypothyroidism, which could hint towards atopic sinusitis.

Fig. 107.1 Trigeminal nerve distribution. The main divisions are 1. ophthalmic, 2. maxillary and 3. mandibular. (Illustrated by Dr Hollie Blaber.)

REVISION TIPS

- Rule of 50s for GCA: Age >50, ESR >50, 50% will have PMR, give 50 mg prednisolone
- Pain in the face can come from the skin, soft tissues, glands, nerves, teeth, mouth, eyes and blood vessels – keep the differential wide
- First-line pharmacological treatment for TN is carbamazepine

108

Altered Sensation, Numbness and Tingling

Louise Mathias, Felix Miller-Molloy, Gregory Oxenham, and Hamish Morrison

EMERGENCY DEPARTMENT, MALE, 40. TINGLING HANDS AND DIFFICULTY WALKING

HPC: For 3 days needs assistance to get out of car, unable to walk, progressive leg weakness: starting in feet and ankles, moving up. Tingling hands/feet bilaterally. No trauma, drug use or change in vision/hearing/speech. **PMHx:** Gastroenteritis 3 weeks ago which self-resolved.

O/E: Obs: HR 80, T 36, BP 120/60, RR 22, 98% on air. **Resp:** Chest clear bilaterally. **Skin:** No rashes/ulcers. **Neuro:** Unsteady gait when assisted with two people. **Tone:** Normal in all limbs. **Power:** 2/5 bilaterally in dorsi/plantar flexion of feet, 3/5 in hip/knee flexors/extensors, 3/5 ab/adduction of fingers and flexion/extension of wrists bilaterally, 5/5 in rest of upper limbs. **Reflexes:** Absent throughout. **Sensation:** Normal joint proprioception and pinprick sensation. Coordination – normal upper limbs, lower limbs too weak to assess. No evidence of CN involvement.

1. List five causes of peripheral neuropathy.
2. Which organism is classically responsible for Guillain-Barré syndrome?
3. What is the inheritance pattern of Charcot-Marie-Tooth disease?

Answers: 1. Remember A–E; A = Alcohol, B = Vitamin B12 deficiency, C = CKD, D = Diabetes, E = Everything else, including vasculitis. 2. *Campylobacter jejuni* (similarity of membrane molecules to peripheral nerve molecules, hence autoimmune reaction). 3. Autosomal dominant.

TABLE 108.1

	Features	Investigations	Management
PERIPHERAL NERVOUS SYSTEM			
Diabetic neuropathy	**RFs:** diabetes (poorly controlled), dyslipidaemia, obesity. **Hx & O/E:** numb/tingling – glove and stocking distribution, worse at night. Risk of ulcer, infection, neuropathic deformity – 'Charcot Joint'	**HbA1c:** regular checks – high. **Test sensation:** with 10 g monofilament. Foot pulses – get ABPI if peripheral vascular disease suspected	**Analgesia:** trial of duloxetine or amitriptyline. Optimal glycaemic control

TABLE 108.1 (Cont'd)

	Features	Investigations	Management
Sciatica	**RFs:** age, obesity, occupation, inactivity. **Hx & O/E:** sciatic roots-L4-S3. Unilateral pain radiates to foot, worse on coughing, lumbar flexion. Numbness in dermatome and weakness in myotome suggest nerve root compression. Damage can be idiopathic or due to pelvic tumours/ fracture	**Clinical diagnosis.** Exclude cauda equina syndrome (see *192. BACK PAIN*). Straight leg raise – positive if pain	Settles in 4–6 weeks. Remain active. Analgesia for lower back pain with caution (± PPI). No evidence for opioids, benzodiazepines, gabapentinoids, anti-epileptics
Guillain-Barré syndrome	**RFs:** 2–3 weeks post *Campylobacter* or virus. **Hx & O/E:** bilateral symmetrical weakness that progresses proximally. Facial or bulbar weakness, hypo/ areflexia, sensory involvement (15%), autonomic dysfunction. Potential progression to respiratory failure. Miller-Fisher variant; triad of ophthalmoplegia, ataxia, areflexia	**Clinical diagnosis** in many. **CSF:** elevated protein, normal WCC. High IgG, ganglioside antibodies. Consider Lyme/ syphilis/HIV. **Nerve conduction studies:** acute demyelinating polyneuropathy. **Lung function:** FVC (need for respiratory support). ECG, serial BP monitoring (if autonomic features)	Respiratory support if needed. Plasma exchange or IV immunoglobulin. DVT prophylaxis. Rehabilitation – may take months
Hereditary motor sensory neuropathy (Charcot-Marie-Tooth disease)	Presents age 5–15 years, adult onset possible. Progressive symmetrical motor/sensory, esp. hands, feet, legs. **Hx & O/E:** high-arched feet (Fig. 108.1), abnormal steppage gait, difficulty walking as child – can delay motor milestones. Leg/distal thigh wasting 'inverted champagne bottle'	**RFs:** FHx of neuropathy – hereditary. **Nerve conduction studies:** various findings. **Genetic testing:** most common PMP22. Nerve US and magnetic resonance neurography	MDT approach including physio, rehabilitation. Orthopaedic surgery may be required, e.g. for pes cavus. Genetic counselling

CENTRAL NERVOUS SYSTEM

	Features	Investigations	Management
Multiple sclerosis	**RFs:** younger patients (20–40s), female, northern latitudes, FHx, history of autoimmune disease. **Hx & O/E:** often starts with one symptom-unilateral optic neuritis, diplopia, ataxia, sensory disturbance and/or weakness in a limb, TGN (see *107. FACIAL PAIN*). Uhthoff's phenomenon (worse when hot), Lhermitte's, internuclear ophthalmoplegia. Three patterns; relapsing/remitting, primary or secondary progressive	**Clinical criteria-based diagnosis,** e.g. McDonald criteria. **MRI:** periventricular plaques, Dawson fingers (lesions surrounding corpus callosum), spinal cord lesions – repeat imaging or addition of contrast can demonstrate dissemination in time. **LP:** oligoclonal bands of IgG present in CSF but not serum	**Acute disabling relapse:** high-dose cortico-steroids, e.g. 1000 mg IV methylprednisolone OD for 5 days. **Disease-modifying drug** (e.g. β-inteferons/ monoclonal ABs such as alemtuzumab). **Symptomatic management:** baclofen/ physiotherapy for spasticity, analgesia targeting neuropathic pain, colonic irrigation, intermittent catheterisation

(Continued)

TABLE 108.1   (Cont'd)

	Features	Investigations	Management
Cauda equina syndrome	See *192. BACK PAIN*		
Stroke	See *101. SPEECH AND LANGUAGE PROBLEMS* **Watershed strokes**: ischaemia from severe systemic hypotension can lead to bilateral weakness/ sensory changes.		
Subacute combined cord degeneration	See *111. UNSTEADINESS*		
Cervical myelopathy	**Hx & O/E:** neck pain, reduced ROM neck, weak/reduced dexterity upper limbs, sphincter disturbance. UMN signs, possibly sensory impairment distally, muscle wasting, gait ataxia	**RFs:** degenerative 'spondylitic' cervical spine, spinal cord tumour/ infection, trauma. **MRI spine:** compression, myelopathy. High T2 signal	Neurosurgery/orthopaedic surgery if appropriate. Physiotherapy walking/ balance aids and exercises

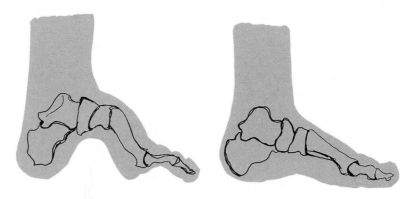

Fig. 108.1 High arched foot in Charcot-Marie-Tooth disease. (Illustrated by Dr Hollie Blaber.)

In the vignette, progressive ascending weakness and sensory loss suggests Guillain-Barré syndrome (GBS). A Campylobacter gastroenteritis is sometimes implicated, and can trigger an autoimmune reaction against peripheral nerves causing lower motor neurone signs (reduced reflexes, flaccidity). Whilst often clinically diagnosed, an LP and nerve conduction studies can be useful. The sub-acute time course and ascending weakness/sensory loss distribution are crucial in diagnosis of GBS. Stroke is a rare cause of acute bilateral leg weakness, but can be caused by single lesions in anatomical variants of the anterior cerebral artery. A parasagittal meningioma could also present with bilateral lower limb weakness.

REVISION TIPS

- Absent reflexes + progressive ascending weakness: consider Guillain-Barré
- The symmetrical distribution and progression of weakness/sensory loss is key in diagnosis
- Know the classic features of MS

109

Fasciculations

Louise Mathias and Harriet Ball

HPC: Small tasks (e.g. buttoning a shirt, writing) more difficult. Recently, tongue twitching, some difficulty swallowing. 2 kg weight loss over 2 months. **DHx:** Ramipril. **SHx:** Ex-smoker with a moderate alcohol intake. No FHx.

O/E: Apyrexial, fasciculations in R bicep/tongue. **Power:** 4/5 R upper limb, 5/5 in L upper limb. **Coordination:** Decreased in R hand. **Reflexes:** Brisk throughout. **Tone and sensation:** Normal throughout. Slight dysarthria. **CVS:** HR 70, BP 135/80, HS I + II + 0. **Ix:** Bloods- no abnormalities detected.

1. What are the main electrolyte abnormalities causing fasciculations?
2. What signs may be observed if the patient experiences bulbar symptoms?

Answers: 1. Hypo/hypercalcaemia, hypomagnesaemia, hypophosphataemia. 2. 'Bulbar' refers to the lower cranial nerves (CN) controlled by the medulla oblongata (Fig. 109.1); bulbar signs include dysphagia/sialorrhea (CN9), dysarthria (CN10), restricted neck movements (CN11), fasciculations/tongue weakness (CN12).

TABLE 109.1

	Features	Investigations	Management
Motor neurone disease	Age 55–75, often no FHx. **Hx & O/E:** progressive LMN (weak/fasciculation) + UMN (brisk reflexes, spasticity) symptoms, with normal sensation. Weight loss from calorie burning/difficulty eating	Rule out electrolyte problem/hyperthyroidism; CK normal or mildly raised. Nerve conduction studies and EMG to detect lower motor neurone lesion. MRI (brain/ cord) to exclude structural cause. Respiratory function tests. Dementia screening (ALS is linked to FTD)	Physiotherapy, OT, nutritional supplement. Muscle cramps; quinine or baclofen
	+ Bulbar symptoms of dysarthria/dysphagia		Unsafe swallow/malnutrition, consider nasogastric or gastrostomy feeding; consider speech and language therapy
	+ Dyspnoea and history of chest infections		Discuss non-invasive ventilation, palliative care. Chest physiotherapy. Antibiotics if chest infection

(Continued)

TABLE 109.1   (Cont'd)

	Features	Investigations	Management
Benign fasciculations	Often post-exertion or stress/ anxiety, high caffeine intake, poor sleep. Not progressive	No UMN signs/weakness. Rule out electrolyte derangement	Explanation; stress management, avoid stimulants
Electrolyte imbalance or drug toxicity	Poor diet, vomiting/diarrhoea, malabsorption, alcohol, long-term steroids, toxins such as lithium	Renal function, calcium, phosphate, vitamin (D/Bs). ECG. GI investigation	Varied diet; supplements-review medications
OTHER EXAMPLES OF COMBINED UMN AND LMN SIGNS			
Combined spinal cord and root/ peripheral nerve lesion	Older age (degenerative disc), trauma; may co-exist with peripheral neuropathy. Often sensory and motor	MRI imaging of the cord and surrounding. Nerve conduction studies	Manage comorbidities such as diabetes. Surgery if impingement of cord/root. See *111. UNSTEADINESS*
Vitamin B12 deficiency	Subacute combined degeneration of the cord; see *111. UNSTEADINESS*		

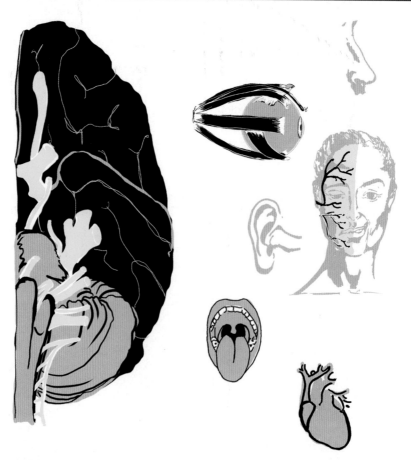

Fig. 109.1 Origins of the cranial nerves. The cranial nerves are numbered according to their origin, from the front of the brain to the bottom of the brainstem. Some of their key functions are illustrated on the right. The "bulbar" cranial nerves (9–12) originate in the medulla oblongata (an old name for which is "bulb"); their functions include motor control of the tongue and pharynx, as well as parasympathetic supply to the body.

Fasciculations are a lower motor neurone (LMN) sign which are most often benign or due to electrolyte abnormality. Combined with upper motor neurone (UMN) signs, such as brisk reflexes or spasticity, and a progressive history, motor neurone disease (MND) should be considered, which is likely in the vignette. There are four clinical patterns to MND; commonest is amyotrophic lateral sclerosis (ALS), which has prognosis from symptom onset of 2–5 years, and with a subset also having fronto-temporal dementia (FTD). Progressive bulbar palsy initially affects the bulbar cranial nerves (9–12), causing fasciculations and weakness of the tongue, and early swallowing difficulty; it has the shortest survival of the four subtypes.

Progressive muscular atrophy presents with lower rather than upper motor neurone signs, and often distal muscles are affected before proximal. Primary lateral sclerosis presents with predominantly UMN signs, and is more slowly progressive than other forms. In each of these four subtypes, sensation is spared.

REVISION TIPS

- Lower motor neurone signs: fasciculations, wasting, weakness, decreased/absent reflexes
- Upper motor neurone signs: brisk reflexes, increased tone, weakness, spasticity, clonus, Babinski's sign

110

Neuromuscular Weakness

Gregory Oxenham and Hamish Morrison

EMERGENCY DEPARTMENT, MALE, 65. UNSTEADY GAIT

HPC: Legs are getting weaker, difficulty walking for a month, struggles rising from chair. Weakness improves when walking around. 5 kg of weight loss over this time; attributed to dry mouth and difficulty chewing food. His COPD symptoms are unchanged, no haemoptysis. Constipated, BO 3 days ago. No altered sensation/tremors/muscle pains. **PMHx:** COPD. **DHx:** Salbutamol, umeclidinium/vilanterol inhalers. **SHx:** Ex-smoker 40 pack years, 20 units/week, lives with partner, independent.

O/E: Appears cachectic, mild SOB at rest without respiratory distress. **Neuro:** Weakness standing from sitting, unsteady gait. Proximal muscle weakness, legs more than arms with global hyporeflexia. Subtle R ptosis and diplopia on right gaze, otherwise normal cranial nerves. **Ix:** CT chest; invasive mass at the right lobar bronchi, extensive mediastinal lymph node involvement.

1. What type of drug is pyridostigmine and why does it help alleviate symptoms of myasthaenia gravis?
2. List some causes of asthenia/fatigue (often called 'weakness' by patients).

Answers: 1. Acetylcholinesterase inhibitor. By inhibiting acetylcholinesterase, pyridostigmine results in more acetylcholine in the synaptic cleft available for neuromuscular transmission. 2. Depression, chemotherapy/cancer, anaemia, heart failure, CKD, hypothyroidism, PE, ILD, fibromyalgia, dehydration – there are many more.

TABLE 110.1

	Features	Investigations	Management
PRIMARILY NEUROLOGICAL WEAKNESS			
Stroke	See *101. SPEECH AND LANGUAGE PROBLEMS*		
Multiple sclerosis	See *108. ALTERED SENSATION, NUMBNESS AND TINGLING*		
Guillain-Barré syndrome	See *108. ALTERED SENSATION, NUMBNESS AND TINGLING*		

TABLE 110.1   (Cont'd)

	Features	Investigations	Management
Lambert-Eaton myasthenic syndrome (LEMS)	RFs: paraneoplastic (n.b. small cell lung Ca) or autoimmune. Hx & O/E: weakness usually LL predominant (gait difficulty often first sign, weak thighs and hip girdle) then bulbar, ± eye involvement. Dry mouth, constipation, impotence (from autonomic neuropathy). Typically no fatiguability or variability. Hyporeflexia and weakness that *improves on exercise* (unlike MG)	Repetitive nerve stimulation: showing an increase in amplitude after stimulation. Anti-P/Q voltage-gated Ca-channel serology (VGCC). CXR ± CT chest (tumour identified in ~50%)	Treatment of underlying malignancy. Often improves LEMS. Paraneoplastic cause should be considered up to 5 years from symptom onset. 3,4-Diaminopyridine. Only licenced symptom treatment in the UK; anticholinesterases can also be used. Prednisolone, steroid-sparing agent, e.g. azathioprine. Intravenous Ig if severe
Myasthenia gravis (MG)	See *102. FACIAL WEAKNESS*		

PRIMARILY MUSCULAR WEAKNESS

	Features	Investigations	Management
Alcohol use disorder	May present confused/withdrawing with muscle weakness. See *169. ADDICTION*		
Glucocorticoid excess (Cushing syndrome or disease)	RFs: long-term steroid use (usually), rarely pituitary/adrenal tumour. Hx & O/E: proximal weakness. Supraclavicular fat pad, striae, osteoporosis, HTN, muscle wasting, T2DM	Creatine kinase: normal. Dexamethasone suppression tests (low and high dose)	Limit exogenous steroids. If Cushing disease, removal of pituitary tumour. Adrenal adenoma; adrenalectomy
Myositis including dermatomyositis	See *160. CHRONIC PAIN*		

TABLE 110.2   UMN and LMN Signs

Table 110.2	Upper Motor Neuron Lesion	Lower Motor Neuron Lesion	Neuromuscular Junction	Musculoskeletal
Inspection	Normal/spastic posture	Fasciculations, muscle wasting	Normal/minimal wasting	Muscle wasting
Tone	Increased (spasticity)	Normal/decreased (flaccid paralysis)	Normal/decreased	Variable
Power	Decreased	Decreased	Fatiguability	Decreased
Reflexes	Increased	Decreased or absent	Normal	Normal

The man in the vignette has features consistent with malignancy, and the CT confirms the suspicions. Many patients with advanced malignancy can appear weak, but generally as asthenia – the general sensation of whole-body weakness/fatigue, as opposed to anything localised to part of the nervous system. However, ptosis, hyporeflexia and weakness localising to proximal muscles are definite neurological findings not c/w generalised fatigue – pointing to a malignant paraneoplastic syndrome. His improvement with movement is a classic reference to the Lambert-Eaton myasthenic syndrome and this is commonly associated with small-cell lung cancer (in exams especially).

REVISION TIPS

- When told a patient has weakness, elicit whether this is true neuromuscular weakness (Table 110.2)
- Questions including a raised CK are likely referring to rhabdomyolysis or myositis; or (if they're being tricky) myocardial infarcts

111

Unsteadiness

Margarita Fox and Hamish Morrison

HPC: Feeling generally fatigued/dizzy, low mood. Progressive tingling, burning and loss of sensation in her feet, feels off balance in the dark. More recently, weakness/stiffness affecting her legs. Getting worse over 3 months. **PMHx:** Coeliac, GORD. **DHx:** Omeprazole. **SHx:** Smoking 10 pack years. **Alcohol:** 10 units/week.

O/E: Neurological: ataxic gait, Romberg's positive (loss of balance with eyes closed), bilateral brisk knee reflexes, absent ankle jerks and extensor plantars. Decreased vibration sense throughout lower limbs. **Ix:** HbA1C: 35 mmol/mol (normal 20–38 mmol/mol), serum B12 90 pg/mL (200–900 pg/mL)

1. A 70-year-old develops abrupt onset unsteadiness. O/E nystagmus, ataxia, pinprick loss in right trigeminal distribution, no facial drooping, light touch intact over face. Loss of pinprick in left upper and lower limbs, power 5/5 throughout. Which vessel territory is responsible for this clinical stroke syndrome?
2. 27-year-old patient with relapsing/remitting MS presents with 3 days of progressive lower limb paraesthesia and unsteadiness. What management is indicated at this stage?

Answers: 1. Lateral medullary syndrome can be caused by posterior inferior cerebellar artery (PICA) territory infarcts. 'Crossed signs' in questions often indicate brainstem pathology (ipsilateral pain and temperature loss over the face, contralateral limb/torso pain and temperature loss, ataxia and nystagmus). 2. MS relapse: consider methylprednisolone 500 mg PO OD 5 days. Admit for IV steroids if PO unsuccessful/severe symptoms

TABLE 111.1			
	Features	**Investigations**	**Management**
Alcohol-related peripheral neuropathy and cerebellar degeneration	**RFs:** heavy alcohol use, and also the RFs for subacute degeneration of the cord. Peripheral neuropathy due to direct toxic effects or reduced B vitamin absorption (predominantly sensory). Cerebellar degeneration: broad-based gait, intention tremor, dysdiadochokinesia, dysarthria. B1 (Thiamine) deficiency – Wernicke's encephalopathy (confusion, ataxia, ophthalmoplegia, nystagmus)	Gamma-GT elevated. AST:ALT >2 suggests alcoholic liver disease. **MRI:** cerebellar atrophy	IV **Thiamine** if Wernicke's suspected. Regular PO thiamine if at risk of ongoing deficiency. Exclude concomitant folate deficiency and treat if required. See *169. ADDICTION*

(Continued)

TABLE 111.1 (Cont'd)

	Features	Investigations	Management
Subacute combined degeneration of the cord	**RFs:** low B12 (diet), malabsorption (IBD, coeliac, pernicious anaemia), medications (PPIs, metformin), frequent nitrous oxide use. **O/E:** classic triad: extensor plantars (UMN); absent knee and ankle reflexes (LMN). Dorsal columns (Fig. 111.1); loss of proprioception/vibration leads to unsteadiness/ataxic gait. Later weak, hyperreflexia, spasticity. Subacute history– months. Romberg's positive: may present with falls due to ataxia	FBC (± macrocytic anaemia), B12 (<200 pg/ml), folate (± co-deficient). Homocysteine and methylmalonic acid (MMA) levels if history of nitrous oxide use. **MRI:** T2/FLAIR hyperintensity in dorsal columns, typically thoracic cord first	Treat B12 deficiency. Hydroxocobalamin 1000 mcg IM alternate days for 2 weeks followed by prolonged oral course. Reversible if discovered early
Multiple sclerosis	See *108. ALTERED SENSATION, NUMBNESS AND TINGLING*		
Guillain-Barré syndrome	See *108. ALTERED SENSATION, NUMBNESS AND TINGLING*		
Posterior circulation stroke – cerebellar	See *101. SPEECH AND LANGUAGE PROBLEMS*		
Cerebellar ataxia; Friedrich's (FA), spinocerebellar ataxia (SCA), paraneoplastic	**RFs:** FHx, certain cancers. **Hx & O/E:** incoordination (gait, fine movement), dysarthria, nystagmus, intention tremor, past pointing. Onset depends on the cause; genetic causes commonly have adult and even elderly onset	**MRI brain** (cerebellar atrophy). **Genetic testing panel.** FBC, U&E, LFTs (exclude EtOH), coeliac screen, vitamin E. Paraneoplastic antibody panel	Treat cause. Supportive; speech and language therapy, physiotherapy, mobility aids. See also *105. TREMOR*

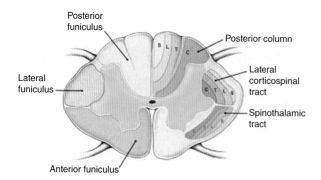

Fig. 111.1 Schematic of posterior column, corticospinal tract and spinothalamic tract in the spinal cord. (Reproduced with permission from Raslan AM. Percutaneous cordotomy and trigeminal tractotomy. In *Youmans and Winn Neurological Surgery*, 4-Volume Set. Elsevier; 2017:Figure 183-1. Copyright © 2017 Elsevier Inc. All rights reserved.)

Maintenance of gait, posture and balance involves several systems; deficit in a patient's cognition, muscle strength, peripheral sensation, vestibular apparatus, vision, coordination or even footwear can lead to 'unsteadiness'. While not mentioned here, some common causes of unsteadiness are osteoarthritis, frailty, infections in cognitively susceptible patients who develop delirium, and diabetic peripheral neuropathy. In the vignette, physical exam, time course, low B12 level and risk factors for poor B12 absorption (coeliac, PPIs) imply subacute combined degeneration of the cord as the diagnosis.

REVISION TIPS

Ataxia: unsteady motion of limbs/torso due to defect in gross coordination of muscle movements
- **Cerebellar** (cerebellar stroke, alcohol, SOL, MS, B12 deficiency, medications, genetic (SCA, FA), paraneoplastic)
- **Sensory** (peripheral, e.g. acute inflammatory demyelinating polyneuropathy, diabetes, B12 deficiency)
- **Vestibular** (labyrinthitis, Meniere's, acoustic neuroma)

112

Sleep Problems

Natalia Hacket, Connie Glover, and Sofia Eriksson

GP CONSULTATION, MALE, 65. **SLEEPINESS**

HPC: Excessive daytime sleepiness for a few weeks. Waking periodically through the night; feels tired during daytime, difficulty concentrating. Wife describes snoring/ 'gasping' during sleep. Otherwise well, denies life stressors. **PMHx:** Hypertension, NIDDM, 15-pack year history. **DHx:** Amlodipine. Tried OTC 'Nytol' for this issue.

O/E: BMI 37, no nasopharyngeal obstruction or craniofacial abnormalities

1. What is your top differential for the vignette?
2. What differential is likely if he describes a burning sensation in his throat when he lies back?
3. What would you suspect if he reported episodes with collapse during the day associated with strong emotions and feeling paralysed as he fell asleep?
4. What would you suspect if he had not slept in 48 hours but felt he had superpowers?

Answers: 1. OSA. 2. GORD. 3. Narcolepsy. 4. Mania/bipolar affective disorder.

TABLE 112.1

	Features	Investigations	Management
Obstructive sleep apnoea syndrome (OSA)	**RFs:** male, obese, older, FHx, alcohol, smoking, adenotonsillar. **Hx & O/E:** excessive daytime sleepiness, irregular breathing and cycles of arousal from sleep	Epworth Sleepiness Scale (Fig. 112.1). Pulse oximetry (overnight oxygen desaturation index), respiratory polygraphy	Respiratory sleep clinic. Lifestyle; weight loss, smoking cessation. CPAP. See also *57. SNORING*
Insomnia	**RFs:** pain, depression, anxiety, mania, dementia, caffeine, medications (e.g. steroids), often no identifiable cause. **Hx & O/E:** difficulty sleeping with enough opportunity to sleep, resulting in impaired daytime function. Normal ENT and neurological examination	Guided by history. Sleep diary	Treat cause, e.g. CBT, antidepressant, analgesia. Sleep hygiene. Hypnotics –short term e.g. benzodiazepine, zopiclone

(Continued)

TABLE 112.1 (Cont'd)

	Features	Investigations	Management
GORD	Gastro-oesophageal reflux disease; see *29. HOARSENESS AND VOICE CHANGE*		
Circadian rhythm disorders	**RFs:** shift work or jet lag disorder	Social history	Sleep hygiene
Restless legs syndrome	Irresistible urge to move limbs, sensations (e.g. pins and needles, burning), worse in the evening, and involuntary jerks	Ferritin, renal function, FBC, TFTs, blood glucose, B12 (can help identify cause)	Treat cause if found
Narcolepsy	Excessive daytime sleepiness, disrupted sleep, vivid dreams, cataplexy, sleep paralysis, hypnagogic hallucinations	Polysomnography. Multiple sleep latency testing. CSF orexin (hypocretin) levels	Sleep hygiene. Stimulants; modafinil (sleepiness) anti-depressant (cataplexy)
Generalised Anxiety Disorder	Worry causing sleeping difficulty, current life stressors	GAD-7 score. TFTs, LFTs, ECG, urine drug screen, glucose whilst anxious, 24 hour urine VMA	Education, self-help techniques, talking therapy, medications. Treat cause
Bipolar affective disorder (BPAD)	Manic episode; irregular sleep-wake cycle, activity at night (unlikely to complain of fatigue)	Collateral history, MSE, physical exam. Bloods (FBC, TFTs, CRP)	Mental health service, psychotherapy, SSRI + antipsychotic, mood stabiliser (lithium)
Depression	See *164. LOW MOOD/ AFFECTIVE PROBLEMS*		
Post-traumatic stress disorder	Hyper-arousal, Nightmares, flashbacks	History	Watchful waiting, focussed CBT, EMDR

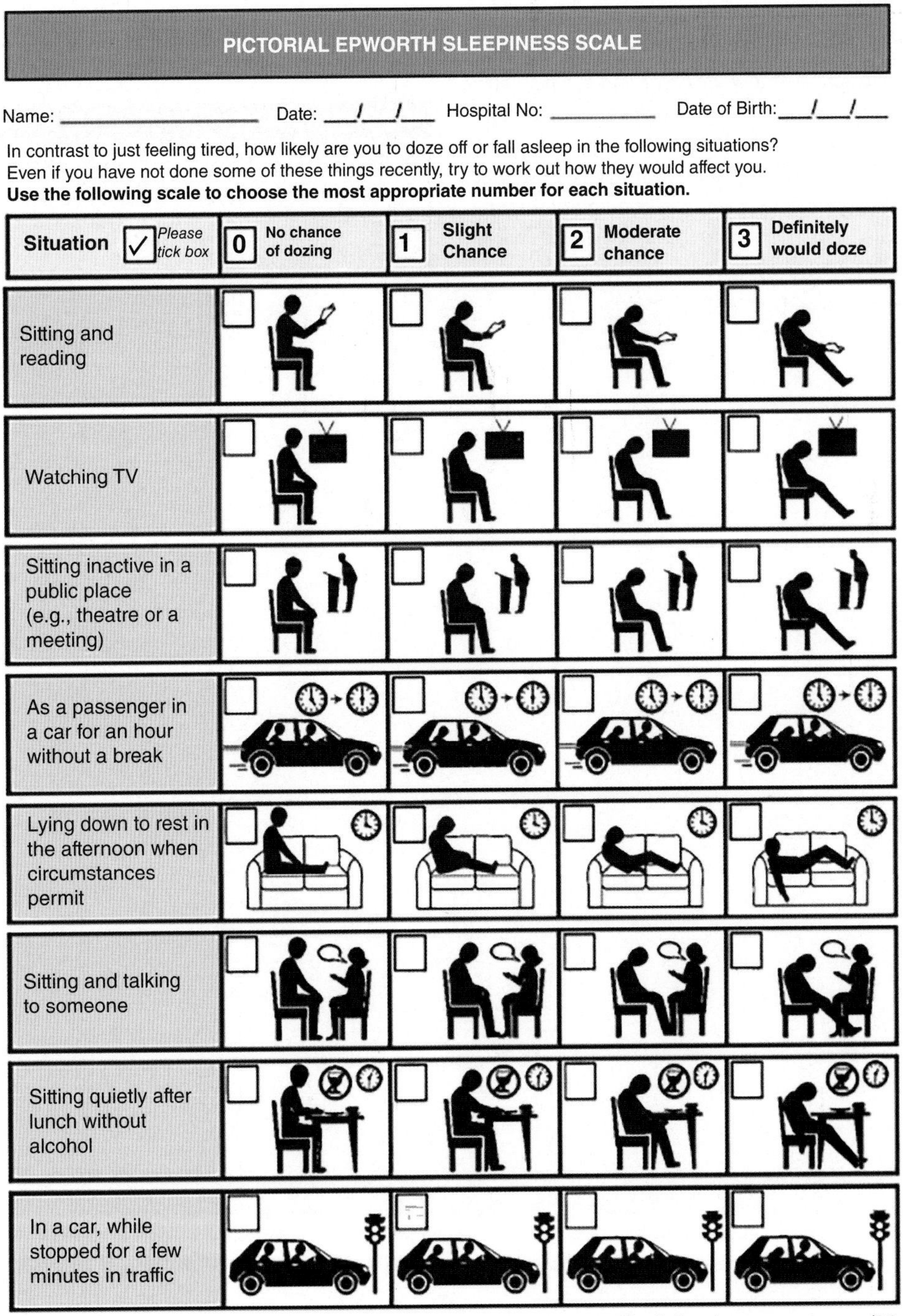

PICTORIAL EPWORTH SLEEPINESS SCALE

Name: ______________ Date: ___/___/___ Hospital No: __________ Date of Birth: ___/___/___

In contrast to just feeling tired, how likely are you to doze off or fall asleep in the following situations?
Even if you have not done some of these things recently, try to work out how they would affect you.
Use the following scale to choose the most appropriate number for each situation.

Situation ✓ *Please tick box*	0 No chance of dozing	1 Slight Chance	2 Moderate chance	3 Definitely would doze
Sitting and reading	☐	☐	☐	☐
Watching TV	☐	☐	☐	☐
Sitting inactive in a public place (e.g., theatre or a meeting)	☐	☐	☐	☐
As a passenger in a car for an hour without a break	☐	☐	☐	☐
Lying down to rest in the afternoon when circumstances permit	☐	☐	☐	☐
Sitting and talking to someone	☐	☐	☐	☐
Sitting quietly after lunch without alcohol	☐	☐	☐	☐
In a car, while stopped for a few minutes in traffic	☐	☐	☐	☐

Total sleepiness score /24

Fig. 112.1 Pictorial Epworth sleepiness scale. (Reproduced with permission from Johns MW. A new method for measuring daytime sleepiness: the Epworth sleepiness scale. *Sleep* 1991;14:540–545.)

History needs to identify if there are symptoms or risk factors of an underlying cause (e.g. depression). Insomnia duration < 3 months is often related to a life event and resolves with time. If >3 months, there is often co-existence of other psychiatric or medical conditions. If no cause is found, keeping a sleep diary and education around sleep hygiene are first steps. For persisting problems, cognitive behavioural therapy for insomnia (CBT-I) is preferred to hypnotics, due to lack of side effects and ongoing benefits.

REVISION TIPS

- Physical (e.g. OSA) and psychological (e.g., anxiety disorders) causes can result in insomnia
- A collateral history, e.g. from a partner, can provide important clues

113

Raised Intracranial Pressure

*Margarita Fox, Berenice Aguirrezabala Armbruster,
and Matthew Boissaud-Cooke*

NEUROLOGY CLINIC, FEMALE, 32.
HEADACHE FOR 15 MONTHS

HPC: 'Troublesome' headache, affects the whole of her head, throbbing pain. For 4 months, worse in the morning, occasionally waking her up, worse with loud noise. Feeling sick, occasionally vomits. Bright lights hurt her eyes, struggling to read, vision is blurred, 'whooshing' sound in her ears. **PMHx:** Previous acne vulgaris, struggles with her weight. COCP, no allergies. Primary school teacher, occasional alcohol, non-smoker.

O/E: BMI 30. Fundoscopy confirms papilloedema. Her visual acuity is reduced. The remainder of her cranial nerve and peripheral nerve examination is unremarkable.

1. 29-year-old with 2-day severe headache, N&V – mother had two unprovoked DVTs in her 30s and is on lifelong anticoagulation. GCS 13 (E3V4M6), difficulty remembering certain words, papilloedema, no focal weakness. What investigation?
2. What are the most common sources of cerebral metastases?

Answers: 1. MR venogram looking for venous sinus thrombosis. 2. Lung cancer, breast cancer, renal cell carcinoma, melanoma, colorectal cancer.

TABLE 113.1

	Features	Investigations	Management
Idiopathic intracranial hypertension (IIH)	**Hx & O/E:** headache worse first thing in the morning and with straining/coughing. N&V. Photophobia, phonophobia, visual disturbance (visual loss/blurring, diplopia), ± papilloedema. Pulsatile tinnitus. Neck/back/radicular pain. Gradual visual deterioration, rarely rapid. Normal neurological examination, ± cranial nerve (CN) abnormalities	**RFs:** obesity, female, social deprivation, working age. **LP:** ↑ opening pressure (>25 cm H_2O) with normal CSF constituents (Table 113.2). Visual fields. **Fundoscopy/OCT:** papilloedema. **Neuroimaging:** to exclude SOL, hydrocephalus, venous sinus thrombosis. Various features possible (empty sella, transverse sinus stenosis, etc.)	Weight loss (reduces ICP/headaches, improves papilloedema/vision). Can induce remission. Acetazolamide, topiramate, analgesics (paracetamol, NSAIDs, triptans, TCAs). Surgery if vision threatened (fulminant): CSF diversion (lumbar drain, ventriculo-peritoneal/lumbar-peritoneal shunt), optic nerve sheath fenestration

(Continued)

TABLE 113.1 (Cont'd)

	Features	Investigations	Management
Cerebral venous (sinus) thrombosis	RFs: young/middle-aged women, OCP, pregnancy. Para-meningeal infections (e.g. sinusitis), cancer. Haematological disorders, PMHx of VTE. Hx & O/E: progressive headache, focal neurology, stroke, seizures. Papilloedema, reduced level of consciousness. *Cavernous sinus:* ocular pain, proptosis. CN palsy (3, 4, 6, 5 (ophthalmic division))	MR/CT venography: to identify venous occlusion. CT head: to identify cerebral oedema/intraparenchymal haemorrhage/hydrocephalus. Bloods: FBC, U&Es, LFTs, clotting, D-dimer, thrombophilia screen, ESR/CRP.	Treat the underlying cause, the thrombosis and complications. • Anticoagulation: start treatment with LMWH or unfractionated heparin, then convert to an oral anticoagulant. Duration depends on aetiology • If seizures – anti-epileptic drugs • In certain select cases, can consider: endovascular mechanical thrombectomy, decompressive craniectomy (large infarction, haemorrhage, cerebral oedema), CSF diversion for hydrocephalus
Brain abscess	RFs: congenital heart disease, endocarditis, pulmonary AVM, sinusitis, dental procedures. Haematogenous, local spread, direct inoculation. Hx & O/E: features of raised ICP, focal neurological deficit, seizures, systemic features of infection (fever, malaise). Quick onset	Inflammatory markers normal or elevated. Blood cultures. CT head + contrast: ring-enhancing lesion, oedema. MRI head + gadolinium/DWI sequences. Consider primary source: CXR, EchoCG, orthopantomogram	Urgent referral to neurosurgery. Consider needle aspiration (MC&S) or excision. Search for (suspected) primary source of infection. Antimicrobial therapy. Risk of seizures: consider anti-epileptic drugs
Brain neoplasm	Clinical features of raised ICP, focal neurological deficit, seizures, endocrine dysfunction (pituitary tumours), incidental finding. Benign/malignant (primary/ secondary)	CT Head ± contrast. MRI head + gadolinium/ DWI sequences: characterise tumour, exclude abscess. CT TAP: to identify primary source of tumour	MDT. Management depends on patient age, performance status, tumour type and location; observation, surgical biopsy/ resection, ± radiotherapy, ± chemotherapy/immunotherapy, ± adjunctive therapy (anti-epileptics, steroids)
Meningitis	See *93. NECK PAIN/STIFFNESS*		
Encephalitis	Headache, fever, altered mental status, focal deficit. Usually viral (HSV-1, VZV), can be autoimmune (anti-NMDA-receptor encephalitis)	Inflammatory. Blood cultures. Serum glucose. Throat swab. MRI head: parenchymal enhancement. Lumbar puncture	Viral: acyclovir. Autoimmune: steroids, IVIG, plasmapheresis, immunosuppress
Aneurysmal subarachnoid haemorrhage	See *49. HEAD INJURY*		

TABLE 113.1 (Cont'd)

	Features	Investigations	Management
COMPLICATIONS			
Visual loss	Papilloedema, optic atrophy, vision loss (peripheral first). Enlarged blind spot	Visual acuity and field testing. Fundoscopy + optic disc photographs	Worsening vision despite medical management; treat the cause (e.g. CSF diversion in IIH)
Herniation (uncal/tonsillar/cingulate)	Depends on aetiology/acuteness of raised ICP; • Stroke • Seizure • Reduced GCS • Neurological deficit (hemiparesis, pupillary abnormalities) • Cushing's response/triad (HTN, bradycardia, irregular respiration) - late sign, brainstem herniation imminent	CT head	Depends on cause: consider emergency decompressive surgery. **Acute raised ICP:** – Head elevation – Osmotherapy (hypertonic saline, mannitol) – ICU hyperventilation

TABLE 113.2 CSF Analysis

CSF Analysis	Normal Adults	Pathology Interpretation
Pressure	Opening pressure 10–20 cmH$_2$O	**Elevated:** • Raised ICP (e.g. tumour, bleed) • CSF flow disruption (e.g. hydrocephalus) **Decreased:** dehydration, shock, intracranial hypotension (iatrogenic, spontaneous)
Appearance	Clear, colourless, not turbid, similar consistency to water	• **Xanthochromic (yellow, orange, or pink):** RBC breakdown • **Cloudy or turbid:** presence of RBC, WBC, protein or bilirubin • **Increased viscosity:** malignancy or meningitis
CSF Glucose	2.8–4.2 mmol/L (or ≥60% of the concentration of plasma glucose)	**Decreased:** presence of cells that metabolise glucose (e.g. bacteria, malignancy, WBC in inflammation)
CSF Protein	0.15–0.45 g/L (or <1% of the serum protein concentration)	**Increased:** infection (bacterial, viral, fungal), malignancy
CSF RBC	No RBC	**Elevated:** SAH, 'traumatic' tap – blood that leaked into the CSF sample during collection
CSF WBC	• 0–5 cells/µL • No neutrophils • Primarily lymphocytes	**Neutrophilia:** bacterial infection **Lymphocytosis:** viral infection, fungal infection, TB infection

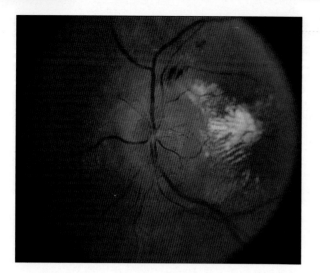

Fig. 113.1 Optic disc oedema. (From Sadun AA, Wang MY. Papilledema and raised intracranial pressure. In: *Ophthalmology*. Elsevier; 2019. Copyright © 2019 Elsevier Inc.)

The most likely diagnosis in the vignette is idiopathic intracranial hypertension (IIH, previously known as: benign intracranial hypertension, pseudotumour cerebri). Headache is the most prominent symptom, which can be accompanied by vision loss, vomiting and tinnitus characterised by a pulsating, rhythmic sound. Ophthalmoscopy may show papilloedema – a sign of raised intracranial pressure (Fig. 113.1). Not everyone with IIH has papilloedema.

REVISION TIPS

- <u>Red flags for raised ICP:</u> morning headaches + N&V, headache increased by Valsalva manoeuvres (cough, straining, bending forward), visual changes, pulsatile tinnitus, seizure, focal neurological deficit, reduced level of consciousness
- <u>Early signs of raised ICP:</u> mental status (irritability, restlessness, confusion), headache, vomiting
- <u>Late signs of raised ICP:</u> Cushing reflex, fixed dilated pupils, Cheyne-Stokes breathing, decorticate/decerebrate posturing, stupor/coma

114

Amenorrhoea

Hannah Clark, Rebecca Newhouse, and Claudia Burton

GYNAECOLOGY CLINIC, FEMALE, AGED 15. AMENORRHOEA AND ABSENCE OF PUBERTY

HPC: Mum concerned about delayed puberty and no onset of menstruation. Healthy and doing well at school. No FHx of delayed puberty.

O/E: Short stature, webbed neck, wide cubital angle. Tanner staging B1 (no breast buds), PH2 (straight pubic hair along labia), A0 (no axilla hair). Height 150 cm (<2nd percentile), weight 56 kg (75th percentile). Mother's height 161 cm; Father's 170 cm

1. List which drugs potentially cause amenorrhoea.
2. What criteria are used for diagnosing PCOS?
3. A 31-year-old woman's periods do not return following post-partum haemorrhage. What may have caused her secondary amenorrhoea?

Answers: 1. Drugs raising prolactin: antipsychotic (phenothiazines, haloperidol), antidepressant (TCA), antihypertensive (methyldopa, reserpine), H2 receptor antagonist (cimetidine, ranitidine, metoclopramide, domperidone). Oral contraception- see commentary below. 2. Rotterdam criteria. 3. Sheehan syndrome; postpartum hypopituitarism due to pituitary necrosis caused by shock – causes varying degrees of anterior pituitary hormone deficiency.

TABLE 114.1

	Features	Investigations	Management
Primary Amenorrhoea			
Constitutional delay of puberty	See *63. PUBERTAL DEVELOPMENT*		
Turner syndrome	See *148. DYSMORPHIC CHILD*. Short stature, webbed neck, widely spaced nipples, wide carrying angle (cubitus valgus). **May not develop normal secondary sexual characteristics**	**Karyotype:** 45XO or mosaic. **Pelvic USS:** 'streak' ovaries	Oestrogen replacement ± growth hormone. Psychological support. Screen: cardiac, renal, ENT, endocrine, autoimmune
Anatomical anomalies including imperforate hymen, absent uterus	**Hx & O/E:** cyclical pelvic pain, dyspareunia or dysuria depending on anatomy	MRI. Renal tract imaging (renal anomalies common)	Referral to specialist

(Continued)

TABLE 114.1 (Cont'd)

	Features	Investigations	Management
Androgen-insensitivity syndrome	Ambiguous genitalia. Breast development, minimal/no pubic hair. Genetically male (karyotype XY), phenotypically female	↑Testosterone. **USS**: absent uterus, undescended testes. **MRI**: often used in addition	Testicular tissue removed due to 5% malignant transformation. Psychological support
Kallmann syndrome (GnRH deficiency)	See *63. PUBERTAL DEVELOPMENT*. Delayed puberty and impaired sense of smell – 'anosmia'	Low serum FSH/LH. MRI brain: no olfactory bulbs	Pulsatile GnRH therapy

Secondary amenorrhoea (Note: these may also cause primary amenorrhoea if they occur before menarche)

	Features	Investigations	Management
Pregnancy	Secondary amenorrhoea is due to pregnancy until proved otherwise	**Beta-hCG urine**	If pregnancy to continue, antenatal support, consider specialist teenage service
Functional amenorrhoea	**RFs**: high stress, excess exercise, weight loss/low BMI, anorexia nervosa/ bulimia. Cycle length >45 days, lack of organic pathology	bHCG (−ve). FBC, LFT, U+E, CRP, TSH, T4, FSH, LH, testost., prolactin. TVUSS	Correct the underlying cause/stressor, modify the stress response with cognitive-based therapy
Polycystic ovary syndrome	Related to: diabetes, FHx. **Hx & O/E**: oligo/ amenorrhoea, obesity, features of androgen excess (hirsutism, acne), possibly subfertility	Rotterdam criteria, ≥2 of: 1. Polycystic ovaries (TVUSS ≥12 ovarian follicles) 2. Oligo/amenorrhoea 3. Hyperandrogenism – raised testosterone, low progesterone	Smoking cessation, weight loss, varied diet. **For menstrual regularity:** metformin (unlicensed use), sometimes COCP is used. **For subfertility:** clomiphene to stimulate ovulation
Hypothalamic dysfunction	Excessive exercise, high stress or eating disorder, low BMI	FSH/LH low or normal. Exclude hypopituitarism/tumour	Advice on diet/stress management. Consider CBT for stress. Osteoporosis risk assessment
Hyperprolactinaemia (various causes, e.g. prolactinoma, see *1. NIPPLE DISCHARGE*)	**Galactorrhoea** (in 30%). If prolactinoma, may also have **visual field defects** (bitemporal hemianopia) and/or headaches	**High prolactin levels** (if >1000 IU/L then do **MRI scan**)	Dopamine agonist to suppress prolactin (cabergoline, bromocriptine). Transsphenoidal resection
Premature ovarian insufficiency (age <40)	See *115. MENOPAUSAL PROBLEMS*		

TABLE 114.1 (Cont'd)

	Features	Investigations	Management
Asherman syndrome (uterine adhesions)	RFs: previous history of certain procedures, e.g. D&C	USS ± hysteroscopy	Hysteroscopy (adhesiolysis), and IUD versus recurrence
Thyroid disease (hyper- or hypo-)	May be asymptomatic/sub-clinical	TFTs	Depends on cause
Chronic conditions	Risk of amenorrhoea and oligomenorrhoea, particularly thyroid disease, diabetes and psychiatric disorders. Management should focus on medication review and treatment optimisation		

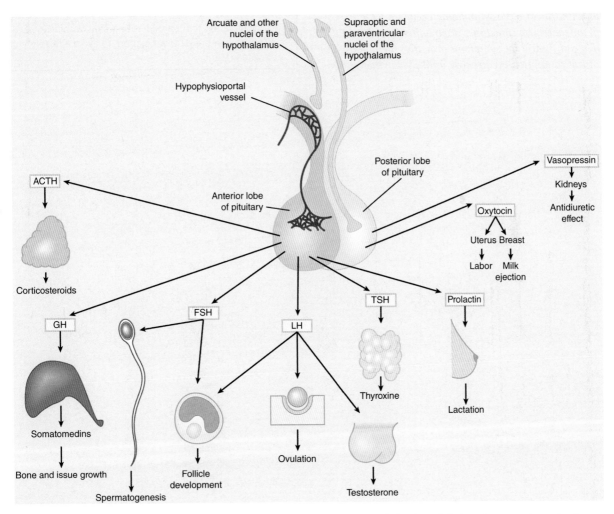

Fig. 114.1 Hypothalamic and pituitary hormones. (Stevens, CW. Chapter 31 Hypothalamic and pituitary hormone drugs. In: *Brenner and Stevens' Pharmacology.* 6th ed., 2022. Elsevier; 363–370.)

Commencement and regularity of menstrual cycles rely on the hypothalamus-pituitary-ovarian axis (Fig. 114.1). Primary amenorrhoea is failure to commence menses, defined as: girls who have not established menstruation by age of 13 and have no secondary sexual characteristics, OR by age of 15 and have normal secondary sexual characteristics. Secondary amenorrhoea refers to loss of menstrual cycle for ≥6 months, after commencement of menarche, where pregnancy is excluded. Some conditions cause amenorrhoea (e.g. genetic conditions, functional causes), but many more common conditions (PCOS, chronic disease) give oligomenorrhoea. Contraception affects menstruation; POP generally causes amenorrhoea, but withdrawal bleeds commonly occur on COCP. Post-pill amenorrhoea sometimes occurs after stopping COCP. HRT can control the symptoms of (early) menopause but natural conception is extremely unlikely. Further options, such as IUD, can provide women with better control. Sudden changes in menstruation, including post-coital bleeding, need 2-week-wait referral to gynaecology. In the vignette, the presentation is primary amenorrhoea with a diagnosis of Turner syndrome. Although familial/constitutional delay of growth and puberty could be a differential, this would normally not present with webbed neck and wide cubital angle.

REVISION TIPS

- Oligomenorrhoea is defined as a break of >35 days between cycles
- Prolactin blood test should not be sent within 48 hours of a breast examination, to avoid a falsely elevated result

115

Menopausal Problems

Alice Parker, Lowri Foster Davies, and Rebecca Newhouse

GP CONSULTATION, FEMALE, 49.
HOT FLUSHES

HPC: Abrupt 5-minute episodes of feeling hot and sweaty. Periods have become irregular, last one 3 months ago – lighter than usual. Mood swings, irritability, low mood, insomnia, fatigue. Sexually active, barrier contraception. Otherwise fit and well. No PMHx, DHx or allergies.

O/E: HR 85, RR 16, SpO$_2$ 100%, T 36.9°C, BP 125/82.

1. What are the differentials for post-menopausal bleeding?

2. What investigations are done for post-menopausal bleeding?
3. What thickness of endometrium is suspicious for endometrial cancer?
4. What are some contraindications to HRT?

Answers: 1. Polyps, fibroids, hyperplasia, endometrial cancer, ovarian cancer, cervical cancer. 2. TVUSS (2WW), endometrial sampling via pipelle or hysteroscopy, examination of external genitalia, speculum. 3. >4mm in post-menopausal women (>4mm is not suspicious pre-menopause). 4. Current/past oestrogen-dependent cancers, e.g. breast, undiagnosed vaginal bleeding, endometrial hyperplasia, unprovoked VTE, raised LFTs, pregnancy, breastfeeding.

TABLE 115.1

	Features	Investigations	Management
Perimenopause and menopause	**Perimenopause:** onset of irregular periods and vasomotor symptoms (e.g. hot flushes, night sweats, poor sleep, urogenital dryness/irritation). **Menopause:** amenorrhoea for 12 months	Average age of menopause in UK is 51. Clinical diagnosis (serum FSH if age >45 years with atypical symptoms, or age 40–45 with menopausal symptoms)	1. Review risks (Table 115.2) 2. Lifestyle modifications 3. SSRI may help vasomotor symptoms 4. Offer HRT (see revision tips) 5. Contraception ≤24 months after last period (<50 years) or 12 months after last period (>50 years) 6. Psychological support if required
Premature ovarian insufficiency	<40 with menopause symptoms. **Causes:** often unknown. Infection (e.g. TB, malaria, mumps), chemo/radiotherapy, autoimmune disorder, chromosomal (e.g. Turner syndrome), FHx. **Protective:** breastfeeding, later menarche, irregular menstruation	FSH >30 IU/L on two blood samples 4–6 weeks apart. **DXA:** bone assessment. (Consider LH, oestradiol, prolactin, testosterone, TSH. Also consider test for adrenal antibodies, karyotype, *FMR1* gene: fragile X syndrome)	

(Continued)

TABLE 115.1   (Cont'd)

	Features	Investigations	Management
Hyperthyroidism	See *58. WEIGHT LOSS*		
Anxiety	Excessive worry about everyday issues, restlessness, insomnia, poor concentration, palpitations, sweating, low mood, irritability	RF: FHx. GAD-7	1. Assess suicide risk 2. CBT 3. SSRIs, SNRIs 4. Monitor
Hypothalamic amenorrhoea	See *114. AMENORRHOEA*		
Endometrial cancer	**RFs:** unopposed oestrogen (e.g. nulliparity, COCP, PCOS, obesity, early menarche), FHx, Lynch syndrome, most age 50–75. **Hx & O/E:** post-menopausal bleeding (PMB). Note, often bleeding can be very light	TVUSS. Endometrial biopsy. CT for staging	Refer for suspected cancer pathway. All women with PMB should be referred on 2WW regardless of age
Secondary amenorrhoea	See *114. AMENORRHOEA*		

TABLE 115.2   Risks and Complications in Menopause and HRT

HRT risks	VTE (HRT tablets), breast cancer (combined HRT), stroke (HRT tablets), endometrial cancer (reduced by a progestogen), coronary heart disease (if started 10 years after menopause)
Post-menopausal complications	Osteoporosis, fractures, CVS disease, stroke, genitourinary syndrome of menopause
Premature or early menopause complications	Osteoporosis, fractures, CVS disease, T2DM, depression, all-cause mortality

The lady in the vignette is experiencing perimenopause. The diagnosis of menopause comes 12 months following her last period. However, the typical presentation shouldn't preclude consideration of other possibilities. The peak age of onset for hyperthyroidism is 20–40 years for women, and other autoimmune disorders or FHx could be relevant. She is sexually active, and barrier methods are not necessarily effective, raising the possibility of pregnancy. However, her periods haven't stopped completely, and pregnancy test is straightforward. Anxiety disorder is harder to exclude. By definition this lady can't have premature ovarian insufficiency as her age is >40.

REVISION TIPS

- Menopause is amenorrhoea for 12 months
- Premature ovarian insufficiency occurs before the age of 40
  HRT. Benefits of short-term HRT usually outweigh risks in most women
- **Composition options:** Oestrogen + progesterone (uterus) or oestrogen only (no uterus)
- **Types:** Cyclical (still menstruating) or continuous (12 months of amenorrhoea, >54 years, or after 1 year of cyclical)
- **Routes:** Oral or transdermal (gel, patch or spray). Progestogen can be given separately (PO or intrauterine)
- **Contraindications:** Endometrial hyperplasia, breast ca, oestrogen-dependent ca, VTE risk, recent MI, deranged LFTs
- **Prescribing options if perimenopausal:** 1 month cyclical, 3 month cyclical
- **Prescribing options if menopausal:** 3 month cyclical, continuous combined, tibolone (must be menopausal >1 year)

116

Contraception Advice – Outline

Emily Vaughan

TABLE 116.1

	Mechanism	Benefits	Side-Effects/Limitations
Hormonal Contraceptive Options			
Combined oral contraceptive pill	Hypothalamic-pituitary-ovarian axis, suppresses FSH/LH mid-cycle surge, inhibits follicle development/ovulation, thickens cervical mucus, thins uterine lining. Break-through bleeding may occur	>99% effective if perfect use. Easy to reverse. Menses can be lighter/less painful. Can control timing, may improve acne. Reduced risk of ovarian, endometrial, colorectal cancer	Temporary; headaches, nausea, breast tenderness, (↓libido). Increased risk of VTE, MI, stroke, breast/cervical cancer. UKMEC Category 3 or 4 (COC should not be prescribed): age >50 years, BMI >35, migraine + aura, smokers + age >35 years, VTE (family or personal history), breast cancer, post-natal + breastfeeding for up to 6 weeks
Progestogen-only contraceptive pill	Thickens cervical mucus, thins uterine lining, inhibits ovulation	Take at same time daily, <3 hours late (12 hours for desogestrel). >99% effective if perfect-use. Easy to reverse. Can use in breastfeeding. Fewer CIs than COC	Irregular menstruation/amenorrhoea. Increased risk of ovarian cysts. Small increased risk breast cancer. UKMEC Cat 4: current breast cancer. UKMEC Cat 3: history of breast cancer, liver tumour
Long-acting Reversible Contraceptives			
Progestogen-only injectable contraceptive	I/m or s/c synthetic progesterone (usually 13 weekly). Suppresses ovulation, thickens cervical mucus, thins uterine lining	Amenorrhoea is common, may help menorrhagia or dysmenorrhoea. Reduced risk of ectopic pregnancy and functional ovarian cysts.	Not quickly reversible. Risk of reduced bone mineral density. Bleeding can be irregular. Weight gain in some. Contra-indication: breast cancer (current or within 5 years)
Progestogen-only subdermal implant	Rod s/c in upper arm. Inhibits ovulation. Thickens cervical mucus and thins uterine lining	Highly effective, lasts ≤3 years. Long duration of action. Reversible. Reduced dysmenorrhoea	Removal of implant may be difficult. May worsen acne (improves in some). May have irregular bleeding

(Continued)

TABLE 116.1   (Cont'd)

	Mechanism	Benefits	Side-Effects/Limitations
Intrauterine contraceptive device (IUD)	Copper device inserted at fundus of endometrial cavity. Lasts 5–10 years. Cytotoxic, spermicidal effect – prevents fertilisation, inhibits implantation. Also inhibits sperm motility	Non-hormonal, rapid return to fertility. Highly effective, reversible + convenient. No evidence IUD increases risk of cervical, uterine or ovarian cancer	CI: PID, recent STI, recent septic abortion/endometritis, pregnant, uterine (bicornuate, <5.5 cm length), gynaecological cancers, copper allergy, Wilson disease. Complications: heavy/painful periods, infection, displacement or expulsion, relative increase in ectopic pregnancy
Levonorgestrel-releasing intra-uterine system (IUS)	T-shaped levonorgestrel; 3 years depending on brand (Mirena 5 years). Reduces endometrial proliferation, prevents implantation. Thickens cervical mucus. In some, prevents ovulation	Low failure rates. Rapid return of fertility. Reduced menstrual loss and dysmenorrhoea. No evidence IUS increases cervical, endometrial or ovarian cancer risk	Menstrual irregularity in first 6 months, some become amenorrhoeic. CI; pregnancy, PID/STI, cervical, endometrial or breast cancer. Complications: acne, breast tenderness, headache, mood changes, relative increased risk of ectopic pregnancy, displacement or expulsion, pelvic infection
Barrier Methods			
Female	Diaphragm (latex or silicone dome on cervix) or cap (smaller, held by suction) – spermicide. Female condom: loose fitting sheath in vagina	Non-hormonal. Female-controlled. Relative sexual spontaneity, as can be inserted prior to intercourse	Not as effective as other contraceptive methods. Do not protect against STI, unlike male condoms
Male condoms	Sheath placed on the penis, usually latex	Protects against STIs	Not as effective as other methods. Risk of malfunction or user error
Natural Family Planning			
Natural	Calendar, temperature, cervical mucus surveillance	No side effects. Conforms to religious requirements for some	Unreliable in those with variable cycle. Less effective than other methods
Emergency Contraceptive Options			
Copper IUD	Inhibits fertilisation/ implantation and sperm penetration through cervical mucus	<1% failure rate, the most effective emergency contraception. Ongoing protection if left in place	As above. Can be fitted up to 5 days after unprotected sex
Levonelle	Inhibits ovulation. Take <72 hours after unprotected intercourse or contraceptive failure	Levonorgestrel synthetic progesterone. <2.6% failure rate. Safe for breastfeeding. Can take more than once in a single menstrual cycle	Side-effects: N&V, breast tenderness, dizziness, menstrual irregularities. Relative CI: levonorgestrel hypersensitivity, acute porphyria, severe liver disease, severe malabsorption syndromes

TABLE 116.1	(Cont'd)		
	Mechanism	**Benefits**	**Side-Effects/Limitations**
ellaOne	Take within 5 days. Ulipristal acetate, progesterone receptor modulator inhibits or delays ovulation, follicle development/rupture. Irregular bleeding	<1.8% failure rate	Contraindications: severe liver disease, uncontrolled asthma. Side effects: N&V, menstrual irregularity including spotting, dizziness, abdo/back pain, myalgia, headache, mood disorders. Avoid breastfeeding for 1 week

UKMEC, UK Medical Eligibility Criteria for contraceptive use.

Hyperemesis/ Vomiting in Early Pregnancy

Hannah Clark and Rebecca Newhouse

**EMERGENCY DEPARTMENT, FEMALE, 24, 8 + 2 WEEKS PREGNANT (G1P0).
PERSISTENT VOMITING**

HPC: Vomiting started at 7 weeks, now vomiting ≤10×/ day, worse mornings and evenings, feels nauseous constantly. Lethargic, weak, not tolerated oral intake for 24 hours. Tried cyclizine, little effect. Dark urine, no pain passing urine. She has not had her booking appointment yet.

O/E: Dehydrated. HR 90, BP 109/66, RR 20, T 36.7°C, SpO$_2$ 98% (air). Mild upper abdominal tenderness. **Ix:** Urine sample shows ketones +2. Mild hypokalaemia on serum bloods.

1. How common is hyperemesis gravidarum (HG)?
2. What gestational hormone is thought to be correlated with HG?
3. Can you name a validated scoring system that can be used to classify the severity of N&V in pregnancy?

Answers: 1. N&V in pregnancy is common (80% of pregnancies), but hyperemesis gravidarum affects only 1.5%. 2. Beta-hCG, since peak concentration in pregnancy coincides with maximal N&V, and increased beta-hCG concentrations occur in twin and molar pregnancies where hyperemesis is common. 3. Pregnancy-unique quantification of emesis (PUQE) score.

TABLE 117.1

	Features	Investigations	Management
Hyperemesis gravidarum	Persistent vomiting in pregnancy, unable to tolerate oral intake, dehydration. Late sign >5% pre-pregnancy weight loss. Starts 4th–7th week, peak 9th week, resolves by 20 weeks. Onset >10 weeks, consider alternative diagnosis	**Urine:** ketonuria indicates dehydration and starvation occur. **Bloods:** electrolyte imbalances. Consider ambulatory care or admission (Fig. 117.1)	IV fluids (replace K deficit). Regular anti-emetic: cyclizine or prochlorperazine (1st line), metoclopramide/ondansetron. Multiple anti-emetics if needed. Consider steroids if intractable. VTE prophylaxis (enoxaparin + TEDS)

TABLE 117.1   (Cont'd)

	Features	Investigations	Management
N&V in pregnancy ('morning sickness')	Troublesome but not severe. Starts 4–7th week, peak 9th week, resolves by 20 weeks. Onset >10 weeks, consider alternative diagnosis	Investigations usually not required. Consider urine sample and bloods	If mild, manage with oral antiemetics. Advise regular sips of fluids and small frequent meals
Gastroenteritis	N&V with abdominal cramps, fever, diarrhoea	Often none, could consider stool culture and bloods.	Supportive, rehydration. Admit if severe
Situations potentially associated with hyperemesis			
Multiple pregnancy	Hx of IVF or previous/FHx of twins. Uterus large for dates	USS to confirm	Specialist referral – consultant-led care
Gestational trophoblastic disease (molar pregnancy)	Irregular PV bleeding (less common; heavy PV bleeding, severe vomiting, first trimester pre-eclampsia)	USS: 'snowstorm', 'bunch of grapes' or cystic appearance. Abnormally high beta-hCG. Excessive uterine size	Removal of molar tissue by suction – histology. Specialist centre follow-up
Key Complications			
UTI	Increased frequency, urgency, dysuria ± haematuria	Urine dipstick/MC&S. Bloods and cultures if suspect pyelonephritis	Always treat in pregnancy. **Avoid trimethoprim in first trimester** (folate antagonist). IV antibiotics if pyelonephritis, sepsis 6 if uroseptic picture
Venous thromboembolism	Dehydration raises haematocrit, hence risk of VTE	Duplex USS for DVT. V/Q scans for PE preferred (due to radiation dose of CTPA)	**Prophylaxis: enoxaparin + TEDS VTE: enoxaparin** (dose based on weight – local guidelines)
Mallory-Weiss tear	Haematemesis (forceful vomiting causes bleeding)	Bloods ± OGD	Resuscitation, treat vomiting. See *50. BLEEDING FROM UPPER GI TRACT/ MELANEA*
Psychological impact	Anxiety, depression, isolation, reduced quality of life	Questionnaires and rating scales	Treat mood/anxiety disorders

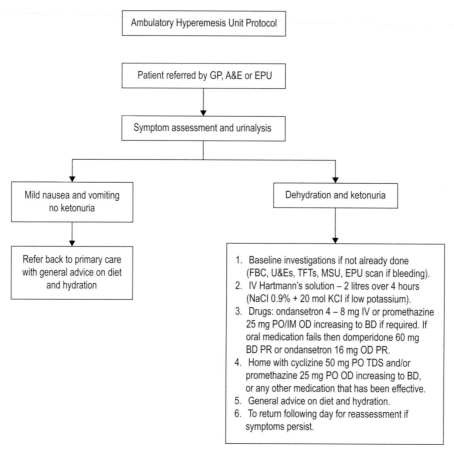

Fig. 117.1 King's College Hospital Ambulatory Hyperemesis Unit treatment protocol. *EPU,* early pregnancy unit. (Reproduced with permission from Ucyigit MA. *Eur J Obstet Gynecol Reprod Biol.* 2020;254:298–301)

The most likely diagnosis in the vignette is hyperemesis gravidarum, suggested by persistent vomiting, inability to tolerate oral intake, ketonuria and hypokalaemia. Differentials to be excluded before diagnosing HG include infection (e.g. UTI), endocrine (e.g. Addison's, thyrotoxicosis), hypercalcaemia, GI (e.g. cholecystitis, pancreatitis, peptic ulcer, gastritis), psychological (e.g. domestic violence, vulnerable patient) and medications.

REVISION TIPS

- The RCOG recommends the following **triad** is present before diagnosing **hyperemesis gravidarum;** 5% pre-pregnancy weight loss, dehydration, electrolyte disturbance

Unwanted Pregnancy and Termination – Outline

Emily Vaughan

The Abortion Act 1967 (amended 1990) applies in England, Wales and Scotland.

Two doctors are required to agree that at least one of the following grounds for abortion is met:

A. Continuance would involve risk to life of the pregnant woman greater than if the pregnancy were terminated

B. The termination is necessary to prevent grave permanent injury to physical or mental health of the woman

C. The pregnancy has NOT exceeded 24th week and continuance of the pregnancy would involve risk greater than if the pregnancy were terminated of injury to the physical or mental health of the pregnant woman

D. The pregnancy has NOT exceeded its 24th week and continuance of the pregnancy would involve risk greater than if the pregnancy were terminated of injury to the physical or mental health of any existing child(ren) of the family of the pregnant woman

E. There is substantial risk that if the child were born it would suffer from such physical or mental abnormalities as to be seriously disabled

For A and B, a second doctor's signature is not required.

TABLE 118.1

	Features	Methods	Additional points
Medical abortion	Can be carried out at any gestation ≤23 weeks + 6 days. If <10 weeks then misoprostol can be administered at home	600 mg oral mifepristone (anti-progestogen), relaxes cervix, stops the pregnancy. 400 mg oral misoprostol (prostaglandin analogue) 36–48 hours later – softens cervix and stimulates uterine contractions	RhD-negative patient with gestation >10 weeks having medical TOP should have anti-D prophylaxis
Surgical abortion	Can be carried out at any gestation ≤23 weeks + 6 days	Cervix priming: mifepristone, misoprostol, osmotic dilator. 1st trimester: cervix dilatation and suction (LA, sedation, deep sedation or GA). 2nd trimester: dilatation and evacuation with forceps (deep sedation or GA)	Rhesus; anti-D as needed. Antibiotic prophylaxis; single dose oral metronidazole. If chlamydia not excluded, doxycycline post-op

Subfertility

Hannah Clark, Berenice Aguirrezabala Armbruster, Rebecca Newhouse, and Aditya Manjunath

FERTILITY CLINIC, FEMALE, 32. UNABLE TO CONCEIVE >12 MONTHS – REGULAR UNPROTECTED SEXUAL INTERCOURSE

HPC: Never been pregnant, partner has two children from a previous relationship. Age at menarche was 11, periods are regular 30-day cycles with 5 days of bleeding. Years of dysmenorrhoea with no definitive diagnosis (never had a laparoscopy). Cyclical bloating, nausea, intermittent deep dyspareunia. **PMHx:** No PID or STIs. **DHx:** Folic acid. **FHx:** Nil. **SHx:** Both non-smokers. She drinks no alcohol, her partner drinks ~10 units per week.
   O/E: Her BMI is 30, partner's is 28.

1. On which day of the menstrual cycle should the mid-luteal progesterone be measured in a patient with a 32-day cycle?
2. With regular sexual intercourse, what percentage of couples will conceive within 1 and within 2 years?
3. Name two risks associated with ovulation induction treatment.

Answers: 1. Day 25 (as mid-luteal progesterone is taken 7 days prior to menstruation). 2. 84% within a year, 92% within 2. 3. Ovarian hyperstimulation syndrome (OHSS). Multiple pregnancy.

TABLE 119.1

	Features	Investigations	Management
Female causes of infertility			
Tubal scarring/ occlusion	Previous ectopic pregnancy or pelvic surgery	Hysterosalpingogram (HSG), hysterosalpingo-contrast-sonography (HyCoSy). Laparoscopy and dye if other pathology (e.g. endometriosis) also needs assessment	Therapeutic laparoscopy – removal of adhesions. Tubal cannulation during HSG to open the fallopian tubes. Consider IVF
Endometriosis	Pelvic pain (>6 months, cyclical/ continuous), dysmenorrhoea, deep dyspareunia, cyclical GI symptoms. May be FHx	**Laparoscopy:** shows ectopic endometrial tissue/ chocolate cyst of ovary (endometrioma). USS ± MRI	Therapeutic laparoscopy. Ablation of endometrial tissue. Consider IVF

TABLE 119.1 (Cont'd)

	Features	Investigations	Management
Pelvic inflammatory disease	Ascending infection due to STIs or uterine instrumentation. Causes adhesion formation within and around fallopian tubes; assess tubal patency (as above). See *133. PELVIC PAIN*		
Polycystic ovarian syndrome	See *114. AMENORRHOEA*		
Premature ovarian insufficiency (POI)	See *115. MENOPAUSAL PROBLEMS* There is still a small chance of conception and contraception should be advised if they wish to avoid a pregnancy. Oocyte donation is an option for fertility in POI		
Hypo/ hyperthyroidism	Hyperthyroidism should be treated prior to pregnancy. Propylthiouracil is the preferred anti-thyroid medication in pregnancy. See *58. WEIGHT LOSS*		
Hypogonadism	**Primary hypogonadism:** (a.k.a. hypergonadotropic hypogonadism) may be caused by genetic disorders (e.g. Turner syndrome) or damage to gonads. **Secondary hypogonadism:** (a.k.a. hypogonadotropic hypogonadism) may be caused by genetic disorders (e.g. Kallman syndrome) or damage to hypothalamus/pituitary	• Baseline bloods to r/o other causes • **Hormone profile:** FSH, LH, testosterone, oestrogen levels to confirm diagnosis • Karyotyping • Consider MRI head	• Multi-disciplinary approach • Consider sex hormone replacement
Prolactinoma	See *1. NIPPLE DISCHARGE*		
Male causes of infertility			
Primary spermatogenic failure/disorder of hypothalamo-pituitary axis/ idiopathic male infertility (40%)	**Congenital:** anorchia, testicular dysgenesis/cryptorchidism, genetic, e.g. AzF microdeletion. **Acquired:** testicular trauma, orchidectomy for torsion/germ cell tumour, varicocele, mumps orchitis	**Normal semen analysis parameters** (WHO): volume >1.5 mL, sperm concentration >15 million/mL, total motility >40%, progressive >32%, morphology >4% normal forms. **Hormone profile:** FSH, LH, testosterone, prolactin. Karyotype	Treat underlying cause. Repeat semen analysis after 3 months of treatment. Surgical sperm retrieval if couple suitable for assisted reproduction, e.g. ICSI. Donor sperm. Varicocele treatment if clinically palpable varicocele **and** abnormal semen
Obstructive azoospermia	Congenital or acquired ejaculatory duct/vas deferens obstruction, e.g. vasectomy	Repeat semen analysis to confirm. FSH, LH, testosterone, prolactin, TSH. Scrotal/transrectal USS. Azoospermia + absent vas deferens, test for cystic fibrosis	Surgical, e.g. vaso-vasostomy. Surgical sperm retrieval for IVF + ICSI or donor IUI; mTESE – microsurgical testicular sperm extraction, PESA – percutaneous epididymal sperm aspiration or TESA – testicular sperm aspiration
Disorder of sperm delivery	Erectile dysfunction, premature/retrograde ejaculation, penile deformity (Peyronie disease, severe hypospadias)		Specialist referral (urology)

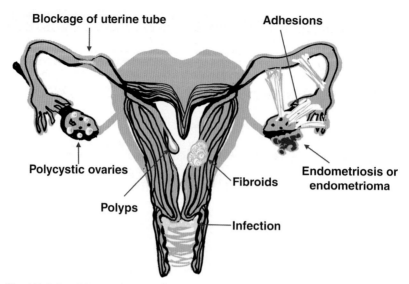

Fig. 119.1 Possible causes of infertility in women. (Illustrated by Hollie Blaber.)

The vignette suggests endometriosis, though formal diagnosis requires laparoscopic visualisation of the pelvis. Other less invasive methods may be useful in assisting diagnosis. Subfertility is a delay in conceiving. Infertility is when a couple is unable to conceive after 1 year of regular unprotected sexual intercourse. Initial investigations in women include mid-luteal phase progesterone (to confirm ovulation), chlamydia screen ± serum gonadotrophins/ progesterone, TFTs and prolactin. Initial investigations in men include semen analysis and chlamydia screen. Causes of infertility include ovulatory (25%), tubal damage (20%), male infertility (30%), and uterine or peritoneal disorders (10%) (Figure 119.1). In 25% of couples a cause for infertility cannot be found. Risk factors include smoking, drugs, alcohol excess, obesity, occupational risks, increasing age in females, and stress. Referral criteria vary between health authorities (check local guidelines) – e.g. refer females <36 years old with normal evaluation including BMI in both partners and unable to conceive for >1 year. Referral is considered in females >35 years old or if evaluation of either partner suggests underlying cause.

REVISION TIPS

- Most cases of infertility are unexplained
- Subfertility may be multifactorial
- Psychological support can also play an important role

120

Normal Pregnancy and Risk Assessment – Outline

Hannah Clark, Alexander Royston, and Manuj Vyas

It is important to have an understanding of the antenatal care that all women should receive during their pregnancy. Much of this centres around assessing for key RFs in pregnancy.

TABLE 120.1

Booking Appointment – Should Take Place Ideally by 10 Weeks	
Full obstetric history	
Any maternal concurrent illnesses	Cardiac, renal, thyroid, respiratory disease, epilepsy, thrombophilia, diabetes, connective tissues diseases. Seek input from specialists.
Assess risk for VTE	RFs: thrombophilia (heritable: e.g. factor V Leiden, protein C/S deficiency; acquired: e.g. antiphospholipid antibodies), medical comorbidities (cancer; heart failure; active SLE, inflammatory polyarthropathy/IBD, T1DM, SCD, nephrotic syndrome), current IVDU, age >35 yo, BMI ≥30, parity ≥3, smoking, gross varicose veins, paraplegia. If high-risk → refer to obstetrics for consideration of antenatal/postnatal LMWH
Assess risk for gestational diabetes mellitus (GDM)	Screen with oral glucose tolerance test at 28 weeks if: • BMI >30 • Previous large baby (>4.5 kg) • Diabetes in first degree relative • Family origin ↑prevalence DM – South Asian, Black Caribbean, Middle Eastern • Previous GDM (screen at 16 and 28 weeks) • 2+ Glucosuria on 1 occasion and 1+ glucosuria on 2 or more occasions
Assess risk factors for pre-eclampsia	**High-risk factors:** • Hypertensive disease in a previous pregnancy • CKD • Autoimmune disease • Type 1 or 2 diabetes • Chronic hypertension **Moderate-risk factors:** • Age ≥40 • Nulliparity • Pregnancy interval >10 years • FHx of pre-eclampsia • BMI ≥35 • Multiple pregnancy **Aspirin** prophylaxis (75–150 mg daily from 12 weeks of pregnancy) for a single 'high risk' factor or ≥2 'moderate risk' factors

(Continued)

TABLE 120.1   (Cont'd)

Maternal mental health	If significant history, antenatal assessment by perinatal mental health team
Domestic abuse	Give women the opportunity to disclose this in a sensitive and secure environment
Substance abuse	Lifestyle advice including smoking cessation and the implications of drug use, smoking and alcohol consumption in pregnancy
Female genital mutilation (FGM)	Pregnant women with FGM should be identified early in antenatal care (through sensitive enquiry) → planning of intrapartum care
Examination Record weight/BMI	
Check BP	Carried out at each antenatal visit (screen for pre-eclampsia)
Clinical	Examine heart, lungs, abdomen
Tests Blood group and antibody screen	**Important to know rhesus D status.** Routine antenatal anti-D prophylaxis should be offered to all non-sensitised rhesus-D negative pregnant women. Screen for atypical red-cell alloantibodies
Hb level	Investigation and treatment for anaemia with iron supplementation if identified
Sickle cell test depending on family origin	All women are screened using the Family Origin Questionnaire. If high risk, offer laboratory screening
Syphilis serology, Hep B virus, HIV test	Should be offered to all pregnant women
Urine sample	Screens for asymptomatic bacteriuria, proteinuria, glucosuria
Mantoux test and CXR	Consider if patient is from area endemic for TB or a TB contact
Chromosomal screening	Offered to all women between 11 and 13 + 6 weeks, mostly with combined screening test: • Nuchal translucency (NT) • βhCG • PAPP-A (Pregnancy associated plasma protein A) ≤1:150 = high-risk ⟶ offer further testing (amniocentesis, chorionic villus sampling or free fetal DNA). Late-booked women: triple or quadruple screening test offered between 15 and 20 weeks. See also *142. WELL-BEING CHECKS- outline*
Dating scan	USS: (10 + 0 weeks – 13 + 6 weeks) ⟶ determines gestational age (usually crown-rump measurement) and to detect multiple pregnancies
Further visits	
16 weeks	Review and discuss results of all screening tests
18–20 weeks	Foetal anomaly scan: ultrasound screening for foetal anomalies should be routinely offered (18 + 0 weeks – 20 + 6 weeks). If placenta extends over the internal cervical os, offer another scan at 32 weeks to see if the placental site has moved
25 weeks	In nulliparous women
28 weeks	Repeat Hb and antibody screen and give 1500iu anti-D if needed
31 weeks	In nulliparous women
34 weeks	Discuss labour, birth and pain relief. **Offer second dose of anti-D to rhesus-negative women (if 500 iu given at 28–30 weeks)**

TABLE 120.1 (Cont'd)	
36 weeks	Discuss breastfeeding, neonatal vitamin K, postnatal care/depression and 'baby blues.' Could **offer external cephalic version (ECV)** to women with an uncomplicated singleton breech pregnancy (exceptions: women in labour, women with a uterine scar, foetal compromise, ruptured membranes, vaginal bleeding and medical conditions)
38 weeks	
40 weeks	In nulliparous women: discuss post-dates pregnancy and its management
41 weeks	Offer membrane sweep. Book IOL by 42 weeks

REVISION TIPS

- Symphysis fundal height is recorded at each antenatal appointment from 24 weeks and then 2–4 weekly
- Should also measure BP and test urine for proteinuria at each antenatal appointment
- RFs for VTE: thrombophilia, medical comorbidities, current IVDU, age >35 yo, BMI $\geq$30, parity $\geq$3, smoking, gross varicose veins, paraplegia

121

Substance Misuse

Gregory Oxenham, Margarita Fox, Alexander Royston,
Katie Turner, Alice Pitt, and Manuj Vyas

HPC: Undergoing CBT to help with mood and ongoing benzodiazepine addiction. She told her midwife about diazepam use; wishes to stop despite multiple failed attempts previously – increased use/dose requirement recently due to anxiety about motherhood. She has concerns for her baby, denies any other substance use. Normal 12-week scan and booking bloods, not yet reporting foetal movements. No vaginal bleeding or abdominal pain. **PMHx:** Generalised anxiety disorder, depression, benzodiazepine misuse disorder, post-traumatic stress disorder.

O/E: Presents with partner. Dressed in baggy clothes, no needle marks. Poor eye contact. Appropriate content of speech, depressed affect, withdrawn, no evidence of psychosis.

1. What is the risk of immediate benzodiazepine reversal in someone with long-term dependence?
2. What is the difference between methadone and buprenorphine in pharmacological mechanism?

Answers: 1. By blocking the GABA receptors, the seizure threshold is reduced. In chronic use, this may provoke seizures which are inherently resistant to further benzodiazepines. 2. Both are used to treat opioid use disorder and both have a longer half-life than injected heroin. Methadone: μ-opioid receptor agonist with higher intrinsic activity than morphine. Buprenorphine: nonselective, mixed agonist–antagonist opioid receptor modulator.

TABLE 121.1

	Features	Investigations	Management
Alcohol misuse disorder (pregnancy)	Foetal alcohol syndrome (FAS): short palpebral fissure, epicanthic folds, thin upper lip, low nasal bridge, indistinct philtrum, micrognathia (Fig. 154.1). Learning difficulties, growth retardation, cardiac defects. Neonate may have withdrawal symptoms, e.g. tremor, irritability, hypotonia	Clinical diagnosis. Screening tests: AUDIT-C/CAGE tests. For FAS prevention: screening questions at booking visit USS: assess growth, cardiac defects	Prevention of FAS: Help the mother stop drinking – behavioural therapy, perinatal mental health services. Early intervention may improve a child's development in FAS. Neonatal follow up at 6 weeks if suspected FAS

TABLE 121.1	(Cont'd)		
	Features	Investigations	Management
Tobacco and smoking (pregnancy)	Women may not disclose smoking due to social pressure not to smoke in pregnancy. **Pregnancy risk:** SGA foetus, miscarriage; increases risk of placental abruption, PROM, pre-term labour and SIDS	Clinical diagnosis. **CO breath test** at booking visit for screening. Explore how much the patient smokes and whether they've considered stopping	Smoking cessation. Stopping prior to 24 weeks means outcomes are similar. Motivational interviewing, behaviour therapy. Nicotine patches/gum – safe in pregnancy, but if still smoking they further increase risk
Cocaine misuse (pregnancy)	Acutely; elation, pressure of speech, agitation, mydriasis, sweating, hypertension, delirium. Long-term mood disorders. Rapid acceleration of cardiovascular disease/coronary artery disease; chest pain/MI. Bloodborne disease in injecting users, chronic lung disease inhaling, and nasal septal perforation in insufflators. **Risk to mother:** pregnancy-induced HTN, pre-eclampsia, placental abruption. **Risk to foetus:** prematurity neonatal abstinence syndrome (NAS), similar effects with amphetamines	**RFs:** early access to drugs/alcohol, childhood family conflict, exposure to drug in peer groups. **Screening questions** at booking visit. Consider bloods for pre-eclampsia – cocaine can cause hypertension. Increased USS frequency	Referral to drug treatment programme. CBT (motivational interviewing, relapse prevention). Specialist midwife services
Opioid misuse (pregnancy)	NAS in foetus (see below)	**Screening questions** at booking visit. Urine analysis for drug screen possible. Severity scoring system for NAS	Opiate substitution treatment: methadone or buprenorphine. Referral to drug treatment programme. Specialist midwife services
Benzodiazepine misuse (pregnancy)	**Foetus:** increased risk of cleft palate if used in 1st trimester. Prematurity and low birth weight. Withdrawal and NAS (sometimes as late as 10 days)	Clinical diagnosis. Urine analysis for drug screen possible	Specialist midwife service. Requires a **slow taper down** in order to stop use – converted to long-acting preparation (usually diazepam)
Key complications Neonatal abstinence syndrome (NAS)	Tremors, irritability/excess crying + high pitch, raised respiratory rate, hyperactive, may have seizures, poor feeding, unstable temperature. Alcohol withdrawal occurs at 6–12 hours	Pre-birth – severity score predicts NAS likelihood. All high-risk infants observed for 72 hours	Regular feeding, quiet room, close nursing. Opiate withdrawal:oral morphine. Seizures: phenobarbitone

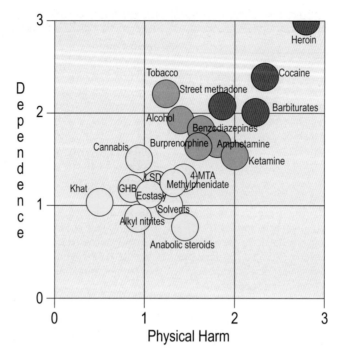

Fig. 121.1 Data showing relative estimated harms of various drugs of abuse. Data from Nutt D, King L, Saulsbury W, Blakemore C. Development of a rational scale to assess the harm of drugs of potential misuse. *Lancet* 2007;369:1047–1053.

Substance misuse in pregnancy is often associated with difficult social circumstances needing specialist care. The patient in the vignette has benzodiazepine dependence, with tolerance to previous dose, unsuccessful attempts to stop and continued use despite perceived harm to her foetus. Multiple prescription medicines risk dependence problems, notably opioids, gabapentanoids, benzodiazepines and Z drugs (zopiclone, zolpidem). Patients on these medications should be reviewed regularly to assess for dependence. Prior to prescribing, doctors should establish a plan regarding duration and intended outcomes. De-prescribing long-term benzodiazepines is difficult for patients and should be undertaken slowly to minimise withdrawal. Table 121.1 focuses on substance misuse in pregnancy and should be used alongside case **169. ADDICTION** (Fig. 121.1).

REVISION TIPS

- Cardiovascular effects of cocaine mimic pre-eclampsia in pregnancy and risk of abruption is increased
- Buprenorphine and methadone are considered comparatively safe in pregnancy but may cause NAS

122

Intrauterine Death and Miscarriage – Outline

Emily Vaughan

AN EMBRYO BECOMES A FOETUS AT 8 WEEKS PREGNANCY

Miscarriage – expulsion of a foetus or embryo at a time when it is incapable of independent survival (includes all pregnancies before 24 weeks, though most are before 12 weeks)

Recurrent Miscarriage – ≥3 consecutive, spontaneous miscarriages in first trimester, with the same biological father

Stillbirth – a child delivered after 24th wiu who did not show any signs of life after delivery

Intra-uterine foetal death – foetus dies in the womb before birth. Death is considered 'late' after 24 weeks
Key signs and symptoms:
- Cessation of foetal movements
- Spotting or per-vaginal bleeding ± pelvic pain
Independent RFs (miscarriage/ late intrauterine death):
- Advancing maternal age, increasing paternal age >45 years
- Previous history of miscarriages
- Smoking, alcohol, recreational drugs
- Poorly controlled maternal diabetic or thyroid disease

Common causes	Risk factors	Investigations	Management
Genetic/structural abnormalities of the foetus	Chromosomal/genetic defects. Teratogens: DHx (thalidomide, valproate, methotrexate, isotretinoin), alcohol, tobacco, recreational drugs. Maternal health (diabetes, PKU). Infectious agents (TORCH)	Karyotype parental blood. Cytogenic analysis	
Uterine abnormalities	Submucosal/intra-mural fibroids. Septate/bicornuate uterus	TVUSS	Treat fibroids. Metroplasty might be considered for septate or bicornuate uterus
Antiphospholipid syndrome (APS)	Up to 15% of those with recurrent miscarriages	Antiphospholipid/ cardiolipin/beta-2-glycoprotein 1 antibodies, lupus anticoagulant	Aspirin or heparin for those diagnosed with APS in pregnancy

(Continued)

Common causes	Risk factors	Investigations	Management
Cervical insufficiency	Premature cervical dilation. **RFs:** previous cervix surgery (e.g. LLETZ, cone biopsy, D&C), Ehlers-Danlos. Often 2nd trimester, can cause premature labour. **Hx & O/E:** pelvic pressure/cramping, loss of mucous plug, vaginal discharge	TVUSS: early cervical shortening (<25 mm) at 16–24 weeks	Progesterone pessaries if cervical shortening. Planned cervical suture: 1. Previous miscarriages or premature births, with cervical shortening. 2. ≥3 late miscarriages or premature births. Emergency cervical suture if membranes are bulging and <24 wiu
Placental problems See *126. BLEEDING ANTEPARTUM*	Placental insufficiency: reduced nutrient/oxygen transfer. Can also lead to pre-eclampsia	USS Doppler of umbilical artery and uterine artery	Placenta praevia/abruption
Infection	Rubella, CMV, vaginosis, HIV, chlamydia, gonorrhoea, syphilis, malaria. Toxoplasma (undercooked meat, cat faeces contamination), listeria (unpasteurised dairy), *Salmonella*	Antenatal screening: hepatitis B, HIV, syphilis at booking appointment. Blood cultures, MSU, swabs, viral screen	Serial USS in foetal medicine with discussion about option for termination if severe malformations

Management of miscarriage

Management	
Expectant	Analgesia. Lasts 7–14 days Expectant management is not appropriate if: • Late first trimester or beyond (increased risk of haemorrhage) • Previous stillbirth • Antepartum haemorrhage • Coagulopathy or unable to have blood transfusion, infection
Medical	Vaginal or oral misoprostol (prostaglandin analogue). Indicated if expectant management >14 days (or not appropriate)
Surgical	Manual vacuum aspiration (LA) or surgical (GA). Indicated if expectant management >14 days or products of conception retained despite medical treatment. Anti-D Ig given to all rhesus-negative women

123

Large for Gestational Age

Hannah Clark and Simon Scheck

FEMALE, 30, 28 + 2 WEEKS PREGNANT.
FOETUS MEASURING ON THE 95TH
CENTILE FOR GROWTH BASED ON SFH

HPC: Birth Hx; G3P2. Previous pregnancies: 1st baby – NVD 7 years ago at 39 + 4 weeks, weighed 3.9 kg. 2nd baby – forceps delivery 4 years ago at 40 + 5 weeks, weighed 4.0 kg. Maternal booking BMI = 29. **PMHx:** Nil. **FHx:** Her sister has T2DM. **Ix:** Recent oral glucose tolerance test, fasting blood glucose of 5.5 mmol/L and a 2-hour glucose of 8.3 mmol/L. USS confirms the estimated weight is on the 95th centile.

1. Why is it important to counsel women about the risks of shoulder dystocia with an LGA baby? Can you think of a legal case that links to this?

2. How is risk of neonatal hypoglycaemia mitigated following birth to a mother with gestational DM?

Answers: 1. Risk of brachial plexus injury or hypoxic injury. Montgomery case/principle; a mother at risk of a macrosomic baby expressed general concerns during antenatal care. Risk of shoulder dystocia was not discussed and planned vaginal delivery was complicated by dystocia, brain damage and cerebral palsy. See commentary below. 2. Immediate feeding (within 30 mins), test neonate's blood glucose, regular feeding (every 2–4 hours), keep pre-feed blood glucose at >2.0 mmol/L.

TABLE 123.1

	Features	Investigations	Management
Constitutionally large foetus	Genetic tendency towards having larger babies. Consider birthweight of any previous babies	USS to exclude polyhydramnios and estimate foetal weight	Serial USS to check growth is staying on the same centile
Gestational diabetes mellitus (GDM) *Pre-existing diabetes will usually result in an LGA foetus too*	**RFs:** BMI >30, previous macrosomic baby ≥4.5 kg, previous GDM, first-degree relative with DM, ethnicity with higher DM prevalence (South Asian, Middle Eastern, Black Caribbean, Pacific Islander). **Presentation:** LGA foetus, polyhydramnios, glucose on urine dip	**Oral glucose tolerance test** at 24–28 weeks. GDM if: fasting glucose >5.6 mmol/L, or 2-hour glucose ≥7.8 mmol/L. If GTT +ve, check HbA1c – can identify pre-existing diabetes	Joint diabetes/antenatal clinic review. Blood glucose monitoring. If fasting glucose <7 mmol/L: trial of diet/ exercise first. If ≥7 mmol/L: insulin ± metformin. If 6-6.9 mmol/L but macrosomia or hydramnios: insulin ± metformin offered. Serial growth scans. **IOL (37-40 weeks):** depending on macrosomia, polyhydramnios, blood sugar control and obstetric risk factors

(Continued)

TABLE 123.1   (Cont'd)

	Features	Investigations	Management
Key Complications			
Shoulder dystocia	Usually due to impaction of anterior foetal shoulder on maternal pubic symphysis (Fig. 123.1). Baby's head will deliver → inability to deliver the body. Risk of brachial plexus injury	RFs: macrosomia, maternal diabetes, multiple pregnancy. Risk higher in diabetic pregnancy (vs same size foetus in non-diabetic). **Obstetric emergency**	Call for help. McRoberts manoeuvre. Suprapubic pressure. Consider episiotomy to allow internal manoeuvres; deliver posterior arm or internal rotation (Rubin's or Wood's Screw manoeuvre), mother onto all fours (Gaskin manoeuvre)
Neonatal hypoglycaemia	Neonatal tremors, sweating, poor feeding, irritability, seizures	Low blood sugar level on routine testing in neonates of diabetic mothers, or macrosomic babies	May require oral or intravenous glucose

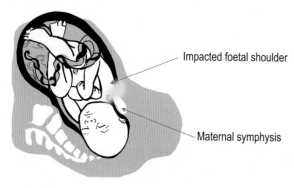

Impacted foetal shoulder

Maternal symphysis

Fig. 123.1 Anatomy of shoulder dystocia. (Illustrated by Dr Hollie Blaber.)

From the vignette we can see that this woman had an instrumental delivery for a relatively large baby, and a family history of T2DM. Here, the foetus is LGA because the mother developed gestational diabetes mellitus, as demonstrated by 2-hour glucose tolerance test level of 8.3 mmol/L. LGA foetuses are associated with a variety of birth complications related to macrosomia, so need referral to a multidisciplinary gestational diabetes clinic. Management should include dietary changes and education and may include metformin or insulin, as maintaining blood glucose within strict parameters will mitigate risk. Women with gestational diabetes or type 1 or type 2 diabetes have increased risk of pre-eclampsia. LGA has increased chance of caesarean section or instrumental delivery due to risk of cephalopelvic disproportion. In Mrs Montgomery's case (see answer 1), the consultant did not discuss shoulder dystocia (with potential significant consequences), as risk was felt to be small and mother had not asked specific questions. Hence Mrs Montgomery was unable to make a fully informed decision on all the options (notably Caesarean section). In 2014, the UK Supreme Court ruled the care was negligent; GMC guidance was reviewed such that it is the doctor's role to provide a patient with all the information to allow them to make a balanced judgement between different options. A risk is judged "material" if a reasonable person in the patient's position would be likely to attach significance to the risk.

REVISION TIPS

- You can remember the diagnostic thresholds for GDM by thinking of it as 5,6,7,8 (for 5.6 and 7.8 respectively)
- Women with GDM have a high risk of recurring GDM in future pregnancies
- Shoulder dystocia is the most concerning complication of GDM

124

Small for Gestational Age

Hannah Clark and Simon Scheck

ANTENATAL CLINIC, FEMALE, 23, 28 + 3 WEEKS. SYMPHYSIS FUNDAL HEIGHT SMALLER THAN EXPECTED

HPC: Plotting the SFH on a growth chart, estimated foetal weight (EFW) below 10th centile. **Background:** G1P0, low-risk pregnancy, midwife-led care, uncomplicated pregnancy so far. Normal screening tests and 20-week anomaly scan. BMI 22. Normal PAPP-A. No symptoms. **PMHx:** Nil. **SHx:** Non-smoker. No alcohol or recreational drugs.

 O/E: T 36.3, HR 76, BP 145/98, RR 14. **Ix:** Urine dip: 2+ proteinuria. Clinic USS; EFW/ abdominal circumference (AC) around the 5th centile.

1. How does the SGA risk assessment affect the monitoring of women during pregnancy?
2. In what circumstances might it not be appropriate to use the SFH as a measurement of foetal growth?

Answers: 1. Women with *one major risk factor on RCOG guidance (Table 124.2) undergo serial ultrasound scans (to check growth) with umbilical artery dopplers from 26 to 28 weeks. Women with three or more minor risk factors have uterine artery dopplers at 20–24 weeks gestation* (abnormal results are predictive of pre-eclampsia and IUGR) – do not confuse with umbilical artery dopplers evaluating placental function. 2. In women with known large fibroids in the uterine cavity, polyhydramnios, twin pregnancy, or high BMI >35 - where measurement of SFH is unlikely to be accurate. Measurement of growth using ultrasound would be indicated in these circumstances.

TABLE 124.1

	Features	Investigations	Management
Constitutionally small foetus	50%-70% of SGA foetuses. **Factors:** ethnicity, foetal sex, parent height. **No pathology is present.** Unlikely to present with any maternal symptoms. Small at all stages but *growth following the centiles*	**USS:** for EFW and/or AC <10th centile. Symmetrically small (i.e. AC centile = head circumference centile) is more likely to be constitutionally small	**Surveillance:** serial ultrasound growth scans and umbilical artery dopplers

(Continued)

TABLE 124.1 (Cont'd)

	Features	Investigations	Management
Foetal growth restriction/intra-uterine growth restriction (IUGR)	RFs: >40 years old, previous IUGR, previous stillbirth, low PAPP-A, low maternal weight, vigorous exercise. Pathological restriction of genetic growth potential. Reduced foetal movements may be reported	USS: for EFW and/or AC. Reduction in AC or EFW. IUGR is more likely in severe SGA foetuses (<3rd centile). Possible reduced amniotic fluid volume and abnormal foetal dopplers	Identify/ address contributory factors. Serial ultrasound growth scans and umbilical artery dopplers. Potentially expedite delivery
Placenta-mediated growth restriction			
Placental insufficiency	Reduced function limits transfer of oxygen/ nutrients to foetus. SGA foetus, increased risk of perinatal mortality	RFs: often none identified, but similar to IUGR. **Umbilical artery doppler:** abnormal flow, reversed flow	As for IUGR above.
Pre-eclampsia (PET)	Develops after 20/40. Hx & O/E: can present with visual disturbance, BP ≥140/90, abdo pain, headache, oedema, N&V, IUGR. Untreated, can lead to eclampsia with seizures. Organ dysfunction – renal, liver, clotting	RFs: *High risk;* HTN in a previous pregnancy, CKD, autoimmune disease, diabetes, chronic HTN. *Moderate;* first pregnancy, >40 yo, pregnancy interval >10 yrs, BMI >35, FHx, multip. Urine: proteinuria /↑PCR. FBC (↓platelets), U&E (↑urea/ creat), LFTs (↑ALT/AST)	Aspirin 150 mg from 12 to 16 weeks to women with RFs for PET- improves placental blood flow and ↓risk of PET/ IUGR. Labetalol/nifedipine for BP control. Routine growth scan surveillance
Maternal smoking/alcohol	Smoking (n.b. ≥11/day)/ alcohol	Carbon monoxide (CO) testing throughout pregnancy. Routine growth scan surveillance	Cessation support – smoking cessation before 15 weeks, reduces risk of SGA to that of non-smokers
Maternal health conditions	Autoimmune disease, renal disease, or thrombophilia	Monitoring during pregnancy	Optimise medical co-morbidities
Non-placenta-mediated growth restriction			
Chromosomal/ genetic abnormalities	Combined/ quadruple test: high-risk results, offer non-invasive prenatal testing (NIPT) – raised risk of baby with Down/Patau/Edwards syndromes	Amniocentesis, chorionic villus sampling or non-invasive testing (free foetal DNA): karyotyping (trisomy 13/18/21, Turner syndrome)	Maternal-foetal medicine (MFM) unit ± genetic counselling. Termination may be offered
Foetal structural anomalies	RFs: isolated or with genetic abnormality. Anencephaly, cleft lip, spina bifida, pulmonary atresia, etc.	May see on 20-week anomaly scan. Detailed anomaly scan- often with foetal medicine unit ± genetic counselling	MFM referral. May require neonatal/neonatal surgical referral (e.g. gastroschisis). Termination may be offered
Congenital infection	CMV, parvovirus, toxoplasmosis, syphilis and malaria	Maternal serological testing. If primary infection → MFM for amniocentesis to test for foetal infection	Treatment depends upon pathogen. MFM for detailed assessment. Neonatal referral

TABLE 124.2   Minor and Major Risk Factors for an SGA Foetus as Defined by the Royal College of Obstetricians and Gynaecologists.

All Women Should Be Assessed for SGA Risk Factors at Their Booking Appointment

Minor Risk Factors	Major Risk Factors
Maternal age ≥35 years	Maternal age >40 years
IVF singleton pregnancy	Smoker ≥11 cigarettes per day
Nulliparity	Cocaine use
BMI <20	Daily vigorous exercise
BMI 25–34.9	Paternal SGA
Smoker (1–10 cigarettes per day)	Previous SGA baby
Low fruit intake pre-pregnancy	Previous stillbirth
Previous pre-eclampsia	Maternal SGA
Pregnancy interval <6 months	Chronic HTN
Pregnancy interval ≥60 months	Diabetes with vascular disease
	Renal impairment
	Antiphospholipid syndrome
	Heavy bleeding similar to menses
	Low PAPP-A (<0.4) – a placental hormone included in routine combined first-trimester screening

In the vignette, the most likely diagnosis is foetal growth restriction from underlying asymptomatic pre-eclampsia. Early onset pre-eclampsia (<34 weeks) has a high chance of progression to severe symptoms, so this woman will require close monitoring for the remainder of her pregnancy, which may be as an inpatient. Antihypertensive medication may be required. Triggers for delivery would include uncontrolled hypertension, deteriorating renal or liver function, eclampsia or foetal compromise.

REVISION POINTS

- SGA refers to any foetus with an EFW or AC below the 10th percentile. Most of these babies are constitutionally small and show normal growth trajectory
- IUGR refers to pathological restriction of growth potential
- IUGR foetuses may have compromise on further investigation (Doppler flow studies, liquor volume)
- Not all growth restricted foetuses are SGA

125

Reduced Foetal Movements – Outline

Hannah Clark, Gregory Oxenham, and Simon Scheck

KEY POINTS

- Foetal movements are a manifestation of foetal well-being and reduced foetal movements (RFM) must be evaluated (Figure 125.1)
- Movements usually first detected 18–20/40 weeks
- Movements tend to increase up to 32 weeks and then plateau but should NOT decrease
- Foetal sleep cycles (where movements tend to be absent) are rarely >90 mins in a healthy foetus
- Strongly encourage women to attend the maternity unit if they experience changes in foetal movements
- When using handheld Doppler, ensure the foetal heart rate is differentiated from the maternal heart rate by feeling the maternal pulse
- 70% of pregnancies with single episode of RFM are uncomplicated. Recurrent, outcomes are poorer

---

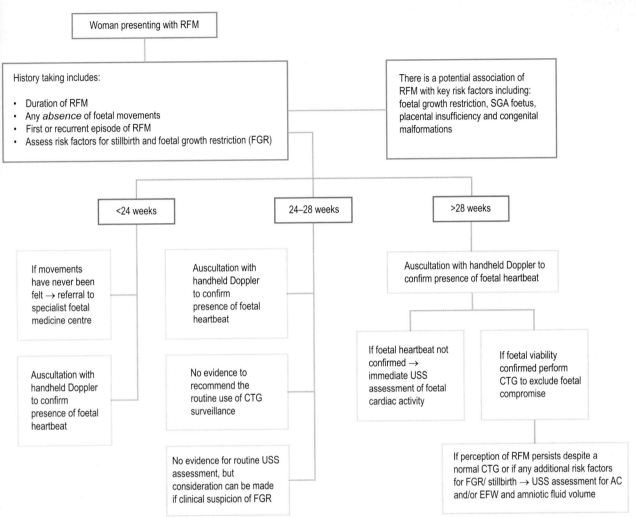

Fig. 125.1 Flow chart adapted from RCOG guidelines on reduced foetal movements. Factors that can lead to decreased perception of foetal movements include; early gestation, maternal stress, maternal obesity, oligohydramnios, anterior placenta, drugs (alcohol, benzodi-azepines, opioids). *AC: abdominal circumference; EFW: estimated foetal weight; FGR: foetal growth restriction.*

126

Bleeding Antepartum

Hannah Clark, Gregory Oxenham, and Simon Scheck

MATERNAL ASSESSMENT UNIT, FEMALE, 28, 36/40 PREGNANT. ABDOMINAL PAIN, VAGINAL BLEEDING AND SHOCK

HPC: 2-hours sudden-onset severe abdo pain (continuous) and bright red vaginal bleeding (soaked three sanitary pads), sensation of reduced foetal movements. No history of trauma. **Birth history:** G2P1. Previous uncomplicated pregnancy/NVD 4 years ago. Current pregnancy: normal scans. Anterior placenta. Rhesus (RhD) negative. **SHx:** Smokes 5–10 cigarettes daily.

O/E: Tense and tender uterus. Cephalic lie. Speculum examination: long, closed cervix, fresh blood in vagina coming from os. HR 115, BP 100/70, RR 20, T 37.2°C.

1. List risk factors for placental abruption.
2. How common is antepartum haemorrhage?
3. What is the Kleihauer test and when/why should it be performed?

Answers: 1. ↑Maternal age, previous abruption, multiparity, smoking, cocaine, pre-eclampsia or hypertensive disease. 2. APH occurs in ~3%–5% of all pregnancies. 3. The Kleihauer test helps to determine the presence and size of foetomaternal haemorrhage (FMH) and is mostly used in rhesus-negative women. Estimating the size of FMH ensures that rhesus-negative pregnant women who have undergone potentially sensitising events (of which APH is one) are given adequate quantities of anti-D.

TABLE 126.1

	Features	Investigations	Management
Uterine sources			
Placental abruption	**RFs:** ↑maternal age, previous abruption, multiparity, smoking, cocaine, pre-eclampsia, hypertensive disease. **Hx & O/E:** sudden-onset, constant abdo pain ± PV bleed (Fig. 126.1). Tense uterus – 'woody hard' if severe. Tachycardia, hypotension – shock may be disproportionate to loss	**Clinical diagnosis.** FBC, U&E, LFTs, coagulation, G&S/CM, Kleihauer test. **CTG:** foetal distress, or absent heartbeat. **USS** limited use – can help assess foetal viability, or to assess size of foetus if extremely premature	A-E resuscitation, fluids and/or blood products. Call for help early ± activate major obstetric haemorrhage protocol. **Emergency caesarean** section. **Anti-D if indicated.** If no obstetric and neonatal care available, urgent transfer

TABLE 126.1   (Cont'd)

	Features	Investigations	Management
Placenta praevia	RFs: previous termination/ praevia/ LSCS; multiple pregnancy, high maternal age, smoking, previous adherent placenta needing manual removal. Usually known low-lying placenta from 20/40 scan. Hx & O/E: painless vaginal bleeding. Soft uterus, non-tender. Abnormal foetal lie/ presentation	Bloods: as above. CTG: foetal heartbeat often normal. TVUSS: to localise placenta site. Note: avoid digital vaginal examinations unless placenta praevia has been excluded on USS	A-E resuscitation, fluids and/or blood products. Call for help early ± activate major obstetric haemorrhage protocol. Give anti-D if indicated. Establish urgency of delivery-usually via CS. If no obstetric and neonatal care available urgent transfer
Lower genital tract sources			
Cervical causes, e.g. polyps, ectropion, malignancy	RFs: malignancy – HSV 16/18, immunosuppression, smoking, prior abnormal cervical smear. Hx & O/E: *ectropion* - post-coital bleeding. *Malignancy* – post-coital/ intermenstrual bleeding, dyspareunia, fatigue. Early disease often asymptomatic	Speculum: for any woman with abnormal PV bleeding to visualise cervix. Colposcopy. CIN far more common than malignancy in pregnancy	Reassurance if ectropion. Management of cervical cancer depends on stage/grade. Do not delay colposcopy if pregnant. See *137. ABNORMAL CERVICAL SMEAR*
Vaginal/ vulval, e.g. vaginitis, infection, trauma	Tend to cause mild bleeding/ spotting or post-coital bleeding. See *136. VULVAL LESION/ ITCH*	Swab: for infection (chlamydia, gonorrhoea, trichomonas)	Antibiotics as indicated. Topical oestrogens never indicated in pregnancy
Key Complications			
Preterm birth	Consider antenatal steroids (<35/40) for foetal lung maturation and magnesium sulphate (<30/40) for neuroprotection. Alert neonatal team, consider transfer or urgent retrieval if neonatal care not available. See *127. LABOUR- OUTLINE*		
Post-partum haemorrhage	See *129. BLEEDING POST-PARTUM*		

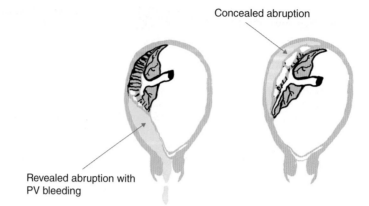

Concealed abruption

Revealed abruption with
PV bleeding

Fig. 126.1 Concealed versus revealed abruption. (Illustrated by Dr Hollie Blaber.)

The most likely differential in the vignette is placental abruption; the PV bleeding leads us convincingly to this diagnosis of abruption. If she had presented without the PV bleeding, it does not exclude placental abruption but widens the important differentials to include renal colic, intrabdominal sepsis and a perforated viscus; pregnant women can be affected by any of the surgical emergencies that may affect non-pregnant women.

REVISION TIPS

- Antepartum bleeding is bleeding from the genital tract after 24 weeks gestation but before birth
- Remember 'concealed' placental abruption; absence of vaginal bleeding does not rule out abruption

Labour – Outline

Hannah Clark

Labour may be defined as the onset of regular uterine contractions with associated cervical dilatation and descent of the presenting part (Table 127.1). Signs of labour include regular and painful uterine contractions, a 'show' (shedding of the mucous plug), rupture of the membranes (but not always) and shortening/dilatation of the cervix.

Foetal monitoring in labour

- Foetal heart rate should be monitored appropriately (Table 127.2)
- Contractions should be assessed every 30 minutes
- Maternal pulse rate should be assessed every 60 minutes
- Maternal BP and temperature should be checked every 4 hours
- Vaginal examination should be offered every 4 hours to check the progression of labour
- Maternal urine should be checked for ketones and protein every 4 hours

Preterm labour (PTL) (Table 127.3)

Induction of labour (IOL)

Around 1 in 5 labours in the UK are artificially induced (Table 127.4). Induction at 41+ weeks aims to reduce stillbirth rates.

TABLE 127.1	Stages of Labour
First Stage	
Latent phase	Cervix effacing (shortening and softening) and thinning. **0–4 cm** dilation
Established phase	Cervix effaced, **4–10 cm** (fully dilated), regular and painful contractions
Second Stage Passive phase	Cervix is completely dilated but no pushing takes place. Allows the baby to descend to the pelvic floor. Often seen with epidural analgesia, where 1–2 hours of passive phase reduces risk of instrumental delivery
Active phase	Maternal **pushing** until the baby is born
Third Stage	Delivery of the **placenta** (usually <15 minutes after delivery of baby). The uterus contracts and the placenta separates. **Active third stage** (IM uterotonics, controlled cord traction), less PPH risk. **Physiological third stage** (waiting for the placenta to deliver naturally)

TABLE 127.2   Foetal Heart Rate Assessments in Labour

Foetal Heart Rate	
Intermittent auscultation	Every 15 minutes during first stage of labour for low-risk women (handheld Doppler). Every 5 minutes during second stage of labour. If any concerns, then for CTG monitoring
Continuous CTG monitoring	Recommended for women with risk factors including induced labour, previous LSCS, multiple pregnancy, abnormal lie, epidural anaesthesia, pre-eclampsia, diabetes, prematurity, small for gestational age, etc. CTG monitoring by abdominal probes or foetal scalp electrode (if factors such as obesity, poor contact of abdominal probe or doubt about source of heartbeat). CTG is sensitive but not specific in detecting foetal hypoxia – foetal blood sampling can improve specificity

TABLE 127.3   Preterm Labour

Definition	Babies born before 37 weeks' gestation
Risk factors	Previous preterm birth, previous cervical procedures (e.g. LLETZ), multiple pregnancy, uterine abnormalities, IUGR, pre-existing medical conditions
Predicting/preventing PTL	Preterm labour clinic for women at high risk 1. USS monitoring of cervical length (vaginal USS) 2. Screening for infections (bacterial vaginosis, chlamydia, gonorrhoea, UTI) 3. Cervical suture. Possible timings: 1. pre-pregnancy, 2. in second trimester following USS evidence of cervical shortening, 3. as a 'rescue' procedure
Diagnosing PTL	Regular painful contractions with cervical change. If no cervical change, tests for PTL risk; 1. USS of cervical length (vaginal USS). 2. Vaginal swabs: **Actim Partus** (from cervical os) or **foetal fibronectin** (from high vaginal swab)
Preparing for preterm birth	**Corticosteroids** if <35 weeks (reduces neonatal respiratory distress/intraventricular haemorrhage. **Magnesium sulphate** if <30 weeks (for neuroprotection)
Trying to stop the birth	**Tocolysis (terbutaline/**nifedipine aiming to stop contractions), ONLY if everything is normal – not if suspected infections, spontaneous rupture of membranes, bleeding or concern for foetal wellbeing

TABLE 127.4   Induction of Labour

Reasons for IOL	**Obstetric** (e.g. prolonged pregnancy, uteroplacental insufficiency, IUGR, pre-eclampsia, oligo-/an-hydramnios) or **medical** (e.g. hypertension, uncontrolled diabetes, renal disease)
Contraindications to IOL	Vasa praevia/placenta praevia, cord presentation/prolapse, foetal distress/malpresentation (e.g. breech), severe foetal growth restriction
Methods for IOL	• Membrane sweep (often referred to as 'stretch and sweep') • Intravaginal prostaglandins (e.g. Propess pessary) • Breaking of waters (amnihook) • Cook balloon • Oxytocin/syntocinon
Risks/considerations with IOL	Uterine hyperstimulation, failed induction, infection, bleeding, cord prolapse (particularly during amniotomy), uterine rupture (rare, higher risk if vaginal birth after caesarean). Instrumental delivery and LSCS rates are higher

Complications of Labour

Hannah Clark and Simon Scheck

LABOUR WARD, 32, G1P0, 41 + 3 WEEKS PREGNANT. ADMITTED FOR ARTIFICIAL RUPTURE OF MEMBRANES (ARM)

HPC: Underwent ARM procedure a few minutes earlier, when she was 3 cm dilated and the foetus was in a cephalic position; clear liquor was drained. Uncomplicated pregnancy so far but known polyhydramnios.

O/E: Following the ARM, the CTG shows variable foetal heart decelerations. On vaginal examination, there is a pulsating mass below the level of the cervix.

1. When counselling women on vaginal birth after section (VBAC) versus elective repeat caesaerean (CS), what is the risk of uterine rupture in VBAC, and what percentage have a successful VBAC?
2. What can be done to try and reduce the risk of severe perineal tears during delivery?
3. Malposition is a cause of delay in labour; what foetal position is most optimal for a vaginal delivery?

Answers: 1. A planned VBAC has a 1 in 200 risk of uterine rupture. VBAC is successful in ~75%. 2. Control of speed and progress of presenting part, manual perineal protection where possible, warm perineal compress, episiotomy when indicated. 3. Cephalic presentation, occiput anterior (OA).

TABLE 128.1

	Features	Investigations	Management
Delay in labour/ failure to progress	RFs: poor uterine contractions (**power**), malposition/ malpresentation of foetus (**passenger**), pelvis/ soft tissues (**passage**). Also exhaustion (2nd stage). *Delay in first stage* if <2 cm cervix dilatation in 4 hours or slowing progress in multip. *Delay in second stage* if primip has been pushing for 2 hours, or if multip has been pushing for 1 hour	**Delay in first stage:** plot partogram – cervical dilatation, descent of foetal head (4-hourly vaginal examination), maternal observations, foetal HR, contraction frequency, status of membranes, presence/colour of liquor and any drugs/fluids given	**Delay in first stage:** offer ARM if membranes not ruptured. If membranes already ruptured, consider augmentation of labour with **oxytocin** infusion. Changing maternal position. Consider CS. **Delay in second stage:** consider instrumental or CS delivery
Shoulder dystocia	See *123. LARGE FOR GESTATIONAL AGE*		

(Continued)

TABLE 128.1   (Cont'd)

	Features	Investigations	Management
Retained placenta	Inability to deliver the placenta during 3rd stage of labour	Clinical diagnosis	Control PPH. If patient stable, try: massage uterus, breastfeeding (stimulates oxytocin), catheter (full bladder causes uterine atony). Manual removal of placenta
Perineal tears	**1st degree:** superficial and involves vaginal skin. **2nd degree:** perineal muscle, anal sphincter intact. **3rd degree:** anal sphincter torn: **3a** <50% of external anal sphincter, **3b** >50%, **3c** into internal anal sphincter. **4th degree:** into rectal mucosa	RFs: instrumental delivery, macrosomia, nulliparity. Clinical diagnosis. MRI: to assess structures if symptoms at 3/12	**1st/2nd degree:** conservative or suturing. **3rd- and 4th-degree tears**, repaired in theatre, routine Abx. Pelvic floor physio for 6 to 12 weeks, consultant follow-up. Hand hygiene advice to reduce secondary infection, laxatives to avoid constipation
Umbilical cord prolapse	**RFs:** malpresentation after 37 weeks, polyhydramnios, unengaged head, prematurity, delivery of second twin. Descent of umbilical cord through cervix below the presenting part after ROM. Abnormal foetal heart rate	Clinical diagnosis. **CTG:** foetal bradycardia or variable foetal heart decelerations. **Obstetric emergency**, call for senior help. **Deliver foetus ASAP** (CS, unless fully dilated with immediate instrumental delivery possible)	**Avoid handling** cord (vasospasm). *Immediate transfer to theatre*-continuous digital elevation to displace the presenting part away from cord. *If no immediate CS available;* patient → left lateral head-down/knee-to-chest position. Catheter to fill bladder and push foetal head up. **Tocolysis** with terbutaline reduces contractions
Uterine rupture	**Hx & O/E:** PV bleeding, unexplained maternal shock ± collapse, cessation of uterine contractions, presenting part disappears from pelvis	**RFs:** VBAC, previous uterine surgery, high BMI, induction of labour, oxytocin. **CTG:** foetal bradycardia or variable decelerations	**Obstetric emergency.** **A–E resuscitation** ± blood transfusion. **Emergency CS** to deliver foetus, control bleeding and repair uterus ± hysterectomy
Amniotic fluid embolism	**Hx & O/E:** acute onset dyspnoea, chest pain, hypoxia, hypotension, reduced consciousness/confusion, possibly seizures, DIC (bleeding from IV lines). Maternal collapse could be the first sign (Fig. 128.1)	**Tends to occur with ROM. DDx:** sepsis, PE, anaphylaxis, epidural anaesthetic toxicity. **Clinical diagnosis.** Exclude other causes of maternal collapse	A-E resuscitation with senior input. No specific treatments, so supportive management is key. Early ICU involvement – high maternal mortality. Consider perimortem CS to optimise maternal resuscitation

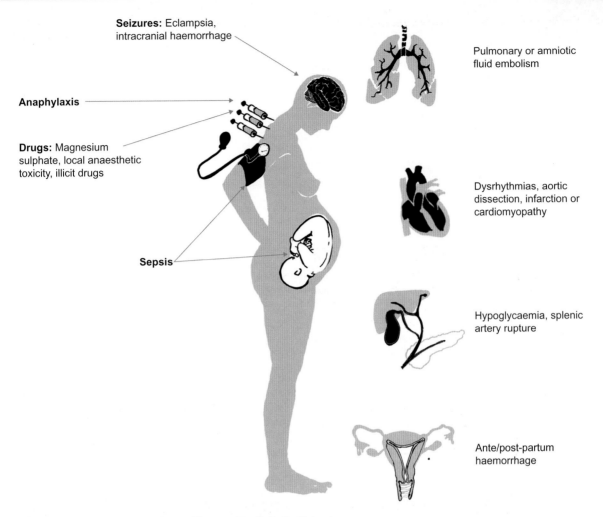

Fig. 128.1 Causes of maternal collapse. (Illustrated by Dr Hollie Blaber.)

The complication of labour being described in the vignette is cord prolapse, recognised by presence of a pulsating mass below the cervix and foetal heart rate variability in the context of a recent ARM. Expedited delivery and alleviating pressure on the cord are vital. Delivery should be by CS, unless the woman is fully dilated and vaginal delivery would be quicker. Transfer to theatre should happen as quickly as possible with digital displacement of the presenting foetal part (to alleviate pressure on the cord) until the CS commences. If relocation is required (e.g. the patient is at home or a birthing centre without obstetric services), the patient should be placed in a position to take the weight of the foetus off the cord and the bladder should be filled with a catheter prior to transfer. Cord prolapse and foetal hypoxia can lead to hypoxic-ischaemic encephalopathy and cerebral palsy, so swift management is essential.

> ### REVISION TIPS
>
> - Remember that the causes of a delay in labour include the 3Ps: Power, Passenger, Passage
> - Shoulder dystocia RFs: macrosomia, maternal diabetes, multiple pregnancy – risk of brachial plexus injury, fetal hypoxia, fracture
> - Mention of ROM followed by maternal collapse should prompt you to consider amniotic fluid embolism, but PE is more common

Bleeding Post-Partum

Anna Ogier, Alexander Royston, and Manuj Vyas

MATERNITY WARD, 31 YEAR OLD, 12 HOURS POST-PARTUM.
ONGOING VAGINAL BLEEDING, FEELING LIGHT-HEADED

HPC: Admitted in active labour at 40 + 2 weeks, G4 P3 (uncomplicated). Uncomplicated labour and delivery, NVD with no instrumentation and first-degree laceration (did not need repair). Placenta delivered intact (spontaneously), estimated blood loss 2 L since delivery. **PMHx:** Nil, no known coagulopathy.

O/E: Pale, shocked. BP 80/60, 115 bpm, CRT 5 secs. RR 24. Uterus feels soft but large. Catheterisation; urine output <15 mL/hour.

1. What are the RFs for post-partum haemorrhage (PPH)?
2. What is given during the third stage of labour to reduce the incidence of PPH?
3. Under which conditions is ergometrine contra-indicated?

Answers: 1. Multiple pregnancy, previous PPH, pre-eclampsia, foetal macrosomia, failure to progress in second stage, prolonged third stage, retained placenta, placenta accreta, episiotomy, perineal laceration, general anaesthesia. 2. Oxytocin (OTC). 3. HTN, ischaemic heart disease, PVD, psychosis, hepatic/renal impairment.

TABLE 129.1

	Features	Investigations	Management
Primary PPH – within 24 hours			
Tone (uterine atony)	**RFs:** multiple pregnancy, polyhydramnios (enlarged uterus), macrosomia, uterine abnormality/infection, prolonged labour, fibroids. **Hx & O/E:** enlarged uterus, boggy when palpated. Generic features of hypovolaemia; tachycardia, hypotension, tachypnoea, oliguria	Most common cause (90%). FBC, clotting screen including fibrinogen, CM ≥4 U. A→E (massive transfusion protocol as necessary), consider ITU (if need for invasive monitoring)	Uterine compression/rubbing (Fig. 129.1), catheter. 1. oxytocin slow injection, 2. ergometrine (CI HTN), 3. consider carboprost (CI: asthma) + misoprostol. **Definitive:** 1st line; intra-uterine tamponade (Rusch balloon). B-Lynch uterine compression sutures. Uterine devascularisation or hysterectomy

TABLE 129.1	(Cont'd)		
	Features	**Investigations**	**Management**
Trauma (vaginal/ cervical laceration)	**RFs:** malposition, instrumental delivery (consider high vaginal tear), tears, episiotomy, cervical laceration, uterine rupture. **Hx & O/E:** presents as per uterine atony (minus enlarged, boggy uterus)	Less common (7%). Examination: inspect vagina/cervix for tears	Initial A→E. Uterine packing/Bakri balloon (tamponade). Surgical repair
Tissue (retained placental products)	**RFs:** prolonged OTC, high parity, preterm delivery, PMHx uterine surgery, IVF. **Hx & O/E:** placenta examined upon delivery seen to be not intact. Retained blood clot	2%-3% of PPH. **USS (pelvic):** diagnostic. **EUA** (theatre)	A→E. Tamponade measures. Manually/surgically remove retained products
Thrombin (clotting abnormalities)	**RFs:** PMHx clotting disorders, HELLP, DIC, DHx anticoagulation. **DIC RFs:** severe PET, sepsis or placental abruption. Shock	Rare. Early recognition vital	A→E. Haematology. Tranexamic acid/Vit K as advised. Correct coagulopathy; FFP (long PT/APTT, or haemorrhaging despite transfusion. **Cryoprecipitate** – ongoing haemorrhage + low fibrinogen. **Platelet concentrate** if low platelets
Secondary PPH – 24 hours-12 weeks			
Retained placenta	As above	USS	
Endometritis	Infection of the endometrium. **RFs:** Caesarean section, HIV +ve, PROM, severe meconium contamination, prolonged labour. **Hx & O/E:** fever, chills, foul discharge, tender abdo/uterus	FBC/CRP (↑inflammatory markers). Blood cultures. **Urine** MSU. **HVS:** gonorrhoea/ chlamydia. (Endometrial biopsy diagnostic, rarely appropriate)	A→E. Sepsis protocol. Broad-spectrum Abx, IVI, O_2 (as required)

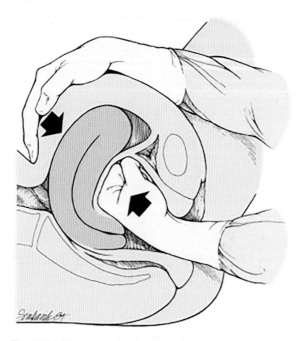

Fig. 129.1 Bimanual massage. Uterine compression and rubbing both stimulate contractions. (From Gabbe SG, Niebyl JR, Simpson JL. *Obstetrics: Normal and Problem Pregnancies*. 4th ed. New York: Churchill Livingstone; 2002:468; with permission.)

The vignette describes significant PPH with shock. The precise cause is perhaps less important than the prompt recognition and treatment. Uterine atony is the commonest cause, and in this case the large soft uterus makes it the probable cause. She has no known coagulopathy, and no instrumentation or significant laceration occurred during delivery. Her previous births have been uncomplicated (although multiparity is an RF for uterine atony, as is passive management of the third stage of labour). She requires urgent fluid resuscitation before transfusion and pharmacological, mechanical and/or surgical management.

REVISION TIPS

- Categories of PPH
  - **Minor (500–1000 mL) or >1000 mL after CS + no shock**. IV access (14 gauge cannula), G+S, FBC, coagulation screen + fibrinogen, Obs (BP every 15 minutes), warmed crystalloid infusion
  - **Major (>1000 mL) and actively bleeding/shock** – 2222 Major Haemorrhage Protocol. A, B, C, flatten patient, fluid resuscitation with blood asap, crystalloid fluids in meantime
- Features (moderate → severe): tachycardia, dizziness, palpitations, weakness, sweating, restlessness, pallor, oliguria, collapse, air hunger, anuria

Difficulty With Breastfeeding

Katie Turner, Alexander Royston, Graham Thornton, and Manuj Vyas

GP CONSULTATION, FEMALE, 32. BILATERAL BREAST PAIN

HPC: 3 days post-partum, breastfeeding. Breasts have felt tender and heavy for the past 2 days, pain is worse just before a feed, baby is finding it difficult to latch.

O/E: Breasts appear swollen and erythematous. On palpation, firm and tender. Nipples appear stretched and flat. Temp 38.0°C, BP 124/62 mmHg, HR 71 bpm, RR 16, SpO_2 99%.

1. What are the main benefits of breastfeeding to the mother?

2. Which bacteria most commonly cause mastitis?
3. Can you name two contraindications to breast-feeding?

Answers: 1. Reduced rates of breast cancer, ovarian cancer and osteoporosis. Reduced incidence of obesity. Amenorrhoea/contraception. Emotional support/bonding. 2. *Staphylococcus aureus* (though can also be caused by *Streptococcus* (*viridans*) and Gram-negative bacilli such as *E. coli*, *Salmonella* spp.). 3. Infants with galactosaemia, maternal viral infection (e.g. HIV), drugs (e.g. lithium, benzodiazepines, aspirin, carbimazole, methotrexate, amiodarone).

TABLE 130.1

	Features	Investigations	Management
Engorgement	**Hx & O/E:** bilateral tenderness, heaviness, swelling, erythema, nipples appear stretched and flat, pain/discomfort worse just before a feed, fever (15%) (Fig. 130.1)	Occurs in the first few days post-partum. Clinical diagnosis	Feed without limitations on frequency or duration, well-fitting bra, non-restrictive clothing, hand express milk, massage breasts after feeds, analgesia
Blocked duct	Unilateral nipple pain when breastfeeding, tender 'pea-sized' lump and 'milk bleb' on nipple tip, erythema, can →mastitis	**RFs:** stress, fatigue, anaemia, immunocompromise. Clinical diagnosis	Feed from the affected breast frequently, well-fitting bra, heat packs/warm showers, gentle massage, analgesia

(Continued)

TABLE 130.1   (Cont'd)

	Features	Investigations	Management
Mastitis	**Hx & O/E:** unilateral, painful, erythematous and systemically unwell (fever/malaise). Usually *Staphylococcus aureus*. Can progress to an abscess	**RFs:** previous mastitis, nipple trauma/ cracking, stagnation during lactation (intermittent/ missed feeds), smoking, obesity, immunosuppression. Clinical diagnosis. **USS:** if abscess-suspected	Reassurance, continue breast-feeding if lactational, analgesia. Consider Abx; symptoms ≥24 hours/ clear signs of infection (usually flucloxacillin). Abscess: USS-guided aspiration (MC&S) ± repeated aspirations
Nipple candidiasis	Bilateral burning nipple pain/ itching/hypersensitivity, worse during/soon after feeds, nipple may be shiny, swollen or fissured, pain may radiate to the breast and chest wall (if ductal infection)	**RFs:** nipple damage, mastitis, recent Abx. Clinical diagnosis	Miconazole cream (mother). Nystatin suspension (infant)
Raynaud disease of nipple	Intermittent pain during and immediately after feeding, blanching followed by cyanosis and erythema, pain resolves when nipple returns to normal colour	**RFs:** PMHx/ FHx of Raynaud phenomenon. Clinical diagnosis	Minimise cold exposure, heat packs after breast-feeding, avoid caffeine, smoking cessation. Persistent: consider nifedipine
Other Important Differentials			
Ankyloglossia (tongue-tie)	**Hx & O/E:** short lingual frenulum, "notched tongue". Inability to latch effectively (may bottle feed better than breastfeed). Poor infant weight gain (paediatrician criteria for concern met)	Congenital anomaly (many asymptomatic). M > F, FHx. Clinical diagnosis	Conservative measures: breastfeeding advice, massaging the frenulum. Surgical division of the lingual frenulum
Cleft lip/palate	Cleft lip apparent at birth, may present with feeding difficulties (nasal milk regurgitation)	**RFs:** sporadic, FHx, maternal smoking, obesity, folate deficiency. 1 in 1000	Surgical repair. Lip: repair at 3 months. Palate: 1 year. Follow-up due to problems with speech, hearing, dentistry

The vignette describes a case of engorgement, consistent with the short period since birth, pain peaking before feeding and bilateral symptoms. Fever is commonly found with breast engorgement (low-grade "milk fever"). Engorgement is caused by distension of the ducts and increased extravascular fluid, and it can cause dysfunctional nursing and nipple trauma: this may lead to early termination of breastfeeding. Differentiating from mastitis is mainly done by the absence of systemic symptoms and because mastitis is rarely bilateral. It is also important to exclude an abscess.

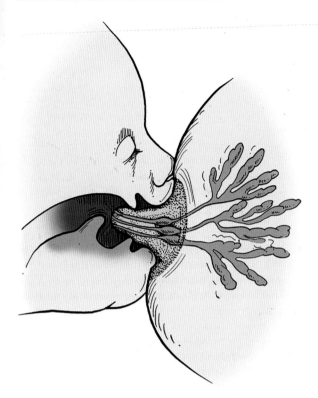

Fig. 130.1 Breastfeeding and engorgement. (From Newton ER, Stuebe AM. *Lactation and Breastfeeding. Gabbe's Obstetrics: Normal and Problem Pregnancies.* Elsevier; 2021.)

REVISION TIPS

- WHO recommends exclusively breastfeeding for the first 6 months
- If a breastfed baby loses >10% of birth weight in the first week of life – refer to midwife-led breastfeeding clinic
- Breast abscess develops in approximately 10% of women with mastitis

131

Pain on Sexual Intercourse (Dyspareunia)

Katie Turner, Alex Digesu, and Alka Bhide

**GP CONSULTATION, FEMALE, 52.
6-MONTH HISTORY OF PAIN DURING
SEXUAL INTERCOURSE**

HPC: Pain is superficial, at vaginal entrance. Complaints of itchiness, burning sensation in the vagina, increased urinary frequency, urgency. Treated for UTI 3 times in last 12 weeks. LMP 9 months ago, has occasional spotting. Nulliparous.

O/E: Pale dry vagina with friable epithelium.

1. Name the two bacteria that are responsible for 25% of cases of pelvic inflammatory disease (PID).
2. Give three complications of PID.
3. What laparoscopic findings are commonly seen in endometriosis?

Answers: 1. *Chlamydia trachomatis, Neisseria gonorrhoeae.* 2. Perihepatitis (Fitz-Hugh–Curtis syndrome), infertility, chronic pelvic pain, ectopic pregnancy, tubo-ovarian abscess. 3. Chocolate cysts, adhesions, peritoneal deposits.

TABLE 131.1

	Features	Investigations	Management
Superficial dyspareunia			
Atrophic vaginitis	Vaginal dryness/pruritis/burning. Mucosa dry, pale/red, petechiae. Discharge (rarely profuse) – white/yellow/blood-tinged. Urinary symptoms, UTIs. Atrophied labia minora/majora	RFs: post-menopausal, nulliparous, smoking, chemotherapy. Clinical diagnosis. Infection screen – if discharge/bleeding. Vaginal pH testing. Vaginal cytology	Vaginal lubricants and moisturisers. Topical oestrogen cream. Systemic HRT – if other post-menopausal Sx
Lichen sclerosus	Shiny, white patches on inner vulva. Scarring, bleeding, dysuria. Age >65 years	Clinical diagnosis. Biopsy if atypical features	Topical steroids and emollients
Candidiasis	See *136. VULVAL LESION/ITCH*		
Bartholin's cyst	Unilateral labial mass. Acute onset of pain. Difficulty passing urine	Clinical diagnosis. Consider biopsy if >40 years to r/o malignancy	If asymptomatic, await spontaneous rupture. Word catheter marsupialisation

TABLE 131.1 (Cont'd)

	Features	Investigations	Management
Deep dyspareunia Pelvic inflammatory disease	See *133. PELVIC PAIN*		
Endometriosis	Cyclical pain, dyschezia, dysuria, dysmenorrhea, subfertility. Fixed, retroverted uterus. See *119. SUBFERTILITY*	Laparoscopy. Pelvic USS	Analgesia. COCP or progestogens. Laser ablation, surgical excision, TAH with BSO
Vaginismus	Involuntary pelvic floor spasm; tightness/pain with intercourse, can prevent penetration (may be impossible). Generalised muscle spasm, breathing cessation. Triggers; fear, history of sexual abuse, relationship problems	Pelvic examination will induce pain. High vaginal swabs, urinalysis – to r/o infection	Usually a long-term issue. Education and counselling. Physiotherapy: pelvic floor relaxation techniques, use of vaginal dilators

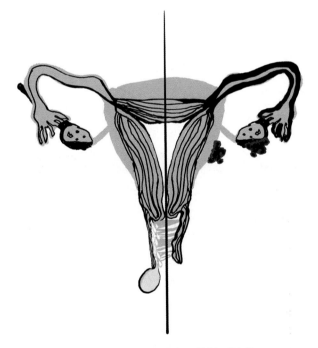

Fig. 131.1 Causes of dyspareunia (see Table 131.1).

Infection leads to inflammation, hence vaginal discomfort is generally seen in candidiasis and PID (Fig. 131.1). PID can be a severe infection, hence prominent pain, malaise, fever. Atrophic vaginitis (menopausal women) and lichen sclerosus (older women) also cause mild inflammation. Each of these can cause vaginal discharge to a varying extent. Endometriosis is due to ectopic uterine tissue causing inflammation at the time of periods, in various potential locations anatomically. Dysuria suggests inflammation close to the external urethral meatus or posterior wall of the bladder and can be seen in candidiasis, atrophic vaginitis, lichen sclerosus, and sometimes in endometriosis. Pain on penetration indicates a problem of the labium (e.g. Bartholin's cyst) or pelvic floor (vaginismus). In the vignette, the most likely cause is atrophic vaginitis, based on age, and clinical features, especially appearance on examination.

REVISION TIPS

- Vaginal atrophy can result from aromatase inhibitors (e.g. tamoxifen) used for breast cancer treatment
- Systemic HRT increases the risk of breast cancer, endometrial cancer, VTE and stroke

132

Vaginal Prolapse

Emily Warren, Alex Digesu, and Alka Bhide

UROGYNAECOLOGY CLINIC, FEMALE, 59.
VAGINAL 'DRAGGING SENSATION'

HPC: Discomfort 'down below' for a few weeks, worse after prolonged standing and during sexual intercourse. Feels well, no weight loss/urinary or bowel symptoms/vaginal bleeding/discharge. **PMHx:** COPD, hypertension. **Obstetric Hx:** Two children, uncomplicated vaginal delivery, one with forceps. **DHx:** Ramipril, formoterol inhaler. **SHx:** Current smoker, 40 pack years, BMI 35, independent ADLs.

  O/E: General inspection normal. With Sims' speculum, the cervix descended into the vagina on straining, close to the hymenal ring.

1. What are the two main classification systems for pelvic organ prolapse (POP)?
2. What are the potential complications of a vaginal pessary?

Answers: 1. POP-Q and Baden Walker. 2. Vaginal discharge, bleeding, difficult removal, pessary expulsion.

TABLE 132.1

	Features	Investigations	Management
Uterovaginal POP	**RFs:** postmenopausal, childbirth, raised intra-abdominal pressure. **Hx & O/E:** dragging/heavy sensation worse if active/standing/intercourse. Severe can externalise (procidentia)	Clinical diagnosis, **bimanual and speculum, exclude UTI.** Pelvic/transvaginal US	Weight loss (BMI > 30), reduce lifting/smoking/constipation, pelvic floor muscle training, pessary. Surgery to restore support (e.g. Manchester repair, sacrocolpopexy, sacrohysteropexy) or hysterectomy
Cystocoele (anterior vaginal POP)	Sensations/RFs as above. May have incontinence or difficulty passing urine	Evaluation as above. Urodynamics if incontinence and planning surgery	Conservative: as above. Surgery: anterior colporrhaphy
Enterocoele (upper posterior vaginal POP)	Sensations/RFs as above. Pulling sensation/low back pain, eases supine	Evaluation as above	Conservative: as above. Surgery: enterocoele repair

TABLE 132.1	(Cont'd)		
	Features	Investigations	Management
Rectocoele (lower posterior vaginal POP)	Sensations/RFs as above. Constipation, incomplete defaecation, incontinence of flatus or faeces, lower back pain	Evaluation as above, with PR examination	Conservative: as above. Surgery: posterior colporrhaphy
Top Differentials Mass of gynaecological origin	For example; fibroid, uterine polyp, ovarian cyst (benign or malignant), cervical elongation, cervical malignancy. See *134. PELVIC MASS* and *137. ABNORMAL CERVICAL SMEAR*		

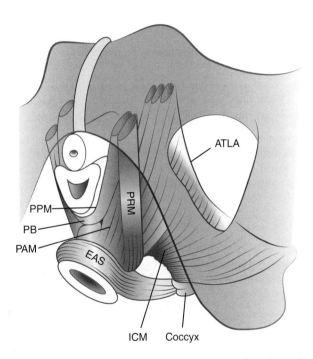

Fig. 132.1 Levator ani (viewed from below after the vulvar structures and perineal membrane have been removed), showing the arcus tendineus levator ani (ATLA), external anal sphincter (EAS), puboanal muscle (PAM), perineal body (PB) uniting the two ends of the puboperineal muscle (PPM), iliococcygeal muscle (ICM) and puborectal muscle (PRM). The urethra and vagina have been transected just above the hymenal ring. (Copyright © DeLancey JO, Kearney R, Chou Q, Speights S, Binno S. The appearance of levator ani muscle abnormalities in magnetic resonance images after vaginal delivery. *Obstet Gynecol.* 2003;101:46–53.)

POP is common, rather varied, and might be identified incidentally. Levator ani (Fig. 132.1) supports the pelvic organs, and childbirth can damage the muscle or its ligamentous support. The compartments are named according to the adjacent pelvic organ that may prolapse; uterovaginal POP indicates either uterine POP or vaginal vault POP (for a woman who previously had hysterectomy). The perineal body behind the vagina may also be affected. Bladder or bowel displacement in a POP may cause incontinence or difficulty emptying; these must be evaluated if planning treatment. Interventional treatment is not needed if asymptomatic, but pelvic floor exercises can be advised. If symptomatic, pelvic floor muscle training (PFMT), known as Kegel exercises, should be supervised by a trained healthcare professional, and maintained. Response should be assessed at 4–6 months. Surgery aims to support the organ, either by attaching it to another structure (e.g. sacrospinous fixation) or by closing the defect (e.g. colporrhaphy). The vignette describes a uterine POP (stage 2, as it is close to the hymenal ring, but not beyond it).

REVISION TIPS

- The common operative repair of cystocoele/rectocoele is anterior/posterior colporrhaphy, respectively. For uterine POP, sacrospinous fixation or hysterectomy, for vault POP (previous hysterectomy) sacrocolpopexy
- Previously mesh was used to close defects, but it is now banned in some countries due to bad complications

133

Pelvic Pain

Claudia Burton, Emily Warren, Berenice Aguirrezabala Armbruster, Sanchita Sen, and Shivam Bhanderi

---

ACUTE MEDICAL UNIT, FEMALE, 28.
TWO DAYS OF LOWER ABDOMINAL PAIN, NAUSEA AND VOMITING

HPC: Blood-stained, thick vaginal discharge. Irregular periods since menarche. Dyspareunia ongoing. No change in bowel habit, some pain on urination. **PMHx:** Anxiety. **DHx:** nil. **SHx:** Independent, no regular sexual partner, DNA for cervical screening, non-smoker.

   OE: pale, clammy. NEWS4 (HR 114, BP 92/50, RR 18, SpO$_2$ 100% on air, Temp 37.8), GCS 15, chest clear, abdomen soft, suprapubic tenderness, bowel sounds present, no neurological concerns.

---

1. What are the key signs of pelvic inflammatory disease (PID)? What follow-up may be required?
2. How is ovarian torsion diagnosed?
3. What are your differentials for pelvic pain in females? What life-threatening diagnosis can be the cause?
4. What causes shoulder tip pain in ruptured ectopic?

Answers: 1. Lower abdo pain, abnormal vaginal discharge, irregular/new sexual partner. Patients with post-coital bleeding or dyspareunia need gynaecological assessment ± cervical screening. 2. Presents with (sub)acute abdo pain, usually localised to RIF, ± N&V, ± adnexal mass. Diagnosis is generally at surgical exploration, with visualisation of a rotated ovary. 3. Key differentials; PID, UTI – ectopic pregnancy. 4. Diaphragmatic irritation from free fluid.

TABLE 133.1

	Features	Investigations	Management
Pelvic inflammatory disease	**RFs:** New sexual partner/no regular partner, STI/PID history, not using barrier contraception, recent surgical intervention/ coil insertion. *Chlamydia trachomatis/Neisseria gonorrhoeae/Mycoplasma genitalium* – reproductive tract infection. **Hx & O/E:** lower abdo pain, dysuria, deep dyspareunia, abnormal vaginal discharge, post-coital bleeding. Cervical motion tenderness- uterine/ adnexal. May present with sepsis. Can lead to infertility, ectopic pregnancy, chronic pelvic pain (higher risk in chlamydia PID)	**Bloods:** baseline (normal), β-HCG (negative). **High and low vaginal swabs:** for STI screen. **NAAT:** for gonorrhoea/ chlamydia/*M. genitalium*. **Urine dip/MSU:** r/o UTI. ±TVUSS. **Laparoscopy:** if severe, or uncertainty	SEPSIS pathway if suspected. Broad-spectrum Abx with anaerobic cover (local guidelines); **Ceftriaxone** 1 g IM once *PLUS* **Doxycycline** 100 mg PO BD 14 days *PLUS* **Metronidazole** 500 mg BD 14 days. Analgesia, counselling (safe sex practice, barrier contraception), contact tracing recommended (from the last 6 months). Treat contacts from *within 60 days* or if >60 days since last sexual contact treat *last sexual partner*.

TABLE 133.1 (Cont'd)

	Features	Investigations	Management
Premenstrual syndrome (PMS)	RFs: ovulatory menstrual cycles, FHx, mood disorders, smoking, alcohol, sexual abuse, trauma, stress, weight gain. Hx & O/E: symptoms mainly in luteal phase, resolve with onset of menses, then symptom-free week. Psychological (e.g. mood swings, irritability, anxiety), physical (e.g. breast tenderness, bloating, headache), behavioural (e.g. reduced cognitive)	Clinical diagnosis. Premenstrual dysphoric disorder (PMDD) is a severe form of PMS	Lifestyle changes. Analgesia. Moderate PMS: consider new-generation combined oral contraceptive and CBT. Severe: consider SSRI off-label use and CBT. Symptom diary, review in 2 months
Ectopic pregnancy	See *67. ACUTE ABDOMINAL PAIN*		
Ovarian or adnexal (ovary + fallopian tube) torsion.	RFs; mass ≥5 cm (neoplasm, cyst), pregnancy, previous torsion. Any age, especially child-bearing. Hx & O/E: N&V, low abdo/ pelvic pain (may be painless), ± mass. Fever/ guarding if necrotic. Discharge if tubo-ovarian abscess. Infants; feeding intolerance, inconsolable	Urinary β-HCG: negative. Bloods: β-HCG (–ve), baseline bloods, G&S/CM, clotting. TVUSS: ± CT (r/o other causes)	A–E. Laparoscopy. Surgical detorsion with adnexal sparing, ± ovarian cystectomy. Salpingo-oophorectomy if necrotic/ malignant cyst/ post-menopausal. After detorsion, ovaries functional in most. Ovarian cyst accident, see *67. ACUTE ABDOMINAL PAIN*
Appendicitis	See *67. ACUTE ABDOMINAL PAIN*		
Key Complications			
Tubo-ovarian abscess/ hydrosalpinx	Hx & O/E: abdo/pelvic pain, discharge, fever, mass (palpable/ tender), can be bilateral	Inflammatory markers. USS: thick-walled mass ± debris. CT or MRI	Antibiotic therapy – often polymicrobial with anaerobes. Surgical drainage may be required
Perihepatitis (Fitz-Hugh-Curtis syndrome)	5%–15% of PID cases (female). Hx & O/E: RUQ/pleuritic pain, N&V	Inflamed liver capsule (Glisson's)/peritoneum. Diagnosis of exclusion, no LFT abnormalities	*Chlamydia + gonorrhoea.* Treat as for PID

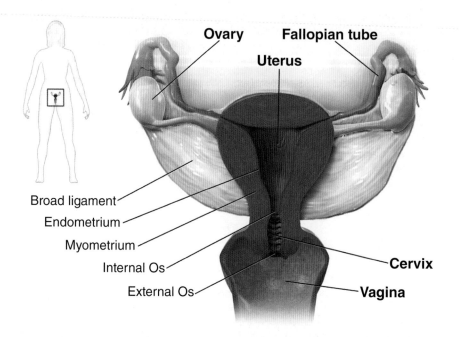

Fig. 133.1 Pelvic inflammatory disease (PID) is an infection of the female reproductive system. (Reference: BruceBlaus, CC BY 3.0 (via Wikimedia Commons.))

*The vignette is in keeping with pelvic inflammatory disease (PID) Fig. 133.1 Whilst sexually transmitted infections can be asymptomatic, picked up on routine screens, PID often presents with abdo pain, abnormal vaginal discharge and pain, or bleeding during intercourse. As with any infections, the most concerning presentation would be sepsis (pyrexia, tachycardia, hypotension). Treatment with broad-spectrum antibiotics should be started even if high and low vaginal swab results are pending. As with any female of child-bearing age, ectopic pregnancy must be ruled out, since it could be life threatening – urinary β-HCG is important in all female patients of child-bearing age presenting with pelvic pain. Endometriosis is described in **119. SUBFERTILITY** and **131. PAIN ON SEXUAL INTERCOURSE (DYSPAREUNIA)***

REVISION TIPS

- Causes of PID: STI (*Chlamydia trachomatis* and *Neisseria gonorrhoeae* are responsible for 25%), recent gynaecological instrumentation (abortion, IUD)
- Treatment – 14-day course of broad-spectrum antibiotics, started prior to swab results.
- Partner tracking to prevent further spread in community

- Risk of tubo-ovarian abscess should be considered in women who are systemically unwell – may require surgical input for drainage
- β-HCG is an essential test for women of child-bearing age in a wide range of presentations

134

Pelvic Mass

Zoe Kay, Leia Alston, and Sanchita Sen

GP CONSULTATION, FEMALE, 26. MENORRHAGIA

HPC: Complaining of heavy, prolonged periods. No inter-menstrual bleeding or dysmenorrhoea. Constipation during the past year, some urinary frequency. Currently trying to conceive with partner, unsuccessful for 2 years.
DHx: Tranexamic acid 1 g TDS for days 1–3 of menstrual cycle and Ibuprofen 400 mg during menstruation. Lives with partner, has never smoked, currently does not drink alcohol.
  O/E: Appears well. HR 88, BP 124/90, RR 12, T 36.6°C, SpO$_2$ 99% (air). Conjunctival pallor, abdominal examination reveals a non-tender pelvic mass extending into abdomen; on bimanual examination, uterus feels large.
Ix: Urinary pregnancy test is negative. Bloods reveal microcytic anaemia.

1. What are the three components of the Risk of Malignancy Index?
2. List risk factors and protective factors which affect ovulations, in relation to ovarian cancer risk.
3. A 24 yo woman is having a scan and histology to investigate the cause for her 3-month abdominal pain. A 6 cm mass is found and the histology reports Rokitansky protuberance. What is the most likely diagnosis?

Answers: 1. Ultrasound score, menopausal status, CA-125. 2. Risk factors (increase the number of ovulations/higher risk of cancer) include early menarche, nulliparity and late menopause. Protective factors (reduce the number of ovulations/lower risk) are combined contraceptive pill use, breastfeeding and pregnancy. 3. Teratoma/dermoid cyst – can contain teeth and hair components and has a high risk of becoming malignant.

TABLE 134.1

	Features	Investigations	Management
Uterine fibroids/ leiomyoma (Fig. 134.1)	**RFs:** increasing age, obesity, black ethnicity, early puberty, FHx. **Hx & O/E:** asymptomatic (most), menorrhagia, dysmenorrhoea, urinary frequency/urgency/incontinence, bloating/constipation, fertility issues, non-tender mass	FBC may reveal anaemia. **Transabdominal and transvaginal USS:** confirm diagnosis. GnRH agonists may be used pre-hysterectomy to shrink a fibroid	Mefenamic/tranexamic acid for pain/bleeding. IUS for menorrhagia. Myomectomy, uterine artery embolisation, total or subtotal hysterectomy

(Continued)

TABLE 134.1   (Cont'd)

	Features	Investigations	Management
Ovarian cysts	RF: premenopausal. Hx & O/E: asymptomatic (most – incidental finding on USS), pelvic pain, palpable mass, bloating, acute complication (haemorrhage, rupture, torsion). Types: functional, mucinous, dermoid cyst, serous cystadenoma, sex cord-stromal tumour. Risk of Malignancy Index: ultrasound score, CA-125, menopause status	TVUSS: confirm diagnosis. No need for further investigation in premenopausal women with simple cyst on USS. CA-125 in post-menopausal women. LDH, α-FP and hCG if <40 with a complex ovarian mass (r/o germ cell tumour)	Ovarian cysts <50mm are usually physiological, do not require further management. Cysts 50–70mm need annual USS follow-up. Larger cysts need further evaluation ± MRI and possible surgical intervention
Ovarian cancer	RFs: increasing age, FHx ovarian/breast ca, endometriosis, genetic (e.g. BRCA), Lynch syndrome, factors increasing ovulations, obesity, smoking. Hx & O/E: persistent bloating, ascites, early satiety, urinary frequency and urgency, abdominal or pelvic pain, PV bleeding	CA-125, LDH, α-FP, beta hCG if <40 with complex ovarian mass (r/o germ cell tumours). Transabdo/TVUSS: confirm diagnosis. CT TAP: staging. Risk of Malignancy Index	Surgery ± adjuvant chemotherapy
Tubo-ovarian abscess (PID)	See *133. PELVIC PAIN*		

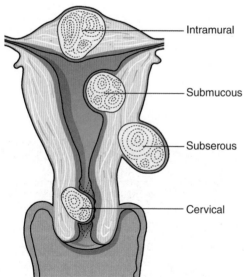

Fig. 134.1 Sites of fibroids throughout the uterus. (Sassarini J, McAllister K. Chapter: 7, Heavy menstrual bleeding, dysmenorrhoea and pre-menstrual syndrome. In: *Clinical Obstetrics and Gynaecology*. Elsevier; 2023. Copyright © 2023 Elsevier Ltd. Published by Elsevier Inc. All rights reserved.)

Labels: Intramural, Submucous, Subserous, Cervical

The top differential in the vignette is fibroids, but differentials like ovarian cyst are important to consider. A key for diagnosis of fibroids is that the pelvic mass is NOT tender. However, fibroids can present with abdo tenderness and fever under the circumstances of 'Red Degeneration'. This is usually secondary to a venous thrombosis of larger fibroids, and pregnancy increases the risk of this happening.

REVISION TIPS

- Triad of ovarian fibroma (benign tumour), ascites, pleural effusion is known as Meigs syndrome – typical MCQ!
- Fibroids can present with abdominal tenderness and fever under the circumstances of 'Red Degeneration'. This is infarction of the fibroid usually secondary to a venous thrombosis. Fibroids >5cm and pregnancy increase likelihood

135

Vulval Lump

Katherine Parker, Sanchita Sen, and Megan Crofts

HPC: Recently noticed a swelling on the left side 'down below', becoming extremely painful 2 days ago. Paracetamol not helping, now painful to walk. No discharge, unusual bleeding or itching. She has two regular partners with whom she usually uses barrier protection, both asymptomatic. No sexual intercourse since symptoms began due to superficial dyspareunia. No recent STI screening. On COCP.

O/E: Mobilising is painful. Mildly pyrexial, otherwise normal observations. **Vulval examination:** Smooth erythematous swelling in the left medial aspect of the labia and introitus. No unusual discharge or evidence of excoriations. Mass feels tense and is tender on palpation. Speculum examination could not be tolerated. No inguinal lymphadenopathy.

1. What is the most likely causative organism of folliculitis?
2. What does VIN stand for and what does it mean?
3. Condylomata lata are a painless lesion that are characteristic of secondary syphilis; apart from the vulva, where else may they develop?

Answers: 1. *Staphylococcus aureus*. 2. Vulval intraepithelial neoplasia; abnormal cells within the epidermis, graded 1–3 in accordance with the depth- premalignant. 3. Other areas of the oral and genital mucosa, and areas of friction: perianal region, under the breasts and axillae.

TABLE 135.1

	Features	Investigations	Management
Painful Vulval Lumps			
Bartholin's cyst/abscess	**RFs:** reproductive age, previous Bartholin's cyst, sexually active. **Cyst:** can be asymptomatic, soft, fluctuant, vulvar lump. **Abscess:** pain, superficial dyspareunia, tense mass with erythema, ± pyrexia, ± discomfort when walking/sitting	Clinical diagnosis. Bloods if abscess: raised inflammatory markers. Biopsy if unclear diagnosis/suspicious	**Cyst:** warm bath, compress to drain. **Abscess:** Abx ± incision and drainage. **Recurrent:** surgery-marsupialisation, balloon (Word) catheter (Fig. 135.1)

(Continued)

TABLE 135.1   (Cont'd)

	Features	Investigations	Management
Folliculitis	**RFs:** recent hot tub/swimming pool, shaving, tight clothing, topical cortico-steroids, DM, immunosuppression. **Hx & O/E:** pain, pruritis, irritation. Multiple erythematous papules/pustules in hair-bearing areas on the border of the labia. Common areas: beard, groin	Clinical diagnosis	**Uncomplicated:** preventative measures (antibacterial soaps, loose clothing). **Complicated/deep/recurrent:** Abx
Vulvar carcinoma	**RFs:** over 60 (though any age), smoker, HPV 16/18, PMHx lichen sclerosus, lichen planus, VIN. **Hx & O/E:** growing nodule/plaque, vulval itching, pain, bleeding, ulceration, discharge	Colposcopy (HPV a risk factor, so also assess for CIN). Examination and diagnostic biopsy	2WW referral. Wide local excision + sentinel node biopsy ± clearance
Painless Vulval Lumps			
Syphilis	**Primary:** solitary, **painless**, indurated ulcer (chancre), lymphadenopathy, non-purulent. Incubation 21 days. 10 weeks later, 25% untreated --> **Secondary:** non-pruritic maculopapular rash on palms of hands and soles of feet, condylomata lata **(moist, broad-based wart-like lumps)**, constitutional symptoms, snail track lesions (mouth), alopecia, early neurological symptoms. **Tertiary:** around 1/3 of untreated patients, up to **40 years** after initial infection. Gumma, CVD, neurosyphilis	**RFs:** unprotected sex, multiple partners, substance use, previous STI. **Swab:** dark-ground microscopy (spirochete), PCR (Treponema DNA). Syphilis serology (treponemal enzyme immunoassay (EIA)/chemiluminescent assay (CLIA))	Referral to GUM clinic – STI screen. IM: benzylpenicillin (doxycycline if penicillin allergic). Counselling: condition, risk factors, complications and prevention
Lipoma	**RF:** FHx. **Hx & O/E:** slow growing, soft, mobile, **painless** (unless compressing nerves/catching on clothing) lump. Usually <5 cm diameter. Within subcutaneous tissue	Clinical diagnosis. Consider imaging if >5 cm (risk liposarcoma)	Watch and wait. Consider excision – cosmetic reasons, compression, uncertain diagnosis
Genital warts	See *139. GENITAL ULCERS/WARTS*		
Molluscum contagiosum	Skin-skin contact; also seen in children. **Hx & O/E: umbilicated**, pearl-like, smooth papules ± swelling, erythema, pruritis	Clinical diagnosis	Infection clears on its own. Treat if affecting quality of life or immune compromise: local (imiquimod cream), cryotherapy
Other benign or malignant lesions	See *17. SKIN LESION*		

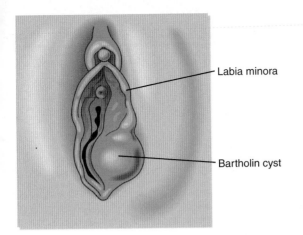

Labia minora

Bartholin cyst

The most likely diagnosis in the vignette is a Bartholin's abscess. A Bartholin cyst is usually painless, but if it grows large it can become uncomfortable, and infection can turn it into a painful abscess. Sometimes a biopsy is recommended to rule out vulval cancer (Bartholin vulval cancer). Consider a suspected cancer pathway referral (2WW) for vulval cancer in women with an unexplained vulval lump, ulceration or bleeding.

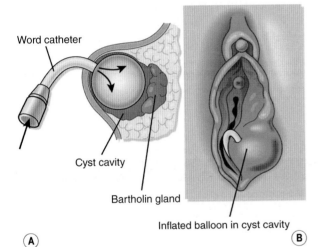

Word catheter

Cyst cavity

Bartholin gland

Inflated balloon in cyst cavity

(A)   (B)

Fig. 135.1 Above: Bartholin cyst in the left labium. Below: use of the Word catheter. (A) Cross section of the catheter in situ. (B) How it lies after placement. (From Adams JG, et al. *Emergency Medicine: Clinical Essentials.* 2nd ed. Philadelphia: Saunders; 2013.)

REVISION TIPS

- 'Gummata' (singular: gumma), seen in tertiary syphilis, are soft inflammatory growths that can develop in any part of the body including within the skin, internal organs and on the skeleton, which may grow to several cm in diameter
- HPV 16 and 18 are risk factors for **anal, vulval, cervical and throat cancer**

136

Vulval Lesion/Itch

Katie Turner, Lowri Foster Davies, Sanchita Sen, and Megan Crofts

GP CONSULTATION, FEMALE, 80.
ITCHY VULVAL LESION

HPC: 2-year history of vulval itching and soreness, failing to respond to topical steroid treatment. The lesion has recently started to bleed.

O/E: A 1.4 cm ulcerated lesion located on the right labium majus. Palpable inguinal lymph nodes.

1. Which HPV subtypes cause cervical cancer?
2. Can you name three infections which may cause vulval itch?

Answers: 1. HPV 16 and 18. 2. *Trichomonas vaginalis*, HSV and *Candida*.

TABLE 136.1

	Features	Investigations	Management
Vulval carcinoma	**RFs:** age >65 yo, lichen sclerosus or VIN. **Hx & O/E:** ulceration, bleeding, irritation. Located on labium majus (Fig. 136.1). Inguinal lymphadenopathy	FBC/U&Es/LFTs may be abnormal. **Biopsy.** **CT TAP:** staging and pre-op MRI may help staging	Surgical excision or wedge biopsy (larger lesion). Lymphadenectomy if >1 mm invasion. Radiotherapy ± chemotherapy
Vulval intraepithelial neoplasia (VIN)	**RFs:** HPV infection, smoking, chronic inflammatory condition (lichen sclerosus, lichen planus). **Hx & O/E:** vulval itch/pain. White or plaque-like lesion	Colposcopy. Biopsy	Excision. Immunotherapy (e.g. imiquimod). Monitor; regular cervical smears ± colposcopy
Lichen sclerosus	**Hx & O/E:** superficial dyspareunia, dysuria. Shiny, white crinkly patches; scarring/bleeding on inner areas of vulva	Age >65 years. Clinical diagnosis. Biopsy if atypical features	Topical steroids, emollients. Advise to use cotton underwear and avoid chemical irritants like perfumed soap
Atrophic vaginitis	See *131. PAIN ON SEXUAL INTERCOURSE/DYSPAREUNIA*		

TABLE 136.1 (Cont'd)

	Features	Investigations	Management
Candidiasis	**RFs:** diabetes, antibiotics, immunosuppression, pregnancy. **Hx & O/E:** non-offensive '*cottage cheese*' discharge, vaginal itch, burning, soreness, dysuria, vulval irritation, erythema, with fissuring + satellite lesions	80% due to *Candida albicans*. Clinical diagnosis. **Vaginal discharge wet mount microscopy:** budding yeast, hyphae (can also be seen on Gram stain). **Vaginal discharge culture.** **Self-swab:** r/o bacterial infection. **MSU** r/o UTI	Advise cotton underwear, avoid irritants (e.g. perfumed soaps). **Local:** clotrimazole pessary 500 mg/1% cream. **Oral:** itraconazole 200 mg twice. Fluconazole 150 mg once
Genital warts (HPV 6 and 11)	See *139. GENITAL ULCERS/WARTS*		
Trichomoniasis	See *138. VAGINAL AND URETHRAL DISCHARGE*		

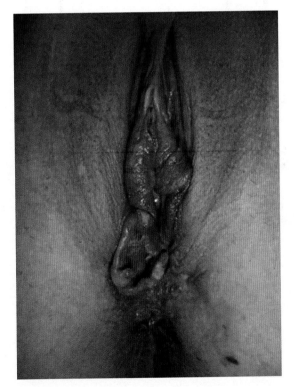

Fig. 136.1 Vulval carcinoma. (Reference: Ljubojevic S, Skerlev M. HPV-associated diseases. *Clin Dermatol*. March–April 2014. Elsevier. Copyright © 2014 Elsevier Inc. All rights reserved.)

The most likely diagnosis in the vignette is vulval cancer. Patients present with a persistent itch, lump, indurated ulcer, bleeding and/or pain. Other causes of vulval itch should be investigated and a skin biopsy should be carried out to confirm the diagnosis. Diffuse genital pruritis in the perimenopause/menopause is commonly atrophic vaginitis – inflammation, thinning and shrinking of the vaginal epithelium, with decreased lubrication, due to lack of oestrogen. It is due to reduced exfoliation of glycogen-producing cells and reduced lactobacilli, hence more alkaline environment, predisposing to vaginitis and UTIs.

REVISION TIPS

- 90% of vulval carcinomas are squamous cell
- 80% of candidiasis is caused by *Candida albicans*
- Both boys and girls aged 12–13 receive the HPV vaccine

137

Abnormal Cervical Smear

Alice Parker and Sanchita Sen

GP CONSULTATION, FEMALE, 45.
ABNORMAL CERVICAL SMEAR

HPC: She received abnormal cervical smear results from her 3-yearly cervical screening test: high-risk HPV (hrHPV): Positive. **Cytology:** High-grade dyskaryosis. She is referred to colposcopy clinic for further investigation.

1. What is management of an inadequate smear test?
2. What are the differentials of post-coital bleeding?
3. What are the differentials of intermenstrual bleeding?
4. When is the HPV vaccine given, and what HPV types does it protect against?

Answers: 1. Repeat at 3 months, if two inadequate samples, refer for colposcopy. 2. Ectropion, cervicitis, vaginitis, polyps, cervical cancer. 3. Endometritis, fibroids, polyps, endometrial/cervical/ovarian cancer, ovulation, cervicitis, ectropion, vaginitis, trauma, adenosis. 4. Boys and girls at age 12–13 years- Gardasil 9 covers 9 HPV types, including 16/18 (cause half of high grade cervical pre-cancers).

TABLE 137.1

	Features	Investigations	Management
Cervical intraepithelial neoplasia (CIN)	Pre-malignant for cervical cancer. **RFs:** HPV, smoking, multiple partners, immunocompromise, COCP. Associated with HPV 16, 18, 31, 33 (Fig. 137.1). CIN 1 = lower basal 1/3 of cervical epithelium. CIN 2 = <2/3 of full epithelial thickness, CIN 3 = >2/3. Screening aged 25–65 years (3-yearly if 25–49, 5-yearly if 50–65)	**HPV primary testing:** if hrHPV+, cytology for degree of dyskaryosis. **If HPV+ and abnormal cytology:** refer for colposcopy. **If HPV+ and normal cytology:** repeat HPV test in 12 months. If now normal, go to standard recall. If still HPV+ and cytology normal, repeat test again in 12 months. If HPV+ in three consecutive smears, refer for colposcopy	For low-grade dyskaryosis, punch biopsy and follow up smears. For high-grade dyskaryosis, LLETZ procedure in colposcopy clinic followed by smear + HPV testing at 6 months to ensure cure

TABLE 137.1 (Cont'd)

	Features	Investigations	Management
Cervical cancer	Most common in women 30–39 years and >70 years. Incidental finding on smear or colposcopy, OR post-coital/post-menopausal/inter-menstrual bleeding, vaginal discharge. O/E: hard/rough ± fixed cervix on bimanual, irregular ± bleeding mass on speculum	Stages 1. Confined to cervix (a: microscopic, b: macroscopic). 2. Upper 2/3 of vagina. 3. Lower 1/3 of vagina. 4. Spread to rectum ± bladder. Colposcopy: irregular surface, vessel formation, abnormal acetic acid uptake. Punch biopsy. Baseline bloods. MRI pelvis and examination under anaesthetic for staging	Early stages (1a): cone biopsy (preserves fertility). Radical trachelectomy. Simple hysterectomy. Late stages (1b+): radical hysterectomy. Radiotherapy ± chemotherapy. Pelvic exenteration

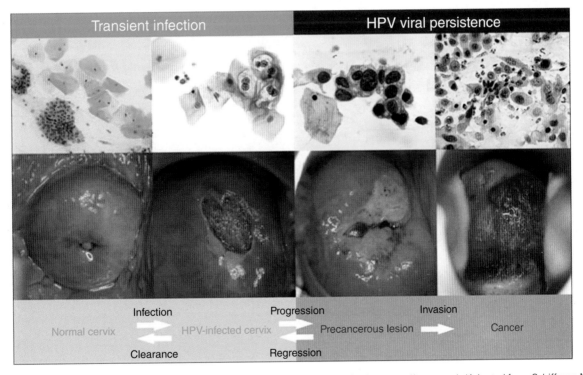

Fig. 137.1 Human papillomavirus and cervical cancer. Cytology (*upper row*) and colposcopy (*lower row*). (Adapted from Schiffman M, Castle PE. The promise of global cervical-cancer prevention. *N Engl J Med*. 2005;353:2101–2104.)

*Dyskaryosis is cervical intraepithelial neoplasia (CIN). CIN describes abnormal cervical cells, which if not treated may develop into cancer. It occurs at the squamocolumnar junction of the cervix, where the vaginal squamous epithelium meets the columnar epithelium of the endocervix. It is graded on a scale of 1–3 (3 is highest grade). The main cause of CIN is human papillomavirus (HPV) infection. It is important to have regular screening tests (see **142. WELLBEING CHECKS – Outline**), as CIN and HPV have no symptoms.*

REVISION TIPS

- The cervical screening programme is for women aged 25–65 years
- Samples from cervical smears are first tested for HPV: if hrHPV is positive, the sample is sent for cytology. If this is abnormal, the patient is referred for colposcopy
- CIN is pre-malignant for cervical cancer

Vaginal and Urethral Discharge

Anna Ogier, Lowri Foster Davies, and Megan Crofts

HPC: 1 week of malodorous, yellow-green discharge with dysuria and itch. She is on POP and has been having unprotected vaginal sex with a new male partner. Three previous partners with whom she had protected sex. No previous STI screen. Cervical smear last month was unremarkable.

O/E: On speculum, cervix appears inflamed with punctate bleeding. Swabs taken for NAAT.

1. What are your differentials for a mucopurulent discharge?
2. What are your differentials for a white/clear discharge?
3. How does management for candidiasis differ if the patient were pregnant?

Answers: 1. Chlamydia, gonorrhoea, trichomoniasis, mycoplasma genitalium. 2. Normal physiological discharge, candidiasis, bacterial vaginosis, ectropion, chlamydia. 3. Pregnant women would be prescribed a clotrimazole 500 mg pessary for up to 7 nights, while first-line therapy for non-pregnant women would be fluconazole 150 mg PO as a single dose. There is potential risk of birth defects or miscarriage associated with fluconazole taken in pregnancy.

TABLE 138.1

	Clinical	Investigations	Management
Trichomoniasis	♀ asymptomatic in 70%–86%. Yellow, green, frothy discharge (10%–30% symptomatic women) + offensive odour, itch, soreness, dysuria, dyspareunia, pruritus, vulval and vaginal erythema. Strawberry cervix. pH >4.5. ♂ asymptomatic in 75% and often transient (<10 days). Urethral discharge + dysuria. Untreated can persist for months	*Trichomonas vaginalis* protozoan. Most common non-viral STI. ♀ swabs: NAAT. Wet mount microscopy: motile trichomonads. Culture. ♂ urethral swab/first catch urine (FCU): culture and NAAT	Treat and **screen** sexual partner(s) from last **4 weeks.** **Metronidazole** 2 g PO stat. Then 400–500 mg BD 5–7 days. Abstain from sexual activity for 1 week

(Continued)

TABLE 138.1   (Cont'd)

	Clinical	Investigations	Management
Bacterial vaginosis	50%–75% asymptomatic. Fishy, grey-white thin discharge. No itch or irritation. ♀ RFs: douching, sexually active, smoking, other STDs, women of Afro-Caribbean descent, women who have sex with women	Anaerobe overgrowth, e.g. *Gardnerella vaginalis*. ♀ Amsel's criteria: clue cells, vaginal pH >4.5, positive whiff test, thin grey discharge. Gram stain: low proportion of lactobacilli	Metronidazole 400–500 mg PO 5–7 days. Can be given to pregnant women. Advice re avoiding vaginal hygiene products
Chlamydia	♀ Often asymptomatic. Cervicitis: yellow, odorous discharge, deep dyspareunia, intermenstrual/post-coital bleed. Cervical motion tenderness. Dysuria-pyuria syndrome/urethritis. ♂ Often asymptomatic. Urethritis (NGU): dysuria, white urethral discharge. Epididymitis: pain ± swelling	RFs: <25 yo, new/multiple sex partners, lack of barrier contraception. *Chlamydia trachomatis*. ♀ Vulvovaginal swab: NAAT. Sterile pyuria. ♂ FCU: NAAT	Doxycycline 100 mg BD 7 days. Avoid sexual intercourse until treatment completed. Test of cure in pregnancy. Advise test for other STIs. Partner contact tracing and treatment. Annual screening: sexually active <25 yo
Gonorrhoea	♀ 50% asymptomatic/ symptoms within 10 days. Cervicitis: increase or altered yellow/green discharge, intermenstrual bleeding, vaginal pruritus. Urethritis (dysuria). Abdo pain/ dyspareunia suspicious for PID. ♂ 95% symptomatic. Urethritis: yellow/green discharge, dysuria, 2–5 days after exposure	*Neisseria gonorrhoeae*. ♀ Vulvovaginal swab: NAAT. ♂ FCU/urethral swab NAAT. MC&S	Ceftriaxone 1 g IM stat. Ciprofloxacin (if sensitive) 500 mg PO stat. Cefixime (PO) 400 mg + oral azithromycin 2 g stat. Screening For STI/HIV. Abstain for 1 week. Partner contact tracing and empirical treatment for gonorrhoea and chlamydia
Mycoplasma genitalium	Asymptomatic (90%–95%) or ♀ Cervicitis: yellow-green discharge, intermenstrual/ post-coital bleeding, dysuria, urinary frequency, dyspareunia, vulvovaginal irritation, cervical motion tenderness. ♂ Non-gonococcal urethritis: dysuria, discharge, urethral itch	RFs: young adult, smoking, recent sexual intercourse, increasing number of sexual partners. ♀ Vulvovaginal or endocervical swab: NAAT. ♂ FCU: NAAT	Doxycycline 100 mg BD 7 days *followed by* azithromycin 1 g PO *then* 500 mg PO OD 2 more days. Abstain for 14 days from start of treatment
Differentials Candidiasis	See *136. VULVAL LESION/ITCH*		

TABLE 138.1 (Cont'd)

	Clinical	Investigations	Management
Genital herpes simplex	Watery vaginal discharge. **Painful genital ulcers,** vesicular blisters, bilateral lymphadenopathy, dysuria. Systemic fever, headache, malaise, myalgia (more common in primary disease). **Tingling, neuropathic pain** in genitals. Recurs to affected dermatome	HSV-1 and HSV-2. Swab/scraping: PCR. Viral **cultures** of lesions	Oral anti-viral *within 5 days of start of episode.* 5 days **Aciclovir** 400 mg TDS or **Valaciclovir** 500 mg BD. Saline baths, analgesia. **Counselling:** recurrence risk. If >6 recurrences in a year consider **daily anti-virals**
Syphilis	See *73. PERIANAL SYMPTOMS* and *135. VULVAL LUMP*		
Chancroid	*Haemophilus ducreyi.* Painful genital ulcer; fluctuant lymphadenitis, travel history	Gram stain. Swab ulcers/bubo culture. PCR	**Azithromycin** 1 g PO. **Trace + Test** sexual partners within 10 days prior to symptoms. **Ceftriaxone** 250 mg IM (pregnant)
Ectropion	Excessive white/clear discharge. Some spotting. **RFs:** oestrogen-containing contraceptives, pregnancy, menstruation	Clinical diagnosis	Stop oestrogen-containing medications. Ablative methods if required
Cervical, vulval or vaginal malignancies	**Red flag features:** weight loss. Lymphadenopathy, **abnormal vaginal bleeding,** offensive white/pink/brown discharge ± blood	Colposcopy/speculum examination + biopsy	2WW cancer pathway
Atrophic vaginitis	See *131. PAIN ON SEXUAL INTERCOURSE/DYSPAREUNIA*		
Normal physiological discharge	No pain or irritation. Can fluctuate with menstrual cycle/ pregnancy		
Key Complications	**Clinical**	**Investigations**	**Management**
Pelvic Inflammatory disease	See *133. PELVIC PAIN*		
Lymphogranuloma venereum	Caused by *Chlamydia trachomatis* (LGV biovar). Painless penile/vulvar inflammation/ ulceration. Chronic inflammation --> scarring, fibrosis --> lymphoedema of genitals. Mainly associated with symptoms of proctitis	Genital or lymph node **swabs** for NAAT. Other STI testing	**Doxycycline** 100 mg PO BD 7–21 days. Aspiration of pus

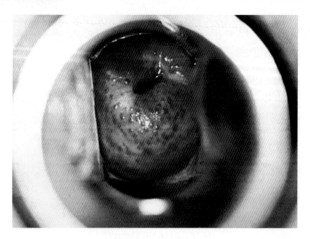

Fig. 138.1 Trichomonas (strawberry cervix). (From Krieger JN, Rein MF. Trichomoniasis. In: Rein M, ed. *Atlas of Infectious Diseases*. Vol V: Sexually Transmitted Diseases. Philadelphia: Churchill Livingstone; 1996:6.5.)

The most likely diagnosis in the vignette is trichomoniasis. Purulent discharge and dysuria, with itch, has several possible causes. However, in combination with the offensive odour and classical 'strawberry cervix' (Fig. 138.1) we are led towards this diagnosis. Most people would be screened for common STIs, alongside a full sexual and contraceptive history, and contact-tracing. Microscopy is quick, although NAAT is more accurate, with culture a reasonable option if this is not available. Bacterial vaginosis is less likely here and would be excluded by lack of clue cells. Counsel on safe-sex practices, including the protective potential of barrier contraception.

REVISION TIPS

- Normal vaginal discharge is around 1–4 mL every 24 hours; transparent, mucousy and white to yellow
- Cervicitis and urethritis are common presentations of STIs, if not asymptomatic
- Other important sequelae include preterm delivery, infertility, reactive arthritis, neoplasia, proctitis and prostatitis

139

Genital Ulcers/Warts

Anna Ogier, Alexander Royston, and Megan Crofts

HPC: New male sexual partner 1 month ago, unprotected penetrative sex. **PMHx:** Successfully treated for chlamydia infection 1 year ago. Current sexual partner does not have symptoms.

O/E: 3mm in diameter solitary growth on shaft of penis. No associated weight loss. No lymphadenopathy. Otherwise well on examination. Chlamydia and gonorrhoea swabs and urine taken at GP surgery are negative.

1. What organism causes syphilis?
2. What is the difference between lichen planus and lichen sclerosus?
3. Which HPV types typically cause anogenital warts?

Answers: 1. *Treponema pallidum* (spirochete bacterium). 2. Both are immunologically mediated dermatoses involving lymphocytic infiltration, with a preference for the genitalia. LP is more likely to involve the mucous membranes including the mouth and vagina; generally harder to treat. 3. HPV 6 and 11.

TABLE 139.1

	Features	Investigations	Management
Anogenital warts (Condylomata acuminata)	**RFs:** Unprotected sexual intercourse, multiple partners, prior STIs, HPV 6/11 (majority cause). **Hx & O/E:** small, individual or multiple, sessile exophytic papillomas. Can be hard and rough (keratinised) or soft, can bleed/become irritated. Often asymptomatic	Clinical diagnosis. Sexual history and examination. STIs screen. **Biopsy:** infrequently required (atypical lesions)	Spontaneous resolution in 1/3. Recurrence common: topical – podophyllotoxin, imiquimod (these weaken condoms). Ablative methods including cryotherapy. Surgical excision is rarely done. Condoms reduce recurrence
Condylomata lata	Secondary syphilis; see *135. VULVAL LUMP*		
Molluscum contagiosum	See *135. VULVAL LUMP*		

(Continued)

TABLE 139.1   (Cont'd)

	Features	Investigations	Management
Pearly papules	Vulva: vestibular papillomatosis. Penis: hirsuties papillaris genitalis. 1–2 mm pearly or flesh-coloured dome-shaped papules typically on sulcus/corona of the penis or labia. Often grow in lines	Clinical diagnosis	Normal anatomical variation: reassurance
Lichen planus	RFs: age (30–60 yo), Hepatitis C. Hx & O/E: itchy, sore papular rash on anogenital skin ± striae. Non-infectious, likely immune-mediated. Hypertrophic warty plaques can mimic neoplasm	Clinical diagnosis. Biopsy (only if uncertain)	Topical steroids (reduce symptoms). Patient education: small increased risk of malignancy
Fordyce spots	Yellow/white spots on head or shaft of penis or on labia	Sebaceous gland without hair follicles	Normal anatomical variation: reassurance

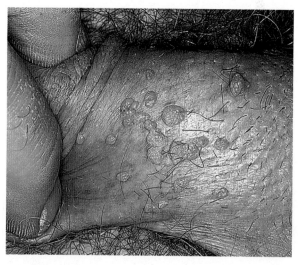

Fig. 139.1 Genital warts. (From Chapman MS. *Sexually Transmitted Infections. Skin Disease: Diagnosis and Treatment.* January 1, 2018:177–202. © 2018.)

carcinoma of the penis may present as a nodule, ulcer or erythematous lesion, which may appear warty, leuko-plakic or sclerotic but the surface is more usually smooth and velvety. This makes discounting penile carcinoma more challenging, but it is largely done on history, presence of risk factors (penile intra-epithelial neoplasia, HPV 16, chronic inflammatory conditions, etc.). Regional lymphadenopathy and red flags, such as weight loss, are important Genital ulcers may result from STI; chancroid (Haemophilus ducreyi), chlamydia, genital herpes, HIV or syphilis. Non-infectious ulcers include aphthous ulcers or Behçet's disease, and also consider penile, vulval or skin malignancy. See *136. VULVAL LESION/ ITCH* and *138. VAGINAL AND URETHRAL DISCHARGE*.

Anogenital warts are typically diagnosed on clinical presentation and history, as in the vignette. As the most common viral STI, the lack of systemic symptoms and appearance of the lesion(s) are important: warts may be morphologically variable but papillomatosis is constant (dermal papillae above the skin producing an irregular undulating surface) (Fig. 139.1). Squamous cell

REVISION TIPS

- HPV 6, 11, 16, 18/Gardasil 9 vaccine currently given to males and females from 12 years old and men who have sex with men up to age 45 years
- 1st line treatment for warts: podophyllotoxin, imiquimod
- Always consider malignancy and review red flag features when presented with a genital growth

140

Prematurity – Outline

Eva Papaioannou, Alexander Royston, and Amber Syed

Self-assessment:

1. What conditions are antenatal IM steroids used prophylactically for?
2. What is the diagnostic investigation for NEC and what does it show?
3. List some common presenting signs of neonatal sepsis.

Answers:

1. RDS (and BPD), NEC and IVH (see Table 140.1)
2. AXR: shows dilated bowel loops, pneumatosis intestinalis (gas in bowel wall), halo sign
3. Temperature instability (fever/hypothermia), change in tone, pallor, ↓feeding, ↓urine output, irritable, cardiorespiratory instability

TABLE 140.1			
	Features	**Investigations**	**Management**
Implications of prematurity (<37 weeks) – SHORT TERM			
Respiratory distress syndrome (RDS)	Surfactant deficiency. Rare >32 weeks gestation (severity↑ as gestation↓). **RFs:** LCSC delivery, hypothermia, perinatal hypoxia, meconium aspiration, FHx of RDS congenital pneumonia, maternal diabetes. **Hx & O/E:** increased work of breathing (WOB), grunting, ↑RR, cyanosis, apnoea	Respiratory + metabolic acidosis, ± renal failure. Monitor: SpO_2. Blood gas. Rule out infection. **CXR:** bilateral, ground-glass appearance (Fig. 141.1)	**Prevention:** IM antenatal corticosteroids. Respiratory support with nasal O_2, CPAP. Intubation + rescue surfactant (via endotracheal tube). Abx (until pneumonia/sepsis excluded). Consider nutrition/fluids
Intraventricular haemorrhage (IVH)	Bleeding from vascular germinal matrix →lateral ventricles. Rare >32 weeks gestation. Asymptomatic (50%), neurological, e.g. seizures	**RFs:** unstable BP, RDS, temperature instability. **ABG:** metabolic acidosis. **CrUSS:** grades I–IV on cranial ultrasound relate to IVH severity	**Prevention:** IM antenatal steroids. Vitamin K IV/IM. Supportive care

(Continued)

TABLE 140.1   (Cont'd)

	Features	Investigations	Management
Necrotising enterocolitis (NEC)	See *141. NEONATAL DEATH*		
Sepsis	See *141. NEONATAL DEATH*		
Anaemia of prematurity	**RFs:** profound prematurity, prenatal hypotrophy (weight <10th percentile), multiple pregnancy, gestosis, anaemia of pregnancy, maternal CVD. **Hx & O/E:** pallor, ↑RR, ↑HR, ↓feeding. May be asymptomatic	Occurs 6–12 weeks after pre-term delivery. **Bloods:** *Consider* FBC, reticulocytes, serum bilirubin level (SBR), LFTs, CRP (infection)	Delayed cord clamping. Limit volume and frequency of blood tests. Iron supplement. Consider blood transfusions. EPO (certain cases)
Retinopathy of prematurity	Ischemic retinal vasculopathy. **RFs:** premature infants, low birth weight, Hx of high-dose supplemental O_2 **Hx & O/E:** strabismus, leucocoria	Regular screening (<32 weeks gestation/LBW). **Fundoscopy:** lack normal vascularisation of peripheral retina	Avoid excessive oxygen (resuscitate in air at birth, titrate oxygen SpO_2: 95%). Referral to ophthalmology. Argon/diode laser. Intravitreal anti-VEGF
Jaundice	Common, usually unconjugated. Physiological in pre-term babies. **RFs:** prematurity (<38 weeks), bruising/haemorrhage, ethnicity (East Asian), breast-feeding, blood group incompatibility. **Hx & O/E:** yellow skin/sclera (daylight), stools mustard yellow colour, urine light yellow. If extreme: altered muscle tone/neurology (seizures, altered crying, drowsiness). Kernicterus	**TBR** (transcutaneous bilirubin): >35 weeks. **SBR** (serum bilirubin): confirmation/<35 weeks. FBC, U&Es, LFTs, CRP, TORCH screen. **Blood group + DAT** (direct antiglobulin test): maternal blood group – assess for incompatibility	Plot on NICE guidelines gestation-specific charts. Monitor SBR frequently. Phototherapy. Severe/refractory: IVIG ± exchange transfusion. Monitor for anaemia. Good hydration, temperature control. Treat underlying factors (infection)

Implications of prematurity – LONG TERM

	Features	Investigations	Management
Bronchopulmonary dysplasia (BPD)	Oxygen dependence at 36 weeks, chronic lung disease. **RFs:** ventilation for RDS, LBW, infection. ↑O_2 requirements, ↑WOB, ↑HR. Lung function impairment can continue through childhood	Continuous SpO_2 monitoring. **Bloods:** baseline, infection. **CXR:** hyperexpansion, diffuse patchy collapse and fibrosis, radiolucent cystic areas	**Prevention:** IM antenatal steroids to ↓risk. Lung protective ventilation. Oxygen (HFNO/CPAP with monitoring). Caffeine for apnoea. Diuretics, corticosteroids, vitamin A, sildenafil. Palivizumab (passive immunity vs RSV)

TABLE 140.1 (Cont'd)

	Features	Investigations	Management
Neurodevelopmental impairment (NDI)	**RFs:** gestation <30 weeks, multisystem malformations, severe asphyxia/IVH, IUGR. **Hx & O/E:** gross motor delay, fine motor impairment, speech and language delay, learning and behavioural. >40% of extremely pre-term infants suffer some form of NDI	**CrUSS:** serially (for basic structures/IVH). **MRI head:** at term, corrected to assess for signs of peri/neonatal injury (periventricular leukomalacia)	Long-term neurodevelopmental follow-up-development assessment (Bayley Scale of Neurodevelopment/ Schedule of Growing Skills (SOGS). Physiotherapy. Support groups

REVISION TIPS

- Premature labour occurs before 37 weeks of pregnancy
- RFs for prematurity: prematurity in previous pregnancies, multiple pregnancy, tobacco/substance use, short inter-pregnancy interval, pregnancy complications
- Pre-term babies have significantly raised mortality rate

141

Neonatal Death

Emmanuella Ikem, David Grant, and Ela Chakkarapani

NICU. 34 + 6 WEEK BABY BOY. INCREASED WORK OF BREATHING AND HYPOTHERMIA

Born 48 hours ago, ventouse-assisted vaginal delivery after preterm premature rupture of membranes (PPROM). Mother had group B streptococcus (GBS) – received intrapartum IV benzylpenicillin. Birth weight 2.9 kg, Apgar scores 5, 8, 10, not requiring resuscitation. On NICU for monitoring.

O/E: ABCDE: Signs of respiratory distress (intercostal, subcostal recession, nasal flaring), RR 90, reduced right-sided air entry, SpO_2 (in 40% FiO_2) 94%; HS I + II, no murmur, HR 180 bpm, capillary refill time >3 seconds, BP 53/22, MAP 26; Drowsy, not alert, equal reactive pupils, glucose 2.6 mmol/L; Widespread mottled skin, no rash, yellow sclera, axillary T 35.2°C. Resuscitation and investigations are initiated, but deterioration leads to cardiac arrest, CPR unsuccessful.

1. What organisms are mostly likely to cause the type of presentation described in the vignette
2. What congenital heart diseases are duct dependent?

Answers: 1. Group B Streptococcus (GBS), *E. coli*, *Listeria monocytogenes*, herpes simplex virus. 2. *Outflow obstruction*: hypoplastic left heart, coarctation of the aorta, interrupted aortic arch; *right to left shunt*: transposition of great arteries.

TABLE 141.1

	Features	Investigations	Management
Congenital heart disease; acyanotic or duct-dependent systemic circulation	2nd day of life, dysmorphic features. Evidence of left ventricular outflow obstruction- shock, heart failure, absent pulses. Cardiac defects may be seen on antenatal foetal ultrasound	Blood gases: metabolic acidosis. CXR: pulmonary oligaemia/plethora. ECG: superior axis – may discriminate likely defects. **Cardiac echoCG** definitive	ABCDE resuscitation. Immediate prostaglandin infusion. Referral to cardiac centre for intervention and surgical palliation or repair

TABLE 141.1 (Cont'd)

	Features	Investigations	Management
Inborn error of metabolism (IEM)	Persistent metabolic acidosis, acute severe illness after symptom free period, hypotonia, unexplained encephalopathy, abnormal Guthrie screen. **RFs:** consanguineous parents, FHx of unexpected death in childhood	One or more of: ↑ bilirubin/ ammonia, hypoglycaemia, deranged electrolytes, metabolic acidosis, raised anion gap. Metabolic screen: urine (organic/amino acids), blood (amino acids, acylcarnitine, DNA storage)	Supportive management. Stop protein feeds and start 10% glucose IV. Correct electrolytes. Seek expert advice. Genetic counselling and screening of siblings
Neonatal sepsis	Early or late. Maternal GBS, chorioamnionitis, prematurity, contaminated line insertion sites. **O/E:** respiratory distress, lethargic, pale, seizures, jaundice, hypo/hyperthermia, circulatory failure	Septic screen. +ve blood culture, ↑CRP, FBC (neutropenia/ neutrophilia). Metabolic acidosis. CXR: patchy shadowing and consolidation. LP: microorganism or raised white cells in the absence of red cells	ABCDE, sepsis. Antibiotics. Early onset: IV benzylpenicillin, gentamicin (± amoxicillin if *Listeria*). Late onset in NICU: IV flucloxacillin, gentamicin. Late onset from home: IV ceftriaxone/cefotaxime
Respiratory distress syndrome (RDS)	Fig. 141.1. See *140. PREMATURITY – Outline*		
Necrotising enterocolitis	Very preterm <34 weeks, perinatal asphyxia, enteral feeding. Distension, gastric/bilious aspirates, bloody stool, absent bowel sounds. High intra-abdominal pressure (reduced venous return, respiratory distress). Sepsis (translocation from gut, perforation). Hypotension/ shock	↑ Inflammatory markers, abnormal clotting, thrombocytopaenia, G&S. Blood cultures: organisms. Metabolic acidosis. AXR: dilated loops, portal vein gas, pneumonitis intestinalis, pneumoperitoneum	Stop enteral feeds, NGT on free drainage. Antibiotics (gentamicin, amoxicillin, metronidazole). If conservative management fails, laparotomy + bowel resection ± anastomosis or defunctioning stoma
Congenital diaphragmatic hernia (CDH)	Antenatal: polyhydramnios. Postnatal: severe respiratory distress, unilateral absent breath sounds/bowel sounds, shifted heart sounds. Other abnormalities (e.g. malrotation)	**Antenatal US:** CDH defect, polyhydramnios. **CXR:** hemithorax bowel loops (air-filled) + mediastinal displacement (Fig. 141.1)	ABCDE at birth, intubation + ventilate, NBM (wide-bore NG tube on free drainage), ± inhaled NO for persistent pulmonary hypertension, surfactant. Surgery once stabilised
Sudden infant death syndrome (SIDS)	Prone sleeping, parental smoking, bed sharing, hyperthermia, head covering, maternal drug use, not breastfed	Post-partum examination, tests for cause of death. Autopsy and coroner's inquest	Support for parents

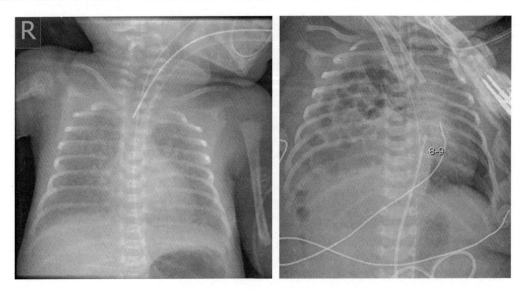

Fig. 141.1 (*Left*) RDS (ground glass appearance). (*Right*) CDH (patient on ECMO). (Left: From Holme N. The pathophysiology of respiratory distress syndrome in neonates. *Paediatr Child Health (Oxford)* 2012;22(12): 507–512, Figure 1. Right: From Badillo A, et al. Congenitaldiaphragmatic hernia: treatment and outcomes. *Semin Perinatol* 2014;38(2):92–96, Figure 1.)

Prematurity remains a major cause of neonatal death and accounts for most conditions seen in NICU. APGAR: colour (Appearance), heart rate (Pulse), reflexes (Grimace), muscle tone (Activity), Respiration – each scored 0–2; normal score 7–10. At 5 mins after birth, APGAR 0–3 has high chance of neonatal mortality, while APGAR 0–6 has raised risk of cerebral palsy. Causes of early death can be complications of prematurity including extensive intraventricular haemorrhage of the brain, pulmonary insufficiency, sepsis, necrotising enterocolitis, congenital malformations, infection, respiratory failure, shock. After discharge home, also consider congenital malformations, inborn error of metabolism (IEM), arrhythmias, congenital heart disease, dehydration, temperature dysregulation, intracranial haemorrhage and non-accidental injury/neglect. Key infections are encephalitis/ meningitis, pneumonia and sepsis. In the vignette, the most likely cause is early onset neonatal sepsis, suggested by the maternal GBS, hypothermia, hypotension (normal neonatal systolic BP is 55–75 mmHg at term, diastolic BP 30 – 50 mmHg), skin mottling with slow CRT (normal <2 seconds) and hypoxia.

REVISION TIPS

- Early onset neonatal infection occurs within the first 72 hours of life. Late onset is from 72 hours to 1 month
- IEM can mimic sepsis; consider if large anion gap, encephalopathy or sudden unexplained infant death
- Although CDH is rare, it has a high mortality rate of approximately 40%

142

Well-Being Checks – Outline

Alice Parker, Kaobi Okongwu, and Simon Thornton

TABLE 142.1			
	Target population	**Investigations**	**Management**
Adult			
NHS health check	Anyone aged 40–74 without a pre-existing condition screened for: CVD, HTN, T2DM, CKD, dementia, risk factors for stroke (FHx of CVD, BMI, smoking, alcohol, physical activity)	BMI, blood pressure. Fasting glucose, HbA1c, cholesterol. Alcohol use disorders identification test (AUDIT). QRISK score	Smoking cessation/weight management service, alcohol intervention services, exercise on prescription, diabetes prevention. Consider statin (QRISK >10%). Anti-hypertensives (NICE guidelines). Dementia awareness
Cervical screening	All women aged 25–65 years; • 3-yearly if 25–49 years • 5-yearly if 50–65 years	HPV testing via cervical smear. **HPV negative:** routine recall. Check cytology if HPV positive	**HPV +ve, normal cytology:** rescreen for HPV in 12 months. **HPV +ve, abnormal cytology:** *137. ABNORMAL CERVICAL SMEAR*
Breast cancer screening	Women aged 50–70 (age X trial covers 47–73), 3-yearly. Women aged ≥40 with BRCA mutation, yearly. >70 can request 3-yearly screening, but not routinely invited	Mammogram. MRI for those with BRCA gene	Suspicious result gets triple assessment; further mammogram, clinical exam, US of relevant quadrant ± needle sampling
Abdominal aorta aneurysm screening	All males, offered at age 65	Duplex USS abdomen	<3 cm: no further action 3-4.4 cm: re-scan **12 monthly** 4.5-5.4 cm: re-scan **3 monthly** ≥5.5 cm or enlarging >1 cm/ year: refer within **2 weeks** to vascular
Colorectal cancer screening	Anyone aged 56, and 2 yearly from 60 to 74 (75+ years old can request)	Faecal immunochemical test (FIT) via post – detects blood in stool	**Normal FIT:** return to regular screening. **Abnormal FIT:** colonoscopy ± biopsy

(Continued)

TABLE 142.1   (Cont'd)

	Target population	Investigations	Management
Diabetic eye screening	Annual eye screening in people with T1DM and T2DM for **diabetic retinopathy.** From 12 years old onwards	**Retinal imaging:** dot and blot haemorrhages, hard exudates, microaneurysms, venous beading, cotton wool spots, neovascular	Ophthalmology if changes near macula or pre-proliferative. Laser photocoagulation
Antenatal screening	Screening for: foetal anomalies; Down syndrome, Edward syndrome, Patau syndrome, anencephaly, spina bifida, cleft lip, congenital diaphragmatic hernia, gastroschisis, exomphalos, congenital heart disease, bilateral renal agenesis, lethal skeletal dysplasia. Blood disorders: sickle cell disease, thalassaemia. Infections: HIV, hepatitis B, syphilis	At booking (8–12 weeks): testing for HBsAg, HIV, syphilis, thalassaemia. Test for SCD in women from high-prevalence areas. 11–13 + 6 weeks: nuchal translucency, PAPP-A, free beta-hCG. 15–20 weeks: *Triple test*; AFP, oestriol, hCG. *Quadruple test* (Down's); AFP, oestriol, hCG, inhibin A. 11 weeks: chorionic villus sampling is offered if indicated. 16 weeks (15–20): amniocentesis is offered if indicated. 18–20 + 6 weeks: anomaly scan	Foetal anomalies – counselling with appropriate specialist. Blood disorders – advice for family planning and treatment as necessary. See also *120. NORMAL PREGNANCY AND RISK-ASSESSMENT- Outline*
Paediatric Newborn blood spot screening	Tests for: SCD, cystic fibrosis, congenital hypothyroidism, PKU, medium-chain-acyl-CoA dehydrogenase deficiency (MCADD), maple syrup urine disease (MSUD), isovaleric acidaemia (IVA), glutaric aciduria type 1 (GA1), homocystinuria	On day 5, blood sample taken from heel of baby	If any positive results, further diagnostic tests done. Treatment commenced if necessary
Newborn hearing screening	4–5 weeks of life. To identify hearing impairment and deafness in babies	Automated otoacoustic emission (OAE) test – sounds to test inner ear response	Normal result = present OAEs. Abnormal result = absent, will require further testing with automated auditory brainstem response to rule out hearing loss

TABLE 142.1 **(Cont'd)**

	Target population	Investigations	Management
Neonatal and infant physical examination (NIPE) screening	Head-to-toe examination. 1st examination is within 72 hours of birth. 2nd examination at 6–8 weeks. Screening for: congenital heart disease, developmental dysplasia of the hip (DDH), congenital cataracts, cryptorchidism, neural tube defects	Head – circumference, anterior fontanelle. Face – dysmorphic features and trauma. Chest – murmurs, breath sounds. Hips – femoral pulses, Ortolani's/Barlow's (DDH). Perineal – hypospadias, imperforate anus, undescended testes. Feet – talipes and abnormal positioning. Back – neural tube defect	Further evaluation according to findings, e.g. echocardiogram, USS for DDH or cranial abnormalities. Surgical referral in suspected neural tube defects and talipes

143

Infant Feeding Problems

Alice Parker, Alexander Royston, and Ciara McClenaghan

GP CONSULTATION, 3-MONTH-OLD MALE BABY. 1-MONTH HISTORY OF EXCESSIVE CRYING AND POOR WEIGHT GAIN

HPC: Appeared to begin after beginning formula feeding. Episodes of crying associated with drawing up of the legs into body. Frequent regurgitation of feeds, diarrhoea (occasionally including blood), not gaining weight.

O/E: Obs. stable and within normal range. Fallen 1 decile on growth chart since last visit, no signs of dehydration or wasting. Eczematous rash on face and limbs.

1. What differential should be considered for frequent, milky, non-bilious, projectile vomiting?
2. What differential is likely in a short history of inconsolable crying, sausage-shaped abdominal mass and redcurrant jelly stool?
3. List some other common causes in an infant with faltering growth.

Answers: 1. Pyloric stenosis. 2. Intussusception. 3. Cystic fibrosis, biliary atresia, inborn errors of metabolism, chronic infections, chromosomal syndromes, congenital heart defects, haematological disorders, emotional neglect or abuse, difficult home environment

TABLE 143.1

	Features	Investigations	Management
Cow's milk protein allergy (CMPA)	RFs: M > F, food allergy, atopic conditions, FHx. Hx & O/E: *IgE*; diarrhoea, pruritis, abdominal pain ± angio-oedema, upper and lower respiratory symptoms (rhinorrhoea, wheeze) <48 hours after cow milk ingestion. *Non-IgE*: delayed onset diarrhoea (bloody or mucus), GORD, colic, perianal redness, atopic eczema	Skin prick testing/ serum IgE if suspected IgE-mediated and severe	*Breastfed babies*: exclude cow's milk and soya from mother's diet with dietician support - trial for 6 weeks, then re-introduce to see if symptoms resolve then re-occur. *Formula fed*: switch to extensively hydrolysed formula for 6-week trial. Consider referral to a specialist allergy clinic or paediatric dietitian, treat eczema, advise parents on use of "milk ladder" to re-introduce milk

TABLE 143.1   (Cont'd)

	Features	Investigations	Management
Colic	Hx & O/E: inconsolable crying, drawing legs up into body, feeding difficulties. Symptoms for >3 hours on >3 days/week. Common, self-limiting, no faltering growth	RFs: maternal smoking, depression, first-born status. Clinical diagnosis	Soothing strategies: gentle motion, holding the baby. Continue breastfeeding, reassure mother, reduce stress
GORD	Weakness in the lower oesophageal sphincter. RFs: neurodevelopmental, duodenal atresia, premature, hiatus hernia, obesity. Hx & O/E: regurgitation/vomiting after feed, failure to thrive (if severe), feeding difficulties, pneumonia	Only if severe or persistent. **24-hour pH impedance monitoring:** frequently pH <4. **Endoscopy:** may see oesophagitis	Reassurance (should be managed conservatively). Diet: small frequent feeds, regulate milk flow, wind part way through feeds, hold upright for 20 mins after. Trial of Gaviscon, ranitidine/omeprazole if severe. Paediatrician if faltering growth or haematemesis
Urinary tract infection	RFs: prematurity, vesicoureteric reflux, (uncircumcised male). Hx & O/E: fever, vomiting, failure to thrive, excessive crying	**Bloods:** FBC ($\uparrow$WCC/Neut), $\uparrow$CRP, U&E. **Urine:** MC&S. Consider USS KUB	Abx as guided by local guidelines and urine culture result
Breastfeeding problems	See *130. DIFFICULTY WITH BREASTFEEDING*		
Older age groups Coeliac disease	RFs: FHx, Down/Turner/Williams syndromes. Hx & O/E: Sx emerge after introduction of wheat, failure to gain weight, diarrhoea (foul stools), anaemia, distension, muscle wasting	FBC ($\downarrow$Hb, $\downarrow$folate, $\downarrow$ferritin), IgA-tissue transglutaminase (IgA-tTg), endomysial antibodies, total IgA	Gluten-free diet
Lactose intolerance	RFs: ethnicity (white: less common), recent gastroenteritis, coeliac. Hx & O/E: abdominal pain, distension, explosive diarrhoea following feeding	Rule out other conditions. FBC ($\downarrow$Hb), IgA-tTG (r/o coeliac disease). Faecal calprotectin (r/o IBD)	Encourage other calcium dietary sources, exclude lactose
Inflammatory bowel disease	Very rare <2 yo, genetic. Hx & O/E: faltering growth, abdo pain, cramping, chronic diarrhoea ± blood/mucus	FBC ($\downarrow$Hb), $\uparrow$CRP/ESR. **Endoscopy**	Need to rule out: allergies, infection, coeliac disease, nutritional/caloric deficits. Urgent paediatrics referral
Other food allergy	See *79. FOOD INTOLERANCE*		

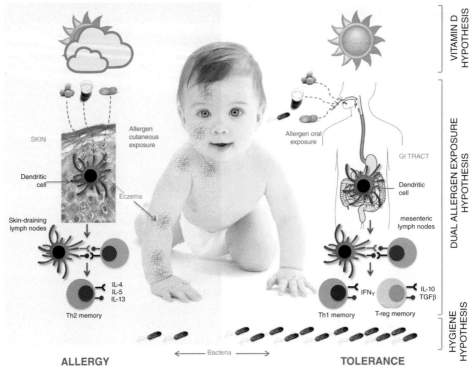

Fig. 143.1 Integration of the vitamin D deficiency, hygiene, and dual-allergen exposure hypotheses. Sufficient levels of vitamin D, a diverse microbiota, and oral allergen exposure collectively support the development of tolerance. Conversely, allergic sensitization is promoted through cutaneous exposure, reduced diversity of microbiota, and vitamin D deficiency. Diminished microbial diversity and vitamin D deficiency are thought to interrupt the regulatory mechanisms of oral tolerance, with the latter also contributing to decreased epidermal barrier function. *GI*, Gastrointestinal; *T-reg*, regulatory T cells. Graphic modified from Lack G. Epidemiologic risks for food allergy. *J Allergy Clin Immunol* 2008;121:1331-6. Copyright © 2008 Elsevier. Reprinted with permission.

The vignette describes cow's milk protein allergy (CMPA). The key pointer is the emergence after switching from breast milk to formula. Episodes of crying associated with drawing up of the legs may suggest colic, but these are common and non-specific symptoms, while the skin rash and occasional blood in the diarrhoea is more specific for CMPA. It is hard to differentiate whether this is IgE-mediated allergy, although on balance it appears to be non-IgE related, given the blood in stools and eczematous rash. A more careful history is required, particularly relating the symptoms to ingestion.

REVISION TIPS

- Infant feeding problems may be caused by infantile colic, allergies, GORD, and breastfeeding issues
- Except following gastroenteritis, infants with symptoms on exposure to cow's milk are more likely to have CMPA than lactose intolerance
- Colic is common and symptoms in infants include crying and drawing up of the legs
- Investigations of failure to thrive include: MSU, coeliac serology, FBC, U&Es, LFTs, TFTs, CRP, glucose, calcium, proteins, immunoglobulins, sweat test, stool MC&S, CXR, skeletal survey, ECG, echo

144

Crying Baby

Emmanuella Ikem and Lindsey Rowley

GP APPOINTMENT. 10-WEEK-BABY BOY.
UNEXPLAINED INCONSOLABLE CRYING

HPC: 1-month history, 3 hours daily on most days. Not associated with feeding, worse in the evenings. Frequent back arching and passage of flatus. Otherwise well, no vomiting, no fevers, no diarrhoea/constipation. Feeding well on breast milk and supplemental formula feeds. Has wet nappies and sleeping well. **PMHx:** Uncomplicated term pregnancy, no complications. Up-to-date with vaccinations (first given 2 weeks ago).
O/E: Obs. HR 130, RR 40, T 37.2, SpO_2 (air) 98%. Well, alert, fixes and follows objects, has social smile, not dehydrated, no rash. No respiratory distress. **Abdo:** SNT, BS present. **ENT:** normal. **Growth:** 50th centile.

1. What system is used to risk-stratify an unwell child?
2. What imaging should be done if a child younger than 6 months has recurrent UTIs?

Answers: 1. NICE traffic light system (see Table 145.2.) 2. USS during acute infection, DMSA/MCUG 4–6 months after.

TABLE 144.1

	Features	Investigations	Management
Teething	Drooling, biting, sucking, irritable, reduced feeding ± mild pyrexia, facial rash	Diagnosis of exclusion	Reassurance. Rub gums with clean fingers/biting on clean/cool objects
Gastro-oesophageal reflux	See *143. INFANT FEEDING PROBLEMS*		
Infantile colic	Thriving baby with random, inconsolable crying, irritability. Drawing up knees/back arching. Not associated with feeding. Frequent excessive flatus	Clinical diagnosis; >3 hours/day on >3 days for at least 1 week	Reassurance. Advice on methods to soothe. Resolves by 3–6 months. Very little evidence behind colic drops

(Continued)

TABLE 144.1   (Cont'd)

	Features	Investigations	Management
Cow's milk protein allergy	See *143. INFANT FEEDING PROBLEMS*		
Constipation	Hard stool, straining with crying, or no stool passage. Streaks of blood on stool or tissue (anal fissure). Palpable faecal mass in lower abdomen, ± abdominal distension, ± dehydration	Clinical diagnosis. Refer if suspect organic cause	Adequate fluid intake. Baby massage. Disimpact with Macrogol 1–2 weeks (± stimulant laxatives). Not impacted- maintain with Macrogol
Post immunisation	Excessive crying for <48 hours post immunisation	Diagnosis of exclusion	Self-limiting
Not to miss ... Intussusception	3–18 months old. May have had recent viral infection. Bile-stained vomit, colic, draws up legs, redcurrant jelly stools, abdo distension, episodic pain. O/E: dehydration, sausage-shaped abdominal mass	**US scan:** 'target sign' (Fig. 144.1). **AXR:** small bowel obstruction.	IV fluid resuscitation. Radiological pneumatic reduction. Laparotomy and open reduction
Non-accidental injury (NAI)	See *155. CHILD ABUSE*		

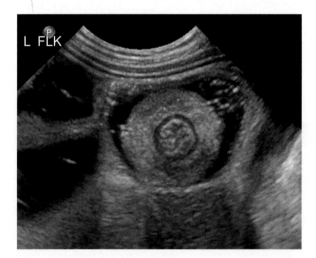

Fig. 144.1 The 'target sign' of an intussusception on ultrasound. Reproduced with permission from Majumder, A., et al. (2021). *J Egypt Natl Canc Inst*, 33(1), 18.

Clinical evaluation must be broad-ranging and fastidious. Babies typically cry for around 2 hours per day, and the amount a baby cries tends to peak at about 4-8 weeks of age. Crying is an important form of communication in young babies to engage their parents' attention and facilitate attachment, but can also be a sign of pain or discomfort. Breastfeeding mothers should be asked about their medications, drugs and diet. In acute uncontrollable crying, surgical and medical causes should be excluded. Conditions to consider include corneal abrasion, occult fracture, urinary tract or other infection, and acute abdomen including inguinal hernia or testicular torsion. Crying can also be a trigger for physical abuse, so non-accidental injury should be considered during examination. In the vignette, the most likely explanation is infantile colic.

REVISION TIPS

- Consolable crying <2 hours/day is common in babies. Premature infants peak crying at 6 weeks corrected age
- Excessive crying in infants is common but usually benign
- Severe inconsolable crying requires a comprehensive clinical evaluation to exclude serious pathology
- Excessive crying can be a trigger for physical abuse

The Sick Child

Gregory Oxenham and Abigail Nye

HPC: Worsening throughout the day; fever, vomiting and aversion to breastfeeding, now not waking up easily. No wet nappy for 12–14 hours. Eight-week vaccines yesterday. **PMHx:** Born at 33/40 by vaginal delivery (single pregnancy), neonatal ICU for 2 weeks (prematurity, suspected infection). Was discharged well, growing as expected. **FHx:** Nil relevant.

O/E: Temp 39.5°C, HR 175, CRT 4–5 seconds centrally, RR65, O_2 94% on air. Cool clammy skin, hands/feet feel cold, thready femoral pulse. Does not wake up, moving four limbs, making intermittent weak cries. Petechiae on soles of the feet, 2 mm purpuric lesion on the big toe. **Ix:** Blood glucose 5.5 mmol/L.

1. What investigations would you send for the infant in the vignette?
2. What antibiotics are indicated to treat this child?
3. What are some longer-term side effects from surviving meningitis?

Answers: 1. CRP, FBC, U&Es blood glucose, blood gas, coagulation screen, multiple blood cultures; urine cultures, lumbar puncture/CSF analysis, whole blood PCR for *N. meningitidis*. 2. Cefotaxime and amoxicillin, given the risk of meningitis. Cefotaxime is also used to treat sepsis of unknown origin in neonates >72 hours old. 3. Deafness, neurological abnormalities, skin scarring from necrosis, psychosocial problems, renal failure, damage to bones and joints, hearing loss.

TABLE 145.1

	Features	Investigations	Management
Infection			
Sepsis	**RFs:** younger age, recent trauma/surgery, impaired immunity, indwelling lines, skin breaches. **Hx & O/E:** presentation often non-specific. Changed behaviour/respiration/ circulation. Parental concern. Evidence of infection (chest, urine, skin). Meningitis more common in younger children	**Blood culture.** FBC (↑WCC, ↑CRP, ↑Neutrophils), U&Es (↑creatinine, ↑urea), clotting (+ fibrinogen–?DIC). **Blood gas:** ↑Lactate, ↓pH. **Urine output.** Identify source. **LP:** infants <1 month with fever; infants 1–3 months who are unwell or have WCC ↑↑/↓↓	Urgent senior paediatric review if sepsis <5 years. Oxygen. **IV Abx:** usually ceftriaxone or cefotaxime - add amoxicillin if <3 months. Benzylpenicillin/gentamicin if <72 hours old. **IV fluid** – guided by lactate but usually a 10–20 mL/kg 0.9% NaCl bolus if shocked, repeated if required. Escalate to critical care/ vasopressors in fluid-resistant shock

(Continued)

TABLE 145.1 (Cont'd)

	Features	Investigations	Management
Viral infection	RFs: contact, winter months, prematurity. Often many of the 'Green' features from Table 145.2. Otherwise, dependent on site of infection: e.g. dry cough, coryza, fever, irritability, sore ear, sore throat, viral rash, poor feeding, reduced UO, parental concern	Based on severity if no clear source. All under 3 month olds with fever should have urine dipstick tested and may need bloods	Often self-limiting. Simple analgesia, fluid intake, return precautions. Abx not indicated unless evidence of bacterial infection, significant illness or <1 month old
LRTI – bronchiolitis	RFs: under 2s, esp. 3–6 months. Winter months. Hx & O/E: coryza 1–3 days, cough, tachypnoea/ chest recession, wheeze/ crackles, fever, poor feeding. *Severe:* apnoea, hypoxia, dehydration, respiratory distress	**Pulse oximetry:** hypoxia requires hospital admission.	Assess severity (Table 145.2). Admit if severe; admit if O_2 sats. <90% for child older than 6 weeks, or <92% for a younger child. **Oxygen** for hypoxia, **high flow or CPAP** if persisting hypoxia or respiratory distress. **Rehydrate** via NGT or IV
LRTI – community- acquired pneumonia	RFs: previous infection, CF, bronchiectasis, prematurity, immunosuppression. Hx & O/E: cough ± sputum, fever, focal crackles on chest, SOB, hypoxia, tachycardia, grunting, chest indrawing, inability to breastfeed or drink, lethargy, altered behaviour/ consciousness	Clinical diagnosis. **X-ray:** if features of severe/ complicated pneumonia. **Bloods:** if severe infection or sepsis	Assess for management in community – clinical judgement + Table 145.2 (for <5 years old). Oxygen. **Abx:** <3 month old – admit for IV antibiotics; >3 month – oral amoxicillin/ clarithromycin/doxycycline. IV if severe/unable to tolerate oral
UTI	Consider in any child <3 months with fever. RFs: instrumentation of urinary tract, congenital renal abnormalities, FHx, constipation. *Infants <3 months*: fever, vomiting, lethargy, irritable, poor feeding. *>3 months*: fever, abdo pain, loin tenderness, vomiting, poor feeding. *Verbal child*: frequency, dysuria, abdo pain, incontinence	**MSU:** clean catch, or 'in-out' catheter sample - MC&S in suspected pyelonephritis, <3 months with fever, positive dipsticks, recurrent UTI	**Review any historic urine sensitivities.** Refer all infants <3 months for IV antibiotics. Lower UTI; PO trimethoprim or PO nitrofurantoin. Bacteriuria + fever (>38°C) or loin pain, treat as **pyelonephritis**; oral cefalexin or IV cefuroxime

TABLE 145.1   (Cont'd)

	Features	Investigations	Management
Bacterial meningitis (including meningococcal meningitis)	**RFs:** extremes of age, neurosurgery. *In neonates –* pre-term birth, ROM for >24 hours prior to delivery, maternal group B strep infection, chorioamnionitis. **Hx & O/E:** presentation variable, may have few specific symptoms. Fever, headache, neck stiffness, photophobia, brady/tachycardia, shock, hypotension, myalgia, non-blanching rash (late finding in meningococcaemia), spreading petechiae, bulging fontanelle (<2 years), hypoglycaemia (infants), altered mental state, seizures	CRP, FBC, U&Es, blood glucose, blood gas, coagulation screen (as for sepsis) – normal CRP/WCC do not r/o meningitis. **Blood culture.** Whole blood PCR: for *N. meningitidis.* **LP:** ↑↑neutrophils, ↓glucose, ↑protein, culture for organism, PCR for organism. Do not allow LP to delay administration of Abx	**IV fluid bolus.** If shocked, 20 ml/kg bolus, repeated if required. **Antibiotics within 1 hour:** <3 months old – IV amoxicillin + cefotaxime; >3 months old - IV ceftriaxone. Suspected meningococcus: pre-hospital, IM benzylpenicillin; in hospital, IV ceftriaxone (cefotaxime if <3 months). Dexamethasone: if bacterial meningitis and >3 months old. Notify Public Health
Endocrine DKA (paediatric)	**RFs:** FHx, autoimmune condition, illness/under-administration of usual insulin in known T1DM. May be first presentation of T1DM. Polyuria, polydipsia, N&V, fatigue, confusion, abdominal pain, Kussmaul breathing (deep laboured gasping). **Cerebral oedema:** headache, agitation, confusion, unexpected bradycardia, HTN, oculomotor palsies, abnormal pupil dilation-more common in <2 years and in more severe DKA	**Glucose:** >11 mmol/L. **Ketones:** >3 mmol/L OR urine >++. **VBG:** pH <7.3, bicarb <15 mmol/L. Assess K⁺. Screen for other causes: e.g. CXR, urinalysis, blood cultures if fever	**IV fluid bolus:** 10 mL/kg 0.9% NaCl (20 mL/kg if shock). Calculate deficit and maintenance fluid – give over 48 hours ± K⁺ supplement. Change to 0.9% NaCl/5% dextrose/40 mmol K⁺ when glucose <14 mmol/L. **Insulin:** 1–2 hours after start of fluid, 0.05–0.10 units/kg/hour. Monitor Na⁺/K⁺/pH/HCO₃⁻/glucose, neurological status. Cerebral oedema: mannitol or hypertonic saline
Malignancy Acute lymphoblastic leukaemia (paediatric)	**RFs:** Down/Klinefelter syndrome, EBV, radiation. Mainly child <5. **Hx & O/E:** hepatospleno-megaly, pallor, bleed/bruising, petechiae, fever, infection, poor feeding, bone pain	↑lymphocyte ±↓Hb, ↓platelets. **Bone marrow:** lymphoblasts. Genetic: Philadelphia chromosome – can alter management	Immediate referral for any child with unexplained **petechiae, hepatosplenomegaly, bone pain.** Chemotherapy: induction, e.g. cytarabine + anthracycline + dexamethasone. Stem cell transplant possible

(Continued)

TABLE 145.1 (Cont'd)

	Features	Investigations	Management
Others			
Inborn error of metabolism	See *141. NEONATAL DEATH*		
Congenital cardiac abnormality	See *152. CONGENITAL ABNORMALITY*		

TABLE 145.2 Risk Stratification in Under 5s

	Green – low risk	Amber – intermediate risk	Red – high risk
Colour (of skin, lips or tongue) Activity	• Normal colour • Responds normally to social cues • Content/smiles • Stays awake or awakens quickly • Strong normal cry/not crying	• Pallor reported by parent/carer • Not responding normally to social cues • No smile • Wakes only with prolonged stimulation • Decreased activity	• Pale/mottled/ashen/blue • No response to social cues • Appears ill to a healthcare professional • Does not wake or, if roused, does not stay awake • Weak, high-pitched or continuous cry

Respiratory	• –	• Nasal flaring
		• Tachypnoea: respiratory rate
		  • >50 breaths/minute (bpm), age 6–12 months
		  • >40 bpm, age >12 months
		• Oxygen saturation ≤95% in air
		• Crackles in the chest
			• Grunting
			• Tachypnoea: respiratory rate >60 bpm
			• Moderate or severe chest indrawing

Circulation and hydration	• Normal skin and eyes
	• Moist mucous membranes
		• Tachycardia:
		  • >160 bpm, age <12 months
		  • >150 bpm, age 12–24 months
		  • >140 bpm, age 2–5 years
		• Capillary refill time ≥3 seconds
		• Dry mucous membranes
		• Poor feeding in infants
		• Reduced urine output
			• Reduced skin turgor

Other	• None of the amber or red symptoms or signs	• Age 3–6 months, temperature ≥39°C • Fever for ≥5 days • Rigors • Swelling of a limb or joint • Non-weight-bearing limb/not using an extremity	• Age <3 months, temperature ≥38°C • Non-blanching rash • Bulging fontanelle • Neck stiffness • Status epilepticus • Focal neurological signs • Focal seizures

(Adapted from NICE Guideline [NG143]. Available at: nice.org.uk/guidance/ng143. Accessed February 2022.)

The baby in this vignette has presented in extremis with evidence of circulatory failure (tachycardia, poor CRT, pallor, cool extremities, reduced urine output) and reduced consciousness, and septic shock is likely. Rapid onset illness, reduced consciousness and spreading petechial/purpuric rash should prompt treatment for meningococcal disease and meningitis. Prematurity here means their corrected age is about 20 days, raising likelihood of severe infection. Vaccination can cause transient fever in infants; this is a diagnosis of exclusion and should not be considered here. Acute lymphoblastic leukaemia may present like this, although unusual in this age. The most important differentials for very sick young infants are sepsis, congenital cardiac disease and inborn errors of metabolism.

REVISION TIPS

- Bronchiolitis – under 2's, coryzal prodrome, widespread crackles/wheeze, respiratory distress
- Parental concern is a valid risk factor for significant illness
- Paediatric infections can be non-specific at presentation, so familiarise yourself with the high-risk features of infections in children

146

Allergies

Emmanuella Ikem and Alexander Royston

**PAEDIATRIC WARD, MALE, AGED 9.
SUDDEN ONSET ITCHY RASH AFTER
ADMINISTRATION OF IV PENICILLIN**

HPC: No respiratory distress, stridor or wheeze.
   O/E: HR 80, RR 22, BP 115/60, SpO_2 (air) 96%. Alert, well perfused, widespread raised erythematous rash on torso, cheeks and limbs. **Resp:** Clear chest, no added sounds. **CVS:** HS I+II+0, CRT <2 seconds.

1. What dose of adrenaline would be administered to this child if anaphylaxis was suspected?
2. How long after the first dose should a second dose of adrenaline be given in an anaphylaxis emergency?
3. What non-sedating antihistamines are useful in allergic reactions?

Answers: 1. For child aged 6 -12, 300 micrograms (0.3 mL) IM adrenaline 1:1000. (<6 yrs: 150 micrograms). 2. Five minutes. 3. Loratadine or cetirizine.

TABLE 146.1

	Features	Investigations	Management
Anaphylaxis. See also *53. ANAPHYLAXIS*	Rapid response. Wheeze, hoarse voice, stridor, respiratory distress, angioedema, urticaria, hypotension, reduced consciousness, shock	Clinical diagnosis. Serum tryptase	ABCDE. Remove trigger. Lay flat, raise legs. IM adrenaline 1:1000. IV chlorphenamine, hydrocortisone, salbutamol. 10 mL/kg IV saline bolus
Allergic angioedema	Immediate response. Swelling commonly affects lip, eyelids, tongue, genitalia, larynx	Clinical diagnosis. Skin prick testing. IgE quantification	High flow O_2. Adrenaline 1:1000. IV chlorphenamine, hydrocortisone
Acute urticaria (Fig. 146.1)	Sudden onset itchy wheals (hives) after triggers (e.g. insect bite, drugs, latex, food allergen), ± angioedema, ± anaphylaxis	Clinical diagnosis. Rash lasting 2–24 hours. Skin prick testing. IgE quantification	Non-sedating or sedating H1 antihistamine (oral). Calamine lotion
Atopic eczema	Symmetrical scaly erythematous patches, dry/itchy, flexural distribution, lichenification, excoriation marks, ± infection	Clinical diagnosis	Avoid allergen. Soap substitute, emollients. Topical corticosteroids/calcineurin inhibitors

TABLE 146.1 (Cont'd)

	Features	Investigations	Management
Asthma exacerbation	Wheeze, cough, increased SOB, chest tightness, tachypnoea. Moderate/severe/life-threatening ± tachycardia	PEFR: % predicted depends on severity	Avoid allergen. Nebulised salbutamol, ipratropium. Oral prednisolone or IV hydrocortisone. IV magnesium sulphate
Allergic contact dermatitis	Itchy, erythematous, scaly rash following exposure to chemicals, nickel, hair dye, fragrance, cosmetics, etc.	Patch testing	Avoid allergen. Emollients. Corticosteroid ointment
Allergic rhinoconjunctivitis	Intermittent or persistent. Seasonal plant pollen. Watery eyes, sneezing, rhinorrhoea ± cough	Clinical diagnosis	PRN topical or oral non-sedating antihistamine. Moderate–severe: regular intranasal corticosteroids
Food allergy	See *143. INFANT FEEDING PROBLEMS*		

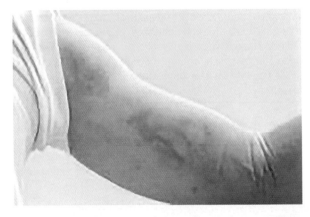

Fig. 146.1 Hives (urticaria). (From Elsevier Patient Education © 2023 Elsevier Inc)

Allergic and drug hypersensitivity reactions are mediated by the immune system and occur after sensitisation and creation of allergen-specific antibodies, T cells, or both. Anaphylaxis is a rapid IgE-mediated systemic allergic reaction that may affect multiple organ systems. Pseudoallergic (anaphylactoid) reactions are fast-acting non–IgE-mediated systemic reactions mediated by mast cells and basophils, which can occur on first exposure. Urticaria is mediated by histamine, causing superficial oedema in upper and mid-dermis, leading to pruritic wheals (hives), and is treated with antihistamines. Angioedema is mediated by bradykinin and causes oedema in deeper layers of mucous membranes and skin. β-lactam–related cutaneous reactions are mostly maculopapular eruptions and urticaria. In the vignette, widespread itchy rash soon after penicillin administration indicates acute urticaria.

REVISION TIPS

- Allergic reactions may be IgE mediated or non–IgE mediated. The former is usually within minutes of exposure, the latter within hours of exposure
- Allergic reactions are mainly caused by inhaled allergens (plant pollens, house-dust mite), ingested allergens (nuts, cow's milk, eggs, soya, wheat), insect bites/stings, drugs, latex
- Chronic urticaria (>6 weeks) is usually intermittent and non-allergic
- Hypersensitivity is an increased sensitivity to allergic stimuli resulting in reproducible signs and symptoms post exposure

147

Abnormal Development/ Developmental Delay

Caroline Bodey and Emmanuella Ikem

GP APPOINTMENT, 22-MONTH-OLD GIRL. DELAYED MOTOR SKILLS

HPC: Never achieved walking. Sat at 9 months. Mobilises by asymmetrical crawling. Reaches for objects with right hand (has done this for 6 months). No feeding problems, no seizures, uses about 20 single words. **PMHx:** Born at 32 weeks, uneventful neonatal course, normal antenatal USS prior to this. Up-to-date with vaccinations. Right-sided squint diagnosed at 12 months. **FHx:** No delayed walking or neuromuscular disease. **SHx:** No safeguarding concerns.

  O/E: Bright and alert, when playing has asymmetrical crawl with left leg stiff and less mobile. When sitting, occasionally falls to left, poor saving reflex with left arm. Uses right arm to grasp toys even when they are presented on her left. When lifted, holds left hand flexed and pronated. Thumb in palm on left. When examined on parent's lap, increased tone in left leg and arm, reflexes easy to elicit on left and positive Babinski reflex on left. **Developmental assessment:** *Gross motor:* Crawls (asymmetric), sits without support. Not pulling to stand. Will step if both hands held. *Fine motor and vision:* scribbles with a crayon using right hand, builds tower of three blocks; *Hearing and language:* responds to her name, understands simple commands, uses 20 words; *Social skills:* finger-feeds self, drinks from lidded beaker, happy for peers to play alongside her but not yet sharing.

1. What are the motor types of cerebral palsy?
2. What pattern of brain injury is more common in preterm babies?
3. What other milestones should you be concerned about when suspecting cerebral palsy?

Answers: 1. Spastic (most common form, from damage to motor cortex), dyskinetic (damage to basal ganglia) and ataxic (rare). 2. White matter damage – periventricular leukomalacia. 3. Impaired motor milestones – not sitting until 9 months, hand preference before 1 year.

TABLE 147.1

	Features	Investigations	Management
Benign variation in locomotion mode	Bottom shuffling – average walking 17 months	History, FHx	Reassurance
Cerebral palsy (Fig. 147.1)	Non-progressive brain injury – before, during or soon after birth (up to 2 years). **Hx & O/E:** abnormal tone, movement, coordination or posture, delayed motor milestones, spasticity, abnormal gait, feeding difficulty. Learning difficulty (45%), seizures	**RFs:** preterm, intraventricular haemorrhage, hypoxic injury, infection, kernicterus, meningitis. **Evaluation:** full history including antenatal and birth. Neurological/developmental examination. **MRI brain**	Multidisciplinary – physiotherapy (orthoses, exercise), OT, SALT, community paediatrics. For spasticity; PO/intrathecal baclofen, botulinum, selective dorsal rhizotomy, splints. Surgical; PEG, scoliosis, hip. Anticonvulsants, analgesia

TABLE 147.1 (Cont'd)

	Features	Investigations	Management
Duchenne muscular dystrophy (DMD)	Male; may present with delayed speech, then motor problems start. Proximal muscle weakness – Gower sign and waddling gait	**Serum CK:** elevated (>10 times normal upper limit). **Genetic testing:** dystrophin gene mutation	Paediatric neurology and community paediatrics. Physiotherapy (mobility), orthopaedics, SALT/OT. Cardiology/respiratory. Genetic counselling
Spinal muscular atrophy	Several different types presenting through childhood, depending on severity. Muscle weakness, hypotonia, absent reflexes	Molecular genetic testing	Multidisciplinary approach with community paediatrics, neurology, therapists (OT, PT, SALT).
Syndromes (e.g. Prader-Willi/Down/ Fragile X)	Global developmental delay, dysmorphic features, hypotonia	Genetic testing	Multidisciplinary approach. See *148. DYSMORPHIC CHILD*
Developmental dysplasia of hip	See *151. LIMPING CHILD*		

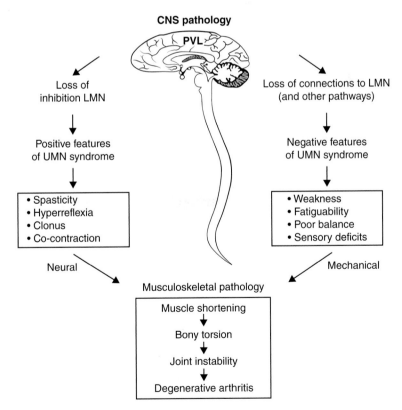

Fig. 147.1 In motor terms, cerebral palsy results in an upper motor neuron lesion, which causes positive and negative features that interact to produce the familiar musculoskeletal pathologic condition. LMN: lower motor neurone; PVL: periventricular leukomalacia; UMN: upper motor neurone. (Courtesy of H. Kerr Graham, MD, The Royal Children's Hospital, Melbourne, Australia.)

In the vignette, the most likely cause of late walking is cerebral palsy. The cause may have been prematurity, although there is often no identifiable cause. Cerebral palsy can be caused antenatally (e.g. preterm birth, twin pregnancy), perinatally (least common cause, e.g. hypoxic ischaemic encephalopathy) or postnatally (e.g. head injury, meningitis). Management of comorbidities in cerebral palsy may need to address: seizures, pain, spasticity (physiotherapy, oral/intrathecal baclofen), excessive salivation, GORD, feeding difficulties, constipation, visual/hearing impairment. Strategies for learning and behavioural difficulties need to be considered as early as possible.

REVISION TIPS

- Bottom shuffling and commando crawling are normal locomotor variant patterns. Walking may occur a bit later than 18 months in these children than those that do ordinary crawling
- Children with joint hypermobility also walk at a later age than average. This can result from hypermobility syndrome, Down syndrome, Marfan and Ehlers-Danlos syndrome

148

Dysmorphic Child

Caroline Bodey, Emmanuella Ikem, and Kirstie Kirkley

HPC: Baby girl born via SVD at term. Feeding difficulties, has yet to pass meconium. Mother, 41 years old, G1P1, had hyperemesis gravidarum, no other significant PMHx/FHx.

O/E: Dysmorphic features include single palmar crease, prominent epicanthal folds and up-slanting eyes. Hypotonic, with pan-systolic murmur, heard best at the left lower sternal border.

1. Match the features with the most likely diagnosis: (a) webbed neck, widely spaced nipples, (b) Brushfield spots, (c) 'rocker-bottom' feet, (d) oligohydramnios.
2. What musculoskeletal/cardiovascular complications are patients with Marfan syndrome (sy.) at risk of?

Answers: 1. (a) Turner sy. in females, Noonan sy. in males or females, (b) Down sy., (c) Edwards sy., (d) Potter sequence. 2. Chest wall deformity (pectus excavatum/carinatum). Aortic (dissection, root aneurysm). Mitral valve prolapse.

TABLE 148.1

	Suggestive Features	Associated Presentations/Abnormalities
Sex chromosome abnormalities		
Turner sy. (45X) (Fig. 148.1)	Females only. Ptosis, high-arched palate. Short stature, webbed neck, wide-spaced nipples, shield chest. Cubitus valgus, short 4th metacarpal, spoon-shaped nails, low posterior hairline	Heart: coarctation of the aorta, VSD, bicuspid aortic valve. GU: hypoplastic streak ovaries, delayed puberty, infertility.
Klinefelter sy. (47XXY) (Fig. 148.2)	Tall stature with long extremities and adolescent gynaecomastia. Micro-orchidism and hypergonadotropic hypogonadism after puberty	Most adult men are infertile. Androgen levels result in variable development of secondary sex characteristics

(Continued)

TABLE 148.1 (Cont'd)

	Suggestive Features	Associated Presentations/Abnormalities
Fragile X sy. (X-linked recessive) (Fig. 148.3).	Males > females. Macrocephaly. Long face with broad forehead, long prominent ears, strabismus, prominent mandible. Hyperextensible finger joints, flat feet	Heart: mitral valve prolapse. GU: macro-orchidism. Development and behaviour: learning difficulties, behavioural difficulties, ADHD, autism spectrum disorder
Trisomy syndromes Patau sy. (Trisomy 13) (Fig. 148.4)	Microcephaly, scalp defects, small eyes, cleft lip/palate, polydactyly	Complex cardiac and renal abnormalities, omphalocele, IUGR, stillbirth
Edwards sy. (Trisomy 18) (Fig. 148.5)	Low set ears, overriding flexed digits, rocker-bottom feet, mandibular hypoplasia, short sternum, small mouth	Complex cardiac, gastrointestinal and renal abnormalities, pulmonary hypoplasia, severe learning difficulties. These are usually life-threatening in infancy
Down sy. (Trisomy 21) (Fig. 148.6)	Flat occiput. Round face, small mouth, protruding tongue, low-set ears, flat nasal bridge, epicanthic folds, up-slanting eyes, Brushfield Spots (pigmented spots in iris). Short neck, single palmar crease, wide sandal gap. Most striking feature in neonates is hypotonia	Heart: AVSD, VSD, PDA, tetralogy of Fallot (ToF). GI: duodenal atresia, Hirschsprung's. Dysplasia of the hip, cataracts, hypothyroidism, leukaemia. Development: global developmental impairment
Micro-deletions Cri-du-chat sy. (Chromosome 5) *5p – deletion* (Fig. 148.7)	Microcephaly. Moon-shaped face, low-set ears, mandibular hypoplasia. Eyes widely spaced, down-slanting	Development: feeding difficulties, global developmental impairment
Di George sy. (Chromosome 22) *22q11.1 microdeletion* (Fig. 148.8)	Down-slanting eyes, wide nasal bridge, cleft palate, small mouth. Frequent infections	Aortic arch anomaly, ToF, VSD. Parathyroid hypoplasia/aplasia, thymus hypoplasia, kidney problems, schizophrenia, hearing loss, autoimmune
Williams sy. (Chromosome 7) *7q11 elastin deletion* (Fig. 148.9)	Peri-orbital fullness, sunken nasal bridge, anterior facing nostrils, full cheeks, wide mouth, wide-spaced small teeth, full lips, small chin. 'Full Elfin face'. 'Starburst' eyes	Heart: supravalvular aortic stenosis, pulmonary stenosis. Hypercalcaemia. Development/behaviour: learning difficulties, very friendly personality, better expressive than receptive language (old term: 'cocktail party speech')
Autosomal dominant Marfan sy. (Fig. 148.10)	*Fibrillin-1 mutation.* Long face with down-slanting eyes, high narrow palate, malar hypoplasia, maxillary/mandibular retrognathia. Tall, slim, long limbs, scoliosis, chest wall deformities, hypermobility, arachnodactyly, ectopic lentil (upward lens dislocation)	Heart: aortic aneurysm, mitral valve prolapse, aortic dissection. Other: pneumothorax

TABLE 148.1   (Cont'd)

	Suggestive Features	Associated Presentations/Abnormalities
Noonan sy. (Fig. 148.11)	*Mendelian – usually autosomal dominant.* Widely-spaced eyes, ptosis, ear abnormalities, webbed neck ('Male Turner syndrome'), widely spaced nipples, cubitus valgus, chest wall deformities	Heart: pulmonary stenosis, ASD, cardiomyopathy. GU: cryptorchidism. Development: mild learning difficulties. Other: bleeding disorders
Non-hereditary chromosomal		
Prader-Willi sy. (Fig. 148.12)	*Deletion in paternal chromosome 15 or maternal disomy.* Almond-shaped eyes, strabismus, thin upper lip, downturned mouth. Significant hypotonia, truncal obesity, short stature	GU: cryptorchidism, hypogonadism, infertility. Development and behaviour: global developmental impairment, behavioural problems. 'Constant, insatiable hunger'
VACTERL sy. (Fig. 148.13)	*No unifying causative gene identified.* Consider VACTERL in child with vertebral and other anomalies; VACTERL association diagnosed when ≥3 listed malformations are present. Intelligence usually normal	<ul><li>V Vertebral abnormalities</li><li>A Anal atresia</li><li>C cardiac defects</li><li>TE Tracheal-esophageal (atresia, stenosis, fistula)</li><li>R Renal and Radial abnormalities</li><li>L Limb abnormalities</li><li>(S) Single umbilical artery</li></ul>
Others		
Foetal alcohol sy. (Figs. 148.14 and 154.1)	Microcephaly, microphthalmia, short palpebral fissures, mid-face hypoplasia, posterior ear rotation, long smooth philtrum, thin upper lip, micrognathia	Heart: ASD, VSD, TOF. GU: urogenital abnormalities. Development: learning difficulties, hyperactivity. Other: alcohol withdrawal
Potter sequence (Fig. 148.15)	Compression due to low foetal urine volume (oligohydramnios). Crumpled low-set ears, recessed chin, depressed nasal bridge, beaked nose, unusual facial creases, abnormal position of hands, talipes equinovarus, joint contractures	Kidney: bilateral renal agenesis. Lung: pulmonary hypoplasia (usually causes death)

TABLE 148.2   Summary of Key Points

	Turner	Klinefelter	Fragile X
Sex chromosomes	*X0*	*XYY*	*X-linked recessive*
General	Pigmented moles	Infertility	Autism, hyperactivity
Intellectual			Impaired
CNS/eyes			Macrocephaly
Head	Webbed or thick neck		Facial
Skeletal	Short stature, cubitus valgus	Tall stature	Joint laxity, scoliosis
CVS	Heart defect		Mitral prolapse
Other organs	Ovarian dysgenesis	Hypogonadism	Macro-orchidism at puberty
	Renal defects, hypothyroid	Gynaecomastia	
	Patau	**Edwards**	**Down**
Trisomy	*13*	*18*	*21*
General		Low birth weight	Hypotonia
Intellectual	Impaired	Impaired	Impaired
CNS/eyes	Brain defect, microphthalmia		Brushfield spots, epicanthic fold
Head	Cleft lip/palate	Wide occiput, small chin	Small mouth/ears, short neck
Skeletal	Polydactyly	Overlapping fingers	Palmar crease, sandal gap
CVS	Heart defects	Heart defects	Heart defects
Other organs	Lung or renal defects	Renal defects	
	Cri-du-chat	**di George**	**Williams**
Deletion	*Chromosome 5*	*Chromosome 22*	*Chromosome 7*
General	High-pitched cry, hypotonia	Autism/ADHD	
Intellectual	Impaired	Impaired	Impaired
CNS/eyes			
Head	Microcephaly	Facial, cleft palate	Facial
Skeletal			Short stature
CVS			Aortic stenosis
Other organs		Impaired immunity	
	Marfan	**Noonan**	**Prader-Willi**
	Autosomal dominant	*Autosomal dominant*	*Non-hereditary*
General			Hypotonia, hyperphagia
Intellectual		Impaired (mild)	Impaired
CNS/eyes			
Head	High palate, retrognathia	Facial, webbed neck	Facial
Skeletal	Scoliosis, hypermobile, tall	Short, pectus excavatum	Impaired growth
CVS	Aortic. Mitral prolapse	Pulmonary stenosis, ASD	
Other organs	Pneumothorax		Hypogonadism

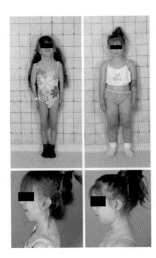

Fig. 148.1 Turner syndrome. (From Saenger P, et al. Turner syndrome. In: Sperling MA, ed. *Pediatric Endocrinology*. 4th ed. Saunders; 2014:664–696, Figure 16.6.)

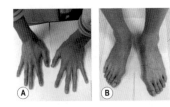

Fig. 148.2 Klinefelter syndrome. (https://www.clinicalkey. com/#!/content/undefined/1-s2.0-S1028455918301438?scroll-To=%231-s2.0-S1028455918301438-gr1)

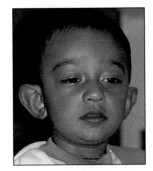

Fig. 148.3 Fragile X syndrome. (From Lissauer T, et al. Genetics. In: *Illustrated Textbook of Paediatrics*. 5th ed. Elsevier; 2018:121–141, Figure 9.13.)

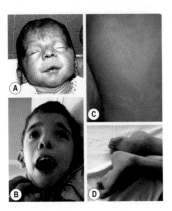

Fig. 148.4. Patau syndrome (trisomy 13). (https://www.clinicalkey. com/#!/content/undefined/1-s2.0-S1769721208000487?scroll-To=%231-s2.0-S1769721208000487-gr1)

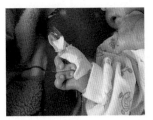

Fig. 148.5. Edwards syndrome (trisomy 18). (https://commons. wikimedia.org/w/index.php?search=edwards+syndrome& title=Special:MediaSearch&go=Go&type=image)

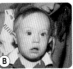

Fig. 148.6. Down syndrome (trisomy 21) (From Curry CJ. Autosomal trisomies. In: Rimoin DL et al., eds. *Emery and Rimoin's Principles and Practice of Medical Genetics*. 6th ed. Academic Press; 2013:1–27, Figure 43.2.)

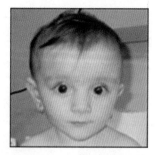

Fig. 148.7. Cri-du-chat syndrome (5p microdeletion). (https: //www.clinicalkey.com/#!/content/undefined/1-s2.0-S176972 1214000305?scrollTo=%231-s2.0-S1769721214000305-gr1)

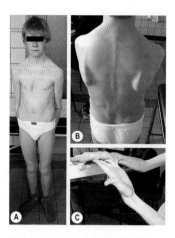

Fig. 148.10 Marfan syndrome. (From Callewaert B, et al. Ehlers-Danlos syndromes and Marfan syndrome. *Best Pract Res Clin Rheumatol.* 2008;22(1):165–189, Figure 3.)

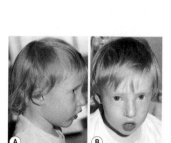

Fig. 148.8. Di George syndrome (22q11.1 microdeletion). (From Radford DJ, Perkins L, Lachman R, Thong YH. Spectrum of Di George syndrome in patients with truncus arteriosus: expanded Di George syndrome. *Pediatr Cardiol.* 1988;9:95.)

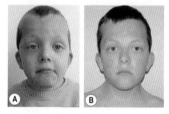

Fig. 148.11. Noonan syndrome. (Chen, Shi, MD; Chen, Liang, MD; Jiang, Yong, MD, PhD; Xu, Haitao, MD, PhD; Sun, Yangxue, MD; Shi, Hao, MD; Li, Shoujun, MD, PhD; Zhang, Jing, MD, PhD; Yan, Jun, PhD. Early Outcomes of Septal Myectomy for Obstructive Hypertrophic Cardiomyopathy in Children With Noonan Syndrome Published May 31, 2022. Volume 34, Issue 2. Pages 655–665. © 2021.)

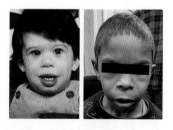

Fig. 148.9. Williams syndrome (7q11 elastin deletion). (A: From Alizad A, et al. Echocardiographic features of genetic diseases: part 6 – complex cardiovascular defects. *J Am Soc Echocardiogr.* 2000;13(6):637–643, Figure 7. B: From Ojha V, et al. Spontaneous pulmonary artery aneurysm in a case of Williams syndrome. *J Cardiovasc Comput Tomogr.* 2020;14(6):e170–e171, Figure 1.)

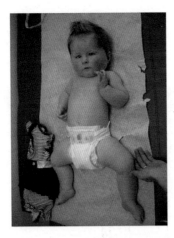

Fig. 148.12. Prader-Willi syndrome. (Reproduced from Hickey SE et al. A case of an atypically large proximal 15q deletion as cause for Prader-Willi syndrome arising from a de novo unbalanced translocation. *Eur J Med Genet.* 2013;56(9):510–514, Figure 1. Copyright © 2013 ElsevierMasson SAS. All rights reserved.)

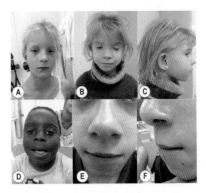

Fig. 148.14. Foetal alcohol syndrome. (From Del Campo M, et al. A review of the physical features of the fetal alcohol spectrum disorders. *Eur J Med Genet.* 2017;60(1):55–64, Figure 1.)

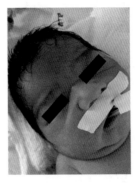

Fig. 148.15. Potter sequence. (https://www.clinicalkey.com/#!/content/undefined/1-s2.0-S2210261221007999?scrollTo=%231-s2.0-S2210261221007999-gr1)

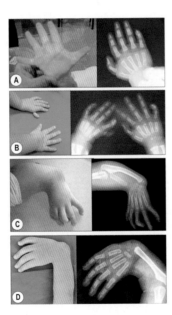

Fig. 148.13. VACTERL. (https://www.clinicalkey.com/#!/content/undefined/1-s2.0-S0022347613012043?scrollTo=%231-s2.0-S0022347613012043-f148-03-9780323847698)

The vignette likely reflects Down sy. (trisomy 21). Failure to pass meconium may indicate Hirschsprung disease, which may affect babies with Down sy. Dysmorphic features can be difficult to determine in babies and may become more apparent later. Additional pointers include behavioural phenotype (e.g. insatiable appetite in Prader Willi sy.) or developmental profile (e.g. difficulty with receptive language in Williams sy.). Causes include chromosomal aneuploidy (such as a trisomy), microdeletion or duplication (e.g. Williams sy.), single gene disorder (e.g. neurofibromatosis), or abnormal imprinting (Prader Willi sy.). History, including FHx over three generations, developmental and pregnancy history, and examination (considering behavioural phenotype), will help guide investigations.Management, including for medical comorbidities, is best led by a paediatrician (often community paediatrician) and a multidisciplinary team.

REVISION TIPS

- Di George sy. **CATCH22**; Cardiac defects, Atypical face, Thymus hypoplasia, Cleft palate/lip, Hypocalcaemia, 22q11.2 deletion
- EDWARDS sy. **EDWARDS**; 18 Trisomy, Digits, Wide head, Affected intellect, Rocker-bottom feet, manDibular hypoplasia, Small jaw
- VACTERL; Vertebral defects, Anal atresia, Cardiac defects, Tracheo-oEsophageal problems, Renal defects, Limb defects

149

Family History of Genetic Disorder

Emmanuella Ikem, Shruthi Sankaranarayanan, and Alexander Royston

CYSTIC FIBROSIS (CF) FOLLOW-UP APPOINTMENT. RISK OF GENETIC DISORDER IN SECOND PREGNANCY

A 4-year-old boy attends with father. Specialist follow-up since diagnosed with CF at birth. Both the father and mother are healthy and have no significant past medical history; father mentions they are trying to have a second child, and they are concerned about the risk of that child also having CF.

1. What is the chance of the hoped-for second child in the vignette having CF?
2. Can undetected cystic fibrosis present symptomatically in adulthood?
3. What is the principal investigation to diagnose CF?

Answers: 1. 25%. A second child having CF requires the abnormal gene to be inherited from both parents: 25% possibility. There is a 50% possibility of the second child being a carrier, and the chance of no abnormal genes is 25%. 2. Yes, CF can be undetected until adulthood: life expectancy is usually higher than if detected at birth. 3. The sweat test.

TABLE 149.1

	Features	Investigations	Management
Cystic fibrosis	**Newborn:** newborn screening, meconium ileus. **Infancy:** jaundice, pancreatic insufficiency, failure to thrive, steatorrhoea, recurrent chest infections. **Child:** bronchiectasis, rectal prolapse, nasal polyps, sinusitis. **Adolescent:** DM, infertility, portal hypertension, cirrhosis, frequent infections: *S. aureus, Pseudomonas aeruginosa, Burkholderia cepacia* complex	**RFs:** FHx (1:4 if both parents carriers). Autosomal recessive (CFTR channel). Mutations: delta F508 (Chr 7). **Preconception screening** (if high risk). **Heel prick:** elevated immunoreactive trypsinogen (IRT). **Sweat test** definitive: chloride >60 mmol/L. **Genetic testing** (if raised IRT/positive sweat test)	MDT approach. Physiotherapy (mucus clearance, mobility, etc.). Increased calories. Fat-soluble vitamin (ADEK) supplements. Saline nebulisers. Abx for frequent LRTI. Lumacaftor (CFTR corrector)/Ivacaftor (CFTR potentiator)- if F508 deletion

TABLE 149.2	Mnemonics for Conditions According to Major Patterns of Inheritance				
Dominant		**Recessive**		**X-linked**	
'DOOMMINANT Heritance'		**'RECCESSIVE PHENOTYPE Group'**		**'X HERITED 6'**	
D	Danlos (Ehlers Danlos)	R	fRiedrich ataxia	X	Fragile X
O	Osteogenesis imperfecta	E		H	Haemophilia
O	Otosclerosis	C	Cystic fibrosis	H	Haemophilia
M	Myotonic dystrophy	C	CAH	E	
M	Marfan	E		R	R/G colour blind
I	Intermittent porphyria	S	Sickle cell disease	I	
N	Neurofibromatosis	S	Spinal muscular atrophy	T	
A	Adenomatous polyposis (FAP)	I	Isovaleric acidaemia	E	
N	Noonan	V		D	Duchenne/Becker
T	Tuberous sclerosis	E			
Heritance	Huntingdon disease	P	PKU	6	G6PDH
	Hypercholesterolaemia	H	Homocystinuria		
		E			
		N			
		O			
		T	Thalassaemia		
		Y	maple sYrup		
		P			
		E			
		Group	Galactosaemia Glutaric aciduria type 1		

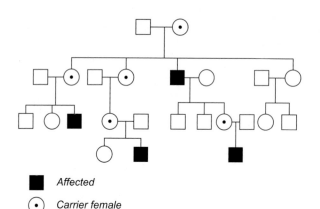

Affected

Carrier female

Fig. 149.1 Pedigree consistent with X-linked recessive inheritance. (From Cook J. Genes in families. In: *Emery and Rimoin's Principles and Practice of Medical Genetics and Genomics.* 7th ed. Elsevier; 2019:201–225. Copyright © 2019 Elsevier Inc. All rights reserved.)

Autosomal recessive conditions commonly feature in exams, notably CF; two copies of the abnormal gene are required to manifest the condition phenotypically. If only one abnormal gene is present then the individual has carrier genotype but is usually asymptomatic, although they can pass the gene to their offspring. Having offspring with CF suggests one of three things: both parents are carriers (as in the vignette); one has the condition and one is a carrier; both parents have the condition. In other patterns of inheritance, autosomal dominant inheritance patterns are easy to calculate the risk for, as only one copy of the abnormal gene is required to inherit the condition. In males, X-linked diseases act like a dominant inheritance pattern, regardless of whether the disease is dominant or recessive, since they have only one copy of the X chromosome. Mnemonics to help remember pattern of inheritance are given in Table 149.2.

REVISION TIPS

- Autosomal dominant inheritance: successive generations affected, male:female proportions approximately equal, both sexes can both be responsible for transmission (usually at least one instance of male–male transmission)

- Autosomal recessive inheritance: females and males affected, usually occurs in only one generation (within a single sibship), parents may be consanguineous
- Conditions with an X-linked inheritance pattern are substantially more likely to affect males

150

Cyanosis

Lucy Andrews, Alexander Royston, Henna Khattak, Ciara Mcclenaghan, Joseph Page, and Viren Ahluwalia

EMERGENCY DEPARTMENT, MALE 8-WEEK-OLD BABY. WENT BLUE ROUND THE LIPS DURING FEEDING

HPC: He went blue around his lips when feeding this morning; this has happened a few times during prolonged crying. Previously healthy, pregnancy/birth uncomplicated. Mother is healthy.

O/E; RS: Chest clear, RR 62. **CVS:** HS I + II + loud murmur. Mild central cyanosis when crying. **Abdo:** SNT, no focal neurology.

1. Which respiratory conditions can lead to cyanosis in adults?
2. What does presence of clubbing suggest in a cyanotic patient?
3. A 74-year-old patient presents with low blood pressure, recent dysuria and they are peripherally cyanosed. What is the most likely cause?

Answers: 1. Acute: PE, pneumothorax, severe pneumonia, acute asthma. Chronic: COPD, fibrosis. 2. It narrows the differential to CHD, suppurative pulmonary disease, right-to-left shunting (cardiac and intrapulmonary). 3. Urosepsis: mottling/cyanosis suggest sepsis (+hypotension). Unwell, with likely metabolic acidosis.

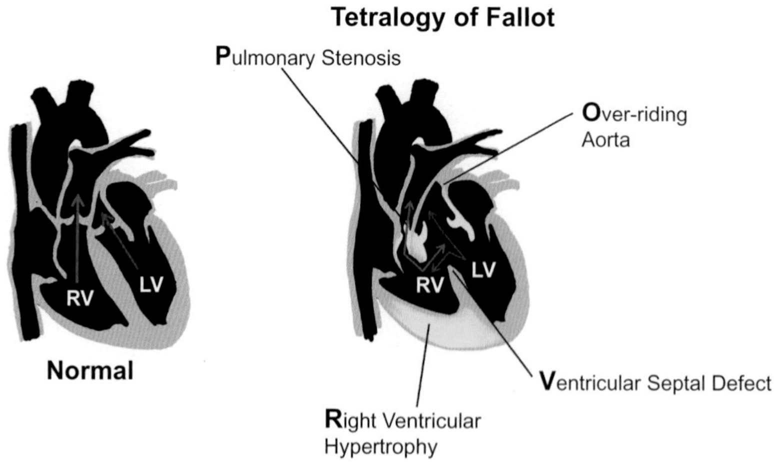

Fig. 150.1 Tetralogy of Fallot. (Illustrated by Dr Hollie Blaber.)

TABLE 150.1

	Features	Investigations	Management
Paediatric cyanosis			
Tetralogy of Fallot (TOF)	'PROVe': Pulmonary stenosis, Right ventricular hypertrophy, Overriding aorta, VSD. **Hx & O/E:** usually presents at 1–2 months with cyanosis and respiratory distress/heart failure. Can present age 1–3 years (milder). Long loud murmur and thrill at left sternal edge, single S2 (pulmonary valve closure inaudible). 'Hypercyanotic/Tet spells': clinical cyanosis when crying/agitated, relieved by squatting (older child) or knee-chest position	**RFs:** FHx (heart defects), retinoic acid, uncontrolled DM, PKU, rubella. **Echocardiogram.** ECG: RVH, RAD. CXR: 'Boot-shaped' heart, reduced pulmonary vascular marking. Microarray: if genetic syndrome suspected. **Cardiac CT angiogram** or **MRI:** delineate anatomy. Cardiac catheterisation: to measure haemodynamics	Prostaglandin to open PDA (neonatal collapse). Diuretic if in heart failure. Surgical repair. β-blockers/morphine/ IV fluids for Tet spells.
Transposition of Great Arteries (TGA)	Neonatal cyanosis: not improved using O_2, collapse, loud single S2, right ventricular heave. (If coexisting VSD, cyanosis less obvious, signs of heart failure)	**RFs:** maternal rubella/ virus, alcohol/smoking/ meds in pregnancy. Poor DM control. **Echocardiogram.** CXR: 'Egg on side' (narrow upper mediastinum)	Prostaglandins: to maintain PDA. Emergency atrial balloon septostomy. **Definitive:** surgery (arterial switch operation) before 4 weeks
Respiratory distress syndrome (RDS)	Surfactant deficiency. **RFs:** prematurity, FHx, LSCS delivery, hypothermia, perinatal hypoxia, meconium aspiration, congenital pneumonia, maternal diabetes. **Hx & O/E:** ↑WOB, grunting, ↑RR, cyanosis, apnoea	Rare >32 weeks gestation (severity ↑ as gestation ↓). **Monitoring:** SpO_2 Blood gases. CXR: 'Bilateral, diffuse, ground-glass appearance'	**Prevention:** IM antenatal corticosteroids. Oxygen, nasal CPAP, ventilation. **Definitive:** surfactant (via ETT). Abx (until pneumonia/ sepsis excluded). Consider nutrition and fluids

(Continued)

TABLE 150.1   (Cont'd)

		Features	Investigations	Management
Adult – Central cyanosis				
Hypoxaemic hypoxia ↓PaO_2	High altitude hypoxaemia (*Low Inspired Oxygen PAO_2*)	**RFs:** altitude, fast ascent (at altitudes >2000 m)/poor acclimatisation. **Hx & O/E:** ↑RR/HR/ BP, fatigue, headache, neurology (ataxia, confusion, coma), cyanosis	**Monitoring:** vital signs, heart murmurs, JVP, crackles may suggest pulmonary oedema. **Complications:** acute mountain sickness (AMS), high-altitude pulmonary oedema (HAPE), high altitude cerebral oedema (HACE)	**Prevention:** slow ascent, O_2. Acetazolamide. Descent from altitude. Hyperbaric O_2. Dexamethasone
	Pulmonary causes (late-sign)	**V/Q mismatch** Pneumonia, pulmonary oedema, PE, asthma, COPD **Hypoventilation (↓PaO_2)** PaO_2 normalises with supplemental O_2, but ↑$PaCO_2$. Causes: opioids, stroke, obesity, hypoventilation, neuromuscular disease, kyphosis, severe COPD **Diffusion impairment** Inflammatory/interstitial lung disease, pulmonary oedema	**Obs:** RR, SpO_2, HR, BP, temp. ABG (↓PaO_2 ±↑$PaCO_2$: ⟶T1/T2RF). FBC (↑inflammatory markers), ↑CRP. Spirometry. **CXR:** pneumonia, oedema. **CTPA** (PE: filling defect) – if D-dimer +ve. **High resolution CT:** (ILD), autoimmune profile	PaO_2 typically normalises with supplemental oxygen. Over-oxygenation risks T2RF in patients with hypoventilation. **Definitive:** cause-dependent; • Pneumonia: Abx • PE: anti-coagulate • PTX: aspirate/chest drain • COPD/asthma: inhaled therapy
	Anatomical shunt	Structural heart disease: de-oxygenated blood passing R⟶L heart. **Hx & O/E:** Eisenmenger syndrome: unrepaired acyanotic heart disease (VSD/ASD/PDA – presents later: commonly teens/ adults) becomes cyanotic as PAH ⟶ RVH ⟶ shunt reversal ⟶ cyanosis	**ECG:** RAD, RVH. **Echocardiogram:** shunt direction. Cardiac MRI. Cardiac catheterisation: assess pulmonary artery pressure	PaO_2 does not normalise when oxygen is given. Immunisations, iron supplementation. Cardiologist with interest in congenital/ structural heart disease
		Pulmonary arteriovenous malformations (PAVM)	**Highly specialised:** FBC, ferritin, PaO_2, imaging	Specialist centres (embolise, resect, transplant)

TABLE 150.1 (Cont'd)

	Features	Investigations	Management
Anaemia or insufficient O_2 carrying capacity	**Conditions:** blood loss, CO poisoning, methaemoglobinaemia, (MetHb), congenital. Drugs causing MetHb: dapsone, local anesthetics, phenacetin, antimalarials	Exclude cardiopulmonary disease of the newborn. Pulse oximetry falsely reassuring (CO/MetHb). **ABG:** normal PaO_2 (room air) but $\downarrow SaO_2$	Education: medications in haemolysis/anaemia. CO poisoning: high flow/hyperbaric O_2. MetHb: stop medications, exchange transfusions, methylene blue, ascorbic acid. Transfusions
Adult – Peripheral cyanosis			
Reduced cardiac output	Acute or chronic heart failure: cardiogenic shock. **Hx & O/E:** mottling, cyanosis, $\downarrow BP$, $\downarrow UO$	**ECG:** ischaemia, dysrhythmia. Inflammatory markers, BNP, ferritin, lactate. **CXR** **Echocardiogram.** **Angiogram:** occlusive coronary disease	O_2 supplementation. Cardiogenic: angioplasty, LVAD, ECMO. Sepsis: Abx, vasopressor support. CCF: diuretics. **Definitive:** treat cause

Other causes: hypothermia, Raynaud's phenomenon, venous obstruction/congestion

In the vignette, the most likely diagnosis is tetralogy of Fallot (TOF), which is the most common cyanotic congenital heart disease (Fig. 150.0). The main murmur is pulmonary stenosis (crescendo-decrescendo systolic ejection murmur, loudest at upper left sternal edge). The mother is describing Tet spells, characteristic of TOF. Finding the typical murmur supports the diagnosis of TOF, as an outflow obstruction is present due to pulmonary stenosis. The child was born at term, which makes respiratory distress syndrome highly unlikely. The differentials for adults and paediatrics with cyanosis vary greatly so the patient's age must be considered. Central cyanosis is generally a late finding in the course of adult illness.

REVISION TIPS

- Cyanosis – a physical sign as a result of hypoxaemia which results in a bluish discoloration to the skin and tissues
- Hypoxaemia – low oxygen in the blood. PaO_2 – arterial oxygen, PAO_2 – alveolar oxygen
- Severely anaemic patients with marked arterial desaturation might not be cyanosed, whereas polycythemic patients develop obvious cyanosis at higher SaO_2
- Central cyanosis is best seen where the epidermis is thin with a good blood supply: the lips, malar prominences (nose and cheeks), ears, and oral mucous membranes (buccal, sublingual)

151

Limping Child

Emmanuella Ikem, Annapurna Jagadish,
Laura Crosby, and Athimalaipet Ramanan

GP CONSULTATION, MALE, AGED 3.
4-DAYS LIMP WITH GROIN AND THIGH PAIN

HPC: Sudden onset limp with constant right groin and thigh pain, unkeen to play. Recent coryzal symptoms, now resolved. Otherwise well.

O/E: Alert and active. HR 110, RR 25, T 37.8°C, SpO_2 99% (air). PGALS (paediatric gait, arms, legs, spine) shows limp, difficulty weight bearing, mild hip pain on active and passive movement, reduced range of movement on abduction and internal rotation.

1. What are the risk factors for developmental hip dysplasia?
2. What endocrinological conditions are associated with slipped upper femoral epiphysis?

Answers: 1. 1st degree FHx, breech presentation, multiple pregnancies, fixed foot deformity. 2. Hypothyroidism, hypopituitarism, growth hormone deficiencies.

TABLE 151.1

	Features	Investigations	Management
Transient synovitis (irritable hip)	Age 3–10, sudden onset limp, recent/concurrent viral illness, ± low-grade pyrexia, no rest pain, reduced internal rotation	Diagnosis of exclusion (rule out septic arthritis)	Reassure. Advise rest and simple analgesia: NSAIDs
Septic arthritis	Acute onset, rest pain, tender palpation, high-grade pyrexia. Red, hot, swollen joint, systemically unwell. Hip held flexed + external rotated. *Use Kocher criteria to assess probability of septic arthritis (see commentary)*	Increased inflammatory markers, positive blood cultures. USS and joint aspiration for MC&S: +ve. **Pelvic XR:** widening of joint space. Consider MRI: rule out associated osteomyelitis	ABCDE + Sepsis 6. Antibiotics (BNF): flucloxacillin 4–6 weeks (check local guidelines). Fluids (if signs of shock). Early orthopaedic referral
Legg-Calve-Perthe disease	**RFs:** 3–10, M > F. **Hx & O/E:** insidious, progressive. Avascular necrosis of femoral head	**Pelvic XR** (AP and frog leg lateral view): femoral head collapse/fragmentation, widening of joint space. XR may be normal; consider MRI	Conservative: rest, analgesia, physiotherapy. Surgery: proximal femoral osteotomy

TABLE 151.1 (Cont'd)

	Features	Investigations	Management
Osteomyelitis	Acute limb pain, difficulty weight bearing/mobilising, swelling over affected site, febrile. Predominantly *S. aureus*	Blood culture: +ve, raised WCC/inflammatory markers. XR may be normal/soft tissue swelling. MRI soft-tissue/joint changes	Antibiotics as per local guidance: initial IV, then oral, total course 4–6 weeks
Juvenile idiopathic arthritis (JIA)	RFs: <16 years, FHx. Hx & O/E: morning joint stiffness, limp, other joints affected (isolated hip rare), ± pyrexia, salmon-pink rash (Fig. 151.1), nail changes, uveitis	Diagnosis of exclusion. ANA and/or RhF are found in a few JIA patients. ↑ Neutrophils, ↓ Hb, ↑ Pts, normal or ↑ESR/CRP	MDT approach. NSAIDs, steroids, DMARDs, biologics. Ophthalmology screening for uveitis.
Developmental dysplasia of the hip (DDH)	F > M, FHx, breech, oligohydramnios, fixed foot deformity. Hx & O/E: spectrum from hip dysplasia, reducible subluxation/ dislocation to irreducible. At 6–8 weeks, Ortolani's/ Barlow's tests may be positive. At >3 months, reduced ROM, leg length discrepancy, Klisic test may be positive. At > 1 year, lumbar lordosis, Trendelenburg gait, toe walking. Assymmetry of thigh folds may be present (Fig. 151.2).	Screening exam at age 6–8 weeks (Barlow's/ Ortolani's). If abnormal: USS hip at age < 6 months, X-ray hip at age >6 months (shallow acetabulum, hypoplastic femoral head, loss of Shenton's line).	*Age <6 months*: Pavlik harness for 6 weeks. *6–18 months*: open/closed reduction + hip spica plaster cast for 3 months. *>18 months*: open reduction, pelvic osteotomy + hip spica for 3 months
Malignancy	Night pain/sweats, weight loss, malaise, pyrexia, palpable mass, pallor, easy bruising, recurrent infections, lymphadenopathy, hepatosplenomegaly	Cytopenia in 1+ cell lines, ↑ LDH, ALP. Blast cells if leukaemia. Urine catecholamines: ↑VMA, ↑ HVA. XR/MRI primary – biopsy	Depends on type of malignancy; chemotherapy, radiotherapy, surgery
Fracture	Trauma; accidental or non-accidental injury (NAI) malignancy	XR	Management varies; fracture type decides treatment options. Safeguarding if suspect NAI, particularly if in a non-ambulant child
Slipped upper femoral epiphysis (SUFE)	RFs: obesity, age 10–13 , hypothyroid, hypopituitarism, growth hormone/ vitamin D deficiencies. Hx & O/E: pain referred to groin/thigh/ knee, reduced hip flexion/ abduction, worse on jumping	Bilateral hip XR (AP and frog leg lateral): wide epiphysis, slipped femoral head	In situ screw fixation ± prophylactic fixation of contralateral hip

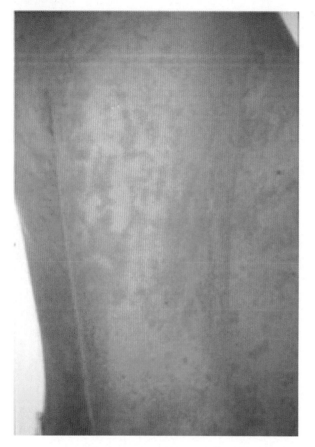

Fig. 151.1 Salmon-pink rash of systemic-onset juvenile idiopathic arthritis. (Reproduced with permission from Lissauer T. Musculoskeletal disorders. In: Lissauer, Carroll eds. *Illustrated Textbook of Paediatrics*. 6th ed. Elsevier;ISBN 9780702081804.)

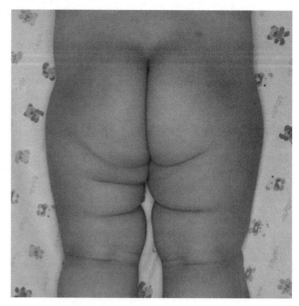

Fig. 151.2 Asymmetrical thigh folds. (Reproduced with permission from MS Kang, GW Han, M Kam and Soo-Sung Park. Clinical significance of asymmetric skin folds in the medial thigh for the infantile screening of developmental dysplasia of the hip. Pediatrics & Neonatology, 60(5) 2019, pp. 570-576.)

determine the probability of septic arthritis based on four parameters (non-weight bearing, Temp > 38.5°C, ESR > 40, WBC >12). The vignette describes a case of transient synovitis, alluding to the recent viral infection. It can be managed conservatively with rest and analgesia.

Musculoskeletal symptoms can reflect JIA, infection, vasculitis or non-accidental injury. Rule out malignancy in children with acute onset limp where there are red flags, such as pain at night, anorexia or bruising. Inflammatory arthritis is associated with chronic conditions, like inflammatory bowel disease, cystic fibrosis or psoriasis. Transient synovitis is the commonest cause of acute hip pain or limp, especially aged 3–10. Consider and exclude septic arthritis, which may need urgent blood cultures and joint aspiration. Use Kocher criteria for septic arthritis to

REVISION TIPS

- Most causes of limp are due to hip pathology, but consider the back, femur, knee, foot and ankle
- Abdominal conditions (appendicitis, inguinal hernia, testicular torsion, UTI) may present as a limp
- A child with transient synovitis can present with a mild pyrexia. Rule out septic arthritis/osteomyelitis if suspicious; septic arthritis is more likely if <3 years old
- Any child presenting with limp **and** pyrexia should be managed in secondary care

152

Congenital Abnormality

Katie Turner, Alexander Royston, and Henna Khattak

1. Can you list the maternal risk factors for congenital heart defects?
2. What chromosomal disorder is most commonly associated with VSD?
3. Which congenital heart defects are associated with Turner syndrome?

Answers: 1. DM, rubella, SLE, alcohol, smoking, drug use. 2. Trisomy 21: Down syndrome. VSD occurs in 45%–50% of cases. 3. Bicuspid aortic valve/VSD/coarctation of the aorta.

TABLE 152.1

	Features	Investigations	Management
Acyanotic			
Ventricular septal defect (VSD)	**RFs:** FHx, trisomy 21, DiGeorge/Turner syndrome, maternal alcohol, diabetes, PKU, lithium, phenytoin, rubella. **Hx & O/E:** heart failure. Hepatomegaly, tachypnoea, tachycardia, pallor, shortness of breath (especially during feeding), sweating, fatigue. Failure to thrive (FTT), chest infections. Pansystolic murmur lower left sternal edge (LLSE): louder in smaller defects ± thrill	*Most common: 30% of CHD.* **ECG:** signs of LVH or biventricular hypertrophy. **CXR:** increased pulmonary vascular markings, cardiomegaly, pulmonary oedema. **Echocardiogram.** **Cardiac MRI:** measure haemodynamic impact	Small: monitor, may spontaneously close. Moderate/large: nutritional support, diuretics, ACEi, consider digoxin. **Definitive:** surgical closure from 3 to 5 months

(Continued)

TABLE 152.1   (Cont'd)

	Features	Investigations	Management
Atrial septal defect (ASD)	**RFs:** maternal DM, ↑CBG, pregnancy: alcohol, smoking, anti-depressants. **Hx & O/E:** usually asymptomatic, heart failure, FTT, chest infections. Ejection systolic murmur upper left sternal edge (ULSE), wide fixed split S2	*5%–10% of CHD.* Investigate as per VSD. **ECG:** tall P wave, RAD, RBBB	If <5mm: should spontaneously close ≤12months. **Diuretics:** if in failure. **Definitive:** surgical closure
Patent ductus arteriosus (PDA)	**RFs:** prematurity, sex (F > M), LBW, rubella infection. **Hx & O/E:** asymptomatic, SOB, chest infections, heart failure, FTT. Continuous 'machinery' left infraclavicular murmur ± thrill, hyperactive precordium, wide pulse pressure	*5%–10% of CHD.* Investigations as per VSD/ASD	Ibuprofen and/or paracetamol promote duct closure-contraindicated in PDA-dependent congenital heart disease. Diuretics if in failure. **Definitive:** surgical closure by PDA ligation
Coarctation of aorta	**RF:** FHx (heart defects). **Hx & O/E:** severe-heart failure/shock in infancy with closure of PDA, weak femoral pulses. Milder-hypertension, headaches, murmur, ↓distal pulses, radio-femoral delay. Mid-systolic murmur: loudest in back below left scapula	**Echocardiogram.** **CXR:** inferior rib notching (Roesler sign). **ECG:** LVH. **Cardiac CT/MRI:** delineate anatomy	Severe neonatal: prostaglandin E1 (Prostin: keeps duct open). Diuretics/inotropes: failure. ACEi, antihypertensives. **Definitive:** balloon angioplasty and stenting. Surgical closure.
Cyanotic			
Tetralogy of Fallot	see *150. CYANOSIS*		
Transposition of Great Arteries (TGA)	see *150. CYANOSIS*		
Key Complications			
Eisenmenger syndrome	Reversal of left-to-right shunt in heart defect (VSD, ASD, PDA) due to pulmonary hypertension. **RF:** unrepaired congenital heart disease in adolescents/adults. **Hx & O/E:** cyanosis, clubbing, right ventricular failure, haemoptysis, 'paradoxical' embolisation, brain abscess. PDA: normal upper limb arterial oxygen saturation (SpO_2 95%); reduced lower limb arterial oxygen saturation (SpO_2 70%)	FBC (erythrocytosis: ↑haematocrit/Hb). **ECG:** RAD, RVH. **Echocardiogram:** shows right-to-left shunt. **Cardiac MRI:** to delineate anatomy. Cardiac catheterisation: assess pulmonary artery pressure	Corrective surgery with defect closure is contraindicated in established ES. Immunisations, iron supplementation. **Definitive:** heart-lung transplantation (end-stage)

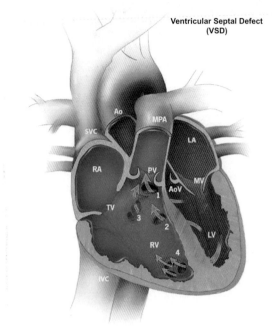

Ventricular Septal Defect (VSD)

RA. Right Atrium	SVC. Superior Vena Cava	TV. Tricuspid Valve	1. Conoventricular, malaligned
RV. Right Ventricle	IVC. Inferior Vena Cava	MV. Mitral Valve	2. perimembranous
LA. Left Atrium	MPA. Main Pulmonary Artery	PV. Pulmonary Valve	3. inlet
LV. Left Ventricle	Ao. Aorta	AoV. Aortic Valve	4. muscular

Fig. 152.1 Ventricular septal defect. Illustration showing various forms of ventricular septal defects. **1.** Conoventricular, malaligned; **2.** Perimembranous; **3.** Inlet; **4.** Muscular. (By Centers for Disease Control and Prevention – Centers for Disease Control and Prevention, Public Domain, https://commons.wiki media.org/w/index.php?curid=29525835)

The vignette indicates a congenital heart defect, and the important distinction is whether this is acyanotic or cyanotic. He is pale and sweaty but not cyanotic, and so a left-to-right shunt is most likely. Well when born, his failing to thrive and pallor/sweatiness can be signs of early heart failure. Ventricular septal defect is the commonest acyanotic CHD, and with the characteristic murmur this history describes a fairly typical case, which usually presents at least 2 weeks post-birth. A small VSD may cause no symptoms but a loud murmur. Other acyanotic conditions may present similarly: ASD and PDA also have distinctive murmurs and are differentiated most accurately using echocardiography.

REVISION TIPS

- Cyanotic – right-to-left shunt results in decreased blood flow through the pulmonary system, leading to lower blood oxygen levels (hypoxaemia)
- Nitrogen wash-out test is used to differentiate cyanotic congenital heart disease from non-cardiac causes of cyanosis
- Use of maternal anti-epileptics (e.g. phenytoin) increases risk of cleft palate formation and congenital heart disease
- Other (non-cardiac) congenital conditions: cleft lip/palate, neural tube defects, talipes equinovarus (clubfoot), developmental dysplasia of hip

Congenital Abnormality, Biliary Atresia – Outline

Marcus Drake

Biliary atresia is due to obliteration of bile ducts, in about 1 in 10,000 infants. Can occur with spleen abnormalities, absent IVC, intestinal malformation. Classified by the most proximal obstruction (Fig. 153.1). Evaluation requires exclusion of TORCH, hepatitis B/C, α1-antitrypsin, galactosemia, CF, tyrosinemia, endocrine abnormalities. Imaging uses ultrasound (atrophic/absent gallbladder, absent intrahepatic ducts), HIDA hepatobiliary iminodiacetic acid scintigraphy (uptake of technetium isotope without emptying into the duodenum), ± MRCP/ERCP.

TABLE 153.1

	Features	Investigations	Management
Biliary atresia	Soon after birth: jaundice, pale stools, dark urine. Advanced: failure to thrive, hepatomegaly, ascites, cirrhosis, portal hypertension	LFTs. Ultrasound, HIDA, ± MRCP/ERCP. Liver biopsy	Hepatoportoenterostomy (Kasai procedure). Liver transplant (10-year graft survival 73%, patient survival 86%)

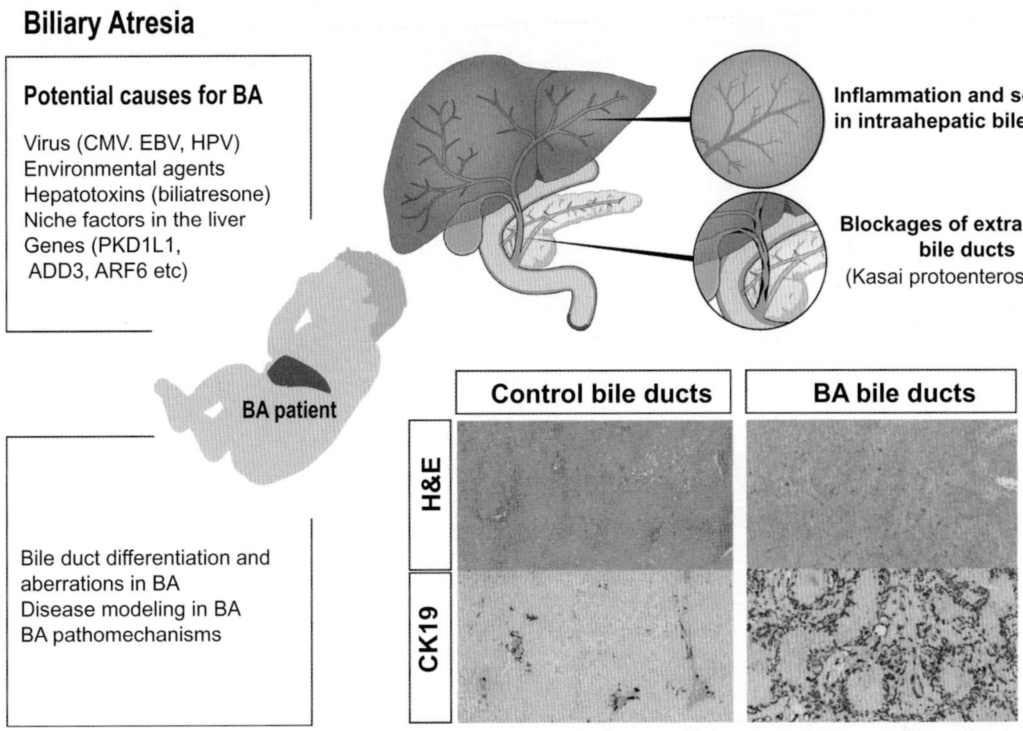

Biliary Atresia

Potential causes for BA

Virus (CMV. EBV, HPV)
Environmental agents
Hepatotoxins (biliatresone)
Niche factors in the liver
Genes (PKD1L1,
    ADD3, ARF6 etc)

BA patient

Bile duct differentiation and
aberrations in BA
Disease modeling in BA
BA pathomechanisms

**Inflammation and sclerosis
in intraahepatic bile ducts**

**Blockages of extrahepatic
bile ducts**
(Kasai protoenterostomy)

	Control bile ducts	**BA bile ducts**
H&E		
CK19		

Fig. 153.1 Schematic depiction of Biliary Atresia. Potential causes for BA are described, as well as the major pathological features of BA, including obstruction of the extrahepatic bile ducts and deterioration of intrahepatic bile ducts. The gallbladder (green) pancreas (beige) and duodenum (light pink) are also shown. Hematoxylin and eosin (H&E) stained and cytokeratin 19 (CK19)-immunostained liver sections from a BA patient and a non-BA control are displayed. At the bottom of the figure, the main topics of the review article are described. Adapted with permission from https://www.clinicalkey.com/#!/content/journal/1-s2.0-S2352396421004837

154

Learning Disability

Katie Turner, Oliver Agutu, and Lindsey Rowley

GP CONSULTATION, MALE AGED 6. CHALLENGING BEHAVIOUR AT SCHOOL

HPC: Mother brings him due to behaviour/meltdowns. School reports show impaired intellectual development. Spends break-times alone. Repetitive behaviours (hand flapping, toe walking). Lines up his toy cars rather than playing with them. Refuses to eat vegetables. Distressed when routines are disrupted. No sense of danger, will speak to strangers. Speech delayed (first words at 32 months, putting words together at 40 months).

O/E: Sat in chair quietly playing on tablet, does not respond when asked a direct question, does not maintain eye contact. Normal physical and neurological examination. 2nd centile growth.

1. Name two conditions often seen in children with autism.
2. What are the risk factors for cerebral palsy?

Answers: 1. ADHD (30%–50%), epilepsy (20%), anxiety, sleep disorders, dyslexia. 2. Low birth weight/prematurity, TORCH infection, perinatal asphyxia, intracranial haemorrhage, neonatal seizures, kernicterus, postnatal infection (e.g. meningitis).

TABLE 154.1

	Features	Investigations	Management
Autism spectrum disorder (ASD)	Affects; 1. Receptive/expressive language (social communication), 2. Developing selective social attachments or reciprocal social interaction, 3. Functional or symbolic play. More common in boys. Monotone voice, stereotyped mannerisms (e.g. hand flapping), rituals/routines, literal thinking, intense specific interests. Impaired social communication including non-verbal cues (e.g. eye contact). Often play alone. Impaired intellect/language. Picky eater. Hypo-/hypersensory awareness	Social communication questionnaires. ADOS (autism diagnostic observation schedule). Speech and language assessment. Consider blood tests including genetics if dysmorphic features or significant learning disability	Educational and behavioural interventions with MDT. Psychology. Speech and language therapy. Occupational therapy (sensory processing). Family support and local support groups

TABLE 154.1 (Cont'd)

	Features	Investigations	Management
Attention deficit hyperactivity disorder (ADHD)	Starting <12 years, symptoms ≥6 months, impact in > one setting (e.g. school and home). Evidence that symptoms interfere with social, school, or work functioning, or reduce their quality. Inattention (forgetfulness, poor listening, difficulty sustaining tasks/following instructions). Hyperactivity/impulsivity (can't wait turn, excessively loud, talk excessively, interrupt, fidgeting)	Full clinical and psychosocial assessment. Rating scales (e.g. Conners questionnaire)	Specialist paediatrician or CAMHS. Refer parents to support group. Medication (age >6 years): methylphenidate, lisdexamfetamine, dexamfetamine, atomoxetine

Other important differentials

Cerebral palsy	See *147. ABNORMAL DEVELOPMENT/DEVELOPMENTAL DELAY*		
Foetal alcohol spectrum disorder	Foetal alcohol syndrome. Facial (Fig. 154.1 and Fig. 148.14): short palpebral fissure, thin vermillion border, smooth philtrum. Cardiac malformations, microcephaly. Learning problems: speech and language, executive functioning, memory, hyperactivity, poor attention, social skills. Higher incidence in children in care	Clinical diagnosis. Facial photographic assessment. Antenatal history – confirmed alcohol consumption?	Multidisciplinary care, lifelong support. Behavioural therapy, education support. Parent training. Medication: stimulants antidepressants, neuroleptics

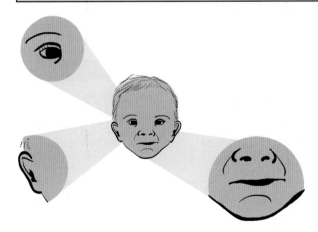

Fig. 154.1 Foetal alcohol syndrome, illustrating distinctive facial features, including small eyes with epicanthal folds, underdeveloped ears ('railroad track'), and a thin, smooth upper lip with thin upper vermillion. (Illustrated by Dr Hollie Blaber.)

Learning difficulties and behavioural issues in children are complex, with many possible causes. Distinguishing features can support a specific diagnosis. Autism is suggested by abnormal social interaction, ritualistic behaviour, sensory hypo/hyper-awareness and altered communication. ADHD is associated with abnormally high energy levels and poor concentration. Consider congenital or acquired abnormalities as possibly contributing to the presence of dysmorphic features, delayed motor milestones and spasticity. There are four types of cerebral palsy: spastic, dyskinetic, ataxic and mixed. The presentation in the vignette is ASD. Educational and behavioural interventions such as applied behaviour analysis (ABA), joint attention and symbolic play are important. Using non-verbal forms of communication, such as communication boards, can help children with ASD to communicate and express themselves. See also 155. BEHAVIOURAL DIFFICULTIES IN CHILDHOOD.

REVISION TIPS

- Children taking methylphenidate need weight and height checked 3–6 times monthly
- Methylphenidate, lisdexamfetamine and dexamfetamine; cardiovascular exam/ECG before treatment, regular BP and heart rate checks

155

Behavioural Difficulties in Childhood

Natalia Hackett, Alexander Royston, Graham Thornton, Kathleen Levick, and Kate McCann

---

GP CONSULTATION, MALE AGED 6.
MOTHER REPORTS THAT HE IS DISRUPTIVE AT SCHOOL

HPC: He gets in fights at school and keeps losing his school shoes. At home he won't listen to her when she asks him to do something and hits his siblings.
PMHx: Normal birth, milestones reached within normal range. Mother is receiving treatment herself for clinical depression.
  O/E: Fidgeting in his chair and then begins playing with items around the room, interrupting his mother and swearing.

1. List six symptoms of inattention or impulsivity.
2. What is important to monitor for children on methylphenidate, and why?
3. What differentials should be considered if this was an 18-year-old male?

Answers: 1. Careless mistakes in school, appears not to be listening when spoken to directly, doesn't follow through on instructions, difficulty organising tasks, loses things, doesn't sustain attention in play, fidgets, leaves seat, runs around/talks excessively, difficulty playing quietly, interrupts others. 2. Height/weight, BP: appetite suppression is a side effect. 3. Antisocial personality disorder, drug misuse, county lines, childhood sexual exploitation.

TABLE 155.1

	Features	Investigations	Management
Childhood trauma	**Hx & O/E:** toxic stress due to adverse childhood experiences (ACEs) in early years/in utero. Challenging behaviour, impaired emotional regulation, reduced concentration. Thorough history and observation essential	**RFs:** poverty, including housing or food insecurity. Exposure to domestic violence/substance abuse. Parental mental health illness/divorce/prison. Physical, sexual, emotional abuse or neglect	Educate parents/child – help to manage emotions. School-based emotional support (trauma-informed approach to understanding the child's needs). Community emotional/parenting support
Child maltreatment	**Hx & O/E:** marked change in emotional/behavioural state (if seen during/soon after maltreatment). Frequent/unusual attendance. Injuries, harmful interactions witnessed, signs of neglect. If presenting with abusive parent, child may exhibit frozen watchfulness, avoidance and not seek appropriate reassurance	**RFs:** as above, sex (M > F), physical disability. If abuse suspected, **seek senior input:** if in hospital – d/w Paediatrics. Childrens Social Care (CSC) with parental consent (unless will put child at risk) to check family background	**Definitive** (certainty/strong suspicion of abuse): jointly managed with CSC to ensure child will be in place of safety. Full child protection medical (paediatrician)

TABLE 155.1 (Cont'd)

	Features	Investigations	Management
ADHD	See *154. LEARNING DISABILITY*		
Autistic spectrum disorder (ASD)	See *154. LEARNING DISABILITY*		
Learning difficulties/ disability See also *154. LEARNING DISABILITY*	RFs: low birth weight, preterm birth, neonatal complications, language delay, epilepsy. Hx & O/E: global impairment of intelligence with social difficulties. Pre-school: developmental delay. Known syndrome or genetic abnormality.	Developmental history. Cognitive assessment (area specific). Functional assessment. FBC, U&Es, LFTs, TFTs, bone profile. EEG (if seizures). Consider genetics	Initial: annual health check, behavioural support. Consider specialist school (dependent on level of LD). Refer to LD team. LD terminology is used for school-age children and is diagnosed by an educational psychologist

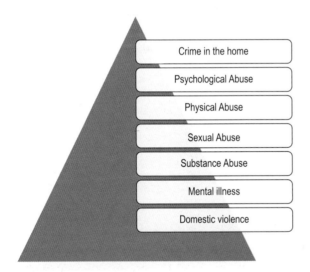

Fig. 155.1 Adverse childhood experience. (From Hustedde C. Primary care: clinics in office practice. 2021;48(3):493–504. Copyright © 2021 Elsevier Inc.)

Although tempting to the clinician, the top differential for the vignette is not ADHD; it is too early for a formal diagnosis, and he is behaving within the spectrum of normal developmental behaviour. The case provides only modest evidence suggestive of exposure to adverse childhood experiences (maternal depression) (Fig. 155.1), but pathologising a normal reaction to challenging circumstances is potentially stigmatising and confers risks of inappropriate treatment or missing an opportunity to safeguard the child. A thorough appraisal of the context should be made – including a consideration of exposure to toxic stress. A formulation favouring the biopsychosocial approach is best practice. The most critical situation to exclude is child maltreatment – which can be difficult.

REVISION TIPS

- **Toxic trio:** exposure to substance abuse, poor (parental) mental health, domestic violence
- Always consider child maltreatment or trauma in your differential
- ADHD – may emerge at 3–7 yo, but if hyperactivity not present, then not typically diagnosed until >7 yo
- Methylphenidate: side-effect of appetite suppression can lead to weight loss/failure to thrive in children

156

Child Abuse

Lindsey Rowley, Katie Turner, and Oliver Agutu

EMERGENCY DEPARTMENT, MALE, 3 MONTHS OLD.
REDUCED MOVEMENT OF LEFT ARM

HPC: Mum says she noticed baby was not moving his left arm this morning, he is unsettled, not feeding well today. Mum does not recall any trauma, but yesterday he was on the floor mat and suddenly started crying whilst she was out of the room. When she came in, he was lying on the mat with his older sister playing nearby, but she wonders if something happened. Born at term, no complications, meeting developmental milestones.
SHx: Lives at home with mum, dad and 3-year-old half-sister. Sister has some speech and language delay. Mum is on anti-depressant medication.
  O/E: Crying, irritable when handled. Not moving left arm, slight swelling upper arm. Three blue bruises noted on one side of his back, one on torso. X-ray shows spiral left humeral fracture. Full skeletal survey; multiple rib fractures, right humeral fracture, at different stages of healing.

1. What triad of symptoms is classically seen in 'shaken baby syndrome'?
2. What is the inheritance pattern of osteogenesis imperfecta?

Answers: 1. Subdural haematoma, retinal haemorrhage, encephalopathy. 2. Autosomal dominant (most commonly).

TABLE 156.1

	Features	Investigations	Management
Physical abuse (non-accidental injury (NAI))	Bruises/burns/bite (human); specific shape, clustered, soft tissue areas, ear. Fractures of differing ages or occult # (rib/spiral/metaphyseal corner). Injury in non-mobile child, intracranial injury in child <3 years. Retinal haemorrhages. Torn lingual frenulum in infants. Multiple injuries	Medical and social history (speak to child alone if appropriate). Examination (document on body map). Exclude coagulopathy or bone disease. Skeletal survey. CT (acute)/MRI (non-acute): brain haemorrhage. Ophthalmology review	Admit for safety and investigations. Inform children's services/child safeguarding lead. Consider safety of siblings. Senior paediatric/child protection review. Medical photography to record injuries

TABLE 156.1 (Cont'd)

	Features	Investigations	Management
Neglect	Non-attendance for medical appointments and school. Poor treatment compliance/hygiene – infections, e.g. scabies, dental caries, developmental delay (n.b. speech/language), faltering growth, inappropriate clothing, injuries from poor supervision (e.g. burns, animal bites)	Medical and social history (speak to child alone if appropriate). Observe interactions with parents. General physical health examination, development assessment	Assess health needs. Senior paediatrician, safeguarding, social services. Support: home visits, local services/resources (e.g. advocates), parenting programmes (e.g. attachment-based interventions)
Emotional abuse	Aggressive, oppositional behaviour. Developmental delay (n.b. language and social skills). Low self-esteem, depression, self-harm, eating disorder. Head banging/body rocking. Enuresis/encopresis, recurrent nightmares	Observe the child and their relationship with parents/carers. Communicate directly with the child, speak to them alone if appropriate	Senior paediatrician, safeguarding, social services. Local services and resources parenting programme (psychotherapy)
Sexual abuse	Recurrent UTIs, STIs, pregnancy. Anal fissures, reflex anal dilatation, torn penile frenulum, vaginal discharge, ano-genital injury, enuresis/encopresis, constipation. Sexually precocious behaviour. Aggression, anxiety, poor school performance, self-harm. Recurring symptoms (e.g. headaches, abdo pain)	Medical and social history (speak to child alone if appropriate). Pregnancy test. STI screen. Urinalysis: for infection. Forensic genital examination	Senior paediatrician, safeguarding, social services. Treat infections. Emergency contraception. Support (for child and family) – independent sexual violence advocates and counselling services
Female genital mutilation (FGM)	Menstrual problems, genital scarring, vaginal discharge, UTIs, urinary stricture/fistulae. Prolonged absence from school. Behaviour changes, depression. Recent travel abroad	Genital examination. Urinalysis: for infection. Sexual health screen	Social services, police. De-infibulation may be indicated in adulthood. Treat infection. Counselling
Other important differentials			
Osteogenesis imperfecta (brittle bone disease)	Genetic disorder of collagen synthesis; key to exclude in NAI. Short stature, fractures from minor trauma, bone deformity. Blue/grey sclera, otosclerosis, deafness, dental imperfections	Medical/FHx. X-rays/bone density scans: osteopenia, thin cortices, deformity, multiple fractures of varying ages. DNA testing. Skin biopsy	Physiotherapy, occupational therapy. Bisphosphonates, vitamin D supplements. Orthopaedic – correct deformity/manage fracture

(Continued)

TABLE 156.1   (Cont'd)

	Features	Investigations	Management
Congenital dermal melanocytosis (previously known as Mongolian blue spot)	Bruise-like birthmark (flat grey/blue pigmented), irregular, indistinct borders. Non-tender. Buttocks/lower back common, can be elsewhere. More common with dark skin. Present at birth or soon after. Usually fade over first few years	May be documented in newborn examination (see in red book). If unsure, review 2 weeks later (bruises will fade in this time, congenital dermal melanocytosis will not)	No treatment needed – typically self-resolves by adolescence

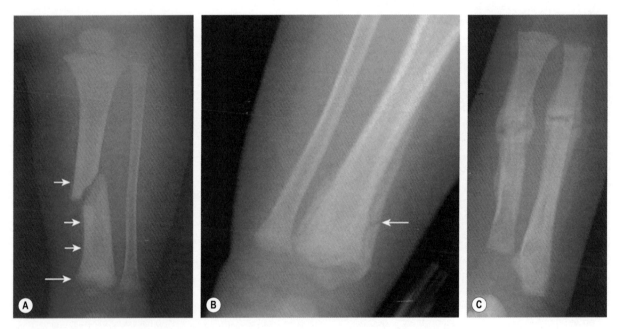

Fig. 156.1 A 3-month-old boy with multiple fractures of differing age. (A) Acute oblique fracture of left tibia; subperiosteal new bone (*short arrows*), irregularity of distal metaphysis (*long arrow*) suggests preceding metaphyseal lesion. (B) Right leg; healing bucket handle fracture with tibial subperiosteal new bone, so injury is >10 days old. Fracture through the subperiosteal new bone (*arrow*) indicates injuries of different age. (C) Left radius and ulna older fractures, with more advanced healing – abundant callus and partially obliterated fracture lines. (https://www.clinicalkey.com/#!/content/book/3-s2.0-B978032349748000143X?scrollTo=%233-s2.0-B978032349748000143X-f143-021ac-9780323497480)

Always perform a thorough but unbiased assessment of any injured child. Detailed history/examination is vital, including clinical details that may suggest genetic or congenital cause, such as blue sclera and deafness (osteogenesis imperfecta), or documentation of bruise-like lesions since birth (congenital dermal melanocytosis). Risk factors for NAI include; age <1 year, prematurity, physical disability, parental mental illness or substance/alcohol misuse, history of domestic abuse. Injury in a non-mobile infant, unusual injury patterns, history inconsistent with the injury, changes to the history from carers, repeat presentations, and injuries of different ages (Fig. 156.1) are suspicious of NAI. Injuries of different ages can occur in osteogenesis imperfecta. In the vignette, NAI through physical violence from the caregiver was the likely cause.

REVISION TIPS

- Developmental delay (particularly language/social skills) can occur in emotional abuse or neglect
- Low self-esteem, depression, self-harm, anxiety or aggression can be seen in all forms of child abuse
- FGM is partial/total removal of external female genitalia or injury for non-medical reasons; all instances in under 18s must be reported to the police

Frailty, Immobility and Struggling to Cope at Home

Alice Parker and Emily Henderson

HOME VISIT, FEMALE, 89.
DECLINE IN MOBILITY AND BALANCE

HPC: Unbalanced when walking at home, several near falls; has fear of falling, so activities are challenging. Antibiotics (community) 3 times in 12 months for lower respiratory tract symptoms. 4 kg weight loss in 3 months, anorexia – can shop and prepare meals, helped by daughter living nearby. **PMHx:** Hypothyroid, HTN, past MI. **DHx:** Amlodipine 10 mg OD, aspirin 75 mg OD, ramipril 5 mg OD, atorvastatin 80 mg, levothyroxine 150 mcg OD. **SHx:** Lives alone in bungalow, no formal carer support.

O/E: Systemically well, difficulty getting out of low chair, low muscle mass, uses walking stick or holds furniture. AMT: 9/10. CVS: HS I + II + 0. RS: Chest clear, equal air entry. Neuro: PEARL, normal power, reduced sensation to light touch in feet. BP 160/80 lying, 134/64 immediate standing, 136/68 1 minute, 148/62 3 minutes with some lightheadedness and 'coat hanger' pain across upper back on standing.

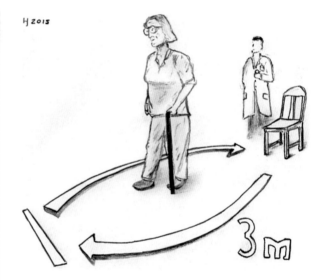

Fig. 157.1 The timed-up and go test. Patients are asked to get up from a chair, walk a distance of 3 m, and sit down again at their normal pace, while the examiner records the time in seconds. Walking aids are permissible. (Reproduced with permission from Gautschi, O. P., et al. (2015). *J Clin Neurosci*, 22(12), 1943-1948

1. What is the likely overarching cause of the patient's symptoms in the vignette?
2. What differentials may be considered in a patient with frequent chest infections?
3. What medications can cause or exacerbate postural hypotension?

Answers: 1. Frailty. 2. Bronchiectasis, COPD, lung cancer, immunodeficiency (e.g. HIV, leukaemia), aspergillosis, cystic fibrosis (young). 3. Antihypertensives, nitrates, beta-blockers, TCAs, alpha-blockers, anti-convulsants, opioids, anti-psychotics, MAO-inhibitors.

TABLE 157.1

	Features	Investigations	Management
Frailty	Sarcopenia (loss of muscle mass and strength), weight loss. Hx & O/E: immobility, incontinence, instability (falls), functional decline. Pressure ulcers, delirium, prone to medication side effects	Comprehensive geriatric assessment (CGA). Frailty score (see commentary). Screening tools, e.g. Clinical Frailty Scale, PRISMA-7 questionnaire. Gait speed (>5 seconds to walk 4 m). Timed up and go test (Fig. 157.1)	Directed at findings from CGA, e.g. PT/OT. Nutritional supplements
Orthostatic hypotension	Common in older adults, and in Parkinsonism. Symptoms occur on standing: dizziness, lightheadedness, fainting	**Lying and standing blood pressure** – diagnostic if fall in systolic >20 mmHg or diastolic >10 mmHg	Lifestyle: adequate fluids, cold water boluses, additional salt/caffeine. Review of contributory medications. Fludrocortisone or midodrine. Full-length compression stockings as tolerated or abdominal binding
Dementia	See *103. MEMORY LOSS*		
Undernutrition	Weight loss, poor appetite; undernutrition is common in older people living alone	Malnutrition universal screening tool (MUST) score	Dietitian support. Nutritional supplements, e.g. Fortisip, vitamins
Sarcopenia	Involuntary loss of muscle mass (quantity) and strength (quality)	Screening tool, e.g. SARC-F (Strength, Assistance in walking, Rise from a chair, Climb stairs and Falls). Timed up and go, gait speed, Short Physical Performance Battery. Dual-energy X-ray absorptiometry	Resistance exercises
Other important differentials			
Labyrinthitis/ vestibular neuronitis	Acute decline in balance. Labyrinthitis: vertigo, hearing loss, tinnitus and nausea. Vestibular neuronitis does not involve hearing loss or tinnitus	Hearing assessment and otoscopy. Head impulse test	Vestibular rehabilitation. Prochlorperazine short-term only (risk of drug-induced parkinsonism)

Frailty is a syndrome characterised as a state of vulnerability whereby physiological reserves diminish and therefore ability to cope with stressors is impaired. There are two approaches to measuring frailty; by phenotype (muscle weakness, slow walking, low physical activity, exhaustion and weight loss) or an index approach, which measures a sum of deficits accumulated. Frailty arises as a result of chronic inflammation with pathophysiological changes across multiple systems. Being frail is independently associated with excess risk of institutionalisation, hospital admission, and death. Frailty is reversible and comprehensive geriatric assessment (CGA) should underpin the approach, identifying risk factors, using exercise to tackle low physical activity and giving nutritional intervention. The objectives should be to improve function, implement care and support to compensate for impairments and improve quality of life. 'Struggling to cope' could be reframed as 'needing more support to cope at home', since provision of adaptations and support can sustain independent living for many.

REVISION TIPS

- Frailty is defined as the reduced ability of the body to return to its normal state following environmental or physiological (e.g. illness) stress, due to the physiological decline in reserves seen with advancing age

- Frailty is associated with many adverse health outcomes including falls, impairment in activities of daily living (ADLs), nursing home admission and mortality

Bone Pain

Alice Parker and Nicole Lundon

HPC: Persistent dull ache, worse on movement, not helped by analgesia. No trauma, sensory loss, weakness or incontinence. 4-months constipation, unintentional weight loss of 8 kg. Denies fevers. **PMHx:** HTN, hypothyroidism, previous Colles fracture. **DHx:** Amlodipine, levothyroxine. **FHx:** #NOF (mother). **SHx:** Sedentary lifestyle. Current smoker, 40 pack years.

O/E: BMI 17, appears dry and frail. **Neuro:** Intact cranial nerves/limb neurology, no urinary retention. Normal anal tone, no saddle anaesthesia. **MSK:** T1/T2 vertebrae tender. **Ix:** Hb 92 (125–155 g/dL), Ca 3.05 (2.25–2.62 mmol/L), creatinine 135 (60–110 mcmol/L), PTH low.

1. Recent onset deafness, and pain in a male patient's legs and back. What is the unifying diagnosis?

2. What bone profile (ALP, calcium, phosphate, vitamin D) results are seen in:
   a. Paget disease
   b. Osteomalacia
   c. Osteoporosis
3. Why does osteomyelitis in children commonly involve the metaphysis of long bones?

Answers: 1. Paget disease – nerve compression due to bony outgrowths causing deafness. 2(a). Paget: raised ALP, normal calcium, PTH, phosphate (PO_4), vitamin D. (b) Osteomalacia: raised ALP, low calcium, low PO_4, low vitamin D. (c) Osteoporosis: normal ALP, PO_4, calcium. May have low vitamin D. 3. The growth plate is present next to the metaphysis portion of bone. This has a very good blood supply which increases the chance of haematogenous spread of infection, leading to osteomyelitis.

TABLE 158.1

	Features	Investigations	Management
Osteoporotic fracture	**RFs:** female, age, low BMI, FHx of osteoporosis, smoking, alcohol, hyperthyroidism, long-term steroids, sedentary/immobility, menopause, rheumatoid arthritis **Hx & O/E:** low trauma fractures, spinal wedge fractures, distal radius fractures, long bone fractures, e.g. #NOF	**X-ray:** commonly spine, distal radius, pelvis. **FRAX score:** to assess fracture risk. Most have normal calcium, phosphate and ALP. May see ↓vit D. **DEXA** (if intermediate risk FRAX) T-score –2.5 or below = osteoporosis	Reduce alcohol, stop smoking, balance/weight-bearing exercise, assess falls risk. Offer vitamin D/calcium supplements (diet calcium is often sufficient). Bisphosphonates if: **T-score <–2.5, >75 + fragility fracture/high risk FRAX/on long term steroids** 1st line = alendronic acid

(Continued)

TABLE 158.1   (Cont'd)

	Features	Investigations	Management
Hypercalcaemia	See *61.HYPERCALCAEMIA*		
Bony metastases (Fig. 158.1)	Commonest: breast, lung, kidney, thyroid, prostate. Persistent bone pain, night pain, tenderness, nerve compression producing neurological symptoms, e.g. spinal cord (UMN), or cauda equina (LMN)	**Investigations to seek primary. Urgent MRI whole spine** if malignant spinal cord compression suspected	Dependent on underlying malignancy. If spinal cord compression, urgent radiotherapy or surgical decompression
Paget disease of the bone	Older male. Commonly affects spine, skull, pelvis, long bones. Hx & O/E: often asymptomatic, or deep boring bone pain, deformity, nerve compression, arthralgia, fractures	↑ALP, normal calcium, PTH and phosphate. **X-ray:** 'cotton wool' skull, sclerosis, coarse irregular trabecular pattern, bone expansion, thick calvarium	Analgesia. Oral bisphosphonates. Surgical fixation in limited cases
Multiple myeloma	**RFs:** age, MGUS, high radiation, Afro-Caribbean. **Hx & O/E:** symptoms of *CRABI*; hyperCalcaemia, Renal dysfunction, Anaemia (plus thrombocytopenia, bleeding), Bone problems (back pain, fractures), Infections	FBC (↓Hb, ↓pts), U&Es (↑urea, creat), ↑Ca, ↑ESR. **Serum electrophoresis/serum-free light chain assay:** paraprotein (monoclonal band). **Urine:** Bence Jones protein. **Marrow aspirate:** plasma cells >10%. X-rays: 'punched out', pepperpot skull, vertebral collapse, pathological #	Analgesia, bisphosphonates, transfusions, antibiotics for infections. Chemotherapy. ± stem cell transplant
Sarcoma	**RFs:** younger age, male. E.g. Osteosarcoma, Ewing's sarcoma, chondrosarcoma. **Hx & O/E:** bone pain, night pain, swelling, pathological fractures	**X-ray:** fluffy/cloud-like lesion, periosteal reaction, 'onion skin', Codman triangle. **CT/MRI:** for staging. **Biopsy**	Excision ± chemotherapy ± radiotherapy
Osteomalacia (or Rickets in children)	**RFs:** vitamin D deficiency, renal failure, FHx. **Hx & O/E:** rickets- 'knock-kneed'. Osteomalacia: bone pain, proximal myopathy, fractures	↑PTH, ↑ALP, ↓calcium, ↓phosphate, ↓vit D. **X-ray:** Looser's zones	Vitamin D and calcium supplements
Osteomyelitis	**RFs:** growth plate (children), DM, IVDU, immunosuppression, open fractures, prosthetics, sickle cell. **Hx & O/E:** gradual onset pain, tenderness, warmth, fever/ systemic signs, reduced ROM	↑CRP, ↑WCC. Blood cultures. **Bone biopsy and culture.** **X-ray:** hazy, sequestra, bone destruction. **MRI:** periosteal lifting, bone destruction, oedema	**IV Abx:** usually 4–6 weeks. **Control source:** drain abscess, debride sequestra. Inadequate treatment risks chronic osteomyelitis

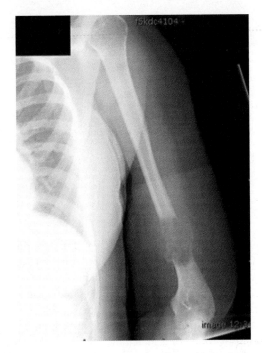

Fig. 158.1 Bone metastasis in a patient with breast cancer. (Steffner RJ, Spiguel AR, Balach T. Chapter: 21, Pathologic fractures. In: *Skeletal Trauma: Basic Science, Management, and Reconstruction.* 2-Volume Set. Elsevier; 2020:Figure: 21.4. Copyright © 2020 Elsevier Inc. All rights reserved.)

In bone pain it is really important to consider any clinical 'red flags' which suggest malignancy. In the vignette, combination of back pain with unintentional weight loss, smoking history and hypercalcaemia does suggest a malignant cause. In addition to this, her renal failure and anaemia would warrant further investigations to specifically look for multiple myeloma. In patients with malignancy and back pain, identifying any features of spinal cord compression is crucial, as emergency treatment is needed. Getting an MRI of the whole spine is important, even if you think you have localised the area, as there are often multifocal sites. Aside from the conditions in Table 158.1, bone pain can also occur in sickle cell anaemia, renal osteodystrophy, Sjögren's and avascular necrosis (AVN). Most common sites for AVN are head of femur/ humerus, knee, talus. RFs include corticosteroids or alcohol misuse. Femoral head AVN causes a dull ache in the groin/ thigh/ buttock; hip ROM reduced in advanced stages. Shown on MRI in early stages, X-ray if advanced. THR if irreversible, age >40 years, large lesion, femoral head collapse/ degenerate acetabulum.

REVISION TIPS

- Symptoms of myeloma can be remembered using CRABI: hyperCalcaemia, Renal dysfunction, Anaemia, Bone problems, Infections
- Hypercalcaemia is initially treated with adequate rehydration
- 'Pathological fractures' commonly refer to fractures through cancerous lesions weakening the bones

159

Acute and Chronic Pain Management – Outline

Alice Parker, David Roberts, and Alexander Reed

Pain definitions:

- Acute pain: Typically lasts up to 7 days (but prolongation up to 90 days is not uncommon). Its duration typically reflects the mechanism; for example, tissue healing may be expected to take longer following major surgery.
- Chronic pain: pain that lasts OR recurs for longer than 3 months. The implication is that there is an ongoing pathological process resulting in continued painful stimulation, or an inappropriate activation of pain pathways.
- Allodynia: the sensation of pain, provoked by a stimulation that should not normally cause pain. For example, light touch on an area distant from a splinter.
- Hyperalgesia: an exaggerated sensitivity to a painful stimulus. A trigger that would normally be sensed as minor pain is experienced as being more severe.
- Nociception: the process by which noxious stimuli are relayed from the peripheral nervous system (PNS) to the central nervous system (CNS). Nociception can occur in the absence of conscious experience, whereas pain cannot.

Analgesic drugs (Table 159.1) act by modulating pain signalling, and by reducing inflammation and sensitisation of nociceptors at the site of actual or potential tissue injury. Acute severe pain, as occurs in many acute diseases, injuries and following surgery, should be managed carefully with opioids and other adjuncts, especially local and regional anaesthetic techniques. Dosing of analgesics should be personalised, due to variations in pharmacokinetics, pharmacodynamics, tolerance and dependence. Opioid dosing requirements consistently reduce with age. Patients who regularly use opioid drugs, either for chronic pain and/or substance abuse, usually have a degree of tolerance and often require higher doses of opioids to achieve effective pain relief.

Regional anaesthesia/analgesia techniques include peripheral nerve blocks, peripheral nerve catheters, fascial plane blocks and catheters, and patient-controlled epidural analgesia. These techniques can provide good relief for a variety of situations, from labour to traumatic rib fracture, and should be utilised to spare the use of other analgesic drugs which all have side effects. They may also reduce the risk of progression to chronic pain.

Multimodal analgesia describes the use of multiple interventions (including medications) that act on different sites along the pain signaling pathway. The intention is to optimise pain relief whilst minimising side effects that occur with increasing doses of a single drug class, e.g. opioids and adverse effects of constipation, nausea, sedation and respiratory depression.

The WHO analgesic pain ladder (Fig. 159.1) is the framework that guides therapy for patients with **chronic pain and in palliative care**. The WHO pain ladder describes a stepwise method of managing chronic pain and pain in palliative care. It is not designed for patients with severe pain at onset, e.g. post surgery.

TABLE 159.1

	Examples
Non-opioid analgesia	Paracetamol, NSAIDs (ibuprofen, diclofenac, naproxen)
Weak opioids	Codeine, dihydrocodeine, tramadol
Strong opioids	Morphine, fentanyl, buprenorphine, oxycodone, methadone
Adjuvants	*Antidepressant drugs*: amitriptyline, duloxetine. *Antiepileptic drugs*: gabapentin, pregabalin. *Other*: topical capsaicin, clonidine, ketamine
Additional options (for severe acute pain in hospital)	Regional analgesia (e.g. nerve block ± catheter, epidural). Lignocaine infusion (needs close monitoring and nursing experience to manage safely)
Non-pharmacological	Group exercise programmes, CBT, acupuncture, TENS

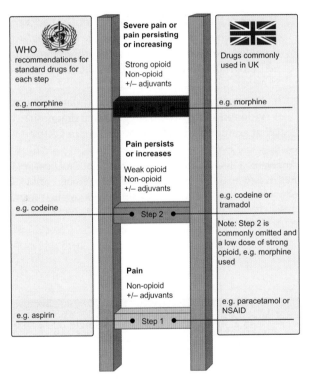

Fig. 159.1 WHO analgesic ladder (Chin C, Moffat C, Booth S. Palliative care and symptom control. In: *Kumar and Clark's Clinical Medicine*. Elsevier; 2021:Figure: 7.3. Copyright © 2021 Elsevier Ltd. All rights reserved.)

REVISION TIPS

- Sedation may signal respiratory depression with opioids. A sedated patient should not be administered further opioid analgesics (exceptions may exist in e.g., palliation, where control of symptoms overrides the risk of precipitating respiratory failure)
- Never combine long-acting with short-acting opioids for acute pain. Neither should opioids be given via different routes simultaneously (e.g. IV and PO morphine being co-administered)
- Codeine is a prodrug that is metabolised to morphine by most people. Some people will fail to convert to morphine and a small number of people are hyper-metabolisers, limiting the utility of this drug
- Tramadol has significant non-opioid actions (e.g. via its serotonergic and noradrenergic pathways) and can be co-administered with other opioid agents
- Methadone is used in opioid abuse disorders but can also be used as an effective analgesic agent by pain medicine specialists. It has strong opioid actions and non-opioid activity including NMDA receptor antagonism
- Ketamine has both pre-emptive (giving prior to painful stimuli leads to less pain) and preventive analgesic properties (even once the medication has worn off, less pain is experienced), making it a highly effective analgesic and dissociative
- Laxatives are prescribed with opioid medications (as a standard of care)

160

Chronic Pain

Alice Parker, Katherine Parker, Emily Warren, and Benjamin Faber

---

GP CONSULTATION, FEMALE, 46.
6-MONTHS PERSISTENT WIDESPREAD PAIN, MAINLY IN JOINTS AND MUSCLES

HPC: Associated morning stiffness, made worse by exercise. Also fatigue, low mood, insomnia – affecting work and social life. **PMHx:** Chronic migraines, depression. **DHx:** Propranolol, sertraline, sumatriptan PRN.

O/E: MSK; Multiple tender points over gluteals, trapezius muscles, supraspinatus. No joint swelling, effusions or restriction of joint movement.

---

1. 75-year-old female, difficulty getting out of bed, very slow dressing, cannot lift her arms due to aching/stiff shoulders, worsening for weeks. No other symptoms, neurologically unremarkable, normal CK.
   a. What diagnosis is most likely?
   b. Development of headaches and darkening of vision in an eye would suggest what diagnosis?
2. What examination features are present in CRPS?

Answers: 1. (a) Polymyalgia rheumatica, (b) Giant cell arteritis (GCA) – 30%–50% untreated lose vision, with 1/3 affected in other eye if still untreated. 2. Allodynia, changes in skin temperature or colour, swelling, abnormal sweating, muscle weakness.

TABLE 160.1

	Features	Investigations	Management
Rheumatology			
Osteoarthritis	See *186. ACUTE JOINT PAIN*		
Rheumatoid arthritis	See *187. CHRONIC JOINT PAIN*		
Fibromyalgia	Chronic widespread pain and tender points. Fatigue, morning stiffness, unrefreshing sleep, depression and memory problems ('brain fog'). Associated: chronic fatigue/irritable bowel syndrome, depression/anxiety, temporomandibular joint pain and chronic migraines	**RFs:** 'Yellow flags' (see revision tips), middle-aged, low income/education attainment, female, previous life trauma (e.g. domestic abuse, sexual assault). No findings of inflammatory joint disease	Educate, reassure CBT. **Graded exercise programmes:** amitriptyline, pregabalin

TABLE 160.1 (Cont'd)

	Features	Investigations	Management
Systemic lupus erythematosus	See *189. MUSCLE PAIN/MYALGIA*		
Polymyositis (PMy)/ dermatomyositis (DMy)	**RFs:** female, other autoimmune *Assoc. with internal malignancy.* **Hx & O/E:** gradual symmetrical proximal weakness, myalgia, dysphagia, dysphonia, arthralgia, constitutional (fever, weight loss, fatigue), Raynaud's, CVS/RS symptoms. Dermatomyositis: as above *plus* photosensitive, heliotrope rash (violaceous/erythematous rash of the upper eyelids ± periorbital oedema), mechanic's hands, Gottron's papules (small purple or red flat papules on knuckles or elbows ± scaling/ulceration)	↑CK (most specific), ↑LDH, ↑ALT, ↑AST, ↑myoglobin. **EMG:** abnormal activity. **Muscle biopsy:** inflamed, atrophy. **Autoantibodies:** ↑ANA (sensitive), Anti-Jo-1 (PMy > DMy, higher risk of interstitial lung disease), anti-SRP (PMy, severe myopathy), anti-Mi-2 (DMy specific), anti-TIF1 (malignancy). ECG, Echo, CXR	Sun avoidance, PT/OT, SALT. **Remission:** 1. Oral/IV corticosteroid. 2. Methotrexate/azathioprine. 3. Consider biologics/IVIG if refractory. **Maintenance.** 1. Methotrexate, azathioprine or MMF. 2. ± IVIG or biologic. Screen for malignancy
Polymyalgia rheumatica	Gradual onset, chronic bilateral shoulder and/or hip stiffness, pain, normal power, constitutional. Associated with GCA	**RFs:** female, >55 years old. **Clinical diagnosis.** ↑ESR (>40)/CRP, rest of bloods normal (including CK)	Oral prednisolone (15 mg OD) – respond in 24–72 hours. + PPI, + bisphosphonates
Complex regional pain syndrome (CRPS)	**RFs:** limb injuries – previous fractures, orthopaedic operations. **Hx & O/E:** dominant, disproportionate pain in one part– often hands/feet. 10% recall no injury. Other features: allodynia, changed skin temperature or colour (Fig. 160.1), abnormal sweating/dysautonomia, swelling, weakness	**Clinical diagnosis.** Consider radiological assessment to r/o underlying injury	Education, analgesia, physical rehabilitation. Psychological therapies (CBT)
Temporomandibular disorder	**RFs:** RA, trauma. **Hx & O/E:** pain of temporomandibular joint ± masseter/temporalis. Worse on palpation, chewing, mouth opening/closing. Jaw clicking, locking or dislocation, headache and otalgia	**Clinical diagnosis**	Self-manage, e.g. soft diet, jaw rest; relaxation techniques, sleep hygiene. Analgesia, ice pack, heat pad. Referral if: symptoms >3 months, worsening, diagnosis uncertain, red flags

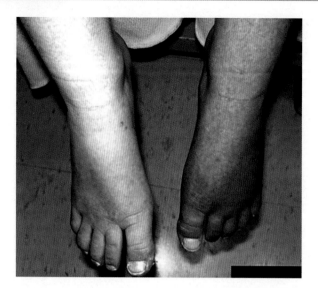

Fig. 160.1 CRPS affecting the left foot and ankle, with cyanosis and mottling. Allodynia was prominent. (Baker R, Szabova A, Goldschneider K. *Chronic Pain Book: A Practice of Anesthesia for Infants and Children*. Elsevier; 2019:Figure: 45.1. Copyright © 2019 Elsevier Inc. All rights reserved.)

In the vignette, widespread pain in joints and muscles with no examination evidence of joint swelling suggests a chronic pain syndrome, the commonest being fibromyalgia. There is widespread muscles tenderness (sometimes referred to as trigger points). Long prodrome (>6 months), concurrent depression and sleep difficulties make fibromyalgia more likely. Prolonged unrefreshing sleep is a common complaint. Relatively young age and the widespread nature of the pain makes osteoarthritis unlikely – in this age group it would generally affect one or two joints. If this were inflammatory arthritis (e.g. rheumatoid arthritis/psoriatic arthritis) examination findings and abnormal investigations (e.g. raised inflammatory markers) are expected. Morning stiffness alone is not diagnostic of inflammatory arthritis.

REVISION TIPS

- Chronic pain syndrome 'yellow flags': belief that pain won't improve, illness behaviour including excessive rest and taking time off work, low mood/anxiety, compensation claims, not actively engaging with treatment, avoiding activity
- Rule out other causes of pain/fatigue before diagnosing fibromyalgia

Death, Dying and End-of-Life Care

Alice Parker, Alexander Royston, and Amelia Stockley

HPC: Diagnosed 3 years ago, no further active treatment options, now in terminal stages. Estimated prognosis of short weeks. She has expressed a wish to die at home and Continuing Heathcare Fast Track funding enabled her to return home with nursing care.

1. What is anticipatory prescribing in end-of-life (EOL) care? What subcutaneous medications are made available 'just-in-case'?
2. A patient on immediate-release morphine 10 mg regularly 4 hourly over several days and two PRN doses of 10 mg every day is now unable to swallow analgesia in the dying phase; what morphine dose is prescribed for a sub-cutaneous syringe driver (SCSD) to replace the oral therapy?
3. What common side effects of opioids can be expected?
4. What are the common signs and symptoms of opioid toxicity?

Answers: 1. Medications prescribed in advance for reliable access if symptoms develop at end of life. Consider an opiate, an anti-secretory, an anti-emetic and an anxiolytic. 2. 40 mg/24 hours by SCSD. Total daily dose of morphine consistently over last few days has been 6× regular (4 hourly) + 2× additional prn 10 mg doses – total = 80 mg. Divide by 2 for subcutaneous equivalence as total daily syringe driver dose. Breakthrough opioid doses are 1/6th of the daily dose. 3. Side effects: drowsiness, N&V, constipation, dry mouth. 4. Persistent sedation (exclude other causes), vivid dreams/hallucinations, delirium, muscle twitching/myoclonus/jerking and respiratory depression.

TABLE 161.1

	Features	Management
Holistic needs assessment	Physical, emotional, psychological, spiritual, religious, cultural, legal and family needs. Take account of prior advance care planning discussions/documents. Consider organ/tissue donation	Agree on realistic levels of intervention. Establish care goals and preferred place of care/death. Multi-disciplinary approach to manage needs (Fig. 161.1). Review medication. Prescribe oral and/or parenteral anticipatory medication for common symptoms, checking most appropriate route for each

(Continued)

TABLE 161.1   (Cont'd)

	Features	Management
Pain	Detailed Pain Assessment (all sources/types); **1.** Disease-related (bone, nerve, liver, ↑ICP, colic) **2.** Treatment-related (chemotherapy, neuropathy, constipation) **3.** Debility (sores/candidiasis/cachexia) **4.** Unrelated illness (arthritis/gastritis) Breakthrough and incident pain. Agree treatment goals, review regularly, pain diary	**Non-pharmacological:** repositioning, equipment review, heat pad, massage, bath, relaxation, distraction. **Pharmacological:** WHO pain ladder (Fig. 159.1); 1. Non-opioid, e.g. paracetamol ± adjuvants, e.g. NSAIDs. 2. Weak opioid, e.g. codeine ± non-opioid ± adjuvant. 3. Strong opioid, e.g. oral morphine ± non-opioid ± adjuvant. Regular laxatives/anti-emetic co-prescribed. Routes of administration individualised to patient. **Parenteral anticipatory prescribing (for when oral or enteral routes are unavailable):** subcutaneous injectable opioid. Opioid choice/dose depends on current prescription, renal/liver function, age/frailty, local guidance/formularies
Nausea and vomiting	**Causes:** 1. *Chemical* (a) Drugs (opioids, cytotoxic, immunotherapy, Abx), (b) Toxins (gut ischaemia, infection), (c) Metabolic (hypercalcaemia/renal) 2. *Gastric stasis* (drugs, peptic ulcer, gastritis, dysautonomia) 3. *Visceral/serosal* (radiotherapy, obstruction, ascites, hepatomegaly) 4. *Cranial* (↑ICP: tumour, infarction) 5. *Vestibular* (opioid/base of skull tumour) 6. *Cortical* (anxiety, pain)	**Non-pharmacological:** avoid aromatic food/triggers, ginger, sea-bands (acupressure), acupuncture, mouth care. **Pharmacological** (Table 161.2): therapeutic approach may be receptor- or cause-directed. Route of administration individualised. **Parenteral anticipatory prescribing:** subcutaneous anti-emetic (depends on previous anti-emetics, cause of nausea, local guidelines and formularies)
Agitation and distress	Reversible causes: delirium, constipation, urinary retention, hypercalcaemia, nicotine/drug/alcohol withdrawal	**Non-pharmacological:** holistic approach required-use ahead of anxiolytics. Physical, psychological, social or spiritual causes of distress. Involve MDT. Complementary therapy. **Pharmacological:** manage delirium-consider reversible causes and/or antipsychotic, e.g. haloperidol, risperidone, quetiapine. Consider oral benzodiazepine/other anxiolytic. **Parenteral anticipatory prescribing:** subcutaneous benzodiazepine (depends on renal and liver function, age/frailty, local guidance and formularies)
Respiratory secretions	Common at end of life	**Non-pharmacological:** positioning, suctioning **Pharmacological:** transdermal hyoscine hydrombromide, hyoscine butylbromide, glycopyrronium, atropine drops. **Parenteral anticipatory:** subcutaneous anticholinergic – prescription based on local formulary and guidance
Breathlessness	Common at end of life. Treatable causes: infection, PE, anaemia, arrhythmia, pleural effusion	**Non-pharmacological:** fan, guided imagery. Fatigue/breathlessness management by OT/PT. **Pharmacological:** opioids, benzodiazepines. Nebulisers – salbutamol (wheeze), NaCl (dry airway)
Further symptoms	Constipation, cough, hiccups	

TABLE 161.2 Anti-emetics in end-of-life care	
Cause	**1st Line Anti-Emetic**
Chemical, e.g. chemotherapy	Ondansetron
Opioid-induced	Haloperidol
↓Gastric motility	Metoclopramide (caution if any suspicion of mechanical obstruction)
Visceral/serosal	Cyclizine
↑ICP	Dexamethasone
Vestibular	Prochlorperazine
Anxiety-related	Benzodiazepine
Multifactorial	**Levomepromazine** (broad spectrum: DEFAULT)

The vignette describes a confirmed diagnosis of an irreversible condition with a rapid deterioration expected with high certainty. Deprescribing should be complete, leaving only medications for symptom control and anticipatory medications PRN. Once at home, domiciliary visits should include symptomatic observations to monitor for signs of distress associated with dying and to guide symptom management plans including non-pharmacological approaches and medication. Syringe drivers can minimise peaks and troughs in medication levels and can be used when an enteral route is no longer available. Monitor for signs of opioid toxicity, but a distinction is made between tolerable side effects (e.g. drowsiness) and dangerous toxicity (e.g. respiratory depression), which might necessitate reversal if indicated.

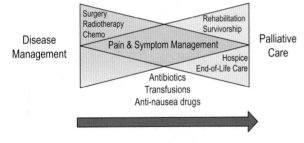

Fig. 161.1 The bow-tie model demonstrating the benefits of early involvement of palliative care. (From Hawley PH. The bow tie model of 21st century palliative care. *J Pain Symptom Manage*. 2014;47(1):2–5. https://doi.org/10.1016/j.jpainsymman.2013.10.009, with permission from Elsevier.)

REVISION TIPS

- Key EOL symptoms: pain, breathlessness, cough, N&V, constipation, agitation, respiratory secretions, hiccups
- Opioids are co-prescribed with a PRN breakthrough (1/6th daily dose), plus laxatives and anti-emetics
- Anti-emetics prescribed depend on the cause of N&V

162

Elder Abuse

Alice Parker, Alexander Royston, and Hannah Podger

HOME VISIT, MALE, 89.
CONCERNS RAISED BY CARER ABOUT NEW ONSET MEMORY PROBLEMS

HPC: Patient denies any problems and answers 'I don't know' to most questions. Appears low in mood, confused. Does not recognise GP despite meeting before.
PMHx: Hypertension, hypercholesterolaemia, aortic stenosis, heart failure. **SHx:** Housebound for 3 years, mobile with frame and assistance, carer helps with bathing weekly. Carer states that daughter helps with other ADLs, but patient hasn't seen her for 4 days.
O/E: Obs stable, AMTS: 6/10. House is cold, unclean and cluttered. Patient sat in a chair, appears unkempt and very thin. Multiple faded bruises on arms. Dry mucosal membranes. Pressure ulcer on sacral region.

1. What is the advised management approach for the situation in the vignette?
2. What is the most clinically concerning part of this presentation?
3. What would the likely diagnosis be if he also had a productive cough/coarse lung crackles?

Answers: 1. MDT approach – involving social services at the outset and escalating to law enforcement authorities as necessary. Even the suspicion of abuse should be reported. 2. Established sacral pressure ulcer – common cause of septicaemia in the elderly. 1-year life expectancy <50%. 3. Pneumonia causing delirium (±elder abuse).

TABLE 162.1

	Features	Investigations	Management
Elder abuse	**RFs** (of perpetrator): stress, past abuse, substance abuse. *Neglect:* carers not visiting, cold house, dehydration, malnutrition, unkempt, ulcers. Missed GP appointments, omitting medications. *Emotional abuse:* low mood, sleep problem, confusion, anxiety/fear, poor appetite, agitation, suicidal thoughts or self-harm. *Physical abuse:* bruising to buttocks, neck, genitals, pattern injuries, black eyes, fractures, internal injuries, injuries with implausible explanations, frequent attendances at hospital	**Clinical photographs**-assessing/recording bruising. FBC (other causes of petechiae, anaemia). Platelet function studies. Basic metabolic profile (including U&Es) – dehydration consistent with abuse/neglect. **X-rays** and search for additional/hidden injuries. Assess for carer burnout	**MDT** – always guarding a patient's dignity and autonomy (full capacity assessment is crucial). Also consider sexual abuse or financial exploitation. **Emergency response:** social services/police as necessary. Housing assistance/convalescent placement. Financial/legal assistance

TABLE 162.1 (Cont'd)

	Features	Investigations	Management
Depression	RFs: prior/FHx depression, recent bereavement, stress, illness. Hx & O/E: low mood, anhedonia, anergia. Pseudodementia in older person: memory loss, tendency to answer 'I don't know'	Consider blood tests (for reversible causes). PHQ-9. Risk assessment. CT brain: normal for age if performed	Consider antidepressants and CBT
Dementia	RFs: age (>75), sex (M > F), ethnicity, genetics. Hx & O/E: gradual onset memory loss, confusion, low mood, difficulties with ADLs. Collateral history (someone who knows the patient). See 103. MEMORY LOSS	Memory: MOCA, ACE-III. Bloods (for reversible causes). CT brain: atrophy, sulcal widening (Alzheimer's), lucencies (vascular), mild atrophy (Lewy body)	Alzheimer's and dementia with Lewy bodies: acetylcholinesterase inhibitors (galantamine, donepezil, rivastigmine), glutamate antagonist (memantine-severe)
Delirium (may be hyperactive or hypoactive)	See 164. LOW MOOD/AFFECTIVE PROBLEMS and 165. ELATION, ELATED MOOD AND PRESSURE OF SPEECH		

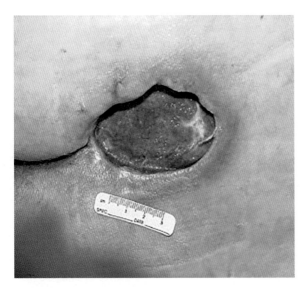

Fig. 162.1 Clean sacral pressure sore. (Reproduced with permission from Levi, B, Rees, R. Diagnosis and management of pressure ulcers. *Clin Plast Surg.* 2007, October 1;34(4):735–748. © 2007.)

The vignette describes a likely instance of elder abuse, but there may be several factors together. There are clinical signs of both neglect (dehydration, pressure sores [Fig. 162.1]) and possible physical abuse (bruising). Also, he is unkempt and thin, and the house is cluttered and unclean. The key is to consider the situation, even though it might be challenging, whilst preserving rapport with those involved whenever possible. When social and life-threatening problems have been addressed (pressure sores, dehydration), screening for depression and/or dementia can take place.

REVISION TIPS

- Elder abuse may involve neglect, emotional abuse, physical abuse, sexual abuse, financial exploitation
- RFs: age >75; dementia; dependence on a carer for personal care; carer depression/mental illness; substance abuse in the older adult or carer; financial dependence of the carer on the older adult
- Pseudodementia is a common feature of depression in the elderly

163

Mental Health Problems in Pregnancy or Postpartum

Natalia Hackett, Alexander Royston, and Aws Sadik

HPC: She feels overwhelmed and helpless, guilty for being a 'bad mother'. Difficulty sleeping (even when baby is). Occasional suicidal ideation, no planning or intent. **PMHx:** Gave birth by NVD 3 weeks ago, normally fit and well, no previous mental health problems.

O/E: Poverty of speech, tearful, impaired concentration, irritable, low affect

1. What are the SSRIs of choice for use in depression for a woman who is breastfeeding?

2. What are the key considerations for starting antidepressants postnatally?
3. What are common symptoms of postpartum psychosis?

Answers: 1. Sertraline, paroxetine. 2. Nature and severity of depression, previous response to treatment, options available and their risk, harms and benefits, the patient's relationships and available support. 3. Severe mood swings, delusions, confusion and hallucinations. Distorted thoughts and behaviour may involve the baby, putting it at risk of harm.

TABLE 163.1

	Features	Investigations	Management
Psychiatric			
Postnatal depression	**RFs:** previous depression, anxiety, recent stress, poor social support. Moderate–severe symptoms for >2 weeks. Often within 1–2 months of birth (can be months postpartum)	**Edinburgh Postnatal Depression Scale** or PHQ-9. **Risk assessment:** suicide, self-harm, risk to infant. FBC, CRP, TFTs – consider	Watchful waiting, psychological therapy, antidepressants (risk-benefit). Specialist input
'Baby blues'	**RFs:** poor sleep, stress. Common. Mild (low mood), onset 2–3 days postnatal, resolve by 5th day	Not required	Review as required

TABLE 163.1 (Cont'd)

	Features	Investigations	Management
Postpartum (puerperal) psychosis	RFs: PMH of BPAD (20% get postpartum psychosis). Rare. Hx & O/E: sudden onset, <2 weeks post-delivery, severe mood swings, delusions, hallucinations, distorted thoughts which may involve the baby – risk of harm	Risk assessment: suicide, self-harm, risk to infant. FBC, CRP, TFTs – consider	Psychiatric/obstetric emergency. Specialist urgent referral – immediate safety of mother and baby. Commonly treated in mother and baby unit
BPAD (postpartum presentation)	RFs: FHx of bipolar disorder, trauma/stress, drugs/alcohol. Hx & O/E: depression and irritable or elevated mood. Likely depressive episode postpartum. A first episode of mania (±psychotic symptoms) after pregnancy would likely be diagnosed as postpartum psychosis	Mental state examination. FBC, TFTs, CRP. Urine: drug screen. CT/MRI	Very short term: benzodiazepine. Mental health service. Psychological therapy, SSRI + antipsychotic. Mood stabiliser (lithium) ± anti-depressant (caution – risk of manic switch)
Generalised anxiety disorder	RFs: F > M (2:1), personality trait, trauma, substance misuse, stress, depression. Hx & O/E: widespread disproportionate worry (no specific trigger). Duration ≥6 months, often prominent physical symptoms. Alcohol: 'self-medication'	GAD7. TFTs, LFTs, CBG. Drug screen. ECG	Stepped care: education, lifestyle advice, SSRI. Psychological therapy (often CBT). β-blockers if physical symptoms problematic (short term)
Obsessive-compulsive disorder (OCD)	RFs: age (<40 yo), genetics, stress, other mental health/neurological illness. *Obsessions* – unwanted (ego-dystonic) intrusive thoughts or images. *Compulsions* – repetitive, stereotyped rituals. Not delusional (patient aware of irrationality)	6 Screening Q's. Assess functional impairment and severity (Yale–Brown Obsessive-Compulsive Scale). Look for other co-morbidity	CBT (including exposure/response prevention), SSRI, clomipramine. Psychiatric services
Post-traumatic stress disorder (PTSD)	RFs: traumatic birth, poor coping, previous trauma/abuse, alcohol. Hx & O/E: intrusive thoughts, avoidance, hypervigilance	History	Watchful waiting. Trauma-focused CBT. EMDR
Organic Iron-deficient anaemia	RFs: blood loss (menorrhagia, UGIB, bowel cancer), dietary deficiency, malabsorption. Hx & O/E: predominant fatigue, SOBOE, pica, restless legs, nail changes	FBC (↓Hb, ↓MCV), ↓ferritin. ↓Transferrin saturation, ↑TIBC. Endoscopy/colonoscopy	Iron supplementation (PO/IV) ± transfusion. **Definitive:** treat cause
Hypothyroidism	Predominant fatigue and cold intolerance	TFTs (↑TSH, ↓T4)	Thyroid hormone replacement

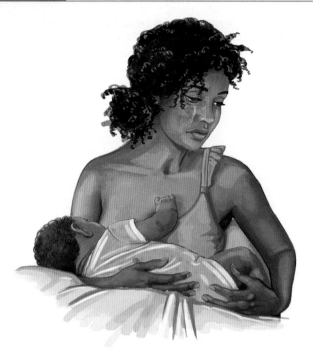

Fig. 163.1 Postpartum depression. (From Smith, RP. *Netter's Obstetrics and Gynecology*. January 1, 2018:492–494. © 2018.)

Low mood is common following delivery, but the features of this case that favour postpartum depression (Fig. 163.1) over 'baby blues' are: symptoms persisting over 2 weeks, symptoms starting within 1 month of birth but not straight away, symptoms more severe including suicidal ideation. This patient lacks the common predisposing risk factors of a previous history of depression or family history of postnatal depression and there is no information about her social situation. Aside from low affect, the absence of any other explicit or implied psychotic symptoms allows one to discount the rare but potentially catastrophic puerperal psychosis.

REVISION TIPS

- Depression in the postnatal period can occur at any time within a year after birth
- Women with BPAD have a 1 in 5 risk of suffering from postnatal psychosis
- Women with severe depression have 40% risk of relapse
- If a woman says to her GP she thinks she has a mental health condition, concerns should not be dismissed
- Valproate not for woman of childbearing age

164

Low Mood/Affective Problems

Alice Parker, Alexander Royston, Jennifer Powell, and Stephanie Upton

GP CONSULTATION, MALE, 40.
PERSISTENT LOW MOOD FOR 9 MONTHS, FOLLOWING SUDDEN LOSS OF FATHER

HPC: Also feelings of guilt, anxiety and worthlessness. Risk assessment: passive suicidal ideation but no plans to self-harm. Protective factors: supportive family (married, two children), religious faith. Eating normally, but insomnia, fatigue, can't focus at work. No PMHx of mental illness. **FHx:** Bipolar disorder (mother). **SHx:** Stopped going to running club, only leaves home for work. Non-drinker.

O/E: Withdrawn with mild psychomotor slowing, quiet and slow speech, flat affect. No thought disorder/disturbed perceptions, no objective evidence of memory problem. Orientated with insight preserved.

1. What severity of depression is this patient likely to have? What is first-line management?
2. What differential should be considered if this patient was elderly?
3. What common physical conditions can mimic depression?

Answers: 1. Severe. CBT or other psychological intervention + SSRI (Fig. 164.1). 2. Dementia. 3. Hypothyroidism, hypercalcaemia, vitamin D deficiency, diabetes.

TABLE 164.1

	Features	Investigations	Management
Psychiatric Depression	Core symptoms: persistent low mood, fatigue/anergia, anhedonia. Others: disturbed sleep, change in appetite/weight gain, poor concentration, thoughts of worthlessness/guilt, slowing of movement, loss of libido, suicidal thoughts/attempts. Can get psychotic symptoms (e.g. derogatory auditory hallucinations or nihilistic delusions of guilt or decaying insides). Severity: ICD-10 criteria	**RFs:** prior depression or FHx. Recent bereavement/stress/illness may contribute. F > M. Consider CBG, U&Es, LFTs, TFTs, calcium, FBC, CRP/ESR (exclude reversible causes). PHQ-9/HADS/BDI-II. **Risk assessment:** improving access to psychological therapies (IAPT)	**Mild:** guided self-help/computerised CBT. Sleep hygiene. **Moderate/severe:** IAPT-CBT or other + SSRI (citalopram, fluoxetine, sertraline), continued 6 months after remission. Referral to mental health team. Consider intensive home treatment. Admit (perhaps under Mental Health Act) if psychotic depression, suicidal intent/plan or self-neglect. **Review:** 2 weeks (if no suicidal ideation). 1 week (if suicidal thoughts or starting SSRIs or 18 – 25yo)

(Continued)

TABLE 164.1   (Cont'd)

	Features	Investigations	Management
Grief reaction	Low mood, may include hallucinations of the dead person. Usually <6 months, improves. Maintained sense of worth + interest in activities. May have suicidal thoughts (wish to join the dead person)	RF: bereavement. Clinical diagnosis	Support, bereavement counselling. Consider psychotherapy
Bipolar disorder	See *165. ELATION, ELATED MOOD AND PRESSURE OF SPEECH*		
Schizophrenia	RFs: FHx. Often presents in young males, early 20s. *Negative symptoms*: low mood, apathy, anhedonia, social withdrawal, self-neglect, poverty of speech and thought. *Positive symptoms*: delusions, hallucinations, thought disorder	Clinical diagnosis. Check organic causes, assess health before treatment; FBC, TFTs, U&Es, LFTs, CRP. ECG	Specialist psychiatric input. 2nd generation antipsychotic (DA antagonist): olanzapine, risperidone, clozapine. Psychotherapy: CBT/psychodynamic
Dementia	RFs: age (>75), sex (M > F), ethnicity, genetics. Hx & O/E: gradual onset memory loss, confusion, low mood, difficulties with ADLs	Collateral history. Memory clinic: MOCA, ACE-III. Bloods (reversible causes). **CT brain:** general atrophy + sulcal widening (Alzheimer's), multiple lucencies (vascular), mild atrophy (Lewy body)	Alzheimer's and dementia with Lewy bodies: **acetylcholinesterase inhibitors** (Galantamine, donepezil, rivastigmine), **glutamate antagonist** (Memantine-severe)
Non-psychiatric			
Hypothyroidism	RFs: PMHx/FHx autoimmune disease, drug-induced. Hx & O/E: fatigue, low mood, weight gain, constipation, dry skin, hair loss, myalgia and arthralgia, intolerance to cold	**Bloods:** TFTs	**Initial:** Levothyroxine
Delirium (hypoactive: typically appears drowsy, quiet, withdrawn, ↓oral intake)	RFs: infection, medication, pain, constipation, urinary retention, stroke, MI, uraemia, hyponatraemia, hypo/hyperglycaemia, hypoxia, alcohol or drug withdrawal, meningoencephalitis or raised intracranial pressure. Hx & O/E: new onset confusion, labile mood, hallucinations, speech impairment and reversal of the sleep-wake cycle	Full examination. FBC, U&Es, LFTs, glucose, ABG. **Septic screen:** lactate, urine output, blood cultures. **CXR.** ECG. Bladder scan	Treat cause. Manage environment (orientate, reduce stimuli). See also *165. ELATION, ELATED MOOD AND PRESSURE OF SPEECH*

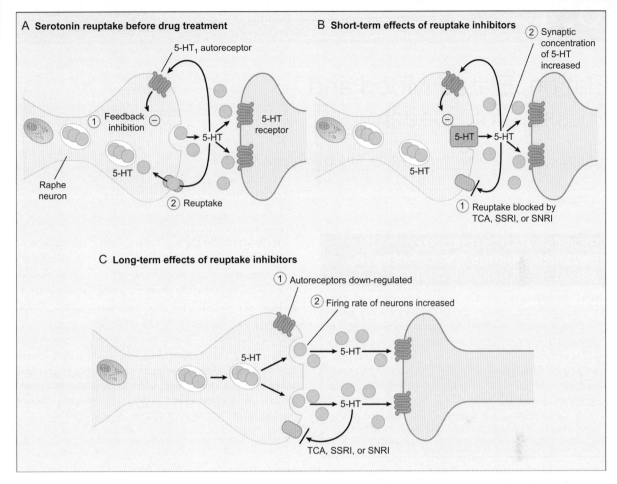

Fig. 164.1 Mechanisms of neuronal reuptake inhibitors. (From Stevens, CW. *Psychotherapeutic Drugs, Brenner and Stevens' Pharmacology*, ed 6. Chapter 22, 243–260. Copyright © 2023 by Elsevier, Inc. All rights reserved.)

The vignette describes a patient suffering from low mood, with a history of recent bereavement. This is not a simple grief reaction, because his symptoms are too prolonged (>6 months, although complex grief is still a possibility after this time) and he has lost his sense of self-worth and interest in normal activities. His feelings of low mood, together with disturbed sleep, poor concentration and fatigue are reasonably diagnostic but rule out an organic condition which may mimic depression (hypothyroidism), and medication side effects. Screening for bipolar disorder by asking about previous hypomanic episodes is important, particularly given his family history.

REVISION TIPS

- Depression core symptoms: persistent low mood, anergia (fatigue) and anhedonia (loss of interest in normal activities)
- Normal grief reaction usually involves low mood for <6 months – longer is abnormal and could indicate depression
- Mental State Exam mnemonic: ASEPTIC
  - A – Appearance/Behaviour
  - S – Speech
  - E – Emotion (Mood and Affect)
  - P – Perception (Auditory/Visual Hallucinations)
  - T – Thought Content (Suicidal/Homicidal Ideation) and Process
  - I – Insight and Judgement
  - C – Cognition

165

Elation, Elated Mood and Pressure of Speech

Natalia Hackett, Alexander Royston, and Nwaorima Kamalu

GP PRESENTATION, MALE, 21.
GIRLFRIEND BRINGS HIM, CONCERNED ABOUT HIS BEHAVIOUR CHANGE

HPC: Partner says patient is not sleeping and has started gambling. Patient doesn't report feeling tired, he feels 'fantastic' and just 'has too much to get done'. Symptoms have increased over several weeks. **PMHx:** Bouts of depression since aged 17. **DHx:** Citalopram discontinued. **SHx:** Lives with girlfriend, works part-time as cashier, recently quit his job for 'bigger projects'. No illicit substance history.

　O/E: Dressed in a bright orange shirt, talkative, pressure of speech, flight of ideas, grandiose delusions of leading a new vaccine project that cures all diseases.

1. What would be the top differentials if the patient:
   a. Was an older hospital in-patient after hip arthroplasty?
   b. Had no history of depression?
   c. Was experiencing chest pain and palpitations?
2. How do you differentiate between a manic, hypomanic, depressive or mixed episode?

Answers: 1a. Delirium. 1b. Possibly a first manic episode (further observation/examination needed.) At high risk of self-harm from depression upon ending the first manic episode. Risk assessment is vital. 1c. Possible cocaine-induced acute coronary syndrome. 2. See Table 165.2.

TABLE 165.1

	Features	Investigations	Management
Psychiatric			
BPAD: manic presentation/ relapse (Fig. 165.1)	*Cognitive*: self-esteem, distractibility, racing thoughts, flight of ideas, speech – tangentiality, clang association, neologisms, word salad. *Behavioural*: pressured speech, decreased sleep, disinhibition, extreme irritability. *Psychotic*: grandiose delusions. Depression/low mood episode. Mania triggered by antidepressant. Can be floridly psychotic, in excess of severity of the affective component	**RFs:** FHx of bipolar, trauma/ stress, drugs/ alcohol. MSE, physical exam. FBC, TFTs, CRP. **Urine:** drug screen. CT/MRI	Benzodiazepine/ sedative (short-term). Mental Health services. Psychological therapy, SSRI + antipsychotic. Mood stabiliser (lithium, valproate – unless woman of childbearing age). Use antidepressants if depressed (with caution due to risk of manic switch)
Schizoaffective disorder	**RFs:** (F > M), FHx of MH illness. Psychotic symptoms in absence of affective symptoms	As BPAD	Specialist mental health. Antipsychotic, psychotherapy

TABLE 165.1   (Cont'd)

	Features	Investigations	Management
Personality disorder (PD). Histrionic and narcissistic traits. Emotionally unstable PD (EUPD)	Present ≥18 yo, wide spectrum of severity. **Histrionic traits: ≥5 of;** 1. Uncomfortable when not the centre of attention 2. Seductive/provocative behaviour 3. Shifting and shallow emotions 4. Appearance draws attention 5. Impressionistic and vague speech 6. Dramatic/exaggerated emotions 7. Suggestible (easily influenced) 8. Considers relationships more intimate than they are **Narcissistic traits:** pervasive pattern of grandiosity, need for admiration, and lack of empathy, with interpersonal entitlement, exploitiveness, arrogance and envy. **Emotionally unstable traits:** dysregulation in this PD is often mistaken for bipolar mania	**RFs:** physical/ sexual abuse, neglect or childhood abandonment, inborn sensitivity to stress, FHx of PD. Screen for depression/ substance abuse. Narcissistic: difficult to diagnose – often high functioning. At increased risk of PTSD, affective disorder, eating disorders	Psychotropics in short term (depending on symptom severity: unlikely to work long term). **Definitive:** supportive psychotherapy dialectical behaviour therapy, mentalisation-based therapy. See also *171. SUICIDAL THOUGHTS AND SELF-HARM*
Cyclothymia	Rare. Persistent mood instability, less severe, not meeting threshold for treatment. Frequently complicated by substance abuse	**RFs:** age (young adulthood), FHx BPAD. As BPAD	Counselling. Mood stabilisers (if unavoidable)
Organic Drug misuse	See *121. SUBSTANCE MISUSE*		
Delirium (hyperactive: typically features restlessness, agitation, wandering)	**RFs:** infection, medication, pain, constipation, urinary retention, stroke, MI, uraemia, hyponatraemia, hypo/ hyperglycaemia, hypoxia, alcohol or drug withdrawal, meningoencephalitis or raised ICP. New onset confusion, labile mood, hallucinations, speech impairment and reversal of the sleep-wake cycle	Full examination. FBC, U&Es, LFTs, glucose, ABG. **Septic screen:** lactate, urine output, blood cultures. **CXR.** ECG	**Initial:** manage environment (orientate, reduce stimuli, etc). **Definitive:** treat cause. See *also 164. LOW MOOD/ AFFECTIVE PROBLEMS*
Frontal lobe disease	**RFs:** poorly understood, genetics. **Hx & O/E:** middle aged, personality and behavioural change, progressive, memory less impacted	History. CT/MRI brain (focal atrophy)	Supportive. Specialist neurology referral. Memory clinic

TABLE 165.2	Distinctions Between Key Episodes
Manic	Abnormally, persistently elevated/irritable mood >1 week, severe enough to impair social function or with psychotic features
Hypomanic	Manic symptoms for <4 days, less severe or no psychotic features
Depressive	2 weeks of low mood, lack of pleasure or loss of interest + 4 more depressive features
Mixed	Alternating manic and depressive symptoms

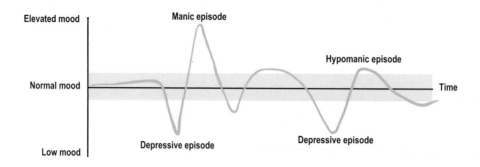

Fig. 165.1 Bipolar affective disorder. (Illustrated by Dr Hollie Blaber.)

The vignette describes a florid manic episode, with many of the hallmark presenting symptoms – pressured speech, flight of ideas, reduced need for sleep, grandiosity, clothing choices and risk-taking behaviour. Particularly diagnostic is the prior history of depression, which suggests a marked fluctuation in affective state. Excluding substance abuse is vital, as an aggravating or precipitating cause. In this age group and gender, it is always important to exclude the presence of overt psychotic symptoms, which might suggest a more schizoaffective disorder. The Cluster B personality disorders (antisocial, borderline, histrionic, narcissistic) are also possible, as there is significant overlap in these conditions – particularly when patients can suffer from co-morbid depression and symptoms may be influenced by substance or alcohol abuse.

REVISION TIPS

- Of the above differentials, BPAD is most commonly associated with pressured speech, e.g. during a manic episode
- Antidepressants can trigger a manic episode

166

Auditory Hallucinations

Natalia Hackett, Alexander Royston, and Sophie Kellman

GP CONSULTATION, MALE, 20.
HOUSEMATES CONCERNED ABOUT ABNORMAL BELIEFS AND SOCIAL WITHDRAWAL

HPC: He reports his housemates are working for the Secret Service. He knew they had turned against him when they bought a new toaster for the kitchen. They comment on everything he does even when they're not in the room, and they are putting thoughts into his head via a computer chip. **PMHx:** Eczema as a child. **D/SHx:** Cannabis use in his teens.

O/E: Good rapport but distracted and displays tangential thinking and delusions

1. List factors that increase the risk of schizophrenia.
2. List the First-Rank schizophrenia symptoms.
3. What types of auditory hallucinations can present with schizophrenia?

Answers: 1. FHx, perinatal factors, social factors (e.g. isolation, unemployment), premorbid schizotypal personality, drug misuse, adverse life events. 2. Auditory hallucinations, delusions of thought interference, delusions of control/passivity phenomena and delusional perception. 3. Thought echo, running commentary, third person (more than one person discussing or arguing about the patient).

TABLE 166.1

	Features	Investigations	Management
Psychiatric Paranoid schizophrenia (Fig. 166.1)	Often young males, early 20s. First-rank symptoms: auditory hallucinations (third person, thought echo and running commentary), delusions of thought interference (insertion/withdrawal/broadcast), delusions of control/passivity phenomena, delusional perception. Negative: low mood, apathy, anhedonia, social withdrawal, self-neglect, poverty of speech/thought	**RFs:** FHx, perinatal/ social factors (isolation, unemployment), premorbid schizotypal personality, drug misuse, adverse life events. Prodromal: anxiety, social withdrawal, erratic behaviour, unmotivated. Exclude organic causes: FBC, TFTs, U&Es, LFTs, CRP, ECG	Psychiatry. Second-generation antipsychotic (DA antagonist): olanzapine, risperidone, clozapine. Psychotherapy: CBT/ psychodynamic

(Continued)

TABLE 166.1 (Cont'd)

	Features	Investigations	Management
Drug-induced psychosis	**RFs:** drug/alcohol, methamphetamine, psychedelics (LSD), MDMA. Related to use or withdrawal. Psychotic symptoms as per schizophrenia – commonly paranoid, can present with fixed beliefs	**Urine:** drug screen. **Bloods:** as per schizophrenia	Psychiatry (include a period of monitoring with no antipsychotics). Specialist drug/alcohol input
Mood disorder (with psychotic symptoms)	Psychotic symptoms can occur in severe depression-derogatory auditory hallucinations and nihilistic delusions (of guilt or decaying insides). BPAD manic patients can be floridly psychotic in excess of the perceived severity of their affective component	**RFs:** as per BPAD/depression. Clinical diagnosis. PHQ9, HADS, BDI-II questionnaires. **Bloods:** as per schizophrenia	Psychiatry
Organic Drug misuse	**RFs:** FHx of addiction, MHI, lack of family, impulsivity, peer pressure, early use. Amphetamine, cocaine. Iatrogenic: steroids, DA agonists	Drug/social history. **Urine:** drug screen	Abstinence. Psychiatric referral if necessary
Temporal lobe epilepsy	Aura with smell/taste deja vu, automatisms	History	Neurology referral
Hearing impairment	Common: patients 'hear' doorbells, telephone rings, music, voices	Audiological assessment	ENT referral – hearing aid, CBT
Other	Brain injury, CNS infection, brain tumour, stroke, HIV, Wilson disease, porphyria, neurosyphilis		

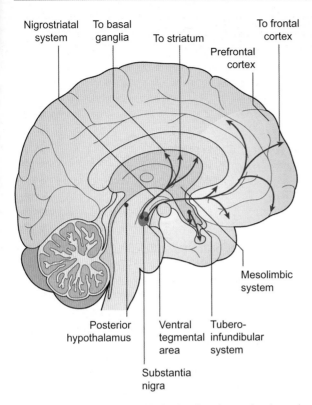

Nigrostriatal system

To basal ganglia

To striatum

To frontal cortex

Prefrontal cortex

Mesolimbic system

Tubero-infundibular system

Ventral tegmental area

Substantia nigra

Posterior hypothalamus

Fig. 166.1 Schizophrenia and bipolar disorder; major dopaminergic pathways in the central nervous system. (From Waller, DG, Sampson, AP. *Medical Pharmacology and Therapeutics.* January 1, 2018:287–296. Elsevier. © 2018.)

Psychotic symptoms, such as auditory hallucinations, are cardinal features of psychotic disorders. First rule out substance abuse, medication side effects and medical disorders (sepsis). Paranoid schizophrenia is the most common condition presenting with these symptoms, made more likely in the vignette by his age and gender, and his previous history of cannabis use. He is past his initial prodromal stage and is now acutely psychotic, suggested by his auditory hallucinations and delusions. Some negative symptoms are reported (social withdrawal), which are also useful diagnostically. Cannabis use is noteworthy as it can be both a risk factor for, and ensuing complication of, paranoid schizophrenia.

REVISION TIPS

- Hallucinations: consider age – younger is more likely to be psychosis, older person is more likely to be dementia or delirium
- Psychosis: consider precipitants – drug use, acute sepsis, high-dose steroids
- Family history is a potent RF, with 85% concordance in twin studies
- Biopsychosocial model of RFs: include adverse childhood events, stress

167

Anxiety, Phobias, OCD

Natalia Hackett, Alexander Royston, and Stephanie Upton

GP CONSULTATION, FEMALE, 20.
CONTINUOUS WORRYING AND DIFFICULTY CONCENTRATING FOR 6 MONTHS

HPC: Feeling irritable, 'on edge', disconnected from her thoughts and experiencing occasional chest tightness with 'missed beats'. **PMHx:** Tension headache, menorrhagia, asthma, excess alcohol intake but not caffeine. **DHx:** Salbutamol PRN.

O/E: Restless, normal chest auscultation, normotensive, mild tachycardia (105 bpm), no signs of hyperthyroidism (goitre, etc.).

1. List the possible physical signs and symptoms of generalised anxiety disorder (GAD).
2. List the possible psychological signs and symptoms of GAD.

3. What would be the top differentials if the patient was unable to leave their house or go to the supermarket due to fear of these situations?
4. A patient with very dry hands due to repetitive washing; when asked why, she says 'she knows it's stupid but she feels her brother might die otherwise'. What is the most likely diagnosis?

Answers: 1. Palpitations, stomach discomfort, dry mouth, nausea, tight chest, loose stool, trembling, tension headache, light-headedness. 2. Poor concentration, sleep disturbance, inability to keep still, worry, derealisation, depersonalisation. 3. Agoraphobia, social phobia. 4. Obsessive-compulsive disorder: often aware of the irrationality, but very difficult to resist impulses to engage in the resulting rituals.

TABLE 167.1

	Features	Investigations	Management
Psychiatric Generalised anxiety disorder (GAD)	Widespread disproportionate worry with no specific trigger. Duration ≥6 months. **Hx & O/E:** often prominent physical symptoms-chest/abdominal pain, palpitations, dry mouth, tension headache (Fig. 167.1). Alcohol (consider 'self-medication')	**RFs:** F > M (2:1), stress, anxious personality traits, substance misuse, comorbid depression. Tests based on clinical features, r/o organic cause; TFTs, LFTs, CBG, drug screen, ECG. **GAD7**	Education, lifestyle advice, SSRI. **Definitive:** psychological therapy (often CBT). β-blockers only if physical symptoms problematic (short-term use)

TABLE 167.1   (Cont'd)

	Features	Investigations	Management
Obsessive compulsive disorder (OCD)	*Obsessions;* unwanted (ego-dystonic) intrusive thoughts or images. *Compulsions;* repetitive, stereotyped rituals. Not delusional –aware of irrationality. Sudden onset in child: consider PANDAS (Paediatric Autoimmune Neuropsychiatric Disorders Associated with Streptococcal Infections)	**RFs:** age (<40 yo), genetics, stress, MH/neurological, pregnancy/postpartum. **6 Screening Q's.** Assess functional impairment and severity (Yale–Brown Obsessive-Compulsive Scale). Consider other co-morbidities	CBT (including exposure and response prevention), SSRI, clomipramine. Psychiatric services referral
Adjustment disorder	Symptoms <6 months, low mood, anxiety, unable to cope, social withdrawal, impact on function	**RFs:** following a stressor-grief, divorce, job loss. As GAD	Watchful waiting. Consider psychotherapy
Panic disorder	Recurrent unpredictable episodes of sudden '100% anxiety', associated with physical features. Feelings of 'loss of control'. 'Pins and needles'	**RFs:** FHx (anxiety), stress, poor coping, physical/sexual abuse. Screen for alcohol withdrawal. Consider excluding cardiac/respiratory/endocrine conditions	Self-help and education. Psychological therapy (CBT). SSRIs
Specific phobias	*Agoraphobia*: a fear of being in situations where escape might be difficult or that help wouldn't be available-too anxious to leave home. *Social phobia*: anxiety limited to social situations. *Specific phobia*: fear of object/situation	**RFs:** F > M, FHx, stress/trauma/illness. As GAD	Relaxation therapy. CBT including graded exposure
Organic Hyperthyroidism	See *10. PALPITATIONS*		
Hypoglycaemia			
Phaeochromocytoma	See *10. PALPITATIONS*		
Drug-induced anxiety	**RFs:** DHx – prescription (salbutamol, antidepressants), recreational (alcohol withdrawal, caffeine), illicit (amphetamines). **Presentation:** as GAD	Depends on drug. **Urine:** drug screen	Medication review. Substance misuse services

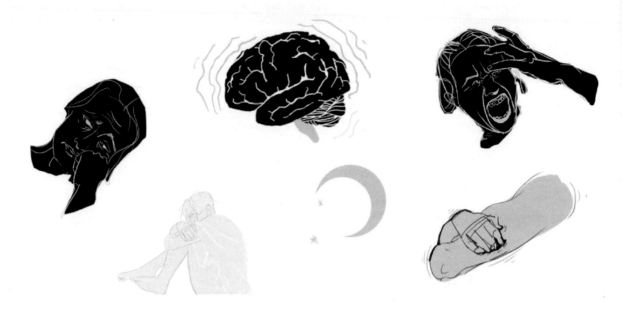

Fig. 167.1 Diagnostic and Statistical Manual of Mental Disorders, Fifth Edition (DSM-5) criteria of GAD; **A.** Excessive anxiety/worry more days than not for >6 months; **B.** Difficult to control worry; **C.** Symptoms, ≥3 of: impaired concentration, irritability, increased muscle tension, sleeping difficulty, restless/on edge, fatigue; **D.** Causes distress/functional impairment; **E.** Not attributable to substance abuse; **F.** Not explained by medical problem or psychoactive substance. (Illustrated by Dr. Hollie Blaber)

The vignette describes a common presentation of GAD. Often without an obvious precipitant, it can be defined as a stress response in the absence of an obvious stressor. Rule out physical causes; in this history there is no obvious hyperthyroidism other than a tachycardia, and caffeine intake is not evidently high. Note that salbutamol can mimic symptoms of anxiety due to adrenergic effects, and excess alcohol intake could be important. Checking substance use is important, as patients may attempt to self-medicate with alcohol, cannabis or street diazepam to manage symptoms.

REVISION TIPS

- Anxiety disorders can present with physical symptoms and organic conditions can cause anxiety
- Anxiety may be 'free-floating' or focused on a particular set of environmental circumstances
- RFs: anxious personality traits, female sex, increased stress, history of physical or emotional trauma, comorbid depression, substance misuse/dependence or other anxiety disorder

168

Somatisation/Medically Unexplained Physical Symptoms

Natalia Hackett, Alexander Royston, and Thomas Nutting

GP CONSULTATION, FEMALE, 32. ONE YEAR INTERMITTENT ABDOMINAL PAIN

HPC: Pain radiates globally, unrelated to food or defecation; she attended clinic twice previously for same complaint. She has excluded dairy/gluten/alcohol/caffeine without improvement, avoiding social events in case of pain. **PMHx:** Lower back pain, headache.

O/E: Clinically stable, obs normal. Abdomen SNT, bowel sounds present, DRE normal.

1. If no organic cause is found, what is first-line treatment for the disorder in the vignette?

2. What would be your top differential after investigations exclude an organic cause, if the patient is:
   a. Convinced they had colorectal cancer when their stomach rumbled?
   b. Reluctant to have a diagnostic laparotomy despite complaining of severe abdominal pain?
3. What disorder is likely if a patient complains of blindness after catching their partner being unfaithful?

Answers: 1. CBT. 2a. Illness anxiety disorder/hypochondriasis. 2b. Malingering. 3. Conversion disorder.

TABLE 168.1

	Features	Investigations	Management
Involuntary Somatic symptom disorder (or bodily distress disorder (ICD11))	Severe and persistent physical medically unexplained symptom(s) for >6 months. Significant disruption of daily life (e.g. affects relationships/academic/occupation/social). Persistent thoughts/anxiety/time devoted to symptoms	RFs: genetic, neglect or sexual abuse, prior chronic illness, poor coping skills, co-morbid MHI (panic disorder). Clinical diagnosis. First exclude organic causes	Psychological input. CBT (primary evidence). Eclectic psychotherapy combination of; CBT, mindfulness, ±short-term dynamic psychotherapy, ±interpersonal/general psychotherapy, ±re-attribution training

(Continued)

TABLE 168.1   (Cont'd)

	Features	Investigations	Management
Illness anxiety disorder (hypochon-driasis)	Preoccupation with having a serious illness for >6 months (illness can change), repetitive behaviours (checking, researching, consulting) causing distress/disruption. Somatic symptoms mild/absent	**RFs:** FHx, serious childhood illness, MHI (depression, anxiety or personality disorder), abuse/past trauma/violence exposure in childhood. Tests: as for somatic symptom disorder	Psychological input. CBT (primary evidence). Potential role for SSRIs or antipsychotics
Functional or dissociative neurological symptom disorder (conversion)	Neurological symptoms (altered motor, sensory or cognitive function) not compatible with recognised organic conditions, e.g. apparent grand mal seizure while responding to commands	**RFs:** F > M, neuro PMHx/FHx, recent ↑stress or emotional/physical trauma, co-morbid MHI (anxiety/dissociative disorder, certain personality disorders), childhood abuse/neglect. Tests: full neurological examination, EEG/MRI	Psychoeducation. Physiotherapy. Occupational therapy. Treatment of co-morbid mental illness. Some evidence for psychotherapies
Psychological factors affecting other medical conditions	Psychological/behavioural factors exacerbate or interfere with condition, raising risk from it, e.g. not taking anti-hypertensives in known HTN (NOT adjustment disorder, which is anxiety after illness diagnosis)	**RFs:** co-morbid depression or anxiety, stressful life events, differences in relationship/coping styles/personality traits. History and examination	Psychological input
Delusional disorder	≥1 delusion persisting >3 months, functioning not obviously impaired (unlike schizophrenia), behaviour not obviously bizarre/odd	**RFs:** age (increasing), immigration, isolation, FHx, sensory impairment. R/o medical cause, schizophrenia, mood disorder	Psychiatric input: psychotherapy. Limited evidence for antipsychotics
Voluntary Factitious disorder (Munchausen's)	Deceptive falsification or induction of signs/symptoms, not solely motivated by obvious external rewards but likely seeking sick role. Has extensive notes, multiple investigations, seen many professionals	**RFs:** childhood abuse/neglect/trauma/illness, alcohol/drug abuse, marriage problems, stress, personality disorder (anti-social PD/EUPD), healthcare worker. Rule out/quantify medical cause	Psychiatry management; treat comorbidity, psychotherapy
Malingering disorder	Discrepancy between claimed disability and objective finding. Seeking secondary gain, e.g. medico-legal financial gain post-accident	**RFs:** medico-legal context, anti-social personality disorder/histrionic traits. Poor compliance with management	Patient will avoid risky investigations or therapy

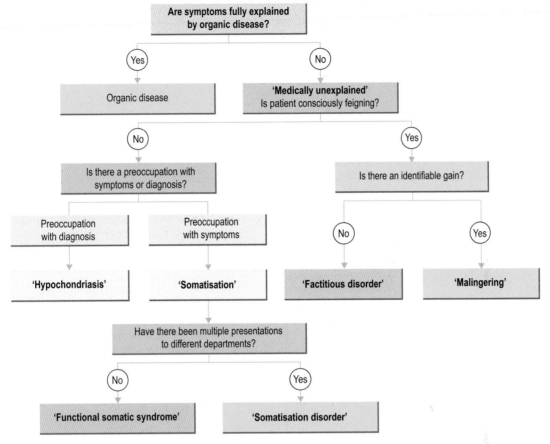

Fig. 168.1 Differential diagnosis of medically unexplained symptoms. (From Steel, RM, Lawrie, SM. Medical psychiatry. In: *Davidson's Principles and Practice of Medicine*, ed. 31. 1235–1261. Copyright © 2023 Elsevier Ltd. All rights reserved.)

The vignette describes somatic symptom disorder (SSD), termed bodily distress disorder (BDD) under ICD11 (one of a group formerly bracketed within 'medically unexplained'). It is a diagnosis of exclusion (Fig. 168.1), as physical symptoms will first be ruled out, sometimes necessitating multiple invasive investigations. Somatic symptom disorder is typified by ≥6 months of symptoms, often severe, that may vary and also affect >1 organ/ system, often with significant life and emotional impact. SSD differs from hypochondriasis, where sufferers have an obsessive interest in their own health and are convinced that mild/normal symptoms are beginnings of severe disease (e.g. "headache means brain tumour"). This field has seen changes, with ICD11 no longer defining somatoform disorders on the basis of the absence of a feature

(a physical or medical cause). Instead significant associated psychological features, and functional impairment, are required for confirming diagnosis.

REVISION TIPS

- Always rule out organic causes first
- Somatic symptom disorder – concentrates on a particular symptom(s)
- Illness anxiety disorder – concentrates on a specific condition
- Functional neurological disorder – neurological symptoms
- Factitious disorder – patient wants patient status
- Malingering disorder – patient wants financial or other gain

169

Addiction

Katie Turner, Gregory Oxenham, and Alice Pitt

GP CONSULTATION, MALE, 48. WANTS TO CUT DOWN ON HIS ALCOHOL INTAKE

HPC: Made redundant 3 months ago, subsequently escalating alcohol intake – needs to drink more to feel the same effects, craves alcohol on waking. ≤8 beers daily, sometimes a bottle of whisky, drinks alone. Hiding his drinking habits from his teenage daughter, but she suspects – negative impact on their relationship. When he tries to cut down he feels sick, anxious and begins to shake. **PMHx:** Depression. **DHx:** Nil. No recreational drug use. **SHx:** Lives alone since divorce. Smokes 20 cigarettes a day.

O/E: Appears sweaty and agitated. Slurred speech. Normal observations.

1. What causes Wernicke-Korsakoff syndrome? What conditions can lead to it?
2. What is the mechanism of varenicline?
3. Which smoking cessation drug is contraindicated in epilepsy?

Answers: 1. Deficiency of vitamin B1 (thiamine) – encountered with chronic alcohol, eating disorders, malnutrition, starvation. 2. Nicotinic acetylcholine receptor partial agonist used for smoking cessation. 3. Bupropion.

TABLE 169.1

	Features	Investigations	Management
Alcohol use disorder	**RFs:** mental health diagnoses, FHx of alcohol use disorder, drinking from an early age. Established pattern of heavy drinking, requires more drinks to maintain same effects, drinking alone/secretly, drinking soon after waking, continuing to drink despite physical/psychological problems Mood swings and personality changes, inability to cut down/stop drinking. *Signs of withdrawal:* tremors, sweating, tachycardia, anxiety. Seizures (7–48 hours). Delirium tremens (48–72 hours). See *172. THREATS TO HARM OTHERS* for acute alcohol intoxication	Clinical diagnosis. Screening tests: AUDIT-C, CAGE tests. Acute intoxication: ↑blood alcohol (not reliable in chronic intoxication). Chronic: deranged LFTs possible - AST >ALT, ↑GGT. FBC – ↑MCV.	Naltrexone (opiate antagonist) – reduces pleasure from drinking. Disulfiram – promotes abstinence. Acamprosate (NMDA partial agonist) – reduces cravings, neuroprotective. **Psychosocial interventions** (relapse prevention). CBT (motivational interviewing, relapse prevention), family/behavioural/social network/environment-based therapy – Alcoholics Anonymous. **Monitor health problems** e.g. cirrhosis, varices, malnutrition

TABLE 169.1 (Cont'd)

	Features	Investigations	Management
Acute alcohol withdrawal	Alcohol excess with sudden cessation: tremors, sweating, tachycardia, anxiety. Can cause **tonic-clonic seizures** (7–48 hours). **Delirium tremens** (48–72 hours): coarse tremor, confusion, hallucination, fever, tachycardia, seizure. **Emergency**	For any seizure: glucose, VBG, FBC, U&Es, magnesium, calcium, ECG. VBG: lactate↑. FBC: macrocytosis. Clinical Institute Withdrawal Assessment for Alcohol (CIWA) score: determine severity of withdrawal, guides treatment	Treat seizure actively and prevent recurrence. **Chlordiazepoxide** (or other long-acting benzodiazepine). **IV Pabrinex.** Then low dose thiamine PO. Drug/alcohol service
Opioid misuse	Needle track marks in IVDU, escalating use of prescription opioids, physical dependence. *Signs of overdose*: respiratory depression, pinpoint pupils, reduced GCS – respiratory acidosis/T2 respiratory failure. *Signs of withdrawal*: dysphoria, lacrimation, rhinorrhoea, tachycardia, N&V	RFs: mental health diagnoses, homelessness, chronic pain, long-term prescriptions of opioids. Urine analysis for drug screen (generally in abstinence programs rather than overdose)	**Emergency management:** naloxone. **Managing dependence** (opiate substitution treatment): methadone or buprenorphine. Harm reduction; needle exchange programmes. Screening for HIV, hepatitis B & C
Benzodiazepine misuse	Escalating use, dependence. *Signs of overdose*; confusion, LOC, slowing of reflexes, incoordination, respiratory depression. *Signs of withdrawal*: agitation, tremor, nausea, tachycardia, tachypnoea, seizures (grand mal), hallucinations	RFs: co-existent mental health diagnoses, chronic pain, long-term prescriptions of benzodiazepines. **Clinical diagnosis.** Urine analysis for drug screen possible	**Emergency management:** observation in overdose – flumazenil occasionally used (caution if chronic use/ seizure disorder, as can provoke seizures which will be resistant to benzodiazepines). Requires a **slow taper down** in order to stop use
Gambling disorder	Needing to gamble with more money to match excitement, continuing despite negative impact on life/responsibilities, gambling when distressed, hiding/lying about it, restless/ irritable when trying to quit	RFs: male, mental health diagnoses, alcohol use, early exposure to gambling, poor academic performance. **Clinical diagnosis**	CBT. Self-help groups. Antidepressants, e.g. SSRIs
Tobacco use disorder	Inability to stop smoking after multiple attempts. Continuing to smoke despite health problems. *Withdrawal symptoms*: anxiety, restlessness, depression, insomnia	RFs: family/friends that smoke, starting at a younger age, mental health diagnosis, other substance misuse. **Clinical diagnosis**	CBT. Nicotine replacement therapy. Varenicline. Bupropion
Key Complications Wernicke-Korsakoff syndrome (Fig. 169.1)	Confusion, nystagmus, ophthalmoplegia, ataxia. Progresses to Korsakoff syndrome – amnesia (mainly anterograde), confabulation, clear consciousness	RFs: alcohol misuse disorder, malnutrition. FBC, U&Es, TFTs, glucose. R/o infectious/metabolic cause. **Neuroimaging**	Thiamine (IM/IV): ensure Mg levels are normal. Avoid IV dextrose unless hypoglycaemic (reduces thiamine levels further)

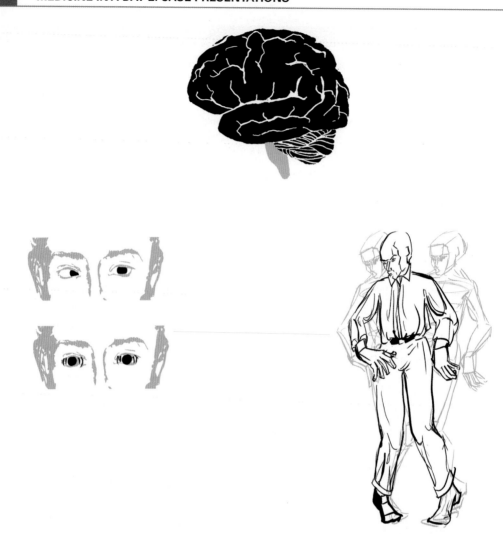

Fig. 169.1 Wernicke encephalopathy – classically a triad of confusion, ophthalmoplegia and ataxia. (Illustration by Dr Hollie Blaber.)

The man in this vignette, with multiple life changes and probable reactive depression, has developed alcohol mis-use disorder. He exhibits several features of dependence, such as tolerance, drinking alone, concealment of intake and withdrawal when he reduces. People with high alcohol intake are susceptible to physical health problems and falls/injuries. Heavy users should be advised to reduce intake gradually to minimise dangerous withdrawal symptoms, the most concerning of which are seizures.

REVISION TIPS

- Disulfiram works by inhibiting the enzyme acetaldehyde dehydrogenase in the alcohol breakdown pathway. The build up of acetaldehyde causes a severe, unpleasant reaction
- Varenicline and bupropion are contraindicated in pregnancy and breastfeeding; note these drugs were withdrawn, and it is not clear if they will be reintroduced

Fixed Abnormal Beliefs – Outline

Greg Oxenham

Fixed abnormal beliefs (delusions) can be found as part of schizophrenia, delusional disorder, severe depression and bipolar affective disorder as well as in drug misuse, acute intoxication and organic causes. Conditions in older adults affect likelihood. For example, Alzheimer's disease can cause paranoid delusions.

Very rarely, patients with delusions may become violent. In most cases this is a reaction intended to protect themselves from the real threat they feel to their safety.

TABLE 170.1

	Considerations
Persecutory delusions	May believe that an organisation or individual intends to harm or kill them
Grandiose delusions	Belief that they have more power or importance than in reality
Capgras syndrome ('imposter syndrome')	Belief that someone they know has been replaced by someone else
Cotard syndrome	Nihilistic delusion where the patient sees themselves as rotting or dead
Paraphrenia	Well-organised paranoid delusions appearing in later life (e.g. a neighbour is trying to break into the house), often with auditory hallucinations (unlike paranoid delusional disorders). Less likely to show negative symptoms of schizophrenia.
Secondary delusions	Brain tumour (malignant glioma, metastases in older patients), head injury, medications, endocrine disorders, infections, complex partial seizures (temporal lobe epilepsy)

Suicidal Thoughts and Self-Harm

Natalia Hackett, Mital Patel, and Hannah Rodgers

EMERGENCY DEPARTMENT, FEMALE, 22. FOUND NEXT TO 5+ EMPTY PACKETS OF PARACETAMOL

HPC: Pale, clammy. Witnessed to vomit by flatmate. Patient disclosed to flatmate she had impulsively taken paracetamol with a bottle of vodka after an argument with her boyfriend; feeling overwhelmed, life not worth living. She then regretted actions and agreed to go to ED with flatmate. Currently distressed, regretful of her actions. Denies further plans of suicide, anhedonia or biological symptoms of depression. Describes chronic feelings of emptiness, shame, suicide ideation, struggling with intense emotions. **PMHx:** Several previous overdoses impulsively after arguments with friends/family/partners. **DHx:** No regular medication. **SHx:** Current smoker (6 pack years).

O/E: Well but distressed. Physical exam unremarkable. **Ix:** Serum paracetamol concentration at 4 hours, LFTs, and PT/INR all within normal range.

1. What are the key features of emotionally unstable personality disorder (EUPD)?
2. What features in the vignette point to a lower risk of future completed suicide?

Answers: 1. SCARS – Self-image unclear, Chronic empty feeling, Abandonment fears, Relationships intense and unstable, Self-harm and suicide attempts. 2. Impulsive action, not planned, patient now regretful of actions with no further suicide plans, no obvious evidence of co-morbid depression.

TABLE 171.1

	Features	Investigations	Management
EUPD	**RFs:** traumatic childhood, neglect, abuse. SCARS (see answer 2). See also *165. ELATION, ELATED MOOD AND PRESSURE OF SPEECH.* Reassurance behaviour, e.g. excess texting, 'leave before they leave me'; finding inconsistency challenging; boundary testing, interpersonal difficulties	Exclude psychiatric co-morbidity (depression) and ongoing risk of harm to self/others. Exclude substance abuse. Check relationships and childhood risk factors	Mental health referral, crisis resolution and home treatment team, Dialectical Behavioural Therapy (psychotherapy). Any admission to hospital should be short with clear goals

TABLE 171.1	(Cont'd)		
	Features	**Investigations**	**Management**
Depression	**RFs:** co-existing mental health conditions, FHx. Low mood with anhedonia (unable to enjoy normal activity), low self-esteem, feeling guilty/tearful, apathy, loss of appetite, lethargy and poor sleep due to early morning wakening, loss of sex drive	Mild: noticeable impact on daily life. Moderate: significant impact. Severe: debilitating, almost impossible to get through daily life (may have psychotic symptoms)	CBT (self-guided/online/in-person/group). SSRI: for moderate–severe depression. Regular exercise can be effective
Post-traumatic stress disorder (PTSD)	Situation where a life was in danger or equivalent – worse if unable to escape/feeling powerless. Four main symptoms: re-living traumatic event (flashbacks, nightmares), avoidance, hyper-arousal and emotional numbing	Diagnosed >1 month after event, up to years later. PTSD checklist – 20-item questionnaire. IES-R (Impact of Event Scale – Revised): assesses subjective distress due to traumatic events	Watchful waiting, trauma-focused CBT, Eye Movement Desensitisation and Reprocessing (EMDR). SSRIs (anti-depressant) sometimes helpful
Bipolar disorder	Periods of mania and depression lasting weeks/months. Manic: feeling euphoric, high energy despite lack of sleep, irregular eating, speaking fast, getting distracted/agitated, uncharacticsly risky/harmful decisions (health, finance). Depressive phase as above	**RF:** FHx. History, collateral history, MSE, physical exam. Rule out infectious/metabolic causes (FBC, TFTs, CRP, etc.). See also *165. ELATION, ELATED MOOD AND PRESSURE OF SPEECH.*	Specialist mental health, psychological therapy, antipsychotic, mood stabiliser (lithium, valproate). Anti-depressants not recommended as prophylaxis for depressive episodes
Other personality disorder (e.g. antisocial personality disorder)	Main types: 1. Suspicious: paranoid personality, schizoid personality, schizotypal 2. Emotional/impulsive: antisocial personality, histrionic, narcissistic (and EUPD) 3. Anxious; avoidant, dependent, obsessive-compulsive	Exclude psychiatric co-morbidity – personality disorder is a diagnosis of exclusion. Assess for concurrent substance abuse	Psychotherapy
Eating disorder	**RFs:** perfectionist personality, FHx, high risk occupation (dancer, model, athlete), ongoing stress. **Hx & O/E:** body image distortions, morbid fear of weight gain. Food restriction with low BMI (anorexia) and/or binging/purging (bulimia)	BMI, BP, pulse, HR. ESR, FBC, TFTs, U&Es, LFTs, CK, glucose, phosphate. ECG if evidence of electrolyte disorder	Eating disorder service. See also *173. ABNORMAL EATING OR EXERCISING BEHAVIOUR*

TABLE 171.2   Self-harm management and the high-/low-risk features of suicide

Self-Harm Management

Initial assessment of physical risk, psychological state, prior mental health conditions and safeguarding concerns, further risk of self-harm or suicide.
Urgent referral to nearest ED if further physical or psychological risk or self-poisoned.
Primary care treatment if minor injury, seek ED consultant advice if unsure.
Primary care review within 48 hours if not presented initially to primary care

Suicide: High-Risk Features	Suicide: Lower-Risk Features
• **Patient:** male, older, single, isolated, low income/unemployed, FHx suicide • **Preparation:** letter, researched, tried to avoid rescue, violent method/high lethality (e.g. firearms, hanging) • **PMHx:** previous suicide attempt, severe depression, anorexia, substance misuse, haemodialysis • **Post event:** resists/tries to evade medical intervention, downplays seriousness of attempt, ongoing suicidal plans, no regret, wishes attempt had been successful	• **Patient:** female, young, good support systems • **Preparation:** nil, impulsive action in response to acute stressors, low perceived lethality, expected to be found, self-rescuing acts (e.g. told someone about attempt, called ambulance) • **Post event:** regretful of act, glad of intervention, no ongoing plans of suicide

The vignette describes EUPD; features must be pervasive and present for as long as the patient can remember. Suicide ideation may be chronic, with self-harm behaviours (e.g. cutting, overdoses) undertaken in times of acute emotional distress, as a way of managing distressing emotions. Assessing ongoing risk to self is vital (Table 171.2), as is excluding any psychiatric co-morbidity, such as depression. It can be helpful to remember the 'ABC of managing EUPD' – promoting Agency, maintaining Boundaries and being Consistent – to help negotiate a management plan with the patient.

REVISION TIPS

- Recommended psychological therapy for PTSD is EMDR or trauma-focused CBT
- Risk assess any patient with a mental health condition (risk to self, to others, to property, risk from others)

172

Threats to Harm Others

Alice Parker, Tom Nutting, and Chetna Kohli

EMERGENCY DEPARTMENT, FEMALE, 32. LIMB LACERATION

HPC: Broke a glass at the pub, cut dorsal aspect of her forearm. Shouted at the nurses, now stumbling up and down the department with clenched fists, threatening others for 'looking at her funny'. Claims she will hurt someone if a doctor doesn't see her immediately. Hospital security called. **PMHx:** None reported.

O/E: Smells strongly of alcohol, is slurring words. 5 cm laceration back of left forearm. No wound soiling/bleeding, no tendon/neurovascular injury.

1. Can you think of any organic medical causes of violence, other than delirium?
2. The patient in the vignette wants to discharge herself. What are your considerations?

Answers: 1. Thyroid dysfunction, dementia, brain tumour, temporal lobe epilepsy, head injury, CNS infection, electrolyte disturbance. 2. Capacity to make the decision – while she has a potential impairment (intoxication), she may have capacity to make the decision to leave without treatment. She must be able to understand the relevant information, retain and weigh it up, and then communicate it. Important information is the risk of infection, bleeding, retained glass and scarring. This injury is not immediately life-threatening.

TABLE 172.1

	Features	Investigations	Management
Acute alcohol intoxication	Slurred speech, ataxia, smell of alcohol, unusual behaviour, stupor, violence. *Withdrawal in chronic use*; nausea, sweating, seizure, delirium tremens (confusion, agitation, hallucinations, tremor, tachycardia, hypertension)	Ethanol levels – a negative finding can rule out alcohol intoxication as a differential. See *169. ADDICTION* for alcohol use disorder/withdrawal	De-escalation ± sedation. Prevent/treat withdrawal/Wernicke's encephalopathy: environment, benzodiazepines + parenteral thiamine. Drug and alcohol team if recurrent issue

(Continued)

TABLE 172.1 (Cont'd)

	Features	Investigations	Management
Anti-social personality disorder	Aggression, violence, frustration, minimal concern for others, impulsivity, criminality	More common in males and incarcerated individuals. Clinical diagnosis	De-escalation ± sedation. Psychotherapy, limited evidence for medication
Delirium	RFs: underlying cognitive impairment, infection, medication, constipation, urinary retention, pain, stress, stroke, MI, uraemia, hyponatraemia, hypo/hyperglycaemia, hypoxia, alcohol/substance misuse or withdrawal. Hx & O/E: acute change in cognition, attention, and consciousness, potential psychomotor disturbances (hyper-/hypo-active), emotional lability, altered sleep-wake cycle, psychotic features (hallucinations, delusions)	Clinical diagnosis. To rule out differentials: • FBC, U&Es, LFTs, glucose • Medication r/v • Bladder scan • Septic screen: lactate, CXR, urine output/cultures, blood cultures • Consider need for CT head	De-escalation ± careful sedation (anti-psychotics or benzodiazepines). Treat underlying cause. Medication review
Substance misuse (Fig. 172.1)	Unusual behaviour, acute psychosis, disturbed perception/cognition/affect, needle track marks, tachycardia, sweating, mydriasis	Usually stimulants: cocaine, amphetamine (patient may not divulge) Consider whether to r/o agitated delirium	De-escalation ± sedation. Benzodiazepines if agitated. Drug and alcohol team if recurrent issue
Psychosis	Hallucinations, thought disorders, delusions, passivity, low mood, anhedonia, flat affect, speech poverty, agitation and distress	Causes: transient psychotic episode, schizophrenia/schizoaffective, depression, bipolar disorder, drug-induced psychosis, delirium	De-escalation ± sedation. Risk assessment and referral to acute MH services. Consider anti-psychotic
Mania	Increased energy, elevated mood, irritability, decreased need for sleep, pressure of speech, flight of ideas, poor concentration, delusions, hallucinations, psychomotor agitation	Clinical diagnosis	De-escalation ± sedation. Risk assessment and referral to acute MH services

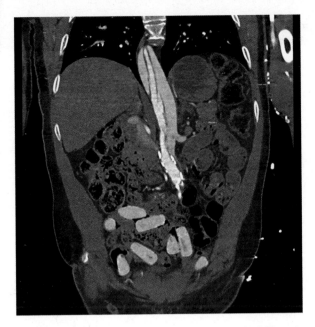

Fig. 172.1 Cocaine packets found in a 'body packer'. There is also an aortic dissection. (From Kévin, M, Dufayet, L, Nicolas, S, Charlotte, G, Dion, E. *Forensic Science International*. Elsevier; October 2021:Figure 2. © 2021 Elsevier B.V. All rights reserved.)

Interactions with violent patients are infrequent but potentially high risk. The vignette describes a laceration for which attempts should be made to give appropriate care (X-ray to exclude retained glass, wound washout/repair), where intervention is prevented. Hence, the primary consideration should be safety of the patient and staff/other patients. Many such patients can be de-escalated with conversation, which also aids capacity assessment for ongoing treatment. Early involvement of senior and security staff helps with safety – sedation is a last resort. The police are called if a violent patient presents a tangible threat to others.

REVISION TIPS

- Organic causes of altered mental state/aggression should always be considered
- Management of violence should initially involve de-escalation techniques – talking with the patient calmly, reassuring them and listening to their concerns, considering environment (noise, light, space, safety)
- Sedation is used as a last resort if patient/staff safety is compromised: lorazepam, promethazine, haloperidol (oral preferred, may require IM)

173

Abnormal Eating or Exercising Behaviour

Katie Turner, Alexander Royston, and Nwaorima Kamalu

HPC: Eating increasingly little for months, skipping meals, making excuses not to eat. Irritable and argumentative for a few months. LMP was 3 months ago (usually regular). Performs well in school, high achiever, but struggling to concentrate. Plays netball and hockey, runs in her spare time.

O/E: Appears thin (64% weight for height). Facial and conjunctival pallor. Thin brittle hair. Skin is dry with yellow tinge. BP 81/60 mmHg, HR 49 bpm. RR 14, SpO_2 98%.

1. How is BMI calculated? What BMI is classed as 'underweight'?
2. What are the risk factors for eating disorders?
3. What complications are most likely to be fatal in anorexia nervosa?

Answers: 1. BMI = weight (in kg) divided by height (in meters) squared. BMI <18.5 is classed as underweight. If anorexia nervosa and age <18, instead of BMI use *% weight for height* from centile chart (<90% is below therapy target). 2. Female sex, puberty, adolescence, obsessive and perfectionist traits, exposure to Western media. 3. Cardiac complications (e.g. arrhythmias, bradycardia).

TABLE 173.1

	Features	Investigations	Management
Anorexia nervosa (AN)	**RFs:** F > M, adolescence/puberty, obsessive/perfectionist traits. **Hx & O/E:** restrictive eating: fear of weight gain, body image disturbance. Low BMI. Constipation, dizzy/fainting, fatigue, cold intolerance, irritability, poor concentration, bradycardia, hypotension, amenorrhoea, hair loss, dry skin, lanugo (fine downy hair), hypercarotenaemia (yellow skin/sclera)	SUSS (SITUP-SQUAT STAND). FBC (pancytopenia), TFTs, U&Es ± ↓↓K (Fig. 173.1), LFTs, CK, CBG, Mg^{2+}, phosphate. Hormones (low, except GH, cortisol). VBG: hypochloraemic metabolic alkalosis (if vomiting). ECG (bradycardia, prolonged QTc, arrhythmias). May need medical monitoring or admission if physically unwell (Medical emergencies in eating disorders (MEED) guidelines- formerly MaRSiPAN)	Anorexia nervosa-focused family therapy for children and young people (FT-AN). Individual eating-disorder-focused CBT (CBT-ED). Maudsley Anorexia Nervosa Treatment for Adults (MANTRA). Specialist supportive clinical management (SSCM). Physical: food/meal plan with dietitian input, be aware of refeeding syndrome (see below). Supplements

TABLE 173.1 (Cont'd)

	Features	Investigations	Management
Bulimia nervosa	Binging then purging (vomiting, laxatives, excess exercise). Normal/overweight BMI. Bloating/fullness, lethargy, GORD, abdo pain, sore throat. Knuckle calluses (Russell's sign), dental enamel erosion, enlarged salivary glands, cardiomegaly	RFs: as anorexia nervosa. Investigate as above	May benefit from high dose fluoxetine (reduces purging frequency). Psychological therapies; CBT-ED. Bulimia nervosa-focused family therapy for children and young people (FT-BN)
Avoidant/ restrictive food intake disorder (ARFID)	Restrictive intake without body image disturbance/fear of weight gain. Nutritional deficiency. Limited range of preferred food: may avoid certain textures	RFs: ASD, ADHD, learning difficulties. Investigate as above	Desensitisation/exposure therapy, CBT, DBT, EMDR. Dietary counselling. Enteral feeding or oral nutritional supplements
'Diabulimia' (ED-DMT1)	Mis- or deliberate under-use of insulin to control weight. Results in frequent DKA	RFs: T1DM and a co-morbid eating disorder (usually AN). CBG	**Initial:** A-E. **Definitive:** MDT approach (endocrine/psychiatric)
Binge eating disorder	Recurrent binge eating (at least once a week) without compensatory behaviours (bulimia). Eating alone, until uncomfortably full, feeling guilt/ embarrassment after	RFs: obesity, FHx, abuse, MHI, frequent dieting. Clinical diagnosis. SCOFF questionnaire	Guided self-help. CBT
Pica	Eating non-food substances (e.g. dirt, stones, hair, paper)	RFs: developmental disabilities, pregnancy, psychosocial stress, malnutrition and hunger. Clinical diagnosis	Behavioural interventions and nutritional rehabilitation. Nutritional supplements
Key Complication Refeeding syndrome	Electrolyte/metabolic disturbance during refeeding. Oedema, tachycardia, seizures, ataxia, rhabdomyolysis. Leads to heart failure, arrhythmias, renal/liver impairment	High risk if little nutritional intake for >10 days or BMI <16. $\downarrow$K, $\downarrow$PO$_4$, $\downarrow$Mg	Monitor and correct U&Es, PO$_4$, Mg, bone profile daily (first 7 days). Forceval PO OD (10 days). Pabrinex 1–2 pairs IV OD (3 days), then thiamine/vitamin B Compound Strong PO

ED-DMT1, Eating disorder comorbid with type 1 diabetes.

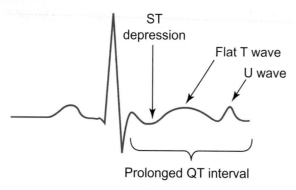

Hypokalemia

Fig. 173.1 Electrocardiographic changes in hypokalaemia. (From Pfennig, CL, Slovis, CM, Corey, M. Electrolyte disorders. In: *Rosen's Emergency Medicine: Concepts and Clinical Practice*, pp. 1525–1542.e2. Copyright © 2023 Elsevier Inc. All rights reserved.)

The vignette describes a life-threatening presentation of anorexia nervosa (exact severity depending on weight, intake, cognitions). The history is typical regarding age, gender, likely perfectionism and participation in sport. No features suggest bulimia (her BMI is reduced, no mention of vomiting/purging). The diagnosis is further supported by the amenorrhoea, irritability and reduced concentration. The finer details of the diagnosis in this case are less important than recognising that she is severely ill and at very high risk of death (indicated by the worrying cardiovascular signs of bradycardia and hypotension).

REVISION TIPS

- In AN, most things are low but G's and C's are raised; Growth hormone, salivary Glands, Cortisol, Cholesterol, Carotenaemia. Glucose; often low, can be high
- AN has the highest mortality rate of any psychiatric disorder

174

Mental Capacity Concerns – Outline

Margarita Fox and Tom Nutting

The Mental Capacity Act provides a legal framework for making decisions on behalf of people who lack the mental capacity to make decisions about their care themselves:

1. **Presume capacity**
2. Do not treat patients as unable to **make a decision** unless they have been fully **supported** in doing so without success
3. A perceived **unwise** decision does **not equate to lack of capacity**/inability to make a decision
4. Any decision made under the MCA on behalf of someone must be in their **best interest**
5. Any decision made must be the **least restrictive** option for a person's rights and freedom

TABLE 174.1

Examples Where Mental Capacity Concerns May Arise	Mental Capacity Act – Assessment of Capacity	Mental Capacity Act – Best Interests
Dementia Delirium Brain injury/stroke, etc. Unconsciousness (e.g. anaesthetic/sudden accident) Mental health conditions Intellectual disability	Capacity is decision and time specific. A person is considered as lacking capacity to make a specific decision if there is disturbance in the mind/brain, which may be permanent or temporary, AND they are unable to do any one of the following: – **Understand** the information – **Retain** the information (long enough to reach and communicate a decision) – **Weigh up** the information as part of decision-making – **Communicate** their decision (by any verbal or non-verbal means, e.g. blinking or squeezing a hand)	Consider: 1. Whether the decision can wait, if the person is likely to regain capacity 2. How to optimise their participation in the decision-making 3. Their past wishes, beliefs and values 4. Views of relevant people (family, carers) **Lasting powers of attorney (LPA):** person may appoint an attorney to act on their behalf and make health decisions should they subsequently lack capacity. **Advance directives:** person (with capacity) can specify treatments they would not want should they lose capacity. Can be verbal unless life-saving (in which case requires written witnessed-signed validation). Cannot demand treatment

(Continued)

TABLE 174.1 (Cont'd)	
How to manage patients who refuse treatment?	
Mental Capacity Act	Used for people who require treatment for physical conditions altering brain function and affecting capacity
Mental Health Act	Used for people who require treatment for severe mental health conditions, but who cannot or do not consent to admission to hospital and treatment for those purposes

REVISION TIPS

- Understand, retain, weigh up, communicate
- Capacity is decision and time specific
- In emergencies, you can perform medical interventions on unconscious (incapacitated) people if it is in their best interests and medically sound
- Attorney is only able to make decisions on life-sustaining treatment if the LPA specifies it

175

Polydipsia and Dehydration

Katherine Parker and Udaya Udayaraj

1. What symptoms would support severe CKD as the cause of polydipsia?
2. In which conditions can HbA1c not be used reliably for assessing diabetes mellitus?

Answers: 1. Anorexia, N&V, fatigue, weakness, pruritis, lethargy, peripheral oedema, insomnia, muscle cramps, nocturia, headache. 2. Those with high RBC turnover rates – haemolytic anaemia, haemoglobinopathies, untreated iron deficiency anaemia, children, HIV, CKD, pregnancy.

TABLE 175.1

	Features	Investigations	Management
Central/cranial diabetes insipidus (DI)	**RFs:** autoimmunity, intracranial tumour/surgery, head injury, granulomatous disease, infection, vascular, radiotherapy, congenital **Hx & O/E:** gradual onset (sometimes quick) polydipsia, polyuria. Dehydrated	Urine output: >3 L in a 24-hour urine collection. Urine dip: rule out DM. U&Es ($\uparrow Na^+$, $\downarrow K^+$), osmolality$\uparrow$, glucose (r/o DM), $\uparrow Ca^{2+}$. Urine osmolality$\downarrow$ Water deprivation test (under endocrinology supervision): failure to concentrate urine. Desmopressin stimulation test	Treat hypernatraemia if present. Desmopressin (PO, SL, nasal) – Na^+ monitoring (risk of hyponatraemia). ± contrast-enhanced MRI brain
Renal/nephrogenic DI	Causes: hypokalaemia, hypercalcaemia, drugs (lithium), relief of chronic urinary retention, cystic renal disease, sickle cell nephropathy, tubulo-interstitial disease (e.g. pyelonephritis), congenital **Hx & O/E:** polydipsia and polyuria, ± features of aetiology. Dehydrated		Acute, treat hypernatraemia if present. Correct underlying cause if possible, e.g. hypercalcaemia. Adequate fluid intake, salt restriction, thiazide diuretics

(Continued)

TABLE 175.1   (Cont'd)

	Features	Investigations	Management
Poorly controlled diabetes mellitus (DM)	*Type 1 (T1DM)* **RFs:** FH, autoimmune. **Hx & O/E:** polyuria, polydipsia, fatigue, unintentional weight loss, recurrent thrush/UTIs, poor wound healing, blurred vision	BM: hyperglycaemia. Urine dip: glucose (G) ± ketones. U&Es, ↑random/fasting G, ketones (↑/normal). Consider VBG (DKA). Diagnosis: symptoms + plasma G >11 mmol/L (random) or >7.0 (fasting) or HbA1c ≥48, *or measurements above on two separate occasions.*	Same-day referral to diabetes team. Education + insulin. RF modification, check complications
	Type 2 (T2DM) **RFs:** age >40, FH, non-Caucasian, PCOS, overweight, inactivity, metabolic syndrome. **Hx & O/E:** asymptomatic, or like T1DM but chronic onset. Maybe complications at presentation. Acanthosis nigricans	If borderline, OGTT. Consider C-peptide - low in T1DM	Education + oral hypoglycemic agents/insulin. RF modification, check complications
Diabetic ketoacidosis (DKA)	**RFs:** infection, physiological stress (e.g. MI, surgery), non-adherence to insulin, drugs (steroids, diuretics, atypical anti-psychotics). **Hx & O/E:** D&V, anorexia, abdo pain, visual disturbance, confusion. Pear-drops breath, Kussmaul breathing, ±shock	Hyperglycaemia, ketosis, acidosis. Urine: 2+ketones, +G. VBG (acidosis pH < 7, ↑K⁺, ↑osmolality), ↑glucose (>11.0), ↑ketones (>3 mmol), U&Es (electrolyte imbalance). ECG: hyperkalaemia (Fig. 175.1) or precipitating MI	Emergency admission. Fluids IV NaCl + insulin (0.1 unit/kg/hr). Monitor serum K⁺ and add to fluids once <5.5 (never in first hour of rehydration). Education
Psychogenic polydipsia	**RFs:** developmental disability, anxiety, psychological co-morbidities, e.g. schizophrenia. **Hx & O/E:** water seeking, excess drinking. Clinically euvolaemic	Urinalysis: NAD. U&Es: hyponatraemia, normal urea, low serum osmolality. Urine low osmolality. Supervised water deprivation test: normal	Behavioural ± ß-blocker, anti-psychotic, ARB (e.g. candesartan). Treat hyponatraemia
Medications	Ecstasy, diuretics, SGLT2 inhibitors (e.g. canagliflozin)		

Key Complications

Dehydration	Poor intake, diarrhoea/vomiting, diuretic. **Hx & O/E:** low skin turgor, dry mucous membranes, hypotension, reduced urine output	U&E: disproportionately high urea, hypo/hypernatremia. VBG: ↑lactate, metabolic alkalosis (vomiting) or acidosis (diarrhoea)	A–E, raise legs. Fluid boluses. ITU support with inotropes

PROTOCOL FOR MANAGEMENT OF ADULT PATIENTS WITH DIABETIC KETOACIDOSIS (DKA)

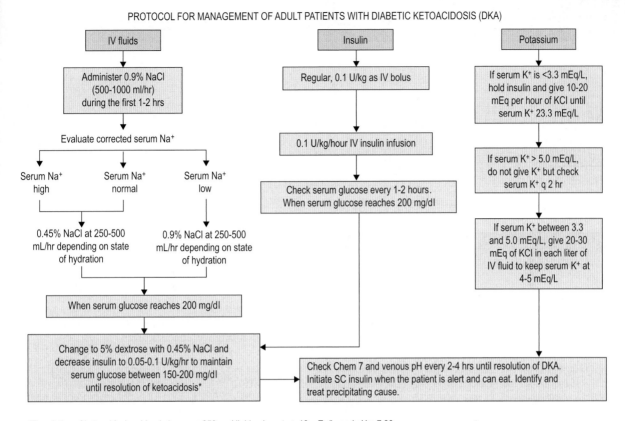

*Resolution of ketoacidosis = blood glucose < 250 mg/dl, bicarbonate > 18 mEq/L, and pH > 7.30.

Fig. 175.1 Protocol for management of adult patients with diabetic ketoacidosis. (From From Pasquel FJ, et al. Hyperglycemic crisis: diabetic ketoacidosis and hyperglycemic hyperosmolar state. In: Jameson JL, et al., eds. *Endocrinology: Adult and Pediatric.* 7th ed. Elsevier;2016:805–15, Figure 46-2.)

In diabetes insipidus (DI) the kidneys cannot concentrate urine and produce copious dilute urine (polyuria), forcing patients to drink large quantities of water (polydipsia) to avoid severe dehydration. The water deprivation test detects inability to concentrate urine; no fluids for 8 hours (or until 3% reduction in body weight), with serum osmolality, urine volume and urine osmolality measured hourly. Urine osmolality normally rises to >700 mOsm/kg, but in DI it remains <300 mOsm/kg with serum osmolality >290 mOsm/kg. Anti-diuretic hormone (ADH), also known as arginine vasopressin (AVP), is normally produced in the hypothalamus and secreted by the pituitary gland (posterior part). Cranial DI is a failure to produce ADH and nephrogenic DI is a failure by the kidneys to respond to it. After desmopressin (ADH analogue) given intramuscularly or intranasally, urine becomes concentrated in cranial DI but stays dilute in nephrogenic. The most likely diagnosis in the vignette is nephrogenic DI secondary to lithium use.

REVISION TIPS

- Patients with diabetes insipidus are at risk of hypernatraemia
- Polydipsia in pregnancy – consider gestational diabetes

176

Acute Kidney Injury and Oliguria

Harriet Diment and Udaya Udayaraj

GENERAL MEDICAL WARD, MALE, 54.
REDUCED URINE OUTPUT FOR 24 HOURS

HPC: Community-acquired pneumonia, admitted 2 days ago with productive cough, temperature 38.5°C. Presented hypotensive, fluid boluses to stabilise BP. Poor oral intake. Catheterised. **PMHx:** HTN. **DHx:** Ramipril 10 mg OD (recently increased from 5 mg), ibuprofen 400 mg QDS, co-amoxiclav 1.2 g TDS IV.

O/E: Reduced skin turgor, dry mucous membranes. BP 115/70. **Ix:** On admission; Urea 7, Cr 100, eGFR 62. 48 hours later; Urea 8, Cr 142, eGFR 37.

1. What is the most likely problem in the vignette?
2. What differentials should be considered if renal failure is identified in a;
   a. 70-year-old man with a history of poor urinary flow and a palpable bladder?
   b. 12-year-old boy with a recent history of cough, presenting with haematuria?

Answers: 1. See commentary. 2a. Post-renal cause of acute kidney injury (AKI) due to BPE causing chronic urinary retention and hydronephrosis. 2b. IgA nephropathy (Berger disease) can follow a viral URTI

TABLE 176.1

	Features	Investigations	Management
Pre-Renal – Impaired Perfusion			
Reduced circulating volume	Haemorrhage. See *42. SHOCK AND LOW BLOOD PRESSURE*		
	Dehydration. See *175. POLYDIPSIA AND DEHYDRATION*		
	Burns injury. See *55. BURNS*		
	Heart failure, cardiogenic shock. See *42. SHOCK AND LOW BLOOD PRESSURE*		
Reduced vascular resistance	**Sepsis:** pyrexia, infection, hypotension (if shock)	**SEPSIS 6:** *Give 3-* high-flow oxygen, IV Abx, fluid challenge; *Take 3-* blood cultures, blood lactate, monitor urine output	
Renal vasoconstriction	**Hepatorenal syndrome:** end-stage liver disease (cirrhosis, liver failure). Jaundice, ascites, encephalopathy. (Exclude spontaneous bacterial peritonitis)	LFTs: ↑↑ALT, ↑ALP (ALT > AST), ↑bilirubin, low albumin. Clotting: ↑PT. Hypoglycaemia	Trial of diuretics, correct electrolytes. Human albumin solution + terlipressin. Renal replacement therapy. Consider liver transplant.
	Drugs: NSAIDs, ACEi, ARB, diuretics	Drug chart review	Stop nephrotoxic drugs

TABLE 176.1 (Cont'd)

	Features	Investigations	Management
Renal – Damage to Functional Units			
Glomerular disease (GD)	**GD with nephrotic syndrome:** proteinuria, oedema (general), hyperlipidaemia, hypoalbuminaemia, thrombosis- high risk. Causes: minimal change disease (MCD), membranous nephropathy (MN), focal segmental glomerulosclerosis (FSGS). **GD with haematuria** (visible or non-visible): thin basement membrane disease (TBMD), IgA nephropathy, Alport sy. **GD with AKI:** post-streptococcal glomerulonephritis (PSGN), rapidly progressive glomerulonephritis. May progress to ESRF	*Kidney biopsy* **GD with nephrotic syndrome:** urinalysis-proteinuria. Hypoalbuminaemia, hyperlipidaemia. **GD with haematuria:** Urinalysis: nephritic sediment. ↑urea/creatinine/CRP. **GD with AKI:** Urinalysis: haematuria, proteinuria. Autoimmune panel	**GD with nephrotic syndrome** MCD and FSGS: oral prednisolone. MN: tacrolimus/ cyclophosphamide/rituximab. **GD with haematuria** TBMD: no active treatment usually. IgA nephropathy: CKD Mx. Consider immunosuppression. Alport syndrome: CKD Mx. **GD with AKI** PSGN: self-limiting. RPGN: cyclophosphamide, rituximab, steroids ± plasmapheresis
Interstitial kidney damage	**Nephrotoxins:** radiocontrast, aminoglycoside, NSAIDs, chemotherapy (e.g. cisplatin), lithium, myoglobin (rhabdomyolysis), PPI (acute interstitial nephritis)	Drug levels (trough and peak). Rhabdomyolysis: ↑ CK, urine may be red-brown	Fluids. Stop drug/titrate to therapeutic range. Steroids in drug-induced interstitial nephritis
	Pyelonephritis: flank/loin pain, rigors, fever, vomiting, dysuria, frequency, urgency	CRP ↑. Urine dip: nitrites, leukocytes. Urine MC&S: culture positive	Fluids, antibiotics (cefalexin/ ciprofloxacin /co-amoxiclav/ trimethoprim)
	Small vessel vasculitis: fever, lethargy, myalgia, anorexia, dyspnoea, haemoptysis	ANCA (anti PR3/MPO), anti-GBM/PR3/MPO. Renal biopsy (crescents, necrotising GN). CXR: pulmonary haemorrhage	High-dose steroids. Plasma exchange + cyclophosphamide/rituximab
	Haemolytic uraemic syndrome. *Children:* haematuria, bloody diarrhoea. *Adults* (atypical HUS: do complement mutation analysis)	Hb <100 (normocytic), ↑LDH, low platelets, low eGFR, low haptoglobins. Urine: proteinuria. Stool: toxigenic *E. coli* O157. Blood film: schistocytes	Supportive: fluids. Renal replacement therapy, plasma exchange/eculizumab for atypical HUS

(Continued)

TABLE 176.1 (Cont'd)

	Features	Investigations	Management
Vessel damage	**Thrombotic thrombocyto-penic purpura:** headaches, seizures, confusion, coma, fever (Fig. 176.1)	Hb <100 (normocytic), low platelets, ↑creatinine. Low ADAMTS13 activity	Haematological emergency. Plasma exchange: replace ADAMTS13. Corticosteroids
	Disseminated intravascular coagulation: bruising, bleeding from venepuncture site	↑PT/APTT/D-dimer, low platelets/fibrinogen. Blood film: schistocytes	Treat cause (malignancy, sepsis, trauma, obstetric emergency). Platelets, cryoprecipitate, FFP
	Malignant hypertension – See *7. HYPERTENSION*		
Post-Renal – Urine Obstruction			
Ureteric obstruction	**Ureteric stone** (stone with single functioning kidney, stone with urosepsis). **Hx & O/E:** colic (loin to groin), N&V, haematuria, anuria	Urine dipstick: +blood, proteinuria, +white cells. Urine MC&S – rule out infection. Non-contrast CT KUB: visualise stones	Fluids, analgesia. Fever – Abx (cephalosporin/ quinolone/gentamicin). Anuric/infected: urgent nephrostomy/stent. Treat stone; see *196. LOIN PAIN*
Urethral obstruction	See *195. ANURIA AND ACUTE OR CHRONIC URINARY RETENTION*		
Key Complication			
Acute tubular necrosis	Prolonged hypoperfusion, nephrotoxicity (drugs, radio-contrast, rhabdomyolysis, lead)	Muddy brown casts in urine	Poor response to fluid challenge. Dialysis

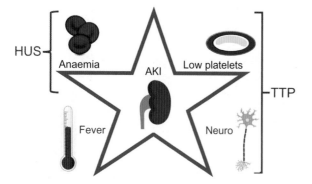

Fig. 176.1 The triad of features of haemolytic uraemic syndrome (HUS) overlaps with the pentad of thrombotic thrombocytopenic purpura (TTP).

In the vignette, sepsis reduces renal perfusion (low vascular resistance/ renal autoregulation redistribute blood, so renal blood flow is less than systolic BP suggests- especially with PMHx of HTN). Dehydration/ ACE-i/ NSAIDs drop glomerular filtration further, causing AKI (tubular necrosis, ± tubulo-interstitial nephritis/papillary necrosis with NSAIDs). In AKI, review medications; 1. Worse AKI (ACE-i, ARB, NSAID, amino-glycoside, diuretic), 2. Drug toxicity (metformin, lithium, digoxin). Aspirin 75 mg (cardioprotective dose) is safe.

REVISION TIPS

- Suspect an AKI in patients with a reduction in urine output and/or a rise in serum creatinine
- Common causes of AKI include sepsis, hypovolaemia and drugs
- Indications for dialysis – remember AEIOU (Acidosis, Electrolytes, Intoxication, Overload, Uraemia)

177

Chronic Kidney Disease

Alice Parker and Laura Skinner

HPC: Tired most of the day, despite adequate sleep. Previously active, no weight loss or red flag symptoms. **PMHx:** Hypertension for 25 years. **DHx:** Amlodipine 10 mg OD, ramipril 10 mg OD.

O/E: HR 72, RR 15, SpO_2 99%, BP 150/95. Appears pale. Chest/abdo unremarkable. **Ix:** Hb 107 MCV 93. ESR 2. eGFR 29, creatinine 137. ALT 20, AST 34, ALP 70, bilirubin 10. Fasting glucose: 5. TSH 4, T4 80. Urine dipstick: protein ++, blood +. MSU: negative for infection. ACR: 24 mg/mmol. 3 months later: eGFR 29, ACR 29 mg/mmol.

1. What are the three types of renal replacment therapy (RRT)?
2. What are the two main clinical signs of hypocalcaemia?

Answers: 1. Haemodialysis, peritoneal dialysis, transplant. 2. Trousseau sign (spasm with inflated BP cuff), Chvostek sign (facial tapping causes spasm).

TABLE 177.1

	Features	Investigations	Management
Hypertension	Long history of hypertension, poorly controlled	Target systolic <140 mmHg and diastolic <90. If ACR is ≥70 mg/mmol, target systolic BP <130, diastolic <80. ACEi/ARB if diabetic with ACR ≥3, or non-diabetic and ACR ≥30, or age <55 years non-black ethnicity. Calcium channel blocker if age >55 or black	
Diabetes mellitus	Most common cause of CKD	Fasting glucose, HbA1c	Optimise glucose control. Target BP <130/80 ACEi/ARB, ± sodium glucose co-transporter 2 (SGLT-2) inhibitor in T2DM (dapagliflozin)
Glomerulonephritis	E.g. Hx of IgA nephropathy, myeloma, SLE, minimal change disease. See *176. ACUTE KIDNEY INJURY AND OLIGURIA*	ANA, ANCA, anti-dsDNA, anti-GBM, anti-phospholipid, paraprotein, complement, cryoglobulin, hepatitis serology. Bence Jones	Treat underlying cause. Manage CKD (see commentary). Consider renal biopsy

(Continued)

TABLE 177.1   (Cont'd)

	Features	Investigations	Management
Renal artery stenosis	Treatment-resistant hypertension, flash (sudden onset) pulmonary oedema	CT or MR angiography	Statins, aspirin, anti-hypertensives. NOTE: in bilateral stenosis, ACE-i/ARB will worsen renal function
Pyelonephritis	History of frequent UTIs	Urine dipstick, MC&S. USS (renal scarring)	Treat UTIs. Manage CKD
Vesicoureteric reflux	May describe loin pain when voiding	USS (hydronephrosis if severe). MCUG	Urological referral
Urinary tract dysfunction	Chronic retention, recurrent bilateral kidney/ureteric stones, neurogenic bladder	USS (hydronephrosis). Urine dipstick, MC&S	Urological referral
Adult polycystic kidney disease	FHx of kidney disease or SAH. Autosomal dominant. HTN, haematuria, UTIs, abdominal mass, flank pain, aneurysms, liver cysts	Abdominal USS. Screening (USS, genetics if indicated)	Manage hypertension/CKD. Consider vaptans, e.g. tolvaptan
Previous acute kidney injury (AKI)	See *176. ACUTE KIDNEY INJURY AND OLIGURIA*		
Nephrotoxic drugs	E.g. ACE inhibitors, ARBs, cyclosporin, tacrolimus, diuretic, NSAIDs, lithium		Review medications
Key Complications Anaemia	Due to reduced EPO. **Hx & O/E:** fatigue, SOB, pallor, palpitations	FBC ($\downarrow$Hb: normochromic, normocytic)	Iron/B12/folate supplementation. Erythropoietin
Hypertension	Kidneys regulate BP control	BP	ACE-inhibitor (or ARB). Target BP <130/80
Cardiovascular disease	Most common cause of mortality in CKD	Lipid profile	Stop smoking, BP control, low-dose aspirin, atorvastatin 20mg
Renal osteodystrophy	Osteomalacia, bone pain, fractures, hypocalcaemia (tetany, lethargy, perioral paraesthesia, depression)	Secondary hyper-PTH ($\uparrow$PTH, $\downarrow$Ca^{2+}, $\uparrow$PO$_4$). X-ray: osteopenia, Looser's zones, salt and pepper skull	Restrict dietary phosphate, phosphate binders. Vitamin D, calcium supplements
Oedema	SOB, peripheral oedema	Pulmonary oedema on CXR ('bat's wing' appearance)	Fluid and sodium restriction. Loop diuretics (increased doses due to resistance)
Acidosis	N&V, anorexia	VBG/ABG	Oral bicarbonate supplements if serum bicarbonate <20mmol/L
Restless legs syndrome	Tingling/aching sensations in limbs, urge to move	Hb, ferritin (iron deficiency worsens symptoms)	Treat anaemia. Dopamine agonist (pramipexole), pregabalin/gabapentin

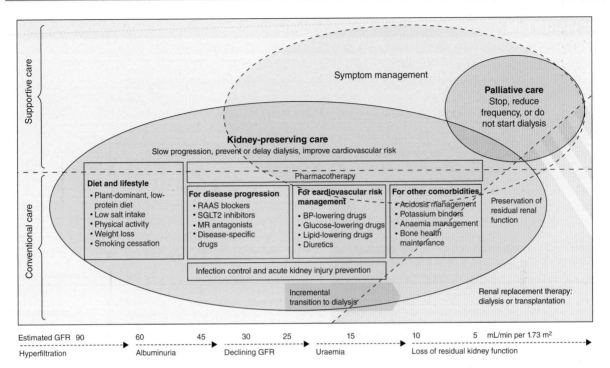

Fig. 177.1 The role of preservative management and its goals (green domain) within the overall conservative management of chronic kidney disease without dialysis (blue zone), and with renal replacement therapy (yellow zone). (Reprinted with permission from Kalantar-Zadeh K, Jafar TH, Nitsch D, Neuen BL, Perkovic V. Chronic kidney disease. *Lancet.* Aug 28 2021;398(10302):786–802.

*Kidney Disease Improving Global Outcomes (KDIGO) define CKD as sustained eGFR of <60 and/or markers of kidney damage, such as proteinuria (including micro- albuminuria, defined by ACR of 3-30mg/mmol, which can be dipstick negative for protein), for ≥3 months. CKD may be asymptomatic until end-stage, then developing lethargy, pallor, oedema, pruritus (see **82. PRURITIS**). Investigations: creatinine, eGFR, urinary ACR, urine dipstick and MC&S. On USS, kidneys are usually small, but hydronephrosis (post-renal mechanism) may be iden- tified. Do renal biopsy if rapidly progressive disease or unknown cause. Congenital causes of CKD include reflux nephropathy, hypoplasia, Alport syndrome and Fabry disease. Treatment; control HTN/ glucose, diet, monitor renal function, exercise/ smoking cessation, review drugs. End stage; statin ± antiplatelet, treat complications. RRT if GFR <10/ refractory. Complications of haemodialysis*

commonly include hypotension, cramps, arrhythmias, arteriovenous fistula problems (thrombosis, stenosis, steal syndrome) and vascular catheter problems (infec- tion, blockage). Rare issues include anaphylaxis, heparin- induced thrombocytopoenia, and those occurring in newly initiated/non-concordant patients, e.g. dialysis disequilibrium syndrome. Complications of peritoneal dialysis include peritonitis, loss of membrane func- tion, hernia or infection of catheter site. Complications of transplant include bleeding, thrombosis, infection, rejection, delayed function or malignancy due to immu- nosuppression. Treatment priorities include kidney pres- ervation and symptom management (Fig. 177.1). In the vignette, investigations identified low eGFR and normo- cytic anaemia; the 3-month timescale enables diagnosis of CKD, eGFR of 44 indicates stage 3B (see REVISION TIPS).

REVISION TIPS

- CKD is sustained eGFR of <60 ± proteinuria (ACR >3 mg/mmol) for at least 3 months
- The most common causes of CKD are diabetes mellitus and hypertension
- IgA nephropathy is Berger disease (not Buerger disease, which is thromboangiitis obliterans)
- Stages of CKD:

Stage	eGFR (mL/min/1.73 m^2)
1	>90 with evidence of kidney damage*
2	60–89 with evidence of kidney damage*
3A	45–59
3B	30–44
4	15–29
5	<15 (indication for RRT)

*Raised ACR, urine sediment abnormalities, electrolyte abnormalities due to tubular disorders, abnormal anatomy or histology, systemic disease or history of renal transplant (KDIGO)

Electrolyte Abnormalities – Overview Table

Zoe Kay and Judith Fox

TABLE 178.1

	Causes	Presentation	Watch out for...
Calcium↑>2.6 mmol/L *Normal adjusted serum calcium: 2.2–2.6 mmol/L (adjusted for albumin level)*	Hyperparathyroidism or malignancy (together cause 90%)	Polydipsia and polyuria. Bone pain, renal calculi. Abdo pain/constipation/ pancreatitis. Depression/psychosis/ decreased GCS	Patients may be severely dehydrated. With low PTH, exclude malignancy. ECG: short QT interval (risk of VF and arrest), Osborne waves
Calcium↓ <2.2 mmol/L	Hypoparathyroidism, transfusion (*citrate in packed RBCs binds Ca²⁺*), vitamin D deficiency (e.g. CRF), hypoalbuminemia	Neuromuscular excitability (**Trousseau/ Chvostek** signs, tetany), seizures	ECG: long QT interval (may lead to torsades de pointes)
Phosphate↑ >1.3 mmol/L *(Normal range 0.8–1.3 mmol/L)*	Renal failure. Drugs: diuretics, laxatives, bisphosphonates. Endocrine: thyrotoxicosis, hypoparathyroidism. Cell lysis: rhabdomyolysis, haemolysis, tumour lysis	Reduced bone resorption, low vitamin D, tetany, hyperreflexia, seizures	Associated with **hypocalcaemia.** ECG: long QT interval (↓Ca)
Phosphate↓<0.8 mmol/L	Malnutrition. Insulin infusion (DKA). Refeeding syndrome. ↑*Losses* /↓*absorption*; diuresis, hyperparathyroid, diarrhoea, burns, sweating, bleeding	Mild: asymptomatic, fatigue. Severe <0.32 mmol/L: SOB, lethargy, cognitive, cardiomyopathy, shock	Cautious nourishment if at risk of refeeding syndrome – usually none
Sodium↑ >146 mmol/L) *(133–146 mmol/L)*	Dehydration, poor urine concentration (DI, renal), primary hyperaldosteronism/Conn syndrome, iatrogenic (e.g. IVI with 0.9% NaCl)	Thirst, lethargy, confusion, ataxia, neurological signs, seizures, coma	**Correct slowly to avoid cerebral oedema.** ECG: nil specific
Sodium↓ <133 mmol/L)	See *179. HYPONATRAEMIA*		

(Continued)

TABLE 178.1   (Cont'd)

	Causes	Presentation	Watch out for...
Potassium↑>5.5 mmol/L (3.5–5.5 mmol/L)	See *180. HYPERKALAEMIA*		
Potassium↓<3.5 mmol/L	**Drugs** (diuretics), **GI losses** (D&V). Other: TPN, poor care during NBM, burns, sweating, refeeding syndrome; renal loss, e.g. Conn syndrome, cellular shifts, e.g. insulin therapy in DKA	Lethargy, weakness, constipation, paralysis, paraesthesia, tetany, cardiac sequelae	Often with **hypomagnesaemia:** predisposes to VF and VT. ECG: large P waves, long PR, ST depression, flat/inverted T waves, U wave formation. Severe: ectopic beats, tachyarrhythmias, VF
Magnesium↑>1.10 mmol/L (0.85–1.10 mmol/L)	**Iatrogenic** (laxative, PPIs, IV supplementation for acute asthma/Torsades), **renal failure** or **transcellular shifts** (rhabdomyolysis, tumour lysis syndrome)	Usually well tolerated. N&V, weakness. Cardiorespiratory arrest (Mg^{2+} >6.0 mmol/L)	Usually self resolves if normal renal function. ECG: PR and QT prolongation. Severe: AV block
Magnesium↓<0.85 mmol/L	**↓Intake/uptake:** TPN, malnutrition, chronic alcohol, PPIs, surgical small bowel removal. **↑Losses:** D&V, diuretics, Gitelman's, burns	Neuromuscular: weakness, tremor, paraesthesia Symptoms of reduced Ca^{2+}/K^+	**Concurrent hypocalcaemia and hypokalaemia.** ECG: PR and QT prolongation. Predisposes to ventricular arrhythmias
Chloride↑>109 mmol/L (96–109 mmol/L)	**Saline infusion,** TPN. Water loss: diabetes insipidus, diuresis, burns, diarrhoea, renal disease	Nil specific	**Often hyperchloremic metabolic acidosis** (normal anion gap). Nil specific on ECG
Chloride↓<96 mmol/L	Drugs: laxatives, diuretics, hypotonic fluids. sweating, diuresis, **vomiting.** Dilution: CCF, SIADH	Usually presents alongside ↓Na: similar symptoms	Associated with **sodium losses** - sodium retained at level of Na+/H+ transporter, so **metabolic alkalosis.** Nil specific on ECG

REVISION TIPS

- Learn the progressive ECG changes in hyperkalaemia, they are easily tested. See *180. HYPERKALAEMIA*
- Hypokalaemia/calcaemia are difficult to reverse in the presence of hypomagnesaemia
- Commonly examined syndromes: hyponatraemia, hypercalcaemia, hyperkalaemia

- In resistant cases of hypokalaemia or hypocalcaemia, **check the magnesium**
- Drugs will <u>not</u> work in hypothermia until the patient is warm
- Be aware of electrolyte movements into cells with **insulin** therapy

179

Hyponatraemia

Katherine Parker and Judith Fox

EMERGENCY DEPARTMENT, MALE, 68. COLLAPSE, NOW CONFUSED AND DISORIENTATED

HPC: Witnessed by daughter; fell to the ground, all four limbs jerking, incontinent of urine, duration <2 minutes, happened 20 minutes ago. Getting forgetful recently, spends much of the day sleeping. **PMHx:** Metastatic lung cancer (small cell), hypertension, hypercholesterolaemia. **DHx:** Statin, ramipril. **SHx:** 70 pack-year history. Retired chef.

O/E: Cachectic, post-ictal. Obs: HR 70, BP 155/86 mmHg, RR 12, PO$_2$ 99% (air), GCS 11 (E3V3M5), T 36.7°C. CVS/Resp: I + II + 0, JVP normal, mucous membranes moist, no oedema, not hypervolaemic. **Ix:** Na$^+$ 117 mmol/L (135–145), K$^+$ 4.0 mmol/L (3.5–5.0), plasma osmolality 245 mOsmol/kg (274–295). Urine: Osmolality 400 mOsm/kg (50–1200 mOsm/kg), Na$^+$ 45 mOsm/kg

1. Which tests should be done to confirm SIADH as the most likely cause in the vignette?
2. Which other paraneoplastic syndromes are associated with small-cell lung cancer (SCLC)? How would they present?
3. What are some of the other causes of SIADH?

Answers: 1. U&Es, uric acid, serum/urine osmolality, thyroid function tests, random/early morning cortisol and review of medications. 2. ACTH: Cushingoid features. Lambert Eaton myasthenic syndrome: limb weakness that improves with exercise. 3. Neurological: GBS, MS, SLE, ICH. Pulmonary: pneumonia, mesothelioma, TB. Other malignancies: oropharyngeal, stomach, pancreas, leukaemia, lymphoma. Drugs: thiazides, SSRIs, ACE inhibitors, loop diuretics.

TABLE 179.1

	Features	Investigations	Management
Pseudohyponatraemia (hypertriglyceridaemia/ hyperproteinaemia [multiple myeloma])	Hyperlipidaemia, diabetes, CVD, raised BMI, xanthoma. Asymptomatic.	Isotonic/normal serum osmolality (275–295 mOsmol/kg). ↑Fasting triglycerides	Artefact: treat root cause, Contact lab to test sample for sodium in a different way
Hyperosmolar hyponatraemia	PMHx DM, or DKA. Head injury patient on mannitol infusion	Hypertonic/high-serum osmolality (>295 mOsmol/kg). ↑Blood glucose, ↑HbA1c	Artefact – none required

(Continued)

TABLE 179.1 (Cont'd)

	Features	Investigations	Management
Hypovolaemic hyponatraemia			
General points	Tachycardia, postural hypotension, dry skin/mucous membranes, low urine output, decreased JVP, reduced skin turgor, thirst. **Serum osmolarity <275 mOsmol/kg.** Repeat to assess rapidity of change. **Urinary sodium: above or below 20 mmol/L.**		
↓Urinary Na – extra-renal losses	D&V, fistula, sweating, burns, cerebral salt wasting, third space losses, e.g. small bowel obstruction (SBO), pancreatitis, sepsis, ± hypotonic replacement of fluid loss	**Urinary sodium ≤ 20 mmol/L.** Consider: ↑lipase/amylase (pancreatitis), abdominal XR for SBO	Acute symptomatic hyponatraemia is an **emergency:** 1. Correct underlying cause 2. Hypertonic (3%) saline to *gradually* correct, monitor Na⁺ 2 hourly. Correction no more than 6 mmol/L in 6 hours <u>OR</u> 10 mmol/L in 24 hours. **Risk of osmotic demyelination if corrected too rapidly**
↑ Urinary Na – renal losses	Primary adrenal insufficiency (Addison's), renal failure, diuretics (thiazides)	**Urinary sodium >20 mmol/L** Consider: short synacthen test, serum renin/aldosterone, urine ACR	
Hypervolaemic Hyponatraemia **General points**	**Interstitial overload/retention:** peripheral, sacral and pulmonary oedema (SOB, crackles, wet cough), fatigue, ascites, weight gain, raised JVP. **Serum osmolarity <275 mOsm/kg:** repeat to assess rapidity of change. **Urine sodium** (low in fluid overload: hyponatraemia often dilution, not loss of sodium)		
Liver cirrhosis	Urine sodium ≤30 mmol/L. LFT (AST/ALT >1), ↑GGT, ↓Albumin, ↑PT, ↓PLT HBV, HCV screening		1. Treat underlying cause 2. Fluid restriction (1000 mL/day) ± diuretic 3. Vaptan (nonpeptide vasopressin receptor antagonist) if fluid restriction fails
Nephrotic syndrome (*aetiology and risk factors vary*)	Urine sodium ≤30 mmol/L. **Urine dip:** protein ++. ↓Albumin, ↑lipids, clotting (may be deranged), FBC, U&Es. Screen for causes		
Chronic congestive cardiac failure	Urine sodium ≤30 mmol/L. ↑BNP. **ECG** (left axis deviation), **transthoracic echoCG,** **CXR** (cardiomegaly, pleural effusion)		
Renal failure	Urine sodium high or low. U/Es, clotting, ↓vitamin D, ↓calcium, ↓Hb		

TABLE 179.1 (Cont'd)

	Features	Investigations	Management
Euvolaemic Hyponatraemia			
Syndrome of inappropriate anti-diuresis (SIAD)	Malignant, neurological, pulmonary, medications. **Diagnosis of exclusion**	Urine sodium >30 mmol/L, osmolality >100 mOsm/kg. Normal thyroid and adrenal function. ↓Uric acid	Fluid restriction (500–1000 mL/day – adults). Consider demeclocycline (ADH antagonist)
Severe hypothyroidism	Urine sodium >30 mmol/L, osmolality >100 mOsm/kg. TFTs (↓free T4, TSH ↓/↑)		Levothyroxine
Secondary adrenal insufficiency	Chronic steroids, anti-psychotics, trauma, radiotherapy, surgery, neoplasm. Hx & O/E: fatigue, weak, anorexia, N&V, weight loss, hypotension, hypoglycaemia	Urine sodium >30 mmol/L, osmolality >100 mOsm/kg. ↓Random/morning serum cortisol, Short Synacthen test	Hydrocortisone. Supportive measures
Medications	Thiazides, SSRIs, carbamazepine, risperidone, sulphonylureas, TCAs	Urine sodium >30 mmol/L, osmolality >100 mOsm/kg	Cessation of medication
Water overload (iatrogenic or psychogenic polydipsia)	Psychiatric history (psychogenic polydipsia), long admission. Nocturia	Urine sodium <30 mmol/L, osmolality 50–100 mosm/L	
Key Complications			
Cerebral oedema and brain herniation	Rapid fall in sodium concentration (<48 hours) leading to symptoms of hyponatraemia. More common in younger patients/children		
Central pontine myelinolysis/ osmotic demyelination syndrome	Rapid correction of hyponatraemia. Risk greater if severe/chronic hyponatraemia. Rapid normalisation of extracellular osmolarity (cell shrinkage, demyelination, irreversible axonal damage); dysarthria, dysphagia, paraparesis, quadriparesis, seizures, confusion, coma		

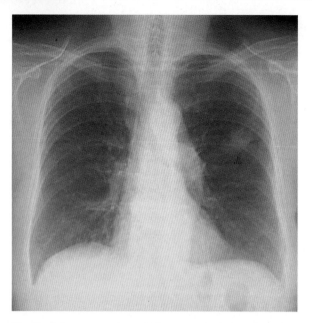

Fig. 179.1 Lung cancer (*arrow*). (From Edward C. Klatt. Chapter 5: The lungs. In: *Robbins and Cotran Atlas of Pathology*. 2020. Copyright © 2020. Elsevier Inc. All rights reserved.)

Hyponatraemia is Na⁺ <135 mmol/L; the most likely cause in the vignette is SIADH due to SCLC (smoker) (Fig. 179.1). He had a seizure, with a new finding of sodium of 117 mmol/L. SCLC originates from neuroendocrine cells, which is why it has a variety of paraneoplastic effects. It commonly metastasises, so CT head is needed to exclude cerebral metastases. Acute management should include hypertonic saline to reduce risk of further seizures.

REVISION TIPS

- Symptoms vary according to severity, **rate of onset**, CNS stability and comorbidities
  - MILD: nausea, vomiting, anorexia, malaise
  - MODERATE: headache, confusion, irritability, ataxia
  - SEVERE: drowsiness, seizures, non-cardiogenic pulmonary oedema, coma, death
- **Acute onset <48 hours**; more severe, greater risk of cerebral oedema
- **Chronic onset** (>48 hours or unknown), less severe
- New diagnosed Addison's is an emergency

180

Hyperkalaemia

Zoe Kay, David Roberts, and Alexander Reed

EMERGENCY DEPARTMENT, MALE, 72. GENERALLY UNWELL

HPC: Malaise, nausea, weakness, breathless, cough, intermittent palpitations. **PMHx:** IHD, CCF, T2DM, hypertension. **DHx:** Ramipril, amlodipine, aspirin, bisoprolol, atorvastatin, furosemide, spironolactone, GTN spray.

O/E: Bounding peripheral pulses with regular rhythm, HR 110, heart sounds quiet. Left lower zone coarse crackles. Abdomen SNT, no ascites. Pitting oedema to mid ankle. Neuro: global hyporeflexia. **Ix:** CXR reveals bronchopneumonia. VBG: pH 7.14, bicarbonate 16 mmol/L. BE−11.1, pCO_2 4.0 kPa, Na^+ 133, K^+ 7.3 mmol/L, lactate 4.6 mmol/L. Other bloods: Hb 124 g/L, creatinine 421 µmol/L, urea 26 mmol/L, Na 131 mmol/L, K 6.9 mmol/L.

1. Which interventions in hyperkalaemia rapidly reduce the serum potassium?
2. What ECG changes are found in *hypo*kalaemia?

Answers: 1. Insulin (combined with glucose to prevent hypoglycaemia), salbutamol and renal replacement therapy. 2. Prominent U waves, T wave flattening, down-sloping ST depression, QTc prolongation.

TABLE 180.1

	Features	Investigations	Management
Acute and chronic kidney disease	**RFs for $\uparrow K^+$ in CKD:** intercurrent illness, sepsis, missed dialysis and commencement of new drugs	Blood gas: look for metabolic acidosis	Emergency management of hyperkalaemia Reduce dietary K^+ and withhold medications that cause hyperkalaemia
Medications leading to hyperkalaemia	Mineralocorticoid receptor antagonists (spironolactone). ACE inhibitor, ARB, beta-blocker, NSAID, digoxin. Blood transfusion	Electrolytes: routinely measure prior to initiating ARB/ACEi/mineralocorticoid antagnoist and monitor regularly afterwards	Stop offending medications. Alternative drug, reduced dose, dietary alterations, patient counselling, changed monitoring regimen

(Continued)

TABLE 180.1   (Cont'd)

	Features	Investigations	Management
Pseudohyperkalaemia	Causes: lysis of RBCs in difficult venepuncture, or taking a sample downstream to potassium-containing IVI	Retake sample, maybe with alternative (e.g. lithium anti-coagulated) bottle. ECG	Avoid unwarranted treatment
Acidosis	*Metabolic* (DKA, AKI, RTA). *Respiratory.* Exchange of H^+ from the ECF drives K^+ efflux from cells, raising the plasma K^+	Blood gas. DKA: ketones/glucose	Treat the cause of acidosis, e.g. insulin infusion in DKA
Cell lysis syndromes – tumour lysis syndrome, rhabdomyolysis	**RFs for rhabdomyolysis:** crush, burns, compartment sy., immobilisation, muscle activity (seizures, extreme exercise, electrocution). **RFs for tumour lysis:** chemotherapy for leukaemia/lymphoma	CK: rhabdomyolysis severity. Myoglobinuria 'Coca-Cola' urine. U&Es. Tumour lysis: hyperuricaemia, hyperphosphataemia, hypocalcaemia	IV crystalloids. Renal replacement therapy if uncontrolled K^+/acidosis or worsening renal function
Adrenal insufficiency	↓Aldosterone reduces renal excretion of K^+. **RFs:** iatrogenic (long-term steroid use), Addison's. Adrenal crisis (illness/surgery): abdo pain, vomiting, shock	↓Na^+, ↑K^+, ↓glucose. ↓9 am cortisol. Short Synacthen test: minimal increase in serum cortisol. TFTs (± hypothyroidism). Adrenal ± pituitary imaging	**Hydrocortisone and fludrocortisone.** Adrenal crisis: hydrocortisone. Increase steroid dosage for stress, e.g. illness/surgery. MedicAlert bracelet/warning card

TABLE 180.2   Management of hyperkalaemia

Severity	Management
Mild (5.5–5.9 mmol/L)	• Treat cause

Moderate (6.0–6.4 mmol/L)	• 12-lead ECG, 3-lead ECG cardiac monitoring, measure baseline glucose
	• Shift potassium into cells with glucose/insulin:
	  • 10 units of Actrapid soluble insulin in 50 mL of 50% glucose over 15 minutes
	  • Consider giving 10–20 mg of nebulised salbutamol
	  • Commence glucose 10% infusion at 50 mL/hr⁻¹ if baseline glucose <7 mmol/L
	• Remove potassium from body:
	  • Consider dialysis if severe AKI/ESRF
	• Prevent recurrence

Severe (≥6.5 mmol/L) or moderate with ECG changes	• 12-lead ECG and 3-lead ECG cardiac monitoring – HDU environment
	• Protect the heart
	  • 10 mL of 10% calcium chloride IV over 2–5 minutes OR
	  • 30 mL of 10% calcium gluconate IV over 2–5 minutes
	• Shift potassium into cells:
	  • 10 units of Actrapid soluble insulin in 50 mL of 50% glucose over 15 minutes
	  • Use 10–20 mg nebulised salbutamol
	  • Commence glucose 10% infusion at 50 mL/hr if baseline glucose <7 mmol/L
	• Remove potassium from body
	  • Consider dialysis if severe AKI/ESRF
	• Prevent recurrence

Cardiac arrest	• Hyperkalaemia is a reversible cause of cardiac arrest • Preceding AKI, CKD and metabolic acidosis increase probability of hyperkalaemia as the cause: **blood gas** • Management as for severe hyperkalaemia ± sodium bicarbonate • The most effective treatment is **dialysis:** disconnect from the dialysis machine prior to defibrillation shocks

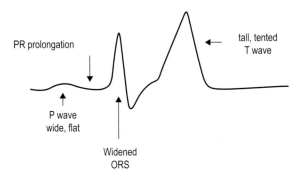

Fig. 180.1 ECG changes in hyperkalaemia. (Illustrated by Dr Hollie Blaber.)

Hyperkalaemia is either asymptomatic or has non-specific symptoms alongside symptoms of the underlying cause, as in the vignette. Hyperkalaemia results in cardiac membrane excitability and spontaneous depolarisation, hence cardiac arrhythmias and potentially cardiorespiratory arrest (pulseless ventricular tachycardia and fibrillation). All patients with high K⁺ level require urgent 12-lead ECG (Fig. 180.1). Therapy addresses ECG changes and serum potassium level. Intravenous calcium, insulin and glucose are key, but may cause subsequent hypoglycaemia. Renal replacement therapy rapidly corrects serum potassium levels and should be considered in severe disease, especially in cardiac arrest. The Renal Association of the UK recommends a 5-step approach to the management of all cases of hyperkalaemia in hospital: (1) protect the heart with calcium salts, (2) drive K⁺ into cells with insulin in glucose solution, (3) remove K⁺ from the body, (4) measure K⁺ and glucose and (5) prevent recurrence (Table 180.2).

REVISION TIPS

- Five steps in hyperkalaemia – protect the heart, drive K^+ into cells, remove K^+ from the body, measure K^+ and glucose, prevent recurrence
- Give calcium gluconate urgently in hyperkalaemia with palpitations or ECG changes, to reduce arrhythmogenesis
- Be aware of drug initiation and monitoring, particularly risk of hypoglycaemia with insulin injection
- Have a low index of suspicion to treat an adrenal crisis presumptively with corticosteroids when no other cause is apparent

181

Investigation Results – Overview Table

Alice Parker, Gregory Oxenham, and Judith Fox

TABLE 181.1

	Sub-Result	Value	Causes
Full blood count	Neutrophils	↑ $>7.5 \times 10^9$/L	Bacterial infection, acute illness, inflammation, myeloproliferative disease, stress, steroids
		↓ $<2 \times 10^9$/L	Post-chemotherapy, drug-induced agranulocytosis, viral infection, Felty syndrome, hypersplenism, bone marrow suppression (e.g. leukaemia)
	Lymphocytes	↑ $>3.5 \times 10^9$/L	Viral infection, lymphocytic leukaemia, inflammation
		↓ $<1.3 \times 10^9$/L	Viral infection, HIV, post-chemotherapy, bone marrow suppression, steroids, autoimmune disease
	Eosinophils	↑ $>0.44 \times 10^9$/L	Parasite or fungal infection, asthma, lymphoma
	Haemoglobin	<130 g/L (male) <115 g/L (female)	*Anaemia* (use MCV to classify)
		>180 g/L (male) >160 g/L (female)	*Primary*: Polycythaemia rubra vera (PRV). *Secondary polycythaemia*, e.g. COPD, altitude, chronic alcohol use, dehydration
	MCV	<76 fL	*Microcytic anaemia*: iron deficiency, thalassaemia, sideroblastic anaemia
		76–96 fL	*Normocytic anaemia*, e.g. chronic disease, acute blood loss, haemolysis, sickle cell anaemia, CKD, pregnancy
		>96 fL	*Macrocytic anaemia*, e.g. B12 or folate deficiency, liver disease, alcohol, hypothyroidism, reticulocytosis
	Platelets	↑ $>400 \times 10^9$/L	*Primary*, e.g. essential thrombocythaemia, PRV. *Secondary*, e.g. bleeding, infection, post-splenectomy, malignancy
		↓ $<150 \times 10^9$/L (thrombocytopenia)	*Increased removal*, e.g. ITP, TTP, DIC, hypersplenism, drug (e.g. heparin, diuretics, quinine, aspirin, alcohol), viral, SLE, HELLP *Decreased production*, e.g. haematological malignancy, megaloblastic anaemia, aplastic anaemia

(Continued)

TABLE 181.1 (Cont'd)

	Sub-Result	Value	Causes
Renal function	Creatinine	↑ >105 µmol/L	AKI (increase in baseline creatinine >26 µmol/L in 48 h/ >1.5 × baseline), CKD
		<59 µmol/L	Pregnancy, low muscle mass/frailty

N.B. – Creatinine depends on the muscle mass and will form part of the calculation for eGFR. Therefore, a single creatinine measurement is not as useful as a trend.

	Sub-Result	Value	Causes
	Urea	↑ >6.7 mmol/L	AKI, CKD, upper GI bleed, dehydration, sepsis, burns, tumour lysis, pancreatitis, increased protein intake
		↓ <2.5 mmol/L	Pregnancy, liver disease, low protein, e.g. malnutrition, alcoholism, anorexia nervosa
	eGFR	↓	*CKD*

Stage	eGFR (mL/min/1.73 m²)
1	>90 with evidence of kidney damage*
2	60–89 with evidence of kidney damage*
3A	45–59
3B	30–44
4	15–29
5	<15

*Raised ACR, urine sediment abnormalities, electrolyte abnormalities due to tubular disorders, abnormal anatomy or histology, systemic disease or history of renal transplant (KDIGO)

	Sub-Result	Value	Causes
	Bicarbonate	↑ >28 mEq/L	*Metabolic alkalosis*: vomiting, NG suction, bicarbonate administration, diuresis *Respiratory acidosis (compensated)*: COPD, obesity hypoventilation, scoliosis
		↓ <22 mEq/L	*Metabolic acidosis*: see ABG results below. **Renal failure** (chronic and acute) can result in acidosis as the kidney is less able to resorb bicarbonate. *Respiratory alkalosis (compensated)*: subacute/chronic hyperventilation/hypoxia, e.g pain, pregnancy (normal), pneumonia, head injury, stroke, hyperventilation while intubated

TABLE 181.1   (Cont'd)

	Sub-Result	Value	Causes
Liver function tests	Bilirubin	↑ >17 µmol/L	*Unconjugated*: haemolysis, Gilbert's, drugs, congestive cardiac failure *Conjugated*: hepatocellular injury, cholestasis *Neonatal hyperbilirubinaemia*: physiological jaundice, prematurity, rhesus disease, TORCH, biliary atresia
	ALT	↑ >35 IU/L	Hepatocellular injury (with raised AST)
	ALP	↑ >300 IU/L	*Cholestasis* (with raised GGT). *Bone causes*, e.g. Paget's, bone metastases or tumours, vitamin D deficiency. *Pregnancy* from second trimester (released by placenta)
	AST	↑ >35 IU/L	Hepatocellular injury (with raised ALT). Muscle damage, cardiac causes
	GGT	↑ >51 IU/L (M) >33 IU/L (F)	Cholestasis (with raised ALP). Heavy alcohol use
	Albumin	↑ (>50 g/L)	Dehydration
		↓ (<35 g/L)	Liver cirrhosis, inflammation, chronic disease, pregnancy, nephrotic syndrome, malabsorption, severe burns

Thyroid function tests		TSH	T4	T3
	Hyperthyroidism	↓↓	↑	↑
	Hypothyroidism	↑↑	↓	↓
	Subclinical hyperthyroidism	↓	Normal	Normal
	Subclinical hypothyroidism	↑	Normal	Normal
	Sick euthyroid syndrome	Normal or ↓	↓	↓

(Continued)

TABLE 181.1   (Cont'd)

	Sub-Result	Value	Causes
Bone profile	PTH	↑ >8.5 pmol/L	*Primary hyper-PTH*: adenoma, hyperplasia, carcinoma *Secondary hyper-PTH*: CKD, vitamin D deficiency, hypomagnesaemia, malabsorption *Tertiary*: hyperplasia after secondary hyper-PTH

	PTH	Ca^{++}	PO$_4$
1°	↑	↑	↓
2°	↑	Normal/↓	↓/↑
3°	↑	Normal/↑	↑

	Sub-Result	Value	Causes
		↓ <0.8 pmol/L	Complication of thyroidectomy. Pseudohypoparathyroidism
	Vitamin D (as serum 25(OH)-vitamin D)	Deficient <20 ng/mL Insufficient 21–29	*Less sun exposure*: darker skin, institutionalised, ageing. *Reduced oral intake*: malabsorption (CF, coeliac, IBD, pancreatic insufficiency) or diet. *Less synthesis*: cirrhosis, renal failure, hyper-PTH
	Total protein (albumin + globulin)	↑ >83 g/L	Dehydration (↑albumin) or ↑globulin (see below) or both
		↓ <60 g/L	Volume expansion (e.g. pregnancy), ↓albumin (see above)
	Globulin Four groups by immuno-electrophoresis: α$_1$, α$_2$, β and γ	↑ >33 g/L	Acute inflammation, severe iron deficiency. *γ fraction; polyclonal increase*: chronic infections, liver disease, connective tissue disease. *Monoclonal increase*: myeloma, Waldenstrom's, monoclonal gammopathy, amyloidosis, lymphoma
		↓ <10 g/L	Immunodeficiency, CLL, nephrotic syndrome, steroid treatment, α$_1$ anti-trypsin deficiency
	Albumin	LFTs. Albumin helps 'adjust' calcium – ionised calcium is inversely related to serum albumin	
	Calcium, phosphate and magnesium	Calcium and phosphate are essential for interpreting the PTH level, while magnesium is vital for maintaining potassium and calcium levels	
Clotting	PT/INR	↑ >16 seconds	Warfarin, liver failure, DIC, pre-eclampsia, sepsis, heparin, low factor II, V, VII or X
	APTT	↑ >45 seconds	Haemophilia A and B, von Willebrand disease, warfarin, heparin, DIC, sepsis, pre-eclampsia, liver disease, low factor II, V, VII, IX, X or XI, anti-phospholipid syndrome (paradoxical)
Cardiac markers	Troponin	↑	Myocardial infarction (MI) (after 4–6 hours). Also; CKD, heart failure, myocarditis, aortic dissection, hypertrophic cardiomyopathy, tachy/bradyarrhythmia, PE, sepsis, chest trauma
	Creatinine kinase	↑	Rhabdomyolysis, MI, vigorous exercise, trauma, surgery

TABLE 181.1   (Cont'd)

Sub-Result	Value	Causes

Other
Lumbar puncture

	Normal	Bacterial	Viral	Fungal	TB
Opening pressure	10–20 cm CSF	↑	Normal or ↑	↑	↑
Appearance	Clear	Cloudy	Clear	Fibrin web	Clear
White cell count	0–5 cells/µL	>100 cells/µL	10–1000 cells/µL	10–500 cells/µL	50–500 cells/µL
Glucose	>60% serum levels	↓ (<40% serum levels)	Normal	↓	↓
Protein	<45 mg/dL	↑	↑	↑	↑

Other:
- Subarachnoid haemorrhage: xanthochromia, raised opening pressure
- Multiple sclerosis: oligoclonal bands
- Guillain-Barré: raised protein, normal WCC

ABG

	pH (7.35–7.45)	$PaCO_2$ (4.5–6.0 kPa)	HCO_3 (22–26 mmol/L)	Causes
Respiratory acidosis	<7.35	↑	Normal. ↑ if metabolic compensation	Respiratory depression, life-threatening asthma, COPD, Guillain-Barré
Respiratory alkalosis	>7.45	↓	Normal. ↓ if metabolic compensation	Hypoxia, anxiety, pain, pulmonary embolism, pneumothorax
Metabolic acidosis	<7.35	Normal. ↓ if respiratory compensation	↓	*Raised anion gap** ($Na^+ – Cl^- + HCO_3^-$): MUDPILES = methanol, uraemia, DKA, propylene glycol, isoniazid, lactate, ethylene glycol, salicylates *Decreased anion gap*: diarrhoea, Addison's, RTA
Metabolic alkalosis	>7.45	Normal ↑ if respiratory compensation	↑	D&V, diuretics, Conn/Cushing syndrome, pyloric stenosis, hypokalaemia

*Anion gap = ([Na$^+$] + [K$^+$]) − ([Cl$^-$] + [HCO$_3$]). Normal anion gap = 7–16 mmol/L. Every 1 g/L fall in albumin decreases anion gap by 0.25 mmol/L. Also affected by paraproteins, lithium.

Note that reference ranges are laboratory specific, as described in "How to use this book" (page xi). See also *178. ELECTROLYTE ABNORMALITIES– Overview Table, 179. HYPONATRAEMIA*, and *180. HYPERKALAEMIA*.

SELF-ASSESSMENT

1. Interpret the following ABG results and think of some possible causes:
   a. pH 7.31, pO_2 9.1, pCO_2 7.9, HCO_3 30
   b. pH 7.27, pO_2 11, pCO_2 3.0, HCO_3 14, Na^+ 134, K 4.2, Cl^- 102
   c. pH 7.52, pO_2 10.3, pCO_2 4.9, HCO_3 29
   d. pH 7.55, pO_2 11.1, pCO_2 3.0, HCO_3 24
   e. pH 7.24, pO_2 7.9, CO_2 9.0, HCO_3 30
   f. pH 7.21, pO_2 8.5, pCO_2 6.5, HCO_3 18
   g. pH 7.49, pO_2 10.0, pCO_2 3.8, HCO_3 30

Answers

a. Respiratory acidosis with partial metabolic compensation, e.g. respiratory depression, COPD, asthma

b. Metabolic acidosis with raised anion gap (= 22) MUDPILES. *If you are given a chloride level they often want you to calculate an anion gap*

c. Metabolic alkalosis – D&V, diuretics, hyperaldosteronism, Cushing's, pyloric stenosis, hypokalaemia

d. Respiratory alkalosis – hypoxia, anxiety, pain, pulmonary embolism, pneumothorax

e. Acute on chronic respiratory acidosis – type 2 respiratory failure, e.g. COPD

f. Mixed respiratory and metabolic acidosis – cardiac arrest, multi-organ failure

g. Mixed respiratory and metabolic alkalosis – liver cirrhosis with diuretics, hyperemesis gravidarum, COPD over-ventilation

182

Stridor

Tejas Netke, Alexander Royston, and Amber Syed

EMERGENCY DEPARTMENT, FEMALE, 3 YEARS OLD. DIFFICULTY BREATHING

HPC: Barking cough, mild rhinorrhoea, worse at night. **PMHx:** Born at term via C-section. Normal development. **DHx:** Up to date with immunisations. **SHx:** Lives at home with both parents and older brother. No pets, non-smoking household.

O/E: Temperature 38.1°C, slightly tachypnoeic, 95% room air (RA), HR 120 bpm, normotensive. Bilateral equal chest expansion, inspiratory stridor at rest. No ENT examinations performed.

---

1. What are the commonest important causes of non-infective stridor in children?
2. In a diagnosis of croup, what are the signs that should trigger an immediate admission?
3. List signs of respiratory distress in a young child

Answers: 1. Anaphylaxis and inhaled foreign body. 2. Apnoea (observed or reported), persistent SpO_2 <92% (RA), inadequate oral fluid intake (<70% of usual volume), severe respiratory distress – grunting, marked chest recession or respiratory rate >70 breaths/minute. 3. Tachypnoea, added sounds, subcostal/ intercostal recession, tracheal tug, head bobbing, grunting, nose flaring. If severe: cyanosis.

TABLE 182.1

	Features	Investigations	Management
Congenital – Children			
Laryngomalacia	Intermittent stridor soon after birth. Hx & O/E: respiratory distress; subcostal/ intercostal recession, tracheal tug, head bobbing. Severe: apnoea, cyanosis. Normal cry (absent cry: vocal cord paralysis; harsh cry: laryngitis due to reflux)	RFs: congenital, M > F, GORD, neurological (generalised or focal hypotonia, cerebral palsy). Do not perform ENT examination – keep child calm to avoid laryngospasm. **ENT referral- flexible laryngoscopy**	Often self-resolves: 90% by 18–20 months. Observation ± GORD treatment. **Definitive:** endoscopic supraglottoplasty

(Continued)

TABLE 182.1   (Cont'd)

	Features	Investigations	Management
Inflammatory – Children			
Croup (laryngotracheobronchitis, Fig. 182.1)	**RFs:** age (6 months–3 years), M > F, parainfluenza 1/3 (autumn/winter), non-immunised. **Hx & O/E:** barking cough, viral prodrome, ± agitation, ± respiratory distress. Generally well child	95% of laryngotracheal infections. Clinical diagnosis	PO corticosteroids: dexamethasone (regardless of severity). Nebulised adrenaline if respiratory distress/agitated/hypoxic. Risk of airway occlusion in severe cases
Epiglottitis	**RFs:** *Haemophilus influenzae* type B (Hib), age < 12 months. **Hx & O/E:** high fever, sore throat, dysphagia, difficulty breathing, irritability, stridor, drooling. Acutely unwell child	**Direct (rigid or flexible) laryngoscopy:** only by ENT.	Calm approach (risk of airway occlusion with laryngospasm). IV access and IV Abx. Urgent senior ENT and anaesthetic– may need to secure airway (direct laryngoscopy ± tracheostomy). Source Difficult Airway kit
Laryngitis	Cough, stridor, hoarse, sore throat, nasal secretions, dysphagia, odynophagia. Fever ± large tonsils ± cervical lymph nodes	**RFs:** URTI (viral), GORD. Clinical diagnosis. Throat swab	Treat empirically. Viral: supportive care. Bacterial: antibiotics (first line: phenoxymethylpenicillin)
Children and Adults			
Anaphylaxis	See *53. ANAPHYLAXIS*		
Supraglottitis *(similar to but distinct from epiglottitis in children)*	**RFs:** unvaccinated (Hib), *Streptococcus pneumoniae*, viruses, trauma, thermal injury, irritant chemicals, recreational drugs (crack), chemotherapy, radiotherapy. Slower onset, more pharyngeal. **Hx & O/E:** dysphagia, odynophagia, drooling, dysphonia, inspiratory stridor, pyrexia, cervical lymphadenopathy, anterior neck tenderness (hyoid)	Urgent ENT referral. **Flexible laryngoscopy:** erythematous, swollen supraglottis. ↑Inflammatory markers, blood cultures. Swab (once airway protected)	**HDU setting:** oxygen, nebulised adrenaline (1:1000 dilution), IV steroids (dexamethasone), empirical IV Abx. Endotracheal intubation or tracheostomy may become necessary

TABLE 182.1 (Cont'd)

	Features	Investigations	Management
Inhaled foreign body	May have localised wheeze, stridor, prolonged coughing, difficulty breathing. Unilateral wheeze: high suspicion	**RFs:** age (<4, >70), bulbar dysfunction, dementia. **CXR:** radio-opaque object, collapse/ consolidation. **Flexible bronchoscopy**	Conscious →encourage coughing, back slaps, Heimlich manoeuvre (small child; abdominal thrusts). Unconscious →start CPR. Flexible bronchoscopy (removal)
Smoke inhalation	**Hx & O/E:** cough, dyspnoea, hoarse, stridor, dizzy, headache, burns, soot around mouth. Tachycardic, tachypnoeic, hypoxia, hypotension, ↓GCS/paediatric GCS/ AVPU	ABG (metabolic acidosis, ↔pO_2). Normal pulse oximetry does not exclude CO poisoning. Consider cyanide (burning plastics/wool/silk). **CXR:** hypoxia (exclude other causes). **ECG:** arrhythmias	A→E assessment. Secure airway as oedema can be rapid (ET tube). CO poisoning: high-flow oxygen. If COHb >20% consider hyperbaric oxygen. Look for: injury, blood loss, burns, evolving lung injury. Analgesia, fluid, wound care

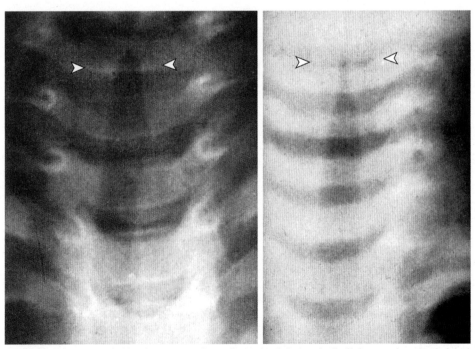

Fig. 182.1 Laryngotracheitis. Anteroposterior radiograph of the neck. (*Left*) A normal tracheal air column (between the arrows). (*Right*) Trachea narrowed (*arrows*) by laryngotracheitis. (From Fuhrman BP, et al. *Pediatric Critical Care*, ed 4. Philadelphia: Saunders, 2011.)

Stridor is a symptom rather than a diagnosis. The top differential for the vignette is croup, with distinctive barking cough, particularly in a young child experiencing severest symptoms at night. As a sign of airway narrowing, stridor is concerning; keep the child calm, with the caregiver, and do not examine throat. Crucial diagnoses to consider are bacterial tracheitis and epiglottitis – life-threatening but rare since introduction of Hib vaccination. If a child has an abrupt onset of stridor without infection, consider anaphylaxis or inhaled foreign body.

REVISION TIPS

	Croup	**Epiglottitis**
Onset	Days	Hours
Preceding coryza	Yes	No
Cough	Severe/barking	Absent/slight
Fever	<38.5°C	>38.5°C
Stridor	Harsh, rasping	Soft, whispering
Voice/cry	Hoarse	Muffled, reluctant

183

Wheeze

Tejas Netke, Alexander Royston, and Joseph Page

GP CONSULTATION, MALE, 30.
SHORTNESS OF BREATH AND WHEEZE

HPC: Symptoms progressed over a week: breathless at rest, non-productive cough, wheeze, struggling to complete sentences. PMHx: Asthma (three admissions, never to ITU). DHx: Salbutamol, beclometasone/formoterol inhalers. SHx: Stone mason, occasional social smoker.

O/E: Sitting upright, pursed lips breathing. HR 110 bpm, RR 26, SpO$_2$ 96% (RA), central trachea, bilateral equal air entry. Chest resonant to percussion, widespread polyphonic wheeze.

1. How do you assess the severity of asthma versus COPD?
2. What ongoing care do patients need post-exacerbation?
3. What is most likely in an older patient, with IHD and previous CABG, getting breathless over a few hours?

Answers: 1. Asthma: based on PEFR. COPD: based on FEV1 and FEV1/FVC (always <0.7: obstructive disease). 2. Monitor PEFR: discharge once PEFR >75% of predicted, continue prednisolone for 5 days. Before discharge: check inhaler technique, have asthma plan in place, follow up with GP/specialist nurse. 3. Acute decompensated heart failure.

TABLE 183.1

	Features	Investigations	Management
Respiratory Acute exacerbation of asthma (Fig. 183.1)	RFs: asthma, atopy (eczema, rhinitis, hay fever), FHx. Exacerbation: viral, exercise, cold, allergen (pollen/dust), work (better at weekends). Hx & O/E: wheeze/chest tight/dry cough (productive = infective), hard to complete sentences, agitation. *Life-threatening:* reduced respiratory effort, hypoxic, loss of consciousness, silent chest, cyanosis	PEFR: severity, reversibility (diurnal variation ± pre- and post-salbutamol). FBC (↑eosinophils/↑WCC), CRP, U&Es (↑↑salbutamol→ ↓K). ABG: assess T1RF, normal or raised ↔/↑CO$_2$ = life threatening – *ITU*. CXR: cause/other pathology (e.g. pneumothorax)	Diary: recent control. ↑Severity →escalate treatment. O$_2$ (aim ≥94%). 2.5–5 mg nebulised salbutamol 'back-to-back'. Ipratropium bromide 0.5 mcg 4–6 hourly. Oral prednisolone 40 mg, IV hydrocortisone if can't swallow. IV MgSO$_4$ (2 g IV over 20 minutes). Aminophylline (senior decision). ITU/NIV/intubate and ventilate. ↓Exacerbations, ↓steroids and improve QoL by reducing allergen exposure, smoking cessation, optimising inhaled therapy

(Continued)

TABLE 183.1 (Cont'd)

	Features	Investigations	Management
Exacerbation of COPD	Exacerbation, see *40. BREATHLESSNESS*. COPD, see *185. COUGH*		
Community acquired pneumonia (CAP)	**RFs:** age, smoking, alcoholism, COPD, immunosuppression, cardio-/cerebrovascular, DM, liver/renal, dementia. **Hx & O/E:** productive cough, wheeze, dyspnoea, pleuritic pain, fever, tachypnoea, localised dull percussion, ↓breath sounds, bronchial breathing. *Complications:* haemoptysis, parapneumonic effusion (33%) ± empyema, abscess, cavitation (*Staphylococcus aureus, Klebsiella, Pseudomonas*)	Observations. FBC (↑WCC), U&Es (↑urea), LFTs (atypical: transient hepatitis), ABG (?T1RF). **Sputum culture:** moderate/high severity CAP (esp. Legionella). **Urine:** Legionella/ pneumococcal antigens. **CXR:** consolidation/ effusion. Repeat 6–8 weeks post-discharge	Clinical judgement: no symptoms are strictly diagnostic. Caution for frail/ vulnerable (↓GCS, delirium, myalgia, abdominal discomfort). CURB-65: guides Mx/Abx. Low severity CAP (scores 0–1) treat home on PO antibiotics (5–7 days). **Definitive:** Sepsis 6. Abx (local guidelines), e.g. amoxicillin/ clarithromycin/doxycycline
Pneumothorax	See *40. BREATHLESSNESS*		
Cardiac/Others Acute heart failure	See *8. PERIPHERAL OEDEMA AND ANKLE SWELLING*		
Foreign body inhalation	Localised wheeze (typically monophonic), prolonged coughing, dyspnoea	**CXR.** **Bronchoscopy**	Encourage coughing, back slaps, Heimlich manoeuvre. **Definitive:** bronchoscopy
GORD	See *185. COUGH*		

CAP, Community acquired pneumonia.

Medication options, to be adjusted for individual patients

	STEP 1	STEP 2	STEP 3	STEP 4	STEP 5
CONTROLLER to prevent exacerbations *Primary options*	As-needed low-dose IGC	Daily low-dose IGC, or as-needed low-dose IGC-ROLA	Daily low-dose IGC-LABA	Daily medium-dose IGC-LABA	Daily high-dose IGC-LABA. Seek expert consultation for additional Rx such as tiotropium, anti-IgE, anti-IL5/5R, anti-IL4R
Secondary options	As-needed low-dose IGC-ROLA	LTRA, or low-dose IGC taken whenever SABA taken	Daily medium-dose IGC or low-dose IGC+LTRA	Daily high-dose IGC, add-on tiotropium, or add-on LTRA	Add oral glucocorticoids at as low a dose as possible
RELIEVERS to treat symptoms	As-needed SABA or low-dose IGC-ROLA				

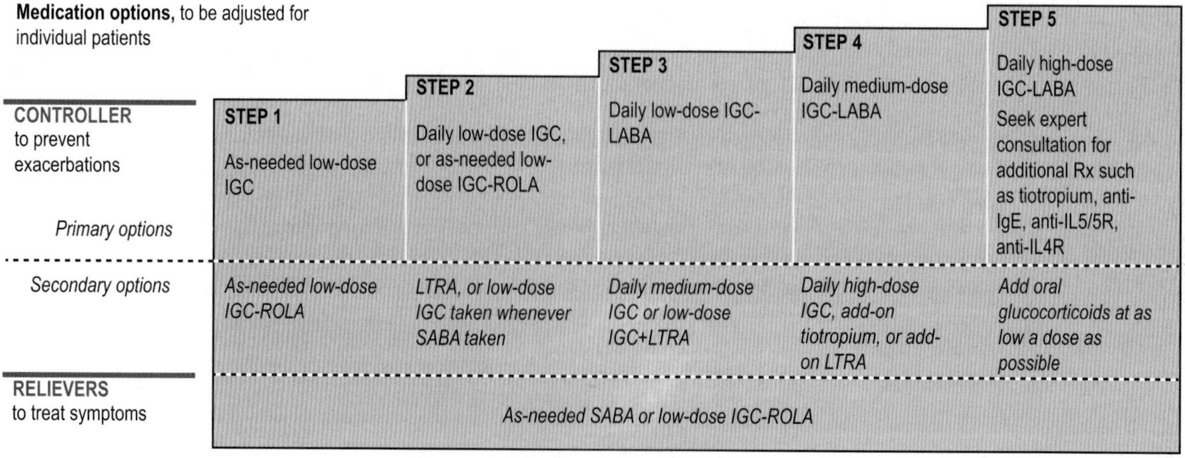

Fig. 183.1 Asthma therapy. *Anti-IL4R, anti-IL5/5 R,* interleukin-4 receptor, interleukin-5/or its receptor *IGC,* inhaled glucocorticoid; *LABA,* long-acting beta2-agonist; *LTRA,* leukotriene receptor antagonist; *ROLA,* rapid onset long-acting beta-2 agonist; *SABA,* short acting beta-2 agonist. (From Jeffrey M, Drazen JM, Bel EH. Asthma. In *Goldman-Cecil Medicine,* 2-volume set. Elsevier; 2020.)

Exacerbations of asthma and COPD can present in a similar manner, and they may co-exist. Asthma exacerbation is more common in younger patients, particularly if there is a history of atopy or childhood asthma. COPD is more likely in older patients (>35) with ≥10 pack-year history of smoking. Pneumonia is unlikely in the vignette, given the absence of fever or sputum production. Acute asthma exacerbation is likely, due to the nature of his symptoms and occupational exposure to dust. A PEFR chart would help identify diurnal variation and reversibility with bronchodilators.

REVISION TIPS

Features	Acute Severe	Life-Threatening	Near-Fatal
SpO_2		<92%	
PaO_2		<8 kPa	
PEFR	33%–50%	<33%	
HR	>110 bpm		
Respiratory	>25/min	'Normal' $PaCO_2$ (4.6–6.0 kPa)	Raised $PaCO_2$
Other features Requiring mechanical ventilation with ↑inflation pressures	Can't complete full sentences	Cyanosis, ↓GCS, hypotensive, exhaustion, silent chest, arrhythmias	

184

Pleural Effusion

Alexander Royston and Joseph Page

GP CONSULTATION, MALE, 72.
WORSENING DYSPNOEA

HPC: Declining exercise tolerance over several months, non-productive cough. No recent infections or fevers, but 1 stone unintentional weight loss. He is fatigued. **PMHx:** Nil. **SHx:** ex-smoker (20 pack years), retired plumber.

   O/E: RR20, SpO$_2$ 92% (room air), HR 80, BP 138/80, reduced air entry left mid zone and dullness to percussion. No palpable cervical lymphadenopathy, no Horner's, no clubbing. **Ix:** CXR left-sided pleural effusion.

1. What are the criteria for exudate versus transudate?
2. What are occupational risk factors for mesothelioma?
3. Name the borders of the 'triangle of safety' when inserting a chest drain.

Answers: 1. Light's criteria – any of the following suggest exudate: pleural total protein/serum total protein ratio > 0.5, OR pleural LDH/serum LDH ratio > 0.6, OR pleural LDH > 2/3 upper limit of the laboratory's reference range of serum LDH. 2. Exposure to asbestos: workers (or their partners) in shipbuilding, mining, car parts manufacturer (brakes), insulation work, plumbing. 3. Lateral edge of latissimus dorsi, lateral border of pectoralis major, 5th intercostal space, base of axilla; this route minimises risk to underlying structures.

TABLE 184.1

	Features	Investigations	Management
Transudative (Light's Criteria)			
Congestive cardiac failure	See *8. PERIPHERAL OEDEMA AND ANKLE SWELLING* Effusions usually bilateral (can present unilaterally). **Pleural aspiration** - only for bilateral effusions or if atypical features/ fails to respond		O$_2$, furosemide, ACEi (or entresto, if severe), β-blocker, spironolactone. SGTL2i: dapagliflozin (not just diabetics). Lifestyle advice, ±diuretic
Hepatic cirrhosis	See *83. ASCITES*. **Paracentesis:** tense ascites (may improve a right-sided pleural effusion)		
Renal failure	See *177. CHRONIC KIDNEY DISEASE*		
Rare causes: constrictive pericarditis, Meig syndrome, hypothyroidism			

TABLE 184.1 (Cont'd)

	Features	Investigations	Management
Exudative			
Pleural malignancy	Any cancer has potential to metastasise to the pleural cavity →accumulation of pleural fluid. **RFs:** smoking history, asbestos exposure, existing cancer diagnosis. **Hx & O/E:** cough, dyspnoea, haemoptysis, weight loss, pain, effusion, clubbing	**CXR:** unilateral pleural effusion (hilar mass, pulmonary metastasis). **Pleural aspiration:** malignancy diagnosed on cytology 2/3 of time. **CT thorax/abdomen/pelvis (with contrast).** **Biopsy:** when pleural fluid cytology non-diagnostic	Repeated pleural aspiration, talc pleurodesis. Indwelling pleural catheter (IPC). MDT (oncology/respiratory)
Pleural mesothelioma	**RFs:** age (60–85 yo), M > F, asbestos exposure, FHx, smoking. Rare. Long latency (30–40 years). Poor prognosis, (presents late). **Hx & O/E:** dyspnoea, pleuritic chest pain, unilateral pleural effusion, cough, fatigue	**CXR:** collapse/↓expansion, effusion (Fig. 184.1), pleural plaques (benign). **CT:** circumferential/nodular pleural thickening, LNs. Thoracocentesis: exudate. **Pleural biopsy** (thoracoscopy/CT guided)	MDT approach. Palliative chemo-/immunotherapy + enhanced supportive care (including legal advice)
Parapneumonic effusion (including empyema)	Uncomplicated (sterile): occur in 20%–40% of hospitalised pneumonia cases. **RF:** recent pneumonia. **Hx & O/E:** dyspnoea, cough, pleuritic chest pain, ↓breath sounds, dullness to percussion, ↓tactile fremitus	FBC, LFTs, CRP, cultures. **Sputum:** gram stain, culture, acid fast bacillix3 (TB). **CXR:** >200 mL of fluid on PA film (blunted costophrenic angle: >50mL). **USS:** complexity of effusion, site for aspiration/drain. **Aspiration:** LDH/protein in pleural fluid (and serum). Red cell count (pleural fluid: if raised, suggests malignancy/pulmonary infarction/ trauma). Microscopy (Gram stain), culture, cytology	Oxygen, diuretics (cause dependent). IV Abx long course. Therapeutic thoracentesis (uncomplicated →can be definitive). Tube thoracostomy. Follow-up CXR (6-8w)
Empyema	Pus in pleural cavity. Mortality ≤20%. **RFs:** recent pneumonia, DM, IVDU, immunosuppression, EtOH, instrumentation. **Hx & O/E:** as above, unwell, longer onset (15/7), swinging fever/rigors, egophony	As above, ↑platelets. **CXR:** loculated effusion, 'D-shaped'. **USS.** **Aspiration:** pH<7.2: infection →chest drain. Light's criteria (high protein and LDH = exudate). CT	Tube thoracostomy. ± Intrapleural fibrinolytics. Surgical: video-assisted thorascopic surgery, thoracoscopy ± adhesiolysis, decortication, open drainage

Less common: TB, PE, RA/serositis/SLE, post-cardiac surgery, pancreatitis, Yellow nail syndrome, drugs (methotrexate, amiodarone, phenytoin, nitrofurantoin)

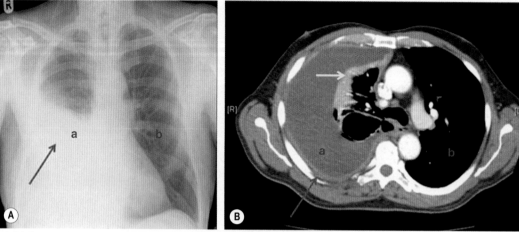

Fig. 184.1 Malignant pleural mesothelioma. The red arrows indicate thickened pleura with an underlying pleural effusion. The yellow arrow indicates thickened mediastinal pleura. (A) Right-sided pleural effusion; (B) Left lung. (From Daunt, M. Malik, M. Malignant pleural mesothelioma and its management. *BJA Education*, 2015-10-01, 15(5):242–247. Copyright © 2015 The Author(s).)

Parapneumonic effusion is an unlikely cause for this patient's dyspnoea in the vignette, due to the absence of infective symptoms. He has no risk factors for liver, renal or cardiac failure. The gradual progression, dry cough, weight loss and smoking history suggest malignancy. The key finding on examination is reduced air entry and dullness to percussion, suggesting an effusion. The patient's occupational history infers likely asbestos exposure, making the diagnosis of malignant pleural effusion due to mesothelioma most likely.

REVISION TIPS

- Bilateral effusion is most likely to be due to cardiac, hepatic or renal failure. Treat the cause
- Other causes of effusions:
  - Transudative: peritoneal dialysis, cardiac (CABG, pericarditis)
  - Exudative: autoimmune (rheumatoid, SLE); abdominal (pancreatitis/pseudocyst, subphrenic abscess); ovarian (Meig's)
- Three stages of empyema: exudative stage, fibrinopurulent stage, organisational stage
- Commonest cause of malignant pleural effusion: lung cancer (>1/3rd), breast cancer (16.8%) and malignant lymphoma (11.5%)

Cough

Alice Parker and Rada Ivanov

1. What type of lung cancer is the patient in the vignette most at risk of?
2. What are the paraneoplastic features of the following:
   a. Small cell lung cancer;
   b. Squamous cell lung cancer;
   c. Adenocarcinoma.
3. What are the differentials for *acute* cough?

Answers: 1. Squamous cell lung cancer due to his smoking history. 2a. Cushing syndrome, SIADH. 2b. ↑PTHrP (↑Ca, but PTH normal/low), ↑TSH, clubbing, hypertrophic pulmonary osteoarthropathy (HPOA). 2c. Gynaecomastia, HPOA. 3. Acute bronchitis, influenza, pneumonia, COVID-19, bronchiolitis, croup, exacerbation of COPD/asthma/CHF, hypersensitivity pneumonitis, whooping cough, inhaled foreign body.

TABLE 185.1

	Features	Investigations	Management
Lung cancer	RFs: smoker, radon/asbestos exposure, occupation (coal dust, diesel fumes). Hx & O/E: cough, SOB, haemoptysis, chest pain, weight loss, voice change, lethargy, clubbing, nicotine stains. Metastases, massive haemoptysis (bronchial artery), pleural effusion, lung collapse, recurrent laryngeal nerve palsy, SVCO, Horner syndrome, phrenic nerve palsy, paraneoplastic	CXR (Fig. 185.1): nodule or mass, hilum enlarged, consolidation (non-resolving), collapse, effusion, bony mets. CT chest ± abdo, PET scan: solid, spiculated, upper lobe, with emphysema in a smoker or ex-smoker. Bronchoscopy or CT-guided biopsy (primary or mets). Sputum/pleural fluid cytology. Markers (e.g. KRAS, EGFR)	Surgical resection if early stage: chemotherapy, monoclonal ABs, TK inhibitors, radiotherapy. Consider palliative airway stenting. Urgent CXR: if >40 yo + smoker + any of cough/fatigue/SOB/weight or appetite loss/chest pain. 2WW referral: if CXR suspicious for lung Ca or >40 with unexplained haemoptysis

(Continued)

TABLE 185.1 (Cont'd)

	Features	Investigations	Management
COPD	**RFs:** cigarette smoke (primary or secondary), occupational, FHx at age <40 (alpha-1 anti-trypsin). **Hx & O/E:** chronic cough, sputum, exertional SOB, frequent chest infections, wheeze. (Exacerbation of COPD, See *40. BREATHLESSNESS*)	**FBC** (↑Hb/secondary polycythaemia), alpha-1 anti-trypsin if early onset. **Blood gas:** ± compensated respiratory acidosis. **CXR:** hyperinflation, flat hemidiaphragm, large pulmonary arteries, reduced vascular marking, bullae. **Lung function:** FEV1/FVC <0.7, low/no reversibility, reduced DLCO	Smoking cessation, vaccinations, pulmonary rehabilitation, mucolytics. SABA/SAMA as required. Add LABA + inhaled corticosteroid (ICS) if asthmatic features. Add a LABA + LAMA if no asthmatic features. **3rd line:** combine LABA + LAMA + ICS. LTOT: based on ABG and pulmonary HTN
Bronchiectasis	**RFs:** previous severe or recurrent infections, impaired mucous clearance (e.g. CF), obstruction, rheumatoid arthritis **Hx & O/E:** large volume productive cough >8 weeks, dyspnoea, fever, poor exercise tolerance, weight loss, haemoptysis. Coarse crackles at lung bases ± wheeze	**Sputum culture:** if purulent/recurrent infection. **High-resolution CT:** tram-track sign, signet-ring sign, dilated peripheral bronchi. QuantiFERON®-TB/CFTR/chloride sweat test: if aetiology unknown	**Pulmonary rehabilitation:** smoking cessation, flu vaccine, immunisations, postural drainage, mucolytics and mucous clearance exercises. Abx for exacerbations and prophylaxis. Lung transplant in limited cases
GORD	**RFs:** obesity, smoking, pregnancy, hiatus hernia. Triggers: supine, post-prandial, alcohol, caffeine, NSAIDs. **Hx & O/E:** heartburn, belching, acid regurgitation, odynophagia, salivation, chronic cough, hoarseness	Consider endoscopy (dysphagia, >55 years + alarm symptoms, treatment-resistant). **Test and treat for *H. pylori***	Weight loss, stop smoking, avoid triggers, small meals, raise head of bed. OTC **antacid**, e.g. Gaviscon. Trial **PPI** for 6 weeks, e.g. omeprazole, lansoprazole. Surgery, e.g. fundoplication
Congestive cardiac failure	See *8. PERIPHERAL OEDEMA AND ANKLE SWELLING*		
Tuberculosis	See *95. HAEMOPTYSIS*		
Postnasal drip	**RFs:** viral infections, sinusitis, allergies, environmental	Clinical diagnosis	Avoid triggers, anti-histamine, decongestant ± nasal steroids
ACE-inhibitor induced cough	Common (4-35%) side effect soon after commencing the medication (onset can take weeks)	Clinical diagnosis	Use alternative, e.g. ARB
Interstitial lung disease	See *40. BREATHLESSNESS*		

TABLE 185.1   (Cont'd)

	Features	Investigations	Management
Sarcoidosis	RF: younger age, African or Scandinavian descent. Hx & O/E: cough, dyspnoea, pain, fatigue, fever, arthralgia, weight loss. *Acute sarcoid:* fever, bilateral hilar lymphadenopathy (BHL), erythema nodosum *(Lofgren syndrome).* *Stages:* I BHL, II BHL and lung infiltrates, III lung infiltrates only, IV pulmonary fibrosis	↑Calcium/ESR, ↑serum ACE (75%). CXR: BHL, upper zone infiltrates. Spirometry: commonly normal or restrictive. Tissue biopsy: non-caseating granulomas	Observation – mild cases usually improve. Steroids if ↑calcium/stage II-III, eye/heart/neuro, fast progression
Asthma	See *183. WHEEZE*		

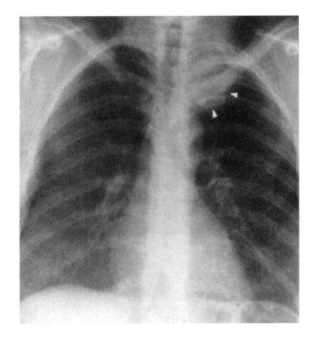

Fig. 185.1 Left superior sulcus lung tumour *(arrows)*. (From Mountain CF. Expanded possibilities for surgical treatment of lung cancer: survival in stage IIIa disease. *Chest* 1990;97(5):1045–1051, Figure 3.)

In the vignette, arguments could be made for this being part of chronic bronchitis and COPD given the smoking history, or LVF since his previous MI – especially given his ongoing hypertension. However, haemoptysis and weight loss may be due to lung cancer, and early diagnosis is essential for outcome. New haemoptysis in someone >40 years of age is an indication for 2WW referral.

REVISION TIPS

- An urgent CXR is needed if >40 years, with 2+ of (1 if smoker): cough, fatigue, SOB, chest pain, weight loss, loss of appetite or if any of: recurrent/persisting chest infections, clubbing, supraclavicular/cervical lymphadenopathy, chest signs suggestive of lung cancer, thrombocytosis
- 2WW referral if there are CXR findings suggesting lung cancer, or >40 years with haemoptysis

186

Acute Joint Pain

Lucy Andrews, Berenice Aguirrezabala Armbruster,
Michael Whitehouse, and Sung-Hee Kim

EMERGENCY DEPARTMENT, MALE, 27.
SWOLLEN, PAINFUL LEFT KNEE, UNABLE
TO WEIGHT-BEAR

HPC: Worsening for the past 24 hours, feels generally unwell. No trauma or joint disorders. Also reports yellowish penile discharge after unprotected sex a few weeks ago. **PMHx:** Eczema.

O/E: Antalgic gait, swollen/erythematous left knee – ROM reduced throughout, passive and active movements extremely painful. Temperature 38°C. No other joints are affected.

---

1. A patient presents with chronic recurrent pustulosis on his feet on a background of 2 weeks of dysuria, a swollen and painful knee and conjunctivitis – what is the most likely diagnosis?

2. A patient presents with a red, hot, swollen finger. You notice small pits in their nails. What is the most likely cause of their joint pain?

3. A patient with an acute painful wrist is positive for RhF and anti-CCP. What is the most likely cause of their joint pain?

Answers: 1. Reactive arthritis – joint pain associated with recent chlamydia or GI infection, e.g. *Campylobacter*. Keratoderma blenorrhagicum, a pustular rash associated with reactive arthritis. Joint aspirate is likely to have ↑WCC but be culture negative. Management is to treat the underlying infection. 2. Psoriatic arthritis – dactylitis and nail pitting. Associated: personal/FHx of psoriasis/psoriatic arthritis, arthritis in RA distribution, eye involvement, ↑ESR/CRP. 3. Rheumatoid arthritis. Anti-cyclic citrullinated peptide (anti-CCP) is more sensitive and specific than RhF.

TABLE 186.1

	Features	Investigations	Management
Orthopaedics			
Septic arthritis	**RFs:** prosthetic joint, recent surgery, IVDU, DM, skin breach, STI immunocompromised. **Hx & O/E:** pyrexia, acute monoarthritis, pain on movement, unable to weightbear (Fig. 186.1)	↑WCC, ↑CRP, blood cultures. **Swab:** from potential source of infection. **Joint aspirate:** crystals negative, leucocyte esterase dipstick, Gram stain, MC&S, ↑/↔ WCC. **XR:** normal in early stages, ± reduced joint space later	**IV antibiotics:** 2 weeks, then 2–4 weeks oral. Check local guidelines. Take joint aspirate before starting Abx. BNF recommends flucloxacillin. Ceftriaxone if gonococcal. May require **surgical drainage and washout**

TABLE 186.1	(Cont'd)		
	Features	**Investigations**	**Management**
Osteoarthritis (flare-up)	Wear and tear mono- or poly-articular (hand), worse on activity, pain improves with rest, morning stiffness <30 minutes, crepitus. *Knee:* pain/tenderness usually over medial aspect. *Hip:* pain/tenderness internal rotation, Trendelenburg's sign. *Hand:* Heberden's (DIP)/Bouchard's nodes (PIP)	**RFs:** age >50, female, obesity, previous joint injury, FHx. **X-ray: LOSS** = Loss of joint space, Osteophytes, Subchondral cysts, subchondral Sclerosis. (DIP – gull's wing appearance)	Lifestyle, exercise, OT, PT, aids and devices. Analgesia (WHO ladder), intra-articular corticosteroid. **Surgical:** consider elective joint replacement
Rheumatology – Crystal Arthropathies			
Gout (flare-up)	**RFs:** male, high purine diet, CKD, drugs (diuretics, ACE-I, tacrolimus), FHx. **Hx & O/E:** hot, red, tender, swollen, painful joint, monoarticular > polyarticular pattern	↑WBC and CRP. **Aspirate:** negatively birefringent needle-shaped crystals. **XR:** para-articular erosions, **'overhanging edges'.** Soft tissue tophi	**Acute:** NSAIDs and/or colchicine. Steroids second line. Lifestyle changes, consider urate lowering – allopurinol or febuxostat
Calcium pyrophosphate (CPP) deposition disease *Pseudogout*	**RFs:** age >60, OA, Wilson's, haemochromatosis or hyperparathyroidism, dehydration. **Hx & O/E:** red, swollen, painful, monoarticular > polyarticular, flares from dehydration or intercurrent infection	↑WBC and CRP. **Aspirate:** CPP crystals. Positively birefringent, rhomboid crystals. **XR:** chondrocalcinosis (knee cartilage, wrist fibrocartilage)	NSAIDs, colchicine, steroids. Anti-inflammatories (or methotrexate if resistant). Optimise hydration, treat any infection. Correct any metabolic cause
Rheumatology – Inflammatory Arthritis With Predominantly Peripheral Joint Involvement			
Rheumatoid arthritis	See *187. CHRONIC JOINT PAIN*		
Psoriatic arthritis	See *187. CHRONIC JOINT PAIN*		
Rheumatology – Inflammatory Arthritis With Axial Involvement			
Reactive arthritis	Arthritis after enteric/venereal infection or Streptococcal throat. **Hx & O/E:** iritis, uveitis, conjunctivitis, circinate balanitis, asymmetrical oligoarthritis, axial arthritis, keratoderma blenorrhagicum	Infectious disease serology. Slit lamp examination. Consider antibody tests, joint aspirate to r/o differentials. **Monitoring:** FBC, U&Es, LFTs	PT. Analgesia, steroid injections. Treat underlying infection. If relapsing/chronic consider conventional DMARDs
Enteropathic arthritis	**RFs:** IBD, coeliac/Whipple disease, intestinal bypass. **Hx & O/E:** asymmetrical large joint oligoarthritis, sacroiliitis, signs of associated enteropathic disease	↑CRP/ESR, ↑WCC. Consider antibody tests, joint aspirate to r/o differentials. **Monitoring:** FBC, U&Es, LFTs	Treat underlying cause. Steroids. PT and OT. DMARDs for remission. Biologic DMARDs if unresponsive to conventional

(Continued)

TABLE 186.1   (Cont'd)

	Features	Investigations	Management
Ankylosing spondylitis	RFs: male, 20–30 yo, FHx. Hx & O/E: spinal involvement (pain relieved by exercise), stiffness, Schober's test positive, question-mark posture, occasional large joint mono/oligoarthritis, extra-spinal	↑CRP/ESR. XR: sacroiliitis, squaring of vertebrae, bamboo spine (late). MRI: sacroiliitis, bone marrow oedema. **Monitoring:** BASDAI, XR, MRI	PT and exercise. NSAIDs. Steroid injections. Anti-TNF agents if NSAIDs fail to control disease. Consider DMARDs for peripheral disease
Rheumatology – Myalgias			
Fibromyalgia	RF: middle-aged female. Hx & O/E: widespread pain >3 months, fatigue, sleep disturbance, cognitive impairment, headache	Clinical diagnosis (fibromyalgia tender points)	Patient education. CBT. Gradual exercise programme. Antidepressants
Polymyalgia rheumatica	>50 yo, bilateral shoulder pain, worse with movement, stiffness, fatigue, normal muscle strength, depression, onset <2 weeks	Clinical diagnosis. ESR >40, ↑ALP (in 30% of patients). Rest of routine bloods usually normal	PO prednisolone (rapid effect – adjust dose for response). Consider DMARDs for recurrent relapses

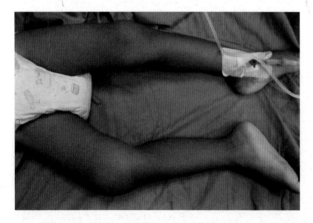

Fig. 186.1 Right knee septic arthritis in a two-year-old boy. There is right knee erythema, flexion deformity and restricted movement (Copyright © 1969, Elsevier. Kurniawan, A., et al. (2021). A rare case of septic arthritis of the knee caused by Salmonella typhi with preexisting typhoid fever in a healthy, immunocompetent child - A case report. *Int J Surg Case Rep*, 78, 76-80.)

The patient in the vignette is young and sexually active, with signs of joint infection and systemic illness. The recent genitourinary symptoms suggest he may have an STI which has led to a joint infection. The most likely diagnosis is Gonococcal septic arthritis.

REVISION TIPS

- Rule out septic arthritis in an acutely hot swollen joint → aspirate joint before giving antibiotics
- Septic arthritis management will differ for patients with prostheses due to biofilm
- If septic arthritis is suspected, treat until an alternative diagnosis is found even if WCC normal/culture negative
- In septic arthritis of a native joint, time is cartilage so early surgical treatment is preferred
- Conventional DMARDs include methotrexate (prescribe with folic acid), sulphasalazine (safe in pregnancy), leflunomide, hydroxychloroquine (safe in pregnancy)

187

Chronic Joint Pain

Katherine Parker and Elizabeth Perry

HPC: Right worse than left, worse in the morning, hard to dress, improves after a couple of hours use. Fatigued and 'under the weather'. Ibuprofen helps. FHx of arthritis. Works as a cleaner, 25 pack-year smoking history.

O/E: Swelling of multiple joints in hands and wrists bilaterally, particularly second/third right PIP/MCP joints; warm and tender. No nail changes. MCP squeeze positive bilaterally. Full range of movement (both active and passive) in all joints, though with some pain.

1. How would your differentials differ if the joint pain was affecting the DIP joint?
2. What five questions can help differentiate inflammatory pain from biomechanical joint pain?
3. When is urgent referral to the rheumatology early inflammatory arthritis clinic appropriate?
4. What are your top differentials for joint inflammation with large lower limb joint involvement and simultaneous lower back stiffness/sacroiliac inflammation?

Answers: 1. Psoriatic arthritis and OA are more likely. 2. Worst time of day? Joint swelling? Relationship to activity? Response to NSAIDs/glucocorticoids? Associated features (systemic)? 3. Persistent symptoms c/w new inflammatory arthritis (e.g. RA or psoriatic) with onset within 6 months and affecting more than one joint, or hands/ feet. 4. Spondyloarthropathies; ankylosing spondylitis, psoriatic arthritis, reactive arthritis, IBD-associated spondyloarthropathy.

TABLE 187.1

	Features	Investigations	Management
Rheumatoid arthritis	**Hx & O/E:** symmetrical polyarthritis, small joints (less DIPs), morning stiffness >1 hour. Boutonniere deformity, Swann neck, Z thumb, ulnar deviation, subluxation (Fig. 187.1). *Extra-articular:* atlantoaxial subluxation, Sjogren's, scleritis, episcleritis, interstitial lung disease, pericarditis	**RFs:** 30–50 yo, F > M, FHx, smoking. ↑CRP/ESR, ↓Hb. **Antibodies:** anti-CCP (highly specific), RhF (60%), ANA (30%). **XR:** 'SPEL' Soft tissue swelling, Periarticular osteopenia, Erosions, Loss of joint space. **USS:** synovitis, effusion. **Monitoring:** DAS-28	Rheumatology with specialist nurse, PT, OT, podiatry, psychology. Analgesia: NSAID. Short-term steroid (PO/IM/intra-articular) for flares. Conventional DMARD monotherapy (treat-to-target strategy, combination if target not achieved). Biological/targeted synthetic DMARDs (e.g. anti-TNF, anti-CD20, IL-6/JAK inhibitor).

(Continued)

TABLE 187.1   (Cont'd)

	Features	Investigations	Management
Psoriatic arthritis	**RFs:** psoriasis, HLA-B27. **Hx & O/E:** may present as distal arthritis of DIP joints, rheumatoid-like symmetrical polyarthritis (may progress to arthritis mutilans), spondylitic pattern, asymmetrical oligoarthritis. *Extra-articular:* psoriatic plaques, nail changes (pitting, onycholysis), dactylitis	↑CRP/ESR – often normal. Seronegative. **XR:** DIP erosion, pencil in cup deformity (late). **PsARC:** for disease monitoring	Rheumatology. Multidisciplinary – PT, specialist nurse, OT, podiatry, psychology. Consider: CVS, fracture, depression. Analgesia: NSAID if not contraindicated. Short-term glucocorticoid for flares. Conventional DMARD monotherapy using a treat-to-target strategy, and add-on combination if needed. Biological/targeted synthetic DMARDs (e.g. anti-TNF, JAK inhibitors) if ≥3 tender joints and ≥3 swollen joints
Osteoarthritis	See *186. ACUTE JOINT PAIN*		
Systemic lupus erythematosus	See *189. MUSCLE PAIN/MYALGIA*		
Polymyalgia rheumatica (PMR)	**RFs:** F > M, age >50. **Hx & O/E:** bilateral shoulder or hip pain, acute or gradual onset, marked early morning/inactivity stiffness, normal power, constitutional symptoms. ± Giant cell arteritis (GCA), see *36. EYE PAIN AND DISCOMFORT*	↑ESR (>40), others normal, ALP may be elevated. CXR and detailed systems enquiry – exclude a paraneoplastic syndrome resembling PMR. If suspect GCA: temporal artery US/biopsy	Oral glucocorticoid (respond in 24–72 hours). If diagnosis uncertain, poor response to treatment or unable to wean glucocorticoid – rheumatology. Urgent rheumatology in line with local GCA pathways if suspected; prednisolone if sight-threatening
Gout	See *186. ACUTE JOINT PAIN*		
Pseudogout	See *186. ACUTE JOINT PAIN*		

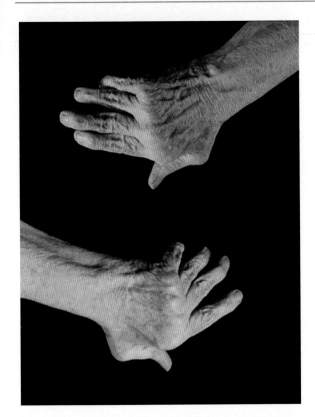

The most likely diagnosis in the vignette is rheumatoid arthritis (RA). The clues are the symmetrical polyarthritis, morning stiffness which lasts >1 hour and improvement with ibuprofen. Family history, smoking and age of presentation are also indicative. Treatment relies on analgesia and anti-inflammatory agents. Conventional DMARDs use treat-to-target strategy, with DAS28 defining the treatment target, and frequent reviews to adjust treatment: methotrexate (with folate supplement), leflunomide, sulphasalazine (safe in pregnancy) and hydroxychloroquine (also safe in pregnancy, monotherapy is only for mild or palindromic disease). In RA, also consider whether the patient is at risk of fracture or depression, or whether there is a cardiovascular risk.

Fig. 187.1 Deformities associated with rheumatoid arthritis – Digits: Swan Neck, Boutonniere's, Z thumb. Wrist: piano key deformity, ulnar deviation. Rachel C. Jeffery. Elsevier. Date: May 2014.

REVISION TIPS

- Key features of inflammatory versus mechanical joint pain
  - **Inflammatory** – younger, morning stiffness >1 hour/inactivity stiffness, small > large joints, joint swelling, systemic features present, positive response to glucocorticoids/NSAIDs <48 hours
  - **Mechanical** – older, insidious/gradual onset, morning stiffness <1 hour, large > small joints, no systemic features, response to NSAIDs minimal, worse on activity

188

Fatigue

Katie Turner, Berenice Aguirrezabala Armbruster, and Elizabeth Perry

GP CONSULTATION, FEMALE, 55. FATIGUE AND LOW MOOD FOR 6 MONTHS

HPC: Unable to sleep at night, excessively sleepy during the day, cannot concentrate – had to reduce her hours working as a ward clerk. No longer going for walks due to physical exhaustion; generalised muscle aches but no specific areas of tenderness. Previously diagnosed with PTSD.

O/E: Pain on lymph node palpation, not enlarged. Bloods (FBC, U&Es, LFTs, glucose, TFTs, ESR, CRP, calcium, ferritin, coeliac serology) all normal.

1. Can you name three causes of hypothyroidism?
2. Can you list the side effects of TCAs?
3. Can you list three possible causes of a microcytic anaemia?

Answers: 1. Hashimoto's, subacute de Quervain's thyroiditis, Riedel thyroiditis, post-thyroidectomy or radioiodine treatment, dietary iodine deficiency, drugs (e.g. lithium, amiodarone). 2. Drowsiness, dry mouth, blurred vision, constipation, urinary retention, prolonged QT interval. 3. Iron deficiency anaemia, thalassaemia, congenital sideroblastic anaemia, anaemia of chronic disease, lead poisoning.

TABLE 188.1

	Features	Investigations	Management
Chronic fatigue syndrome (CFS)/myalgic encephalomyelitis	Persistent fatigue for ≥6 weeks (worse with activity), post-exertional malaise, unrefreshing/disturbed sleep, cognitive	RFs: female, associated chronic condition/psychosocial condition. Clinical diagnosis (Fig. 188.1)	CFS service. Manage any stress, anxiety and/or depression. Pacing/energy management. CBT. Sleep hygiene advice
Depression	See *164. LOW MOOD/AFFECTIVE PROBLEMS*		
Obstructive sleep apnoea	**RFs:** male, obesity, adenotonsillar hypertrophy, macroglossia, other comorbidities (e.g. TIA, hypothyroidism). **Hx & O/E:** excessive daytime sleepiness, snoring, fatigue, apnoea. **Associated conditions;** obesity, depression, hypertension, stroke disease	Clinical diagnosis. Collateral history from partner can be helpful where possible. Screening questionnaires can be helpful to assess the extent and severity of symptoms, e.g. STOP-BANG, Epworth Sleepiness Scale. Sleep studies	**Adults:** 1. Assess any impact on driving/work-related safety 2. Referral to sleep clinic 3. Intra-oral devices 4. CPAP 5. Upper airway surgery **Children:** 1. Consider adenotonsillectomy 2. Consider CPAP

TABLE 188.1 (Cont'd)

	Features	Investigations	Management
Hypothyroidism	**RFs:** FHx, co-existent autoimmune disease, thyroid damage (e.g. surgery), iodine deficiency, female, pregnancy, increased age. **Hx & O/E:** tiredness, weight gain, constipation, depression, muscle aches, cold intolerance, dry skin, menstrual irregularities, carpal tunnel disease, hair loss. **Consider secondary hypothyroidism,** e.g. cerebral malignancy, head trauma, surgery, pituitary gland disease	TFTs, thyroid antibodies. Consider FBC, HbA1c, coeliac serology, lipid profile. **ECG** (may show arrhythmias in elderly). Consider neck USS	Emergency admission if serious complication, e.g. myxoedema coma. Arrange urgent endocrinology referral if secondary hypothyroidism suspected. Levothyroxine (T$_4$)* monotherapy for uncomplicated primary hypothyroidism *Seek urgent specialist guidance if any features of adrenal insufficiency – thyroid hormone replacement in adrenal failure can precipitate adrenal crisis*
Iron-deficiency anaemia	**RFs:** pregnancy, menorrhagia, NSAID use (risk of GI bleed). **Hx & O/E:** SOB on exertion, headaches/ dizziness, fatigue, palpitations, conjunctival/ facial pallor, glossitis, koilonychia (spoon-shaped nails)	FBC (↓Hb), iron studies (↓iron/ferritin, ↑TIBC). Consider B12/folate and coeliac serology. **Blood film:** target cells and pencil poikilocytes	Address underlying cause. PO ferrous sulphate. If intolerance, consider parenteral iron. Consider blood transfusion. Monitor Hb/FBC to assess response to treatment

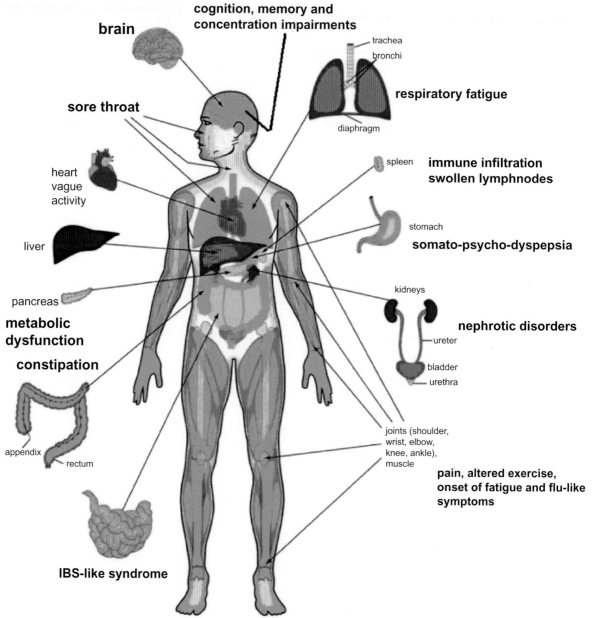

Fig. 188.1 The involvement of human body organs in chronic fatigue syndrome. (Reproduced with permission from; Bjorklund, G., et al. (2019). Chronic fatigue syndrome (CFS): Suggestions for a nutritional treatment in the therapeutic approach. *Biomed Pharmacother*, 109, 1000-1007).

The most likely diagnosis in the vignette is *chronic fatigue syndrome*, based on the clinical presentation and the exclusion of differentials. A battery of tests may be considered, including FBC, U&Es, LFTs, bone profile, CRP, ESR, TFTs, ferritin, CK, HbA1c, IgA tissue transglutaminase, myeloma screen, urinalysis. It is important to treat any associated symptoms of anxiety or depression.

REVISION TIPS

- Fatigue must persist for at least 4 months and affect mental and physical function to diagnose CFS
- Be aware of red flags – significant weight loss, altered bowel habit or urinary symptoms, blood loss, SOB, jaundice, acute onset or long-term duration
- Always consider the possibility of malignancy

189

Muscle Pain/Myalgia

Katherine Parker and Elizabeth Perry

HPC: 3 months joint aches, muscle pain which is difficult to localise – fatigue and mouth ulcers. Ibuprofen minimal improvement. Similar episode 12 months ago. Stressed at work, worried this is causing her hair to fall out. **PMHx:** Nil. **DHx:** Nil. **FHx:** Asthma.

O/E: Obs normal. 2 × 1.5 cm scaly plaques on the scalp, with hair loss. Face: symmetrical, non-tender erythematous rash across the nasal bridge and cheeks, sparing the nasolabial folds. MSK: no muscle wasting, diffuse tenderness on palpation of the upper/lower limbs, normal sensation, power 5/5. Otherwise normal.

1. Which drugs can trigger SLE?
2. Early systemic sclerosis may present with fatigue, arthralgia and myalgia; what other features would indicate this diagnosis?
3. Which baseline blood tests should be performed prior to starting a statin?

Answers: 1. Phenytoin, isoniazid, carbamazepine, terbinafine, sulphasalazine. 2. Raynaud's, sclerodactyly, GORD, dysphagia, digital ulcers, telangiectasias, pulmonary involvement. 3. HbA1c/fasting glucose if risk of DM, lipid profile, LFTs, U&Es, TSH, CK- see commentary below.

TABLE 189.1

	Features	Investigations	Management
SLE (Fig. 189.1)	**RFs:** Afro-Caribbean/Asian descent, F > M, age 15–45. FHx, medication (e.g. hydralazine), UV exposure. **Articular:** symmetrical polyarthritis, **non-deforming**. Morning stiffness, relapsing/remitting course. **Extra-articular:** myalgia, photosensitive (malar) rash, oral ulcers, alopecia, Raynaud's, Sicca syndrome, pleuritis, endocarditis, pericarditis, seizures, psychosis, renal. Antiphospholipid syndrome	**Immune:** ANA, anti-dsDNA, anti-Smith, low complement, anti-histone (drug induced). Antiphospholipid antibodies (e.g. lupus anti-coagulant and anti-cardiolipin). ↓Hb, ↓WBC, ↓pts, ↑APTT, ↑CRP/ESR. **XR:** no bony changes, ± capsule inflammation (Jaccoud's arthropathy). **CXR:** ± pleural effusion, cardiomegaly. Tests of other systems	Rheumatology- urgent if concerns of organ involvement. Sun avoidance, manage CVS risks. **Hydroxychloroquine** for skin/MSK/systemic. Short-term steroid for flares. **Azathioprine** or **methotrexate** may be used for maintenance. **Cyclophosphamide** or **mycophenolate mofetil:** for organ threatening. Biologics, e.g. anti-BLyS, anti-CD20 may be used in treatment-resistant

(Continued)

TABLE 189.1 (Cont'd)

	Features	Investigations	Management
Influenza	See *25. NASAL OBSTRUCTION*		
Lyme disease *Borrelia burgdorferi*	See *54. BITES AND STINGS*		
Polymyalgia rheumatica	See *187. CHRONIC JOINT PAIN*		
Polymyositis, dermatomyositis	See *160. CHRONIC PAIN*		
Fibromyalgia	See *160. CHRONIC PAIN*		
Statin muscle-related adverse events	**RFs:** high-dose steroids, PMHx/FHx muscular disorder, alcohol, liver disease, CKD, hypothyroidism, low vitamin D, medications increasing plasma levels (e.g. amiodarone, clarithromycin, amlodipine). **Hx & O/E:** muscle pain, tenderness or weakness after starting statin	CK in unexplained muscle pain (baseline CK should be <5× normal limit <u>prior</u> to initiation of statins). **Investigations to identify reversible aetiologies:** TSH, vitamin D, LFTs, U&Es. If muscle symptoms or raised CK persist despite stopping the statin, consider EMG and muscle biopsy, HMGCR antibody	Discontinue statin and wait for CK to return to baseline. Address reversible aetiologies, e.g. drug interaction, hypothyroid, vitamin D deficiency, ARF. If reversible and symptoms resolved, retrial with close monitoring. If no reversible aetiology, switch to pravastatin or fluvastatin

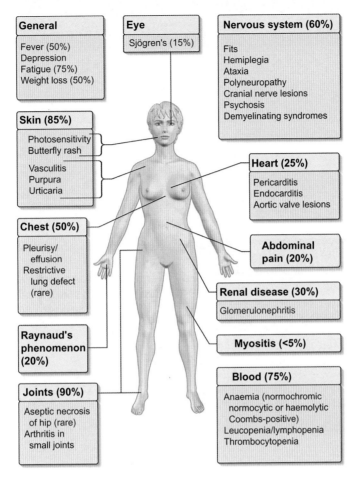

General

Fever (50%)
Depression
Fatigue (75%)
Weight loss (50%)

Eye

Sjögren's (15%)

Nervous system (60%)

Fits
Hemiplegia
Ataxia
Polyneuropathy
Cranial nerve lesions
Psychosis
Demyelinating syndromes

Skin (85%)

Photosensitivity
Butterfly rash

Vasculitis
Purpura
Urticaria

Heart (25%)

Pericarditis
Endocarditis
Aortic valve lesions

Chest (50%)

Pleurisy/
   effusion
Restrictive
   lung defect
   (rare)

**Abdominal
pain (20%)**

Renal disease (30%)

Glomerulonephritis

**Raynaud's
phenomenon
(20%)**

Myositis (<5%)

Joints (90%)

Aseptic necrosis
   of hip (rare)
Arthritis in
   small joints

Blood (75%)

Anaemia (normochromic
   normocytic or haemolytic
   Coombs-positive)
Leucopenia/lymphopenia
Thrombocytopenia

Fig. 189.1 Clinical features of SLE. (Kumar, DPJ, Clark, ML. Chapter 8, Rheumatology. In: *Kumar & Clark's Cases in Clinical Medicine.* Elsevier; 2021.)

The most likely diagnosis in the vignette is SLE. The key things to notice are the extra-articular signs such as malar rash and myalgia. Further testing will be required to confirm the diagnosis. When starting a statin, check HbA1c or fasting blood glucose in people at high risk of diabetes mellitus. Also check the lipid profile and LFTs (ALT, AST – exclude statin if these are >3× upper limit of normal). U&Es should be checked, and the dose adjusted if there is impaired renal function. TSH is important, as hypothyroidism can cause dyslipidaemia, and there is increased risk of statin-induced myopathy if not treated. CK is also checked if there is myalgia or a high-risk of muscle-related adverse events.

REVISION TIPS

- Dermatomyositis can be associated with internal malignancy. Screening should be performed at onset AND for the next 3 years
- New onset Raynaud's in an adult can be indicative of an underlying connective tissue disorder – e.g. systemic sclerosis, SLE, dermatomyositis. Low threshold for early rheumatology opinion
- Chronic fatigue syndrome is typically more fatigue than myalgia, while myalgia predominates in fibromyalgia
- For SLE, think SOAP BRAIN MD; Serositis, Oral ulcers, Arthritis, Photosensitivity, Blood disorders, Renal, Antinuclear antibodies, Immunological, Neurological, Malar rash, Discoid rash

190

Fit Notes

Alexander Royston and Jennifer Powell

GP PRESENTATION, MALE, 36. LOWER BACK PAIN, REQUESTING A FIT NOTE

HPC: Reports injuring his back at work and also complains of shooting pains down one leg, but denies symptoms of saddle paraesthesia or sphincteric dysfunction. **PMHx:** Backache, erectile dysfunction. **DHx:** Ibuprofen PRN. **SHx:** Smoker (10 pack years), moderate alcohol. Works in a manual profession.

O/E: Obs stable, clinically well. DRE declined. Back examination reveals pain on lumbar extension/flexion, positive straight leg raise. Neurological testing otherwise all normal. Schober's test negative.

1. What is the procedure for absence from work inside the first 7 days?

2. Is a GP's assessment or advice binding on the patient's employer?

3. If a patient has a personal or social problem and is asking for a fit note (for example, caring for relatives), what should the doctor do?

Answers: 1. To claim Statutory Sick Pay for illness of 7 days or less, the patient may self-certify using the appropriate form. **2.** No, it is classed as advice and it is for employers to determine whether or not to accept. **3.** Doctors can issue fit notes only to cover the patient's own health condition. If a personal issue is causing them stress resulting in ill health, it may be appropriate to issue a fit note – this will depend on clinical opinion.

TABLE 190.1

	Features	Investigations	Management
Prolapsed intervertebral disc (PID)	**RFs:** age 35–50, male, physically demanding work. **Hx & O/E:** seizing pain worse on bending/twisting, radiating to buttock/leg (sciatica). According to affected root(s); myotome weakness, diminished reflexes, altered sensation, root tension (Fig. 190.1). Exclude cauda equina syndrome (see *192. BACK PAIN*)	MRI spine	Rest, analgesia, physiotherapy. Lumbar microdiscectomy ± laminectomy

TABLE 190.1 (Cont'd)			
	Features	Investigations	Management
Mechanical lower back pain	**RFs:** age >30, lack of exercise, overweight. **Hx & O/E:** non-specific pain, worse on movement. No cause identifiable. Chronic if >4 weeks, may have 'yellow flags'	**Bloods:** only if >4 weeks/red flags. X-ray (consider). **CT/MRI** (consider if >4 weeks)	Analgesia, CBT, physiotherapy. Suggest amended duties, instead of 'not fit for work'
Depression	**RFs:** prior/FHx of depression. Recently bereaved/ill. Stress. **Hx & O/E:** low mood, poor appetite/sleep, anhedonia, anergia	PHQ-9. Risk assessment. Bloods (for reversible causes)	First line – talking therapies. Consider anti-depressants
Malingering disorder	**RFs:** socio-economic. Wants secondary gain, e.g. financial gain post-accident	Patient will avoid risky investigations	
Somatic symptom disorder	**RFs:** stressful/traumatic life events, anxiety/depression. **Hx & O/E:** severe persistent physical medically unexplained symptoms >6 months. Significant disruption of daily life. Persistent thoughts/anxiety/time devoted to symptoms	Exclude organic causes, depending on symptoms and signs, before clinical diagnosis of somatic symptom disorder	Psychological input. Eclectic psychotherapy; CBT, mindfulness, and/or short-term dynamic psychotherapy, interpersonal/general psychotherapy, re-attribution training

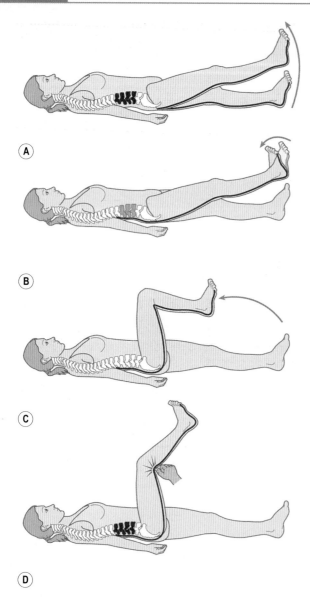

Fig. 190.1 (A) Straight-leg raising limited by the tension of a sciatic nerve root over a PID. (B) Tension is increased by foot dorsiflexion (Bragard test). (C) Tension is relieved by knee flexion. (D) Pressure on the popliteal fossa tenses the posterior tibial nerve, causing pain locally and in the back. (Reproduced with permission from Gibson, J, Brenkel, I. The musculoskeletal system. In *Macleod's Clinical Examination*, ed 14. 251–282. © 2018 Elsevier. All rights reserved.)

NHS GPs are required to issue, free of charge, a Statement of Fitness for Work to patients for whom they provide clinical care. Although the patient in the vignette has declined a rectal examination, this is common behaviour and there is no compelling concern for cauda equina syndrome. While psychosocial barriers can develop around chronic back pain that limit people returning to work, concerns over malingering would need a longer time period, further presentations and more yellow flag symptoms. In chronic back pain and with long work absence, depression can be both cause and effect, and it should be screened for. Generally, patients do not do well with long periods off work (mental/physical health, well-being and finances). They can begin to conform to the sick role, with future reintegration back into work then becoming difficult. Signing a patient off work completely must only be for short periods and with appropriate follow-up arranged (should only continue if being seen to engage with physio/psychotherapy, etc.)

191

Soft Tissue Injury/Minor Trauma

Marie-Louise Lyons, James Miller, and Michael Whitehouse

EMERGENCY DEPARTMENT, MALE, 24.
INJURY TO THE ANKLE WHILST PLAYING FOOTBALL

HPC: Was tackled by another player and twisted ankle. Generally fit and well, no other injuries.

O/E: Swollen ankle, unable to weight bear, pain on palpation over lateral malleolus, superficial laceration over medial malleolus. Obs: normal. **Ix:** X-ray shows no fracture.

1. What are the Ottawa ankle rules?
2. What are the 6 P's used to identify compartment syndrome?

Answers: 1. Ottawa rules recommend radiographs for ankle/midfoot injuries if pain and tenderness over the posterior 6 cm or tip of the lateral or medial malleolus; midfoot pain and tenderness over the navicular or base of fifth metatarsal; ankle or midfoot pain and unable to take four steps straight after injury and in the ED. Clinical discretion also applies. 2. Pain (e.g. pain out of proportion, pain on passive stretch, poor response to opiate analgesia), Paraesthesia, Paresis, Pulseless, Pallor, Persistent Cold.

TABLE 191.1

Differentials	Clinical	Investigations	Management
Soft tissue injury	**RFs:** sport, inversion injuries (85%), eversion – court games and team sports. **Hx & O/E:** restricted range of motion, tenderness, pain. Bruising, difficulty or unable to weight bear	**XR:** Ottawa ankle rules determine if XR required. AP (mortise) and lateral views, to rule out fracture (Figs. 191.1 and 191.2). XR will not identify ligament damage. **MRI:** to exclude ligament injury, and to grade muscle strains	Analgesia. **R.I.C.E** - Rest, Ice, Compression, Elevation. Reassure-6 weeks to 6 months recovery. **Partial ligament tear:** gentle mobilisation, physiotherapy. **Complete tear:** persistent instability with pain/limited function, consider surgery. Physiotherapy

(Continued)

TABLE 191.1 (Cont'd)

Differentials	Clinical	Investigations	Management
Closed bone injury	RFs: sports, forced eversion, trauma, osteoporosis, fall, RTA. Hx & O/E: swelling, bruising, pain, inability to weight bear, tender, deformity. Pain on palpation, crepitus	Neurovascular (NV), skin. XR: AP (mortise) and lateral. Stability and Weber classification guide treatment of lateral malleolar fractures. CT	Analgesia. Reduce promptly, splint in POP backslab, reassess distal NV status, check XR. Unstable # (disrupted syndesmosis) often needs fixation. Stable: mobilise full weight-bearing in cast/walking boot. Fracture clinic at 2 and 6 weeks. NV deficit may recover when reduced. If not, urgent CT angio, vascular surgery – explore ± fasciotomy
Open bone injury	Hight impact trauma, crush injury. Hx & O/E: painful, swollen, unable to weight bear, deformed joint, wounds. Look for other injuries. Compartment syndrome - see *45. PAINFUL SWOLLEN LEG*	ATLS Vascular/nerve/skin examination. Repeat after reduction and splinting. ABG/VBG: lactate. FBC, U&E, clotting, G&S. XR: AP and lateral views. CT scan. If not in major trauma centre, transfer to orthoplastic unit.	Follow BOAST guideline. IV Abx: follow hospital guidelines. Remove gross contamination. Wound photography, saline gauze, occlusive dressing. Tetanus – give vaccine if needed. Analgesia, NBM, urgent realignment and splinting. Emergency wound debridement by combined orthopaedics/plastics. Internal/external fixation. Soft tissue closure/reconstruction within 72 hours. Amputation – MDT decision unless life-saving
Nerve injury	Due to the initial trauma, or surgical complication. Impaired power/sensation distal to the injury	XR. MRI for soft tissue injury. Nerve conduction studies	Analgesia, specialist review <24 hours. Immediate reduction if associated dislocation. Surgery- plastic and orthopaedic
Tendon injury	*Achilles (calcaneal) rupture/ tendinopathy.* RFs: sports, systemic steroids, quinolone, DM, hypercholesterolaemia. Hx & O/E: sudden pain and 'pop', can't raise heel off floor, dorsi-flexed, poor walking, swollen bruised calf	Simmonds/Thompson test: reduced plantar flexion when calf is squeezed. Simmonds triad: calf-squeeze, tendon gap, abnormal angle of declination. MRI: complete vs. incomplete – diagnostic. US if no MRI	R.I.C.E., analgesia, gently mobilise weight bearing if incomplete. POP slab in plantar flexion if complete. Physiotherapy. Boot with heel wedges or range of motion boot locked in plantar flexion, progressively reduced. Surgical: open vs. percutaneous repair
Vascular injury	RFs: trauma, fracture. Hx & O/E: hypovolaemia if haemorrhage. Weak or absent pulses. Ischaemia distally. Compartment syndrome – 6 Ps	Vascular/neuro examination. FBC, G&S, U&Es. Lactate: to identify limb ischaemia. Intracompartmental manometry. CT angiography	ATLS assessment, IVI. Major haemorrhage protocol. Direct pressure/tourniquet. Re-align and splint. Revascularise within 4 hours/ amputation. Compartment syndrome: fasciotomy within 1 hour

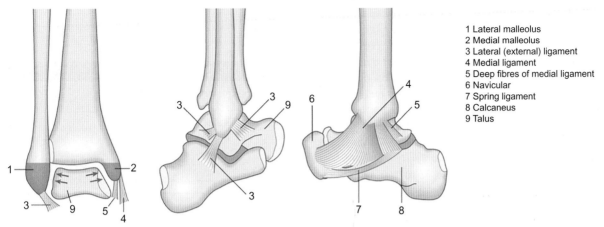

1 Lateral malleolus
2 Medial malleolus
3 Lateral (external) ligament
4 Medial ligament
5 Deep fibres of medial ligament
6 Navicular
7 Spring ligament
8 Calcaneus
9 Talus

Fig. 191.1 Ankle ligaments (From Jane Gibson, Ivan Brenkel. The musculoskeletal system. In: *Macleod's Clinical Examination*. 2018. Copyright © 2018 Elsevier Ltd. All rights reserved.)

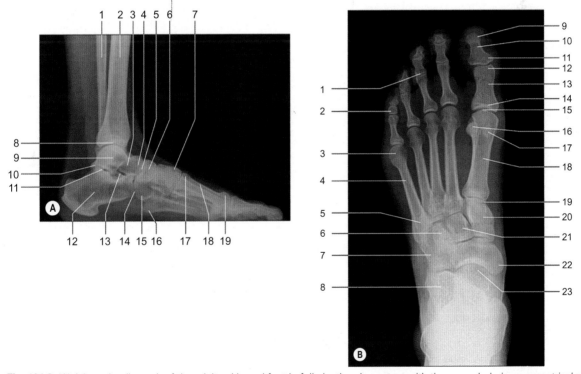

Fig. 191.2 (A) A lateral radiograph of the adult ankle and foot in full plantigrade contact with the ground, during symmetrical standing. Key: 1, fibula; 2, tibia; 3, talar neck; 4, talar head; 5, talonavicular joint; 6, navicular; 7, medial cuneiform; 8, talocrural joint; 9, talar body; 10, posterior process of talus; 11, subtalar joint; 12, calcaneus (note the trabecular pattern); 13, tarsal sinus; 14, calcaneocuboid joint; 15, cuboid; 16, styloid process of the fifth metatarsal; 17, base of the first metatarsal; 18, shaft of the first metatarsal; 19, head of the first metatarsal. (B) A dorsoplantar radiograph of the adult foot in full plantigrade contact with the ground, during symmetrical standing, in a male aged 24 years. Key: 1, interphalangeal joint; 2, middle phalanx; 3, head of fifth metatarsal; 4, shaft of fifth metatarsal; 5, base of fifth metatarsal; 6, lateral cuneiform; 7, cuboid; 8, calcaneus; 9, head of distal phalanx; 10, shaft of distal phalanx; 11, base of distal phalanx; 12, head of proximal phalanx; 13, shaft of proximal phalanx; 14, base of proximal phalanx; 15, first metatarsophalangeal joint; 16, lateral (fibular) sesamoid; 17, medial (tibial) sesamoid; 18, shaft of first metatarsal; 19, first metatarsocuneiform joint; 20, medial cuneiform; 21, intermediate cuneiform; 22, tuberosity of navicular; 23, talar head. (Courtesy of New York College of Podiatric Medicine, New York, NY.) (Ankle and foot. Book: Gray's Anatomy. Author: Susan Standring. Publisher: Elsevier. Date: 2021. Copyright © 2021 Elsevier Ltd. All rights reserved.)

In the vignette, a soft tissue injury such as an ankle sprain is likely, as is common in sports such as football. Most likely he has torn his lateral ligament complex by 'twisting his ankle'/over-inverting his ankle – perhaps if his medial malleolus was stood on. Ankle inversion is the most common 'ankle sprain', due to relative weakness on the lateral side. The superficial laceration to the medial malleolus is unlikely to be an open fracture. Furthermore, nothing suggests he has a tendon, nerve or vascular injury. The Ottawa ankle rules indicate his inability to weight-bear and the malleolar pain meant an X-ray was appropriate to exclude a fracture.

REVISION TIPS

- Fracture management principles, the 4 Rs: Resuscitation, Reduction, Restriction (immobilisation) and Rehabilitation
- In minor trauma you should examine joint, peripheral vascular, nervous system and skin integrity
- Most ankle fractures involve some degree of rotation – see the Lauge-Hansen classification system

192

Back Pain

Alice Parker, Berenice Aguirrezabala Armbruster, and Matthew Boissaud-Cooke

EMERGENCY DEPARTMENT, MALE, 55.
LOW BACK PAIN AND RIGHT LEG PAIN, FOR FOUR MONTHS

HPC: Onset while walking, constant lumbar back pain and electric shock-like pain radiating to right buttock/foot. Worse on prolonged sitting. GP commenced paracetamol and naproxen, with only initial benefit. For 4 weeks, sole of his right foot 'feels different', with intermittent pins and needles. Mobility reduced, no weakness/left leg pain/bowel or bladder symptoms/saddle anaesthesia. **PMHx:** Nil of note, no other regular medication, office worker.

O/E: No spinal deformity or tenderness. Limited forward flexion/extension. Lower limbs: tone normal, power 5/5 in all myotomes except 4/5 right plantar flexion, absent right ankle reflex, altered sensation sole of right foot. Nerve root tension sign present; right straight leg raise (SLR) 15 degrees of elevation. Hip examination is unremarkable.

1. What diagnosis should be considered in gradual onset back pain and PMH of tuberculosis?
2. A patient presents to A&E with back pain, fever and a limp. Supine, the left leg is flexed at the knee and externally rotated at the hip. Extending the hip makes the pain worse and you note a painless lump above the inguinal ligament. What is the likely diagnosis?
3. What is the most common causative organism in discitis?
4. What pathologies can lead to cauda equina syndrome?

Answers: 1. Spinal tuberculosis (Pott disease). 2. Psoas abscess. Extension of the hip causes pain as the psoas muscle is stretched. 3. *Staphylococcus aureus*. 4. Lumbar prolapsed intervertebral disc, trauma, epidural haematoma or abscess, tumours, neuropathies, ankylosing spondylitis.

TABLE 192.1			
	Features	**Investigations**	**Management**
Prolapsed intervertebral disc	Hx & O/E: onset after physical strain, pain worse on bend/twist, radiates to buttock/leg (sciatica). According to affected root(s); myotome weakness, diminished reflexes, altered sensation, root tension (SLR)	MRI lumbo-sacral (L/S) spine (CT myelogram if MRI contraindicated)	Analgesia, physiotherapy. Lumbar microdiscectomy ± laminectomy

(Continued)

TABLE 192.1   (Cont'd)

	Features	Investigations	Management
Lumbar spinal stenosis	**Causes:** ligamentum flavum hypertrophy, bulging disc, facet joint cysts/hypertrophy, spondylolisthesis, osteophytes. **Hx & O/E:** lumbar back/ leg pain (neurogenic claudication- worse on walking, relieved by rest), helped by walking uphill/ leaning forward. Weakness / sensory disturbance.	MRI L/S spine. **Lumbar radiographs** (flexion/extension view) – dynamic instability	Analgesia, lifestyle modifications (weight loss, exercise). Decompressive laminectomy (for spinal canal/intervertebral foramina) ± instrumented fusion
Metastatic spinal cord compression	Primary neoplasia, metastases, myeloma, lymphoma. **Red flags:** age <18 or >50, gradual onset, pain at night-time/rest, worse on straining (coughing), thoracic pain, localised spinal tenderness, not improving despite analgesia, weight loss. LMN signs at level of lesion, UMN signs below level, bowel/bladder dysfunction	PMH breast/lung/GI/ prostate/renal/thyroid cancer. FBC (↓Hb), ↑ESR, LFT, bone profile, myeloma screen. **Urgent MRI spine.** **CT TAP**	Options include high-dose steroids, radiotherapy, surgery (decompression, tumour debulking), chemotherapy. Refer to neurosurgeons/oncologists
Cauda equina syndrome	**Red flags:** bilateral sciatica, severe/ progressive bilateral lower limb weakness. **Hx & O/E:** urinary symptoms (difficulty initiating urination, decreased urinary sensation, incontinence). Bowel symptoms (loss of sensation of rectal fullness, incontinence). Saddle paraesthesia/anaesthesia. Sexual dysfunction	**Urgent MRI L/S spine**	Nil by mouth. Analgesia. Urgent referral to neurosurgery or spine surgeons for consideration of surgery to treat cause (a large herniated disc is most common)
Spinal fracture	**RFs:** major trauma- can be minor trauma (older/steroids/osteoporosis). **Hx & O/E:** structural spine deformity (i.e. palpable step between vertebrae), contusion/abrasion, point tenderness	**CT spine.** **MRI spine:** if neurological deficit. FRAX score ± DEXA if suspect osteoporosis	Local spine services; non-operative vs operative (depends on fracture type, stability, neurology, etc.). Exclude other traumatic injuries, or pathological/ insufficiency fractures
Spine infections	**Red flags:** fever, TB/recent UTI, DM, IVDU/immunocompromised, pain at rest. **Types:** discitis, spondylitis (vertebral osteomyelitis), spinal epidural abscess. **Hx & O/E:** , fever, **pain,** ±neurological deficit	CRP, ESR, blood cultures. MRI spine (neurological compromise), CT/ XR (bony destruction, instability). Search for primary source	Find infection source, sample/cultures, Abx - involve microbiology. Local spine services. **Surgery:** for sample, drain abscess, decompress, treat instability (late, rare)

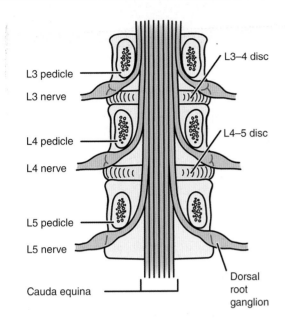

Fig. 192.1 Coronal schematic view of the exiting lumbar spinal nerve roots. Each lumbar spinal nerve root is named for the vertebra above it. Note that because of the way the nerve roots exit, L4–L5 disc pathology usually affects the L5 root rather than the L4 root. (Redrawn from Borenstein DG, Wiesel SW, Boden SD. *Low Back Pain: Medical Diagnosis and Comprehensive Management.* Philadelphia: WB Saunders; 1995:5.)

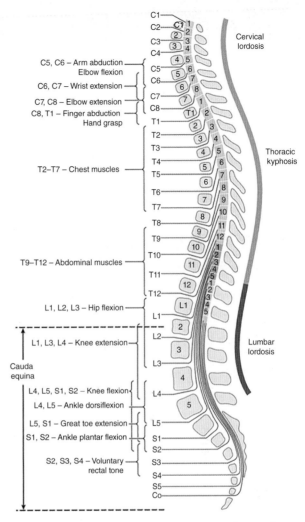

Fig. 192.2 The normal spinal curves and root innervations. (Gibson J, Brenkel I. Chapter 13, The musculoskeletal system. In: *Macleod's Clinical Examination.* Elsevier; 2018. Copyright © 2018 Elsevier. All rights reserved.)

*The most likely diagnosis in the vignette is an L5/S1 prolapsed disc compressing the right S1 nerve root (hence the distribution of sciatica, gastrocnemius weakness, absent ankle jerk). See Fig. 192.1 for a representation of the lumbar spine nerve roots. Fig. 192 shows nerve root levels for various motor functions. The adult spinal cord (usually) finishes at L1/2 vertebral level, so the lower spinal cord segments are not co-located with their associated vertebral level; nerve roots from low thoracic segments and below must pass caudally to reach their associated vertebral level. Sciatica, see **108. ALTERED SENSATION, NUMBNESS AND TINGLING.***

REVISION TIPS

- Always ask about red flag symptoms/signs and document clearly
- Cauda equina syndrome should always be ruled out in a patient presenting with back pain. If suspected, an urgent MRI should be arranged

193

Musculoskeletal Deformity

Ioan Llwyd Hughes, James Miller, and Michael Whitehouse

EMERGENCY DEPARTMENT, MALE, 70. KNEE PAIN AFTER A FALL

HPC: Turned, knee gave way, 'pop' sound and he fell – rapid swelling in left knee.

O/E: Painful swollen knee, unable to weight bear. Able to straight leg raise, but feels knee is unstable. No erythema, subtle bruising around the knee. Lateral joint line tenderness; Thessaly's and McMurray's tests positive.

Ix: XR no fractures, suprapatellar effusion.

---

1. What is the most common imaging modality for suspected bony injuries?
2. Medial knee tenderness with instability on valgus stress- what is the most likely diagnosis?
3. Is intra-articular involvement of a fracture in a joint more likely to be managed non-operatively or surgically?
4. For suspected soft tissue injury in the knee where X-ray reveals no pathology, what is the next appropriate investigation?
5. For a broken leg with increasing foot pain made worse by stretching the great toe – what is the diagnosis and what needs to be done?

Answers: 1. X-ray (think "bones X-ray, soft tissue MRI"). 2. Medial collateral ligament (MCL) injury. 3. Surgical management. 4. MRI. 5. Compartment syndrome and emergency fasciotomy of all four compartments.

TABLE 193.1

	Features	Investigations	Management
Adult Lower Limb MSK Deformity Secondary to Trauma			
Ligament injury (Fig. 193.1)	LCL: tender lateral aspect, laxity on varus stress testing. MCL: tender medial aspect, laxity on valgus stress testing. ACL: Lachman/anterior drawer test. Pivot shift test. PCL: pain around back of knee, posterior sag test	X-ray: possible suprapatellar effusion/lipohaemarthrosis, avulsion fracture (#) of tibial spine or Segond #. MRI. CT: rarely necessary	Analgesia, RICE, immobilise (cricket pad splint/hinged knee brace). PT/rehab. Arthroscopic/open ligament repair. Initial bracing (external fixation) followed by staged repair (high energy, complex, dislocated)

TABLE 193.1 (Cont'd)

	Features	Investigations	Management
Meniscal injury	Twisting injury on semi-flexed, weight-bearing knee (younger adults). Older: degenerative meniscal tears from less severe stress. **Hx & O/E:** pop sound, pain on loading, joint line tenderness. Thessaly/McMurray tests. Apley grind test	**X-ray:** suprapatellar effusion. **MRI:** diagnosis and pattern, r/o concomitant injuries	RICE, analgesia, immobilise (hinged knee brace), PT, quads rehab. Intra-articular local anaesthetic/steroid (degenerative tear). Arthroscopic meniscal repair ± meniscectomy
Patellar fracture	Direct trauma to anterior knee. Unable to straight leg raise, palpable defect	**X-ray:** #, lipohaemarthrosis. **CT:** complicated/comminuted fracture, check articular congruity	Hinged knee brace/cricket pad splint, immobilising in extension, full weight-bearing. ORIF
Distal femoral fracture	Direct trauma or twisting injury in low-energy fragility #. Pain of distal femur, worse with movement. Unable to weight-bear	**X-ray:** #. **CT:** surgical planning, evaluate intra-articular involvement	Hinged knee brace. External fixation initially if swollen/difficult to control. ORIF osteoporotic #. Retrograde intramedullary nail, beware intra-articular split. Nail-plate combination in unstable/fragility-type #. Arthroplasty (distal femoral replacement poor bone stock).
Tibial plateau fracture	High-energy trauma in young patients. Can be low energy in older. Tender on palpation/movement. Soft-tissue swelling or fracture blisters	**X-ray:** #. **CT:** #, configuration, surgical planning. **MRI:** with CT when suspect multi-ligamentous injury	Hinged knee brace, NWB in minimally displaced #. External/Ilizarov fixation for swelling/comminuted #/high-risk soft tissues. ORIF. If needed, arthroplasty is usually after bony union
Paediatric Lower Limb MSK Deformity			
Ricketts	**RFs:** vitamin D deficiency, renal failure, drugs (e.g. anticonvulsants), liver disease, FHx. **Hx & O/E:** bow-legged, bone pain, craniotabes, osteochondral swelling, Harrison sulcus	Normal/↑PTH, ↑ALP, ↓calcium, ↓phosphate, ↓vit D. XR: loss of cortical bone, Looser's zones, cupped metaphysis. Monitor calcium levels	Calcium and vitamin D supplementation
Congenital talipes equinovarus	**RFs:** FHx, male, neuromuscular disease. **Hx & O/E:** hindfoot in varus, adducted forefoot, ankle in equinus and cannot be dorsiflexed, sole of foot points medially	Clinical diagnosis. XR may be used to assess severity	Manipulation and casting using Ponseti method. Nightly brace for 3 years for maintenance. Surgery for fixed deformity involving Achilles tenotomy

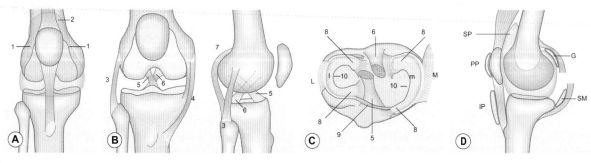

Key

G	Bursa under the medial head of gastrocnemius	1	Extension of synovial sheath on either side of patella	7	Posterior ligament
IP	Infrapatellar bursa	2	Extension of synovial sheath at upper pole of patella	8	Horns of lateral (I) and medial (m) menisci
L	Lateral tibiofemoral articulation	3	Lateral ligament	9	Connection of anterior horns
M	Medial tibiofemoral articulation	4	Medial ligament	10	Unattached margin of meniscus
PP	Prepatellar bursa	5	Anterior cruciate ligament		
SM	Semimembranosus bursa	6	Posterior cruciate ligament		
SP	Suprapatellar pouch (or bursa)				

Fig. 193.1 Structure of the right knee. (A) Anterior view, showing the common synovial sheath. (B) Anterior and lateral views, showing the ligaments. (C) Plan view of the menisci. (D) Bursae. (Gibson J, Brenkel I. Chapter 13, The musculoskeletal system. In: *Macleod's Clinical Examination*. Elsevier; 2018. Copyright © 2018 Elsevier. All rights reserved.)

High-energy and sports-related injuries can point towards ligamentous and bony injuries in the young but degenerative conditions predispose to similar injuries for older patients. In the vignette, it is a low-energy injury, whilst the feeling of instability suggests structural instability in the joint anatomy. Examination then involves a "LOOK, FEEL, MOVE, Special test" approach, emphasising neurovascular check distally, plus checking joints above and below, and the contralateral side. Lack of bony injury on X-ray makes acute fracture unlikely. With a pop sound upon injury and joint line tenderness it could be ACL with associated meniscal injury. Cruciate injury is unlikely (check with Lachman/pivot shift/sagging of tibia on femur). Absence of pain behind the knee makes ruptured Baker's cyst or popliteal aneurysm unlikely.

REVISION TIPS

- Use history to determine high-energy or low-energy fragility type
- Intra-articular bony injuries are more likely to need surgery, to reduce the risk of arthritis later on
- Rapid swelling within a joint could be caused by a ligamentous or meniscal injury
- 6 P's of compartment syndrome; Pain, Poikilothermia, Paresthesia, Paralysis, Pulseless, Pallor. Worsening pain, pain on passive stretch or pain out of proportion must get serial assessment and senior review to decide on emergency fasciotomy

194

Trauma in Children

Emmanuella Ikem, Berenice Aguirrezabala Armbruster,
and Michael Whitehouse

EMERGENCY DEPARTMENT, MALE, AGE 5. SWOLLEN, PAINFUL RIGHT ELBOW

HPC: Witnessed fall on outstretched arm whilst climbing. Unable to mobilise elbow, pain, swelling, constantly crying. Otherwise well. **PMHx:** nil. No social concerns.

O/E: Swollen, immobile, deformed right elbow, no breach to skin, tender palpation, normal neurovascular assessment. No other injuries. Obs: RR 22, SpO$_2$ 98% (air), HR 110, BP 110/60, T37°C.

1. What neurovascular tissues are at risk in the type of fracture described in the vignette?
2. What hand presentations result from nerve damage from this fracture?
3. What is the difference between buckle and greenstick fractures?
4. In which supracondylar fractures should you check the distal neurovascular status?

Answers: 1. Brachial artery and median nerve (anterior interosseus nerve). 2. Lack of pincer grip and sign of benediction. 3. In buckle fracture, there is an incomplete cortical disruption resulting in a bulge. In greenstick fracture, there is a unilateral cortical breach. 4. All of them.

TABLE 194.1

	Features	Investigations	Management
Supracondylar fracture	Peak age 5–7 years. Fall on outstretched arm with hyperextended elbow. Posterior displacement (95%) creates 'S'-shaped deformity. Pain, swelling, deformed elbow, immobile, reduced ROM ± bruising/puncture, ± neurovascular	Check distal pulses, CRT, individual nerve function. **Gartland classification:** types I–III (Fig. 194.1) **X-ray:** distal humerus #, ± displacement (lateral view), anterior/posterior fat pads	Depends on displacement/ Gartland classification. *Non-displaced:* above elbow cast with 90 degrees flexion/neutral rotation for 3 weeks. Check XR at 5–7 days. *Displaced:* closed reduction, percutaneous K-wire fix
Radial head subluxation (pulled elbow)	Caused by axial pulling. **Hx & O/E:** slightly flexed elbow, pronated forearm, tender at radial head. No swelling/deformity	Clinical diagnosis, elbow held in extension and will not permit to be moved. **XR:** if uncertain/suspected fracture. No obvious changes for pulled elbow	Closed reduction with supination and then flexion of the elbow – radial head reduces with a snap. Parent education, screen for NAI

(Continued)

TABLE 194.1   (Cont'd)

	Features	Investigations	Management
Open fracture	Breached skin ± neurovascular compromise. Gustilo Anderson classification I–IIIc (post-debridement). May have associated injuries	Pre-surgery FBC and U&Es. Consider G&S (intended surgery), CM (arterial injury) and blood cultures. If major trauma, then full trauma CT	ATLS + neurovascular assessment. IV Abx as per local guidelines. Initial wound care: saline + dressing ± tetanus booster. Reduction, splinting, post-reduction XR. Surgical debridement. Fixation when overlying skin closure or soft tissue coverage is achievable
Growth plate fracture	Growth plate tenderness, swelling, deformity. May occur through any of the growth plates. In the distal humerus can be either condyle or entire distal humeral epiphysis	AP and lateral X-ray. Salter-Harris classification: Mnemonic SALTER; I – Straight through growth plate II – Above growth plate III – Lower growth plate IV –Through everything V – Ruined growth plate	*Non-displaced:* above elbow cast. *Displaced:* • I – Closed reduction, percutaneous K-wire fixation • II – Closed reduction, screw fixation, supplemental cast • III, IV, V – ORIF with screws + supplemental cast Orthopaedic follow-up
Greenstick fracture of radius	Fall on arm or direct hit. **Hx & O/E:** swelling, deformity, pain	**AP and lateral X-ray:** one cortex broken, the other plastically deformed but not broken	Angulation <10 degrees: below elbow cast 3 weeks. Angulation >10 degrees: consider reduction; if struggling to control, consider above elbow cast
Torus/buckle fracture of humerus	Fall on outstretched arm. Low energy impact. No obvious clinical deformity	**AP and lateral X-ray:** usually distal metaphyseal fracture	Removable splint or bandage. Discharge with no further review

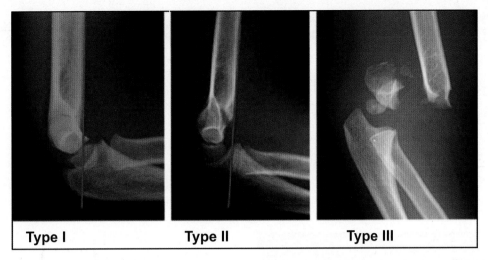

Type I　　　　　Type II　　　　　Type III

Fig. 194.1 Lateral radiographs demonstrating the modified Gartland classification of supracondylar humeral fractures. Type I: non-displaced fractures. The anterior humeral line (*red*) intersects the capitellum. Type II: loss of cortical continuity anteriorly and intact posterior cortex. The anterior humeral line (*red*) does not intersect the capitellum that is displaced posteriorly. Type III: complete loss of anterior and posterior cortical continuity. These fractures are unstable. (From Douglas RR, Ho CA. Fractures of the pediatric elbow and shoulder. In: Abzug JM, Neiduski R, Kozin SH, eds. *Pediatric Hand Therapy*. Elsevier; 2020:Figure 19.2.)

The most likely diagnosis in the vignette is supracondylar fracture of the humerus, the most common childhood fracture. Complications include nerve injury, vascular compromise, compartment syndrome and malunion. BOAST guidelines are used as standards of practice. Document radial pulse, digital capillary refill time and radial, median (including anterior interosseous) and ulnar nerve functions individually. Surgery is normally performed on the same day of injury – urgent/night-time surgery is occasionally required (absent radial pulse, impaired perfusion to hands/fingers, open injury or threatened skin viability). Vascular impairment usually resolves on fracture reduction. Post-operatively there is need for neurovascular monitoring. Routine long-term follow-up is not usually required.

REVISION TIPS

- Supracondylar fractures carry risk of vascular or nerve damage
- Non-displaced paediatric fractures can be managed with splints/casts; displaced fractures may require closed/open reduction with internal/external fixation depending on articular surface involvement
- If a fracture is potentially unstable, the position should be checked at around 5 to 7 days
- Intra-articular fractures would usually require open reduction and internal fixation (ORIF)
- 75% of growth plate fractures are Salter-Harris type 2
- Always consider NAI in children presenting with fractures

195

Anuria and Acute or Chronic Urinary Retention

Tejas Netke, Emma Gull, and Jonathan Cobley

EMERGENCY DEPARTMENT, MALE, 84.
LOWER ABDOMINAL PAIN

HPC: Severe increasing suprapubic pain, constant and dull in nature, not radiating. Nausea, no vomiting. No fever, haematuria, dysuria. No loss of appetite or change in bowel habit. Several months of urinary frequency, nocturia and poor flow; today unable to pass urine.
PMHx: T2DM. **DHx:** Tamsulosin 400 mcg OD, metformin 500 mg OD.
   O/E: Lower abdominal distention, dull to percuss. DRE: enlarged, smooth prostate gland. **Ix:** Normal U&Es.

1. What are the potential causes of falsely elevated PSA levels (i.e. not due to cancer)?
2. Which medication types can precipitate acute urinary retention (AUR)?
3. Why is it important to check U&Es and serum creatinine in AUR patients?

Answers: 1. BPE, UTI/prostatitis, instrumentation, urinary retention (possibly ejaculation or exercise). 2. Anticholinergics, opioids, benzodiazepines, calcium channel blockers, TCAs. 3. To exclude acute-on-chronic retention, as risk of electrolyte imbalance/ post-obstructive diuresis.

TABLE 195.1

	Features	Investigations	Management
Benign prostate enlargement (BPE), due to prostatic hyperplasia	Asymptomatic or causes lower urinary tract symptoms (LUTS); voiding LUTS (hesitancy, slow stream), post-voiding LUTS (dribble, incomplete emptying), storage LUTS (urgency, frequency, nocturia; *overactive bladder syndrome*). Palpate for distended bladder. DRE to assess size/shape of prostate – BPE versus cancer	Symptom score, e.g. International Prostate Symptom Score (IPSS). Urinalysis: exclude UTI. Flow rate test and post-void residual bladder volume. USS: hydronephrosis may indicate chronic urinary retention (CUR). Impaired U&Es: may indicate CUR	*AUR*: immediate urethral or suprapubic catheter. Analgesia. *CUR*: catheterise and observe for post-obstructive diuresis. Urology for TWOC/TURP. *Voiding LUTS*: tamsulosin (alpha-1 adrenergic antagonist). Finasteride/ dutasteride (5α-reductase inhibitor). *OAB*: antimuscarinic (tolterodine, oxybutynin), beta-3 agonist (mirabegron).
Prostate cancer	**Hx & O/E:** often asymptomatic. Voiding LUTS ± weight loss ± bone pain ± palpable lymph nodes. DRE: enlarged, uneven and asymmetrical prostate	PSA, U&Es, creatinine, FBC, LFTs (ALP abnormal if metastasised to bone). Transrectal prostate biopsy; graded using Gleason scale. ± Multi-parametric MRI	*Observation* if low-risk/life expectancy <10 years, or *surveillance* (>10 years). Radical prostatectomy/ radiotherapy: high-risk, organ-confined disease, life expectancy >10 years. Goserelin/degarelix for high risk

TABLE 195.1 **(Cont'd)**

	Features	Investigations	Management
Phimosis (Fig. 195.1)	*Phimosis*: preputial meatus restricted, e.g. BXO. *Paraphimosis*: retracted prepuce constricts glans. Any age, catheterised patients greater risk	Clinical diagnosis	*Phimosis*: circumcision. *Paraphimosis*: reduction to replace prepuce, followed by circumcision at a later date
Urethral stricture	**RFs**: previous instrumentation, urethritis	Clinical diagnosis. Cystoscopy	Dilation, stricturotomy, urethroplasty
Differentials – Women			
Pelvic organ prolapse	**RFs**: increased age/BMI, vaginal deliveries, smoking. Anterior POP (cystocoele) can distort the urethra, hence voiding difficulty. Vault or posterior POP rarely affect urethra. See *132. VAGINAL PROLAPSE*	Post-voiding residual volume. Urodynamic studies may be used to see if there is also stress urinary incontinence	Observation + pelvic floor muscle training. Surgical cystocoele repair if symptomatic (sensation of lump, visible bulge). Pessary if not fit for surgery
Pelvic mass	Benign or malignant. See *134. PELVIC MASS*	Imaging according to suspected cause	According to identified cause
Differentials – Both			
Blocked catheter	Recent (difficult) catheter, blood in catheter bag	Palpable uncomfortable bladder	Flush, reposition or reinsert the catheter
Neurological, e.g. cauda equina syndrome, spinal metastasis	Prolapsed intervertebral disc (central), trauma, malignancy. **Hx & O/E:** back pain, saddle anaesthesia, weakness, incontinence (urinary and/or faecal). PAINLESS urinary retention	Whole spine MRI	Immobilise (supine), urgent neurosurgical review, decompressive surgery. *Spinal metastasis*: urgent surgery (decompress and stabilise)/ radiotherapy/ IV methylprednisolone/ Dexamethasone, with PPI

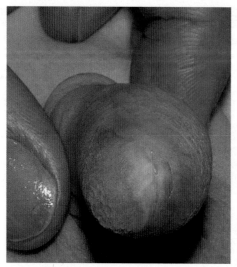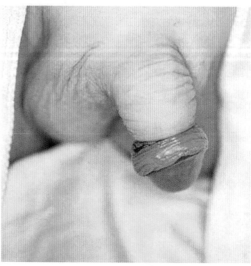

Fig. 195.1 BXO causing a severe phimosis (*left*). Retracted foreskin causing paraphimosis (*right*). (Reproduced with permission from Charles Keys and Jimmy P.H. Lam. Foreskin and penile problems in childhood. *Surgery*, 2013, 31 (3) Pages 130-134 Elsevier).

AUR causes a painful distended bladder, and BPE is by far the commonest cause. Medications (especially if anticholinergic) may be relevant, due to impaired bladder emptying; polypharmacy increases risk of AUR. Prostate-specific antigen (PSA) becomes difficult to interpret, as it can be elevated by BPE, AUR, urinary tract infection or prostate malignancy. Some patients with chronic retention may develop AUR ('acute-on-chronic retention'); this necessitates regular observations and fluid monitoring after catheterisation, due to risk of post-obstructive diuresis. The potential severity of the diuresis that can result from catheterising someone in chronic retention is often underestimated, risking severe dehydration and electrolyte disturbance (e.g. hypokalaemia, hypo-/hypernatraemia, hypomagnesaemia). In AUR caused by cauda equina syndrome, the bladder is painlessly distended in conjunction with back pain. Anuria with unilateral loin pain can result from ureteric obstruction in someone with a single (functioning) kidney. In the vignette, the cause of AUR is likely to be BPE, and the normal U&Es means chronic retention is unlikely.

REVISION TIPS

- Obstruction can occur at any part of the urinary tract; the most common cause is BPE, phimosis is common, but ureteric obstruction (in a patient with only one functioning kidney) is rare
- Acute urinary retention is an emergency and the bladder must be urgently decompressed with a catheter
- Be wary of acute-on-chronic retention and monitor these patients closely for post-obstructive diuresis

196

Loin Pain

Katherine Parker, Marcus Drake, and Jonathan Cobley

EMERGENCY DEPARTMENT. MALE, 65.
2 DAYS CONSTANT LEFT LOIN PAIN

HPC: Gnawing character, radiating to lower back, increasing severity. Nauseous. No aggravating or relieving factors. No urinary or bowel symptoms. **PMHx:** HTN, anxiety. **DHx:** Amlodipine, atorvastatin, sertraline. **FHx:** MI. **SHx:** Smoker (40 pack years), heavy drinker.

O/E: BMI 34, pallor, apyrexial. **CVS:** HR 96, BP 120/80, HS I + II + 0. **Abdomen:** Central pulsatile, expansile mass. No renal angle tenderness. Bowel sounds present. **Ix:** Dipstick haematuria.

---

1. When is immediate hospital admission indicated in patients with renal colic?
2. How would an acute renal infarction present?
3. What are your differentials for pleuritic loin pain?

Answers: 1. Shock, infection, pre-existing kidney disease, bilateral obstruction, poor oral intake, uncertain diagnosis. 2. Asymptomatic or loin pain with N&V, in a vasculopath with new onset HTN and non-visible haematuria. 3. Lower lobe pneumonia (also fever, cough), pulmonary embolism (SOB, tachycardia, VTE risk factors).

TABLE 196.1

	Features	Investigations	Management
Nephrolithiasis/ renal colic	**RFs:** male, obese, chronic dehydration, FHx, anatomical abnormalities, diet (oxalate, urate, salt, animal protein). **Hx & O/E:** acute, unilateral, loin to groin pain, N&V, haematuria. Renal angle tenderness	Urinalysis: haematuria. Pregnancy test: βhCG -ve. Urgent (<24 hours) low-dose **non-contrast CT KUB** (USS if pregnant or <16 yo). Aetiology: bloods (calcium, urate, PTH). Stone analysis	Analgesia (diclofenac), fluids, anti-emetic (ondansetron). Stone in mid/distal ureter: <5 mm watch and wait, <10 mm medical expulsion: alpha-blocker (tamsulosin). Proximal/large/persistent: ESWL, PCNL, ureteroscopy
	+ Ureteric obstruction: severe pain + hydronephrosis	Monitor urine output. U&Es (↑creat if single functioning kidney or bilateral). Renal USS	Urgent admission, urology. Decompression (percutaneous nephrostomy/ stent)
	+ Infection: fever, dysuria. Can rapidly progress to sepsis	Urinalysis: nitrites ± blood, leukocytes. MC&S. FBC (↑WCC), ↑CRP	Urgent admission, urology. Hourly Obs, IV antibiotics + decompression

(Continued)

TABLE 196.1   (Cont'd)

	Features	Investigations	Management
Acute pyelonephritis	**RFs:** recurrent UTIs, DM, immunosuppression, catheterised, anatomical abnormality, pregnancy. **Hx & O/E:** unilateral loin/back pain. Fever, rigors, N&V, myalgia, flu-like symptoms. Renal tenderness, ↑HR, ↓BP	Dipstick (not advised age >65 or indwelling catheter). MSU: MC&S. FBC (↑WCC), U&Es (± ↑creat), ↑CRP. Blood cultures, USS if septic	Admission: sepsis, obstruction, structural abnormality, AKI, treatment failure, pregnant. Antibiotics (7–10 days). Men, non-pregnant women: PO cefalexin, ciprofloxacin. Pregnant: PO cefalexin. IV cephalosporin
Renal cell carcinoma (RCC)	**RFs:** smoking, male, >55, obese, HTN, family history. >50% asymptomatic. May present with triad of haematuria, flank pain, palpable mass (uncommon)	Urinalysis: blood. ↓Hb/↑RBC, ↑LDH (paraneoplastic). US abdomen: renal mass. CT abdo/pelvis: mass, lymphadenopathy, mets	Watch and wait (small mass/frail patient)/cryotherapy/surgery (radical nephrectomy or partial nephrectomy)/chemotherapy/radiotherapy/immunotherapy
Vital Differentials			
Ectopic pregnancy	See *67. ACUTE ABDOMINAL PAIN*		
Ruptured AAA	See *44. TRAUMA AND MASSIVE HAEMORRHAGE*		

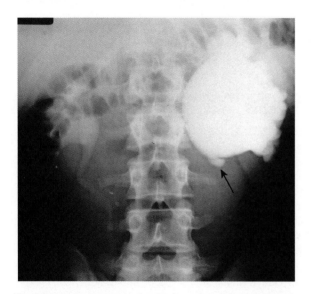

Fig. 196.1 IVU of left pelvi-ureteric junction (PUJ) obstruction (*arrowed*). PUJO can present with loin pain at any age (usually young), when a narrowed PUJ is insufficient for a rise in rate of urine production (e.g. patient overhydrates or recently started a diuretic). Acute treatment is drainage (nephrostomy or stent); definitive treatment is laparoscopic pyeloplasty. (Reproduced with permission from M. Magdi Yaqoob and Neil Ashman. Kidney and urinary tract disease. Kumar and Clark's Clinical Medicine, 36, 1339–1408).

Loin pain is commonly renal/ureteric colic due to a stone, but can be blood clot or papillary necrosis (analgesic/diabetic nephropathy, pyelonephritis, sickle cell). For radio-opaque stones, shock-wave lithotripsy (ESWL) is a treatment option, even if there is some hydronephrosis or acute ureteric obstruction; however, infection is a contra-indication to ESWL. Rare causes; acute obstruction of the join between the renal pelvis and the top of the ureter (young adults) (Fig. 196.1), iatrogenic blockage (e.g. ureteric trauma from gynaecological, urological or colorectal surgery) or retroperitoneal fibrosis (older adults, bilateral). Danger issues are pyrexia (sepsis is rapid if UTI complicates an obstructing stone) or anuria (stone in a person with only one functioning kidney). Urine output and renal function are monitored for both reasons. Urgent drainage is needed for pyrexia with obstruction: nephrostomy (for impacted distal ureteric stone, patients too unwell for GA, or if stent not technically feasible) or retrograde ureteric stent (proximal stones, presence of coagulopathy, or interventional radiology unavailable). Stones analysis: calcium oxalate (common), struvite (associated with UTI) or urate (metabolic syndrome). Preventing stone recurrence: high fluid (2.5–3 L/day), low salt (<6 g), balanced diet, normal calcium intake (700–1200 mg/day), fresh lemon juice and avoid carbonated drinks. Consider potassium citrate for calcium oxalate stones. If salt is <6 g/day, consider off-label thiazide for calcium oxalate stones with hypercalciuria. RCC is often an incidental finding; it can cause paraneoplastic abnormalities (e.g. hypercalcemia, non-metastatic hepatic dysfunction) or constitutional symptoms (fever, cachexia, weight loss). In the vignette, the presentation implies a stone, but is a rupturing AAA. AAA and ectopic pregnancy are life-threatening, and must be considered in a presumed stone presentation until diagnosis is confirmed.

REVISION TIPS

- Renal stones on X-ray: calcium visible, cystine partly visible, urate and xanthine radiolucent
- Causes of acute pyelonephritis: *E. coli*, *Klebsiella*, *Proteus*, *Pseudomonas*, *Enterobacter* spp.

197

Scrotal/Testicular Pain and/or Lump/Swelling

Natalia Hacket, Lelyn Osei Atiemo, and Jonathan Cobley

HPC: Pain since waking, not helped by paracetamol. No dysuria, discharge, vomiting. Nauseated. 'Pain attacks' a month ago after minor scrotal trauma during rugby game – resolved. **PMHx:** Nil. **SHx:** Not sexually active.

O/E: Apyrexial. Left testicle tender, swollen, transverse lie. Negative Prehn sign, no solid lump, no transillumination.

1. What would be your top differential/first-line management if the patient:
   a. Presented after 3 days of scrotal pain associated with urethral discharge?
   b. Was a 35 year old who had noticed a painless 1 cm lump in his testicle?
2. How is a 60 year old with 'scrotal heaviness' found to have a left-sided varicocoele initially investigated?

Answers: 1a. Epididymitis. Treat with Abx (e.g. ceftriaxone/doxycycline), consider STI screen. 1b. Testicular cancer. Arrange USS, 2WW referral (tumour markers, radical orchidectomy). 2. Kidney USS to exclude left renal carcinoma.

TABLE 197.1

	Features	Investigations	Management
Testicular torsion	**RFs:** 'bell clapper' testis, undescended testis. Any age, peak 12–18. Twisting occludes the spermatic cord, hence ischaemia. **Hx & O/E:** sudden severe pain – swollen, red, elevated testicle, no cremasteric reflex, -ve Prehn sign	If torsion suspected, seek immediate surgical review. Decision to operate is made on clinical basis. Imaging is not done, due to the risk of testicular loss associated with any delay	Keep patient NBM. Immediate hospital referral for surgical exploration. **Bilateral** testicular fixation (restore perfusion and prevent subsequent torsion on either side)
Epididymo-orchitis (epididymitis)	**Hx & O/E:** acute unilateral pain, swelling, Prehn sign, scrotal erythema, dysuria, discharge, pyrexia. Consider UTI or STI. Parotid swelling; mumps orchitis	STI screen. Urinalysis. Saliva swab for PCR ± serum antibodies if possible mumps	Abx for UTI (e.g. ofloxacin) or STI (e.g. doxycycline for chlamydia, ceftriaxone for gonorrhoea) with same-day sexual health referral

TABLE 197.1 (Cont'd)

	Features	Investigations	Management
Indirect inguinal hernia (Fig. 197.1)	RFs: male, older age, connective tissue disorder, FHx, smoking. Hx & O/E: episodic painless inguinal swelling, bigger on cough/Valsalva. Can't get above swelling, ± reducible. Risks: incarceration, strangulation, intestinal obstruction.	Exclude strangulation (acutely painful, firm irreducible mass) or obstruction (vomiting, constipation, abdominal pain and distension)	Infant/young to be seen within 2 weeks, others routine. Strangulation/obstruction; immediate admission. Adults/older child refer urgently if (partially) irreducible
Hydrocoele (Fig. 197.1)	Common in neonates. Can usually get above swelling, not reducible, transilluminates, may be larger at end of the day	USS to confirm diagnosis. Adults may need urgent USS to exclude malignancy	Infants, surgical ligation if persisting at age 2 years. Hydrocoele repair in adult (not aspiration)
Varicocoele (Fig. 197.1)	Chronic, 'bag of worms', scrotal heaviness, worse on standing. Can cause decreased fertility. Nutcracker syndrome (compression of left renal vein by superior mesenteric artery)	USS with flow Doppler imaging if diagnosis unclear. Left-sided varicocoele --> get kidney USS for renal cell carcinoma (cancer extension in renal vein towards IVC)	Most need no treatment. Scrotal support for discomfort. Specialist review if infertile and wishing for children. Urgent referral if new onset age >40, or stays tense when supine
Haematocoele	Blood in tunica vaginalis after trauma (rarely chronic with testis cancer): tender swelling, does not transilluminate	History and examination. Scrotal USS – urgent if chronic/no trauma	Admit if acute trauma. Conservative management, sometimes surgical if large or painful
Epididymal cyst (spermatocoele)	Middle-aged, PCKD, cystic fibrosis. Hx & O/E: chronic, smooth, non-tender cyst on epididymis. Transillumination varies, can be 'Chinese lantern'.	Can be multiple and bilateral. USS if diagnosis unclear	Reassurance (common, harmless). Bothersome symptoms: routine urology review
Testicular cancer	RFs: FHx, cryptorchidism, white ethnicity, infertility, Klinefelter's. 25–40 years, lymphoma if age >50. Hx & O/E: non-tender, lump in body of testis (Fig. 197.1). Rare: haematospermia, hydrocoele. Supraclavicular lymphadenopathy, weight loss, gynaecomastia. Dyspnoea if lung metastasis	USS. Tumour markers; AFP, chorionic gonadotrophin (hCG), LDH. CT chest, abdomen, pelvis	Urgent (2WW) urology. Radical orchidectomy, radiotherapy, chemotherapy

AFP, Alpha-foetoprotein; LDH, lactate dehydrogenase.

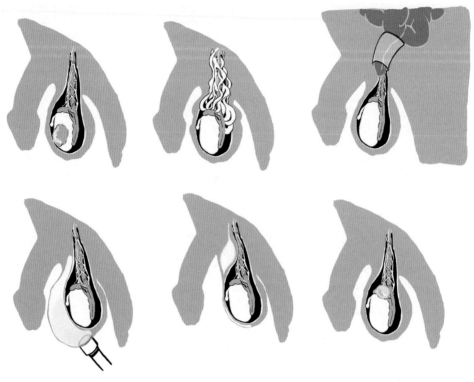

Fig. 197.1 *Top left*, Testicular tumour; *top middle*, varicocoele; *top right*, indirect inguinal hernia. *Bottom left*, Hydrocoele ('non-communicating' as the communication to the peritoneal cavity has atrophied – in infants, there may be communication requiring surgical ligation); *bottom middle*, encysted hydrocoele of the spermatic cord; *bottom right*, cyst in the head of the epididymis.

In the vignette, the presentation is typical for testicular torsion. Suspicion for torsion is always needed in severe testicular pain. Immediate surgical exploration takes precedence over many cases on the emergency list, due to necrosis risk from 4 hours (duration of full ischaemia is uncertain from history, so pain present for longer is still explored urgently). The age distribution of torsion is bimodal (peaks neonatally and puberty), but it can occur at other times. Testicular cancer is usually not painful, unless there is inflammation (hence secondary hydrocoele); incidence rises from age 12, peaking at 25–40 years old (34–39 for seminoma, 26–31 for non-seminoma germ cell tumour, such as teratoma). Lymphoma more likely if older than 50. Prehn sign (pain relief by elevating testis) suggests epididymo-orchitis, which sometimes follows UTI (instrumentation/catheter) or STI (sexually active, urethral discharge). Left testicular vein arises from the left renal vein, which may be blocked by the superior mesenteric artery (nutcracker syndrome) or intraluminal extension of renal tumour. Right testicular vein comes off the IVC.

REVISION TIPS

- Torsion versus epididymitis – low threshold for suspecting torsion, especially if attend <6 hours after onset, previous pain attacks, N&V, absent cremasteric reflex or abnormal testicular lie
- STIs are a common cause of epididymo-orchitis, as a result of urethritis

198

Abnormal Urinalysis

Lara Yorke and Alex Ridgway

HPC: Feels well. Pregnancy uncomplicated. **PMHx:** IDDM. **DHx:** Insulin (detemir and aspart). **SHx:** Non-smoker, no alcohol.

 O/E: HR 88, BP 162/112, HS I + II + 0. Soft, non-tender abdomen, mild pitting oedema. **Neurology:** Grossly intact. Obstetric: symphyseal-fundal height 23 cm, longitudinal lie with cephalic presentation. **Ix:** dipstick proteinuria +++, negative ketones, negative glucose.

1. What is the likely diagnosis in the vignette?
2. In general, over what age does urinalysis become less reliable diagnostically?

Answers: 1. Pre-eclampsia, 2. >65 years old.

TABLE 198.1

	Features	Investigations	Management
Leucocyte esterase (interpret at 2 minutes)	Leucocyte enzyme, so WBCs are present. +ve = UTI, malignancy, stone, contamination	**UTI:** MSU – MC&S. **Urinary tract malignancy:** imaging, endoscopy, biopsy. **Stone:** U&Es, imaging	**UTI:** Abx (local guidelines). **Malignancy:** as per type/stage/grade. **Stone:** As per site/size
Nitrites (60 seconds)	Almost all gram-negative bacteria. Nitrites +ve = UTI	**UTI:** MSU – MC&S to identify organism	**UTI:** antibiotics (local guidelines)
Urobilinogen (60 seconds)	Bilirubin broken down in intestine, enters portal circulation, excreted by kidney. Normal: 0.2–1.0 mg/dL. Increased: haemolytic anaemia, cirrhosis, hepatitis. Decreased: biliary obstruction, cholestasis	**Haemolytic anaemia:** FBC, reticulocytes, bilirubin, serum LDH, direct Coombs test, peripheral blood smear. **Cirrhosis/hepatitis:** LFTs, hepatitis markers, transient elastography. **Biliary:** LFTs (ALP), US/CT/MRCP	**Haemolytic anaemia:** steroids, rituximab, splenectomy. **Cirrhosis/hepatitis:** Lifestyle, manage symptoms/complications. **Biliary obstruction:** treat cause, cholecystectomy

(Continued)

TABLE 198.1   (Cont'd)

	Features	Investigations	Management
Protein (60 seconds)	+ve (>150 mg/day) = pre-eclampsia, CKD, nephrotic syndrome, UTI, dehydration, strenuous exercise	**Pre-eclampsia:** albumin:creatinine ratio (ACR ≥8 mg/mmol) or protein:creatinine ratio (≥30 mg/mmol), blood pressure, FBC, U&Es, LFTs, foetal heart auscultation, US, CTG. **Nephrotic syndrome/CKD/dehydration:** U&Es, ACR, renal ultrasound	**Pre-eclampsia:** as per severity; admit, anti-hypertensives, corticosteroid, expedite delivery. **Nephrotic sy:** ACE-I/ARB, steroids, immune-suppress, plasma exchange, albumin. **CKD:** treat cause/complications, nephrology
pH (60 seconds)	Normal pH 4.5–8. Low: DKA, metabolic acidosis, e.g. sepsis. High: UTI, metabolic alkalosis, e.g. vomiting	**DKA:** emergency admission, VBG (serum glucose and pH), HbA1c, ketones. **Sepsis:** FBC, CRP, VBG (lactate), blood culture, urine output. **Vomiting:** VBG (pH), U&Es. **Renal tubular disease:** VBG (serum pH, electrolytes, anion gap), renal ultrasound	**DKA:** A–E assessment, IV fluids, potassium, insulin infusion. **Sepsis:** fluids, antibiotics, oxygen. **Vomiting:** anti-emetics, fluids. **Renal tubular disease:** alkali treatment, vitamin D, control potassium levels
Ketones (45 seconds)	Produced in liver from fatty acid metabolism. +ve = DKA, ketogenic diet, starvation		
Glucose (30 seconds)	Glomerular filtration > tubular reabsorption. +ve = DM, medications (SGLT2 inhibitors), tubular disease, e.g. Fanconi syndrome		
Blood (60 seconds)	Presence of myoglobin/haemoglobin. Significant ≥1+. +ve = UTI, malignancy, nephritic syndrome, pyelonephritis/cystitis, stone, rhabdomyolysis, trauma	**Bladder malignancy:** cystoscopy ± TURBT, CT. **Nephritic syndrome:** U&Es, BP. **UTI:** FBC, CRP, MSU. **Rhabdomyolysis:** creatine kinase. **Renal calculi:** U&Es, FBC, CRP, calcium, urate, non-contrast CT	**Malignancy:** as per type/stage/grade. **Nephritic sy:** ACE-i/ARB, steroid, antibiotic, plasma exchange, cyclophosphamide. **UTI:** Abx, analgesia, hydration. **Rhabdomyolysis:** fluids, alkalinisation, diuretics, haemodialyse. **Stone:** as per site/size

TABLE 198.1 (Cont'd)

	Features	Investigations	Management
Specific gravity (45 seconds)	Relates to osmolality. Normal: 1.001–1.035. Low (dilute) = diabetes insipidus (DI), diuretics. High (concentrated) = SIADH, dehydration, glycosuria	DI: urine osmolality, water deprivation test, desmopressin test, serum glucose. SIADH: serum osmolality (low), urine osmolality/sodium (high/high). Glycosuria: HbA1c, glucose, ketones	DI: desmopressin. SIADH: manage cause, fluid restrict, tolvaptan. Glycosuria: treatment dependent on cause
Bilirubin (30 seconds)	Haemolysis product. +ve: biliary obstruction	Biliary: LFTs (ALP), US/CT/MRCP	Biliary: treat cause, cholecystectomy

TABLE 198.2 Aetiology of false positives in urinalysis

Component	False Positive
Leucocyte esterase	Vaginal/penile contamination, sexually transmitted infections
Nitrites	Improperly stored dipsticks. False negatives more common (see commentary)
Urobilinogen	Azo dyes (textiles/paint industry, some medications)
Protein	Visible haematuria, presence of semen/mucus, pH >7
Ketones	Medication (penicillamine, captopril, levodopa)
Glucose	Incorrect storage of test strips
Blood	Menstrual blood, dehydration, exercise
Specific gravity	IV radiopaque contrast media, proteinuria, dextran
Bilirubin	Medications (phenazopyridine [Pyridium] or Etodolac [NSAID])

New hypertension (>140/90 mmHg) at >20 weeks gestation PLUS any of proteinuria (≥1+), organ dysfunction (raised creatinine or LFTs/thrombocytopenia/DIC/haemolytic anaemia) or placental dysfunction (foetal growth restriction/abnormal doppler) indicate pre-eclampsia. Proteinuria goes against pregnancy-induced hypertension. BP >160/110 is a medical emergency. The negative ketones and glucose indicate her IDDM is controlled. Nitrites result from bacterial conversion of endogenous nitrates to nitrites and have a high specificity for urinary tract infection. This test has low sensitivity, as sufficient time is needed for nitrite reductase to work, and sometimes UTI is due to a bacterium which does not express the enzyme. Leucocytes indicate inflammation, often UTI or contamination (e.g. vaginal flora if failing to obtain clean catch midstream specimen), but potentially malignancy or urinary tract stone. Older/catheterised patients can have asymptomatic bacteriuria without an infection, leading to a positive dipstick and potentially harmful overtreatment with antibiotics. Glycosuria is sugars (glucose, galactose, fructose) in the urine- glucosuria is most common. All these tests have some risk of false positives (Table 198.2).

REVISION TIPS

- **Sensitivity**: the ability of a test to correctly identify patients with a disease. **Specificity**: the ability of a test to correctly identify people without the disease
- **True positive**: the person has the disease and the test is positive. **True negative**: the person does not have the disease and the test is negative

Haematuria

Emily Warren and Marcus Drake

HPC: 24 hours haematuria with increased urinary frequency, dysuria, blood mixed in with the urine, every time she passes urine. Nothing similar previously. Feels well, no abdominal pain, fever or N&V. No change in bowel habit.

O/E: Comfortable and stable. HS I + II + 0, well perfused, 65 bpm, lungs clear. Abdomen soft, slightly tender suprapubically, active bowel sounds. **Urine dip:** Positive for blood and nitrites.

1. If someone presented with proteinuria, haematuria and had *COL4A5* mutation, what would the diagnosis be?
2. What are the chemical compositions of common kidney stones?
3. What are the common causes of haemoglobinuria?

Answers: 1. Alport syndrome. 2. Calcium, struvite (magnesium ammonium, phosphate), uric acid, cystine. 3. Acute nephritis, severe burns, malaria, transfusion reaction, sickle cell anaemia, strenuous physical activity.

TABLE 199.1

	Features	Investigations	Management
Cystitis/ pyelonephritis (UTI)	**Hx & O/E:** dysuria, blood in urine, increased urinary frequency, urgency. Vomiting/fever may suggest pyelonephritis. Causes; *E.coli, Staph. saprophyticus, Klebsiella, Proteus, Pseudomonas.* spp. Also consider candida (old/ young, DM, hospitalization/ ITU, immunosuppressed, recent broad-spectrum Abx, recent surgery, catheterisation, transplant).	Urine MC&S. FBC (raised WCC in infection), U&Es, CRP (raised in infection). Blood cultures if pyelonephritis/ sepsis.	*Cystitis:* Abx (local guidelines, e.g. female nitrofurantoin/ trimethoprim 3 days. Nitrofurantoin 7 days if pregnant or male). *Pyelonephritis:* Abx (local guidelines, e.g. PO cefalexin/ ciprofloxacin. IV amikacin/ ceftriaxone/ciprofloxacin. Pregnant: PO cefalexin/IV cefuroxime)

TABLE 199.1 (Cont'd)

	Features	Investigations	Management
Nephrolithiasis (Fig. 199.1)	Peak age 20–40, male > female **Hx & O/E:** excruciating pain, unable to stay still, haematuria. Increased frequency, dysuria. Fever suggests infection: urgent drainage needed. See *196. LOIN PAIN* *Recurrent stones:* risk increased by high protein low fibre diet, inactive/ bed-bound, FHx, recurrent UTIs, antiretrovirals	Non-contrast **CT KUB:** visualise stone(s), hydronephrosis. Urine MC&S (exclude UTI). FBC, U&Es, uric acid, CRP, calcium, glucose (exclude sepsis or renal failure). Stone composition analysis. 24 hour urine analysis (recurrent stones/ children)	Analgesia ± IV fluids. Stones <5 mm in lower ureter: 95% pass spontaneously. Stones >5 mm/pain not resolving/failure to pass: alpha blocker (off label). ESWL, ureteroscopy or PCNL. *Obstructed infected kidney:* Abx (as for pyelonephritis) and urgent stent or nephrostomy to resolve infection before stone removal
IgA nephropathy	Haematuria during URTIs. **RFs:** FHx IgA nephropathy/ vasculitis (HSP), Asian/ European ethnicity. Male teens to 30s. ESRF 12% at 5 years; HTN, crescents, proteinuria, glomerulosclerosis, tubulointerstitial fibrosis	Urinalysis; blood and protein. Dysmorphic RBCs and casts. Exclude other causes of glomerulonephritis (e.g. lupus, vasculitis). Renal biopsy: Oxford IgAN (MEST-C) classification	Weight loss, salt reduction. ACEI/ARB: target BP <125/75 mmHg if proteinuria >1 g/day or <130/80 mmHg if less. Statins
Bladder cancer	Transitional cell cancer (TCC) of urothelium. **RFs:** smoking, chemicals, cyclophsophamide. Age >40, M>F. **Hx & O/E:** painless haematuria, frequency, dysuria	Urine: MC&S (sterile pyuria), cytology. Cystoscopy + biopsy (transurethral resection of bladder tumour: TURBT). CT urogram (to exclude upper tract TCC)	*Low risk superficial TCC:* TURBT. *Stage T1:* TURBT, intravesical BCG. *T2/3:* radical cystectomy with urinary diversion (e.g. urostomy). *T4:* palliative chemo/ radiotherapy.
Renal cancer	**RFs:** age >50, male, haemodialysis, obesity, smoking, HTN, tuberous sclerosis, von Hippel-Lindau. 85% are renal cell cancer. **Hx & O/E:** asymptomatic. Mass, weight loss, loin pain fatigue. Pyrexia/ sweating. (Left varicocoele)	FBC (polycythaemia), U&Es. **USS:** renal mass. **CT:** mass/ metastases. CXR: 'cannonball mets' (Fig. 199.1)	Radical nephrectomy (partial nephrectomy for small RCC). Cryotherapy/radiofrequency ablation if small, or unfit for surgery
Prostate cancer	**RFs:** age >50, FHx, African-Caribbean **Hx & O/E:** initially asymptomatic. LUTS, haematuria, haematospermia, impotence, tenesmus. DRE (normal in early stages): asymmetry, firm nodule. Mets: bone pain, lymphadenopathy, weight loss	FBC, U&Es, CRP, LFTs, PSA. Transrectal ultrasound biopsy (Gleason scoring system). MRI scan. Suspect mets: bone scan, XR	Low risk: active surveillance (PSA). Localised: radical prostatectomy, brachytherapy/ radiotherapy. Advanced/ mets: androgen deprivation/ androgen receptor targeted therapy, chemotherapy, symptom control

(Continued)

TABLE 199.1 (Cont'd)

Key Differential	Features	Investigations	Management
Menorrhagia	Heavy, painful periods. Known fibroids, polyps, endometrial pathology. Blood in toilet can be mistaken for haematuria	Bimanual + speculum. FBC, clotting screen, TFTs. Hysteroscopy ± biopsy. Pelvic USS/TVUS	No or <3 cm fibroids: intrauterine system (Mirena), tranexamic acid, COCP or desogestrel pill. Uterine artery embolisation. Fibroids >3 cm: GnRH, myomectomy, hysterectomy

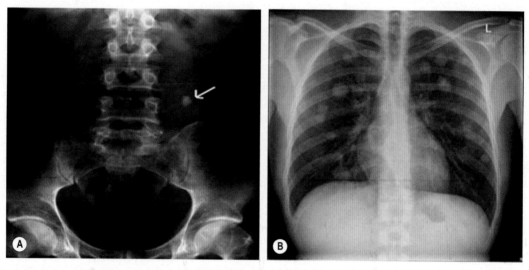

Fig. 199.1 (A) Kidneys, ureters and bladder X-ray (*KUB*) showing left ureteric stone. (B) Chest X-ray showing cannonball metastases from a renal cell carcinoma. Nadir I. Osman and Richard D. Inman. Urological diagnosis, history and investigation. Surgery, 31 (7), 337–345, 2013.

The vignette describes cystitis. Also consider other infections (pyelonephritis, tuberculosis, cytomegalovirus, prostatitis in men), tumours (renal, bladder, prostate), vascular (arteriovenous malformation, renal vein thrombosis, infarct, sickle cell disease), coagulopathy/anticoagulants, trauma (e.g. catheterisation, radiation) and papillary necrosis. Visible haematuria is uncommon with renal disease except IgA nephropathy, and sometimes autosomal dominant polycystic kidney disease (due to cyst rupture) or glomerular disorders (IgA vasculitis/ Henoch-Schönlein purpura, thin glomerular basement membrane disease, lupus nephritis and post-infectious nephritis). Blood at the start or end of the stream may have prostatic or urethral origin. Blood in the toilet pan might be mistaken for haematuria, hence consider menorrhagia. Eating beetroot can colour the urine red.

REVISION TIPS

- Painless haematuria suggests malignancy, haematuria with pain suggests stone or UTI
- Bladder cancer RFs: tobacco, environmental (paints, dyes, metals, arsenic, petroleum), age
- *Escherichia coli* and *Staphylococcus saprophyticus* cause ~80% of community-acquired uncomplicated UTIs in women

200

Urinary Symptoms and Incontinence

Emma Corke, Christian Aquilina, and Marcus Drake

GP CONSULTATION. FEMALE, 63.
12 WEEKS OF URINARY URGENCY WITH URINARY INCONTINENCE

HPC: Urgent need to pass urine, little warning, leaks before reaching the toilet. Changes incontinence pad twice daily. Increased voiding frequency, nocturia. No dysuria, no fever, otherwise healthy. **PMHx:** HTN, OA. **DHx:** Amlodipine, ibuprofen. **FHx:** Nil. **SHx:** 15 units of alcohol per week, non-smoker, drinks four cups of tea per day.
  O/E: Obs – normal. Vaginal examination NAD. Urine dipstick negative.

1. What are the contraindications for anti-muscarinic medications?
2. What are the red flag symptoms of cauda equina syndrome?
3. What are the differentials for dysuria?

Answers: 1. Closed-angle glaucoma, cognitive impairment, post void residual (PVR) >300 mL, significant bowel disease, myasthaenia gravis. 2. Bowel/urinary incontinence, PVR, saddle anaesthesia, bilateral leg weakness. 3. UTI, urethritis, sexually transmitted infections, vaginitis, dermatological conditions, e.g. lichen sclerosus.

TABLE 200.1

	Features	Investigations	Management
Overactive bladder syndrome (OAB)	OAB is urgency, increased frequency and nocturia with or without urgency urinary incontinence. **RFs:** older age, obesity, neurological disease	OAB symptom score, bladder diary. Urine dipstick to r/o UTI. Flow rate test + PVR scan. (Urodynamic studies)	Reduce caffeine, bladder retraining. Anti-muscarinic (trospium, solifenacin, tolterodine, oxybutynin), beta-3 agonist (mirabegron). Botox bladder injection
Stress urinary incontinence (SUI)	↑Intra-abdominal pressure (e.g. laughing/coughing). Female: obstetric, older age, post-menopausal, obesity. Male: radical prostatectomy	Abdominal ± vaginal examination. Symptom score. (Urodynamic studies). Consider neurological disease in both sexes	Weight reduction, PFMT. Surgery, e.g. colposuspension/urethral bulking in women, artificial urinary sphincter in men
Retention with overflow	Chronic urinary retention in men, dribbling incontinence	See *195. ANURIA AND ACUTE OR CHRONIC URINARY RETENTION*	
Urinary tract infection	See *199. HAEMATURIA*		

(Continued)

TABLE 200.1   (Cont'd)

	Features	Investigations	Management
Benign prostate enlargement (BPE) causing lower urinary tract symptoms (LUTS)	Older male with BPH. Asymptomatic or voiding LUTS (hesitancy, slow stream), post-voiding LUTS (dribble, incomplete emptying). Can be associated with storage LUTS (urgency, frequency, nocturia; OAB). **DRE:** exclude palpable malignancy/ prostatitis.	Symptom score (IPSS). Flow rate and PVR scan. MSU (r/o UTI). PSA (after counselling), renal function. **USS:** hydronephrosis may indicate chronic urinary retention (impaired U&Es)	Tamsulosin if bothered by voiding LUTS. Finasteride if prostate volume large (>40 mL). Urological review if still bothered: TURP or minimally invasive alternatives
Urethral stricture (Fig. 200.1)	Male, history of urological procedures/STI. Voiding symptoms	Urinalysis. Flow rate and PVR scan	Urological review; dilation, urethrotomy or urethroplasty
POP	See *132. VAGINAL PROLAPSE*		

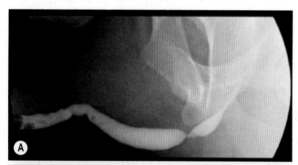

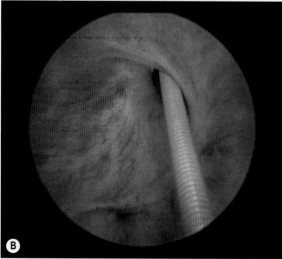

Fig. 200.1 Cystoscopy view and contrast urethrogram showing a urethral stricture as a result of previous instrumentation in the male urethra. Mitchell Tublin, Joel B. Nelson, Amir A. Borhani, Alessandro Furlan, Matthew T. Heller and Judy Squires, Imaging in Urology, Urethral Stricture, 2018, 258–259.

SUI is caused by impaired sphincter function, due to obstetric history, surgery or neurological disease. Pelvic floor muscle training (PFMT) for women should be supervised by a healthcare professional, e.g. physiotherapist or continence advisor. Midurethral tapes (e.g. TVT) were the most common interventional treatment, but complications from vaginal mesh surgery have led to their current withdrawal from NHS use. OAB syndrome is defined by presence of urgency, which can lead to urgency incontinence (OAB wet), and can be associated with other urinary 'storage' symptoms, i.e. increased frequency and nocturia. OAB is more prevalent in older age groups and in neurological disease. Dysuria is a burning urethral discomfort typical of UTI, though urethral symptoms can be caused by a stricture, a distal ureteric stone, or irritation of the bladder base ('trigone'), e.g. by a bladder stone. Voiding symptoms indicate that there may be a blockage in the urethra, such as BPE or a stricture. In men DRE is mandatory, to assess enlargement, and because prostate cancer is prevalent in older men (though it is a rare cause of voiding symptoms). Weakness of the bladder's 'detrusor' muscle means incomplete emptying, i.e. a post-void residual (PVR), caused by chronic obstruction, ageing or neurological disease.

REVISION TIPS

- Do not prescribe anti-muscarinic drugs to patients with poor bladder emptying, cognitive decline, closed angle glaucoma, myasthaenia gravis
- Diuretics can push older people into urinary incontinence, especially if their mobility is poor

201

Erectile Dysfunction

Katherine Anderson and Anna Ogier

GP CONSULTATION, MALE, 58. POOR ERECTIONS

HPC: Two years of difficulty obtaining and maintaining erections. Good libido. **PMHx:** NIDDM, HT. **DHx:** Metformin, ramipril. Current smoker (20 pack years). Occasional alcohol, no recreational drugs/anabolic steroids.

O/E: Raised BMI. **CVS:** BP 154/80, weak pedal pulses. **Neuro:** Reduced pinprick sensation in feet. **GU:** Normal size testes, no testicular masses, normal phallus without deformity, retractile foreskin, no penile plaques. DRE: Small prostate.

1. How do phosphodiesterase type-5 (PDE5) inhibitors work?
2. When are PDE5 inhibitors contraindicated?

Answers: 1. Reduced cGMP breakdown, so penile vascular relaxation/increased blood flow. 2. Nitrate use, severe cardiovascular disease, hypotension, recent CVA, non-arteritic ischaemic optic neuropathy.

TABLE 201.1

	Features	Investigations	Management
Vasculogenic	**RFs:** increased age, HTN, CVD, hyperlipidaemia, DM, BPH, increased BMI, alcohol misuse, smoking, recreational drugs. **Hx & O/E:** normal libido, gradual onset, middle age, multifactorial	Total testosterone (T), U&Es, LFTs, TFTs, HbA1c, LH, FSH, lipids. Sexual/psychological history and cardiac risk stratification	Glucose control, smoking cessation, weight loss. PDE-5 inhibitor (e.g. sildenafil, tadalafil). Refer to urology if oral options fail, cardiology if intermediate or high risk
Medications	Anti-depressants (nb SSRIs), anti-hypertensives (nb beta-blockers, diuretics), anti-psychotics, recreational drugs (anabolic steroids, cannabis, cocaine)	Medication and drugs history including illicit substance and anabolic steroid use	Change medication to a different class if possible
Neurological	Parkinson disease, multiple sclerosis, multiple system atrophy, spinal cord disease	Full neurological examination	As above, plus treatment of underlying condition
Psychosexual	Sudden onset: stress, major events or psychiatric illness. Loss of/premature ejaculation. Nocturnal erections normal	Psychological history	Psychosexual therapy. PDE-5 inhibitor may help short term. Mental health referral if severe distress

(Continued)

TABLE 201.1   (Cont'd)

	Features	Investigations	Management
Hormonal	Hypogonadism, hyper- or hypothyroid, hyperprolactinaemia, e.g. prolactinoma (bitemporal hemianopia, galactorrhoea, decreased libido), Cushing syndrome	Total T, FBC, U&Es, LFTS, TFTs, LH, FSH, prolactin. Thyroid US. Hyperprolactinaemia: visual field testing, MRI	Refer to appropriate specialty for specific treatments
Peyronie disease	Painful erections, penile curvature	GU examination: fibrous scar tissue palpable	NSAIDs for pain. Refer to urology
Iatrogenic	Surgery/radiotherapy, e.g. prostatectomy, spinal surgery		PDE5 inhibitors. Refer to urology if refractory
Aortoiliac disease (Leriche syndrome)	Triad of buttock/thigh claudication, decreased femoral pulses, erectile dysfunction. See *4. LIMB CLAUDICATION*		

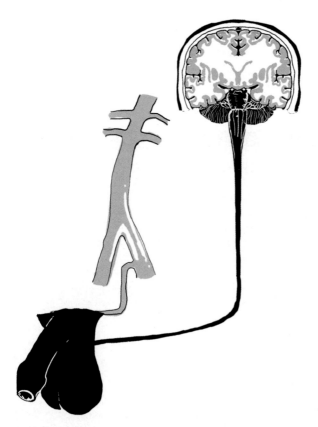

Fig. 201.1 Mechanisms affecting erectile function; innervation and blood supply are crucial, while psychological concerns can be detrimental.

The penis contains spongy tissue that becomes rigid when filled with blood, thus creating an erection. Vascular, neurological and hormonal abnormalities may lead to erectile dysfunction (ED) (Fig. 201.1). ED generally affects men >50 years of age. Small vessel vascular disease is most common, but Leriche syndrome suggests large vessel stenosis needing priority referral to vascular surgery. Lifestyle modifications are smoking cessation, moderating alcohol, optimising weight by healthy diet and exercise. PDE5 inhibitors are first-line oral therapy, but are contraindicated in severe cardiac disease, hypotension, recent stroke/MI or nitrates use (e.g. GTN, ISMN). They can cause reversible impairment of blue-green colour discrimination. If this fails, options include vacuum erection device, and alprostadil (intracorporal injection or intraurethral pellet of prostaglandin E1). Peyronie disease causes penile curvature, with pain initially - surgery may be offered once the curvature has stabilised. Severe prolonged priapism may cause fibrosis, hence intractable ED for which penile implant (inflatable or semi-rigid) may be needed. The diagnosis in the vignette is erectile dyfunction, and the mechanism is probably vasculogenic.

REVISION TIPS

- ED can be caused by vascular, neurological and endocrine health conditions
- Common medications causing ED; anti-depressants, anti-hypertensives and anti-psychotics
- Psychogenic ED differs from organic causes as onset is quick and morning erections are preserved

INDEX

Note: Page numbers followed by *f* indicate figures; *t*, tables; *b*, boxes

591